Introduction to
MEASUREMENT
in Physical Education and Exercise Science

Introduction to

MEASUREMENT

in Physical Education and Exercise Science

MARGARET J. SAFRIT, Ph.D.

Henry-Bascom Professor
University of Wisconsin
Madison, Wisconsin

Second Edition

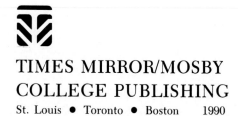

TIMES MIRROR/MOSBY
COLLEGE PUBLISHING
St. Louis ● Toronto ● Boston   1990

Editor: Pat Coryell
Editorial assistant: Loren Stevenson
Production editor: Amy Adams Squire
Book design: Candace Conner
Editing/production: CRACOM Corp.

Library of Congress Cataloging-in-Publication Data

Safrit, Margaret J.
    Introduction to measurement in physical education and exercise
science/Margaret J. Safrit.—2nd ed.
        p.   cm.
    Includes bibliographical references.
    ISBN 0-8016-3298-6
    1. Physical fitness—Testing.   I. Title.
GV436.S223   1990
613.7′1—dc20   89-12916
                                                CIP

C/D/D   9   8   7   6   5   4   3   2

To my parents—
Margaret Cline and the late Ernest Crawford Safrit, Sr.—
with grateful appreciation for their
constant support and encouragement
during my years as a student and
throughout my career in academia.

Preface

Preparing the second edition of this textbook has been a challenging task. Because the first edition has been well received, there was no reason to make drastic changes in the overall format of the book. However, new information has been published in the field of measurement and evaluation in physical education and exercise science since the release of the first edition. This material, particularly in the context of physical fitness testing, warranted the preparation of a new edition. For example, efforts to consolidate national fitness test programs failed; consequently, the Health-Related Physical Fitness Test and the popular Youth Fitness Test are no longer endorsed nationally. The American Alliance for Health, Physical Education, Recreation and Dance now sponsors the Physical Best program, which incorporates a fitness test as a part of its educational program. At least five other major fitness tests have been revised since the publication of the first edition. Physical education teachers and fitness specialists must be able to make educated decisions about the appropriate test to use in their setting. Recent research associated with fitness testing is summarized to aid the user in making good decisions.

New additions to the book include a section on testing motor performance in the aging population, new problems and answers in the statistics chapters, expanded material on the development and use of rating scales, the inclusion of step-by-step approaches to calculating statistics, and a greatly expanded chapter on grading. A computer diskette containing programs (e.g., basic statistics, measurement of change, body fat estimation, and grading) has been improved and now includes a menu for the convenience of the user. An instructor's manual continues to be available for the course instructor. A series of laboratory experiences can also be obtained by writing to the author.

This textbook was written to prepare the undergraduate student in physical education or exercise science to use measurement and evaluation techniques effectively. The basic principles of measurement are exemplified in both school and nonschool settings, since many students are now preparing for careers in nonschool settings. Numerous examples of tests are provided throughout the book.

FOCUS

In the fields of physical education and exercise science, two concepts assume universal significance—measurement of motor behavior and evaluation of the performance of physical skills and the effectiveness of educational programs. Teachers of physical education should be able to select good tests, administer them properly, and use the results to improve student achievement. Although tests of motor behavior are of predominant interest to the teacher, knowledge tests and tests of affective behavior—such as sportsmanship—are also used. Further, the evaluation of instruction, curriculum, and program cannot be ignored. Specialists in fitness and sports centers have similar needs. The status of incoming clients should be evaluated. The effectiveness of the center, both programmatically and financially, must be assessed. Indeed, without the tools of measurement, indicators of attainment would be limited to totally subjective judgments.

FEATURES

- One of the prominent features of this book is its *straightforward presentation of measurement and evaluation concepts*. It is based on 25 years of author experience in teaching measurement to undergraduate physical education majors and provides a clear, accurate discussion of issues appropriate at this level of instruction.
- Another strong point is the inclusion of two chapters on the use of *microcomputers* along with the use of several programs that can be used by both students and faculty. These chapters have been moved so that they now follow the statistics chapters. As mentioned earlier, the software has been improved and is available on a diskette.
- An important and timely feature of the book is its *representativeness of the field of physical education and exercise science* as it exists today. No longer are most majors in physical education or kinesiology or exercise science preparing to teach or coach physical education. Many students are interested in alternative careers in a nonschool setting such as a fitness center. A practical approach to testing in this type of setting is included.
- The organization of the book provides a *practical presentation* for learning. After a general introduction to measurement and evaluation in physical education, the technical section of the book is introduced with an overview of basic statistics, microcomputers, and measurement concepts. The next section of the book encompasses easy-to-locate material on testing and types of tests. The latter portion of the book deals with typical problems associated with the measurement of motor skills and abilities.

ORGANIZATIONAL FEATURES

The book is divided into ten parts. Part One presents an overview of measurement and evaluation, including an up-to-date coverage of the importance of these concepts in school and nonschool settings in physical education and exercise science. In Part Two statistical techniques that can be used to describe test scores are presented in a straightforward manner, with step-by-step examples and problems/answers for the student. The material is written in a simplified manner for those who have only the most basic arithmetic skills. In Part Three emphasis is placed on the use of microcomputers in our field. This part can be followed easily by students with no previous experience on a microcomputer. Part Four focuses on concepts in measurement, presented in understandable and accurate terminology. Both norm-referenced and criterion-referenced measurement are covered. The latter approach to measurement has become even more important now that several of the national fitness tests use criterion-referenced standards. The textbook becomes even more practical in Part Five with a detailed description of test construction techniques for both sports skills and knowledge tests. In Parts Six and Seven many examples of tests of physical performance are presented and analyzed. These include tests of sports skills, health-related physical fitness, performance-related physical fitness, muscular strength and endurance, balance and flexibility, motor ability, and affective behavior. A variety of unique measurement concerns in physical education are covered in Part Eight: measurements of physical performance, including a sampling of sports skills tests and tests for strength, endurance, and motor ability. The appendixes include statistical tables, microcomputer programs, and sources for a wide variety of sports skills tests.

PEDAGOGICAL FEATURES

Extensive author experience in teaching undergraduate students in measurement and evaluation has been used to design a book that is a genuine aid to student learning.

Key Words: Each chapter begins with a list of the most important terms that students should learn while reading the chapter.

Introduction: A description of the purpose of the chapter prepares the student for each chapter's application of information to both physical education and exercise science.

Tables, Drawings, and Photographs: Tables and illustrations are used throughout to provide additional information and to clarify concepts and activities.

Summary: Summaries at the close of each chapter carefully reiterate its major points of content.

References: Presenting the most complete and up-to-date documentation, the references provide sources for further study.

Annotated Readings: Selected resources are provided with annotations to enhance the learning process.

Learning Experiences: A set of learning experiences concludes each chapter and provides student exercises to reinforce the material in the text. When appropriate, answers are provided.

Glossary: The text concludes with a comprehensive glossary in which each key word shown at the beginning of the chapter is listed and defined.

SUPPLEMENT

An Instructor's Manual and Test Bank are available for instructors using the textbook. The manual contains supplementary information to be used at the discretion of the instructor. Included in the manual are chapter objectives; chapter overviews; additional learning experiences; microcomputer programs modified for the Commodore and the IBM; additional sample tests; 21 transparency masters of important drawings, tables, and charts; and over 660 multiple choice, true/false, matching, and essay test questions. Separate answer keys are provided. The manual is perforated for convenience.

ACKNOWLEDGMENTS

No textbook can be completed without the assistance of many others, and this has certainly been true for this book. Their support is gratefully acknowledged.

Many authors and publishers granted permission to reproduce material in this text. The American Alliance for Health, Physical Education, Recreation and Dance was especially generous. Several colleagues—Michael Pollock, Timothy Lohman, Janet Seaman, and Dale Ulrich—kindly granted permission to reproduce several of their photographs.

Sincere appreciation is expressed to Linda Spraker for the artwork and Jerry M. Capps for the photography. The models for the photography were of great assistance. Several were undergraduate students at the University of Wisconsin–Madison: Daniel McCourt, Sharon Novak, Spencer Kurtz, Kenneth Siedenberg, and Laurie Rabideau. M. Glaucia Costa, Linda M. Hooper, Terry M. Wood, Long-guang Gao, and Weimo Zhu deserve special recognition for their contributions to the preparation of both the text and the Instructor's Manual. Thanks are extended to two of my colleagues—Bonnie Chalmers-Ballsrud, Adapted Physical Education, and Francis J. Nagle, Biodynamics Laboratory. Finally, the photography sessions could not have been completed without the indispensable assistance of Kay Harty, principal, and Christine J. Harper, physical education teacher at Midvale Elementary School, and Jack Horton, principal, and the physical education staff at Orchard Ridge Middle School in Madison, Wisconsin, as well as the cooperation of the children in both schools.

Reviewers were selected by the publisher to evaluate the first edition of the textbook. Their reviews were extremely helpful in revising the text and, without question, contributed to improvements in the original version. A very special debt of gratitude is conveyed to these individuals for their thorough and conscientious analysis of the book:

Donald Steele
University of Maryland–College Park

Steve Edwards
Oklahoma State University

Emma Gibbons
Texas A & M University

Joy Hendrick
State University of New York at Cortland

Mary Ford
Winthrop College

Sincere thanks are also expressed to Judy Hillmer and Donna Camesi for assistance in preparing the Instructor's Manual. Their efficiency is hereby acknowledged.

Finally, a well-deserved recognition is extended to the staff of Times Mirror/Mosby College Publishing for supplying sound direction to the preparation of the text. Michelle Turenne was invaluable in the development of the first edition, and the assistance of Pat Coryell and Loren Stevenson in preparing the second edition is greatly appreciated. Their aid contributed significantly to the quality of the final product.

Margaret J. Safrit

Contents

Appendixes

Part One

An Overview of Measurement and Evaluation

1

The Value of Measurement and Evaluation

KEY WORDS *Watch for these words as you read the following chapter:*

achievement

competency-based evaluation

criterion-referenced test

evaluation

formative evaluation

improvement

mastery test

measurement

norm-referenced test

qualitative measurement

quantitative measurement

summative evaluation

test

test user

Title IX

The field of physical education has changed. From its inception to the early 1970s, the majority of students majoring in physical education planned to teach physical education in a school setting and perhaps coach one or two sports. During the 1970s the interests of some students began to vary. As the emphasis on health and fitness mushroomed in the United States, careers other than teaching in schools became available to physical education majors. For instance, as fitness clubs sprang up around the country, managers and instructors trained in physical education were sought. How has this changed the field of physical education? Even though many of the basic scientific principles taught to physical education teachers are germane, for those choosing other career options in the motor behavior area, the application of these principles may vary. Thus every area of specialization in physical education has been affected, including the measurement and evaluation area. For example, tests are sometimes used to motivate students in a school setting. Some students may be motivated because they realize their test score will be used in determining unit grades. In nonschool settings, such as private fitness clubs, private sports clubs, corporate fitness centers, the Young Women's Christian Association (YWCA), and the Young Men's Christian Association (YMCA), tests will not be motivating because of grades, at least in the traditional sense. On the other hand, a test may stimulate individuals to improve their performance in both school and nonschool settings. The underlying principles of measurement are the same in both settings, but the application of these principles may differ depending on the clientele and the predetermined objectives.

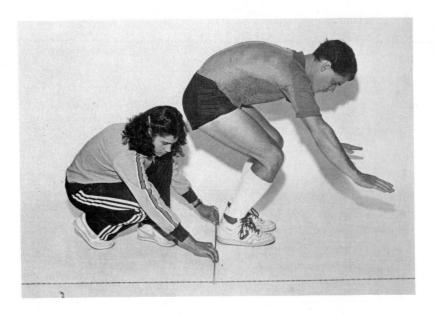

Measurement is also essential in developing the skills and abilities required for other career options in physical education and exercise science. Every type of career, whether it involves education, business, sports medicine, or research, requires expertise in measurement. For example, athletic trainers use a variety of measurement and evaluation procedures. Many of the competencies listed by the National Athletic Trainers' Association for certified athletic trainers require a background in measurement and evaluation. A career in sports management involves constant evaluation of personnel and programs. An exercise scientist engaged in research uses principles of measurement throughout the process of designing and conducting studies.

Measurement and evaluation are also vital aspects of instruction. The importance of these processes is not diminished if the instruction takes place in a non-school setting. Many of the measurement principles used by physical education teachers are useful for exercise specialists and instructors in sports clubs.

This book focuses on the use of measurement and evaluation of motor behavior in school and nonschool settings. The basic measurement concepts are applicable no matter where a test is administered. However, the way in which test scores are used may vary, depending on the setting.

Suppose an individual joins a fitness center. Before prescribing an exercise program for the client, an instructor administers a battery of fitness tests. These tests might be identical to those used in physical education classes in local high schools. Yet in the private club context, the constraints surrounding the measurement process can be quite different from the public school situation. In the private club, testing is often individualized. The age and needs of the client may differ from those of the high school student. Attention must be paid to appropriate motivational strategies. Techniques that are effective in the fitness center may not have the same impact in the high school, and vice versa. The importance of prior medical approval is magnified in the older population. Since private clubs are often able to administer tests on a one-to-one basis, the use of laboratory-type testing procedures is more feasible in this setting than in the schools.

Most students reading this textbook will have already spent many years in physical education classes in the school system. Can you recall whether tests were used in these classes? If so, when were tests usually administered during a unit of instruction? Did testing seem important to your physical education teacher? How were the test scores used? Were test results used for any purpose other than determining grades? The use of tests probably varied from unit to unit. The same situation exists in nonschool settings. In some instances no tests are used at all, and in others the testing program is of high quality. In subsequent chapters several of these testing programs are described. Measurement practices in both school and nonschool settings are included, with material directed to the budding exercise specialist or private sports club instructor as well as the future teacher of physical education, athletic trainer, and so forth. Since the nonschool and school settings encompass so many potential career options, each with a different title, the term **test user** will be used in a generic sense throughout this textbook to refer to an individual who selects and administers a test, regardless of his or her job title.

MEASUREMENT AND EVALUATION DEFINED

Measurement and evaluation are closely related processes. From a practical standpoint, **measurement** takes place when a test is administered and a score is obtained. If the test is **quantitative,** the score is a number. If the test is **qualitative,** the score may be a phrase or a word such as *excellent,* or it may be a number representing a phrase or word. A more precise definition of measurement is the process of assigning a number to an attribute of a person or object. According to this definition, measurement is a quantitative and not a qualitative process. If body fatness is the attribute of interest, it can be measured by determining skinfold thickness. The number assigned to this attribute represents skinfold thickness reported in millimeters (mm). Such a score would fit the universal definition of the term *measurement.* Throughout this textbook, however, measurement is interpreted in the broadest sense as encompassing both quantitative and qualitative indicators.

The process of **evaluation** involves the interpretation of a score. Once skinfold thickness has been measured, what does the score mean? If the sum of tri-

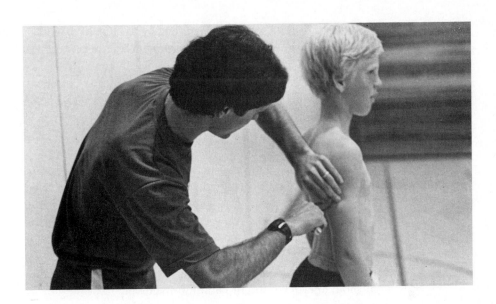

ceps plus calf skinfolds is 18 mm for a 10-year-old boy, is this a reflection of a desirable amount of body fatness? The score must be interpreted to have true meaning. In the strictest sense of the word, measurement is an objective, non-judgmental process, whereas evaluation requires judgments.

USE OF TESTS

Throughout this textbook *test* will be used synonymously with the noun *measure*. For example, a measure of maximal oxygen uptake has the same meaning as a **test** of maximal oxygen uptake. Tests have many uses in school and non-school settings. A test may be administered for one purpose or for multiple purposes, as determined by the test user. Usually the rationale for using a test encompasses more than one purpose. The following are a few of the uses of tests in physical education and the exercise sciences.

Motivation

Tests are frequently administered for motivational purposes. A skills test might be administered in a physical education class to encourage students to improve their skills further. In a corporate fitness center, skinfold measures might be used to motivate overweight employees to lose weight. When a performance standard must be met in a public service setting, examinees are sometimes motivated to work toward meeting the standard by taking a test. The advance knowledge of an upcoming test can motivate students to practice a skill with greater intensity. When a test is administered more than once, students are usually interested in the extent to which they have improved. They like to compare their current score with a previous score, which, in itself, can be a motivational factor. The use of tests for motivation is most effective if scores are viewed in the context of areas needing improvement rather than in a punitive sense. In other words, the test should be used as a positive factor in performance before, during, and after the test's administration.

Achievement

One of the most common uses of tests is the assessment of achievement. How much has an individual achieved during a specified period of time? If most of the clients in a center are below average in their levels of fitness after a year of participation in a fitness program, this points to insufficient achievement by the participants. Do students achieve a higher level of skill in several sports after participating in a physical education program year after year? Do employees in a corporate fitness center achieve the targeted amount of weight loss? **Achievement** should not be confused with **improvement.** Improvement is the difference in performance from one point in time to another. These points may or may not coincide with the beginning and end of the course. Achievement in and of itself encompasses only the final ability level at a designated time and is sometimes relative to a standard or criterion.

Improvement

The idea of measuring improvement is near and dear to the hearts of many professional physical educators and exercise scientists and understandably so. The rationale is that individuals lacking in skill cannot be expected to achieve the level a highly skilled group can attain; thus, the beginning ability level of each participant is considered and the extent to which the individual improved beyond that point is assessed. Similarly, individuals with initial low levels of fitness will be unable to achieve the same level of fitness upon completion of a training program as those who are highly fit. These are valid concerns. Nonetheless, a number of factors make the desired amount of improvement difficult to obtain when dealing with sports and other forms of physical activity. In a school setting units of instruction are often too short to bring about desired levels of improvement. The background of the student or client can also affect the amount of improvement during a unit. Those who have an adequate understanding of the underlying principles of movement can sometimes learn new skills in a shorter period than those without this knowledge. On the surface, measuring improvement seems to be a reasonable solution to the problems associated with fairly assessing individuals with varying skill levels. However, inherent problems exist in the measurement of improvement and are discussed in Chapter 9.

Diagnosis

One of the most important uses of measurement in physical education is to diagnose weaknesses in performance. What is wrong with a student's tennis serve? Why does a racquetball club member have an ineffective backhand? Why has an individual's running performance failed to improve? In other words, the diagnostic process helps the participant learn more efficiently. Furthermore, the teacher is able to *teach* more effectively. Diagnostic procedures can be particularly potent when assessing knowledge of principles and concepts in our field. In this case errors in responding to individual items or clusters of items can pinpoint gaps in the examinee's knowledge of specific content. For example, a student in a badminton class may answer incorrectly many of the test items dealing with rules specific to the singles game in badminton. This suggests a need to review that particular section of the rules book. Of course, tests are not the only means of diagnosing weaknesses, but they are extremely useful in this respect. Some diagnostic tests can be self-administered, allowing the instructor to spend more time meeting other instructional needs. Diagnosis is a major component of the athletic trainer's job. The correct assessment of injuries and the identification of an appropriate treatment are typical expectations of a trainer. This requires knowledge of a variety of measurement techniques as well as the correct test protocol under various circumstances. Many other personnel, such as exercise specialists and sports management specialists, must make diagnoses on a daily basis.

Prescription

Once weaknesses have been diagnosed, the test user formulates a prescription for correcting these weaknesses. *Exercise prescription* is a widely used term for prescribing the appropriate exercise program for an individual. Adapted physical education teachers frequently prescribe corrective activities for students even though the term *prescription* might not be used. This usage of tests is not limited to exercise programs. Athletic trainers may prescribe treatment in a whirlpool or tape an injured body part to treat the athlete. When an area needing improvement has been identified on the basis of test results, a prescription for correction is appropriate regardless of the form of sport or physical activity. Sometimes students can generate their own prescription for improving performance, based on test results.

Grading

Grading is a practice that occurs in almost all physical education programs throughout the United States. Sound grading practices are based on the use of well-developed objective and subjective tests, because grades represent symbols of achievement. Moreover, once a teacher makes a decision on grades for a given unit, the impact on students is immediate, long-lasting, and usually irreversible. Even though the importance of grades is obvious, they are not always determined on the basis of tests. The stark reality is that grades are still determined subjectively by many physical education teachers and are frequently based on behavioral assessments such as wearing proper uniforms, effort, and sportsmanship, rather than physical performance. The use of measurement to determine grades is certainly appropriate, but to administer tests solely for the purpose of determining grades suggests a limited view of the value of measurement.

Evaluation of Unit of Instruction

In planning a unit of instruction, a set of objectives is typically set forth. At the end of the unit, an effort is usually made to determine whether the objectives have been met. Making this judgment is difficult without administering tests, especially if the evidence must be submitted to someone else such as the school principal, club manager, or corporation president. Test data can also be used to demonstrate the effectiveness of programs in a nonschool setting to potential members.

Evaluation of Program

The evaluation of individual units of instruction, along with an assessment of the overall program, provides evidence of the effectiveness of a total program. Perhaps one or two teachers in a school met the predetermined objectives in their classes, but overall the school might have fallen short in this respect. A system-wide program evaluation can include the evidence from this unit as well as broader evaluation procedures encompassing the program in the entire system. All the franchises for a fitness corporation might be evaluated on the ability of the corporation as a whole to meet program objectives and financial goals. Program evaluation forces examination of the total picture rather than narrowly focusing on an isolated unit in a single location.

Classification

Over the years tests have been used to place individuals into groups on the basis of their ability level in motor performance, allowing those with the same or similar classifications to be grouped for purposes of instruction or work-outs. The underlying assumption is that both learning and instruction are more efficient if the learners have similar ability levels.

Prediction

One way in which tests have been used with increasing frequency is as predictors of various aspects of motor behavior. For many years coaches have been interested in tests to predict success in their sport. Sport psychology has blossomed as an area of specialization in physical education, and there has been considerable interest in attempting to predict success in a variety of physical activities using measures of psychological and physiological parameters. In some instances the prediction involved Olympic athletes; other efforts were directed to the college athlete. Efforts have also been directed to predicting long-term involvement in physical activity. In exercise physiology, scores on a fitness test might be used to estimate maximal oxygen uptake. The percentage of one's body fat can be predicted using indicators such as skinfold thickness tests. These are merely a few examples of the widespread use of tests as predictors in physical education and exercise science.

NORM-REFERENCED AND CRITERION-REFERENCED MEASUREMENT

Just as a test can be used for various purposes, it can be designed by the test developer to perform different functions. One of these functions is to measure *individual differences*. For many years sport psychologists have been interested in studying an athlete's traits, such as self-motivation. To be able to study self-motivation, it must be possible to measure it. Thus if a sport psychologist plans an experiment on self-motivation, a test would be administered to the athletes at some point during the experiment. If all athletes obtained the same score on the test, how would the results be interpreted? It would be logical to suggest that all athletes participating in the experiment had the same level of self-motivation, yet this outcome is not very likely. A group of athletes—in fact, any group of individuals—would be expected to have differing levels of a trait. The test of the trait, in other words, is expected to detect *individual differences* in the trait. In the early part of the twentieth century, most of the advances in measurement were made by individuals interested in this approach.

Educators have also been interested in this function of measurement. One way of knowing how much a student has achieved is to examine his or her score in relation to the scores of others on the same test. In essence a student's score is compared to other students' scores. Here again, individual differences are anticipated because some students are expected to perform better than others. This function identifies the test as a **norm-referenced** test. The score is compared to a set of norms. For example, scores on the fitness test sponsored by the Amateur Athletic Union may be compared to the national norms for the participant's gender and age group. Generally the educator is interested in the performance of the students in relation to other students.

Although educators are aware that students differ in many ways, they are, however, sometimes unconcerned about individual differences. Suppose, for example, a physical education teacher identifies a cardiorespiratory function objective for his or her classes and plans to use a test of the mile run to measure this objective. A standard that reflects a satisfactory level of cardiorespiratory endurance is also set for the test. For example, a standard of 7 minutes and 30 seconds is set for 16-year-old boys. In other words, the goal for each 16-year-old boy in all classes is to run the mile in 7:30 by the end of the school year. This type of test is called a **criterion-referenced** test. A standard of performance is set that all or most students are expected to meet. The standard assumes importance because it is *referenced to a criterion behavior.* In the above example the criterion behavior is a satisfactory level of cardiorespiratory function. Students who meet the standard are labeled *masters* and those who do not are labeled *nonmasters.* Another name for a test performing this type of function is a **mastery test.** There are no restrictions on the number of students who master the test. The question of interest is whether the student was able to meet the predetermined standard. In a norm-referenced context, the question of interest concerns how the student's score compares with the scores of others. Several of the recently revised national physical fitness tests use criterion-referenced rather than norm-referenced standards. These standards are presented in Chapter 16. Competency exams, such as those used by the American College of Sports Medicine to certify exercise specialists, represent a prime example of criterion-referenced tests.

Each of these types of measurement, norm-referenced and criterion-referenced, provides a valuable approach to testing. To suggest that one function is better than another is not meaningful because one approach may be more desirable in a specific context. Most of the published tests in physical education are norm-referenced measures; however, interest in criterion-referenced testing has increased in recent years, especially in the schools. This interest should lead to an increase in the development of new mastery tests.

FORMATIVE AND SUMMATIVE EVALUATION

A number of new terms are being introduced in this chapter that will be used throughout this textbook. The term *evaluation* was defined in a previous section as the interpretation of a score. The process of evaluation can take place at any time during a program or unit of instruction. In an aerobic dance class, for instance, an informal self-evaluation often takes place several times during each session of an instructional unit. The participant engages in vigorous physical activity, stopping to measure heart rate at periodic intervals. Evaluation of the heart rate is accomplished by judging whether the rate is high enough to provide the desired physiological benefits. When evaluation occurs *during* the training period or instructional unit, it is known as **formative evaluation.** This type of evaluation is not uncommon in physical fitness units, where performance is often monitored on a daily basis. Formative evaluation is also appropriate for other aspects of the physical education curriculum in the schools but has been used less frequently in this setting. More typically, tests are administered at the end of the unit. When evaluation takes place solely at the end of a unit, it is referred to as **summative evaluation.** For example, the last 2 days of a tennis unit might be devoted to administering one or two skills tests, a written test, and a test of playing ability. The test scores are usually used to evaluate achievement. In a physical education class this may be translated to a unit grade. In a private tennis club, and perhaps in a school setting, these test scores might be used as an indicator of the effectiveness of instruction.

When only summative evaluation takes place, it is often too late to correct problems that have already been identified. In a school setting students move to another unit of instruction; thus if the objectives of the previous unit were not met, it is too late to remedy the situation. Had evaluation taken place during the unit of instruction, deficiencies could have been addressed in a more positive way. The teacher could have prescribed activities to correct these deficiencies. Should formative evaluation be used in a nonschool setting? Yes, the provision of feedback to clients on an ongoing basis helps them understand their strengths and weaknesses. In fact when exercise is the primary mode of physical activity, it is only through regular evaluation that the instructor can monitor the appropriateness of the exercise. When the physical activity involves a sport, private clubs are less likely to engage in formal evaluation, either formative or summative. Formative evaluation is equally important in athletic training. If the strengths and weaknesses of athletes are tested periodically, perhaps a significant number of injuries can be avoided.

Although formative evaluation has been emphasized in this section of the book, one should not assume it is superior to summative evaluation. Sometimes one approach is more appropriate than the other, depending upon the reasons for evaluation. Formative evaluation is stressed here simply because it has been neglected in the past. Using either approach exclusively is not necessary. To maximize the effectiveness of evaluation procedures, both formative and summative evaluation should be used.

BRIEF HISTORY OF MEASUREMENT

In the late 1880s a number of prominent physical educators were also medical doctors. They were primarily interested in body symmetry and proportion and prescribed exercise to modify body size. Thus anthropometric measures were used extensively during this period. In 1861 Edward Hitchcock of Amherst, Massachusetts, developed standards of age, height, and weight; chest, arm, and forearm girths; and strength of the upper arm. He was the leading authority in anthropometry between 1860 and 1880. Because of his contributions in the area, Hitchcock is often called the father of measurement in physical education. In 1878 Dudley Sargent of Harvard University developed similar tables of standards. Strength tests were also used during this early period. Sargent was an active contributor in this area as well as in anthropometry, developing the Intercollegiate Strength Test in the 1870s.

Widespread usage of both strength and anthropometric measurement lagged in the early 1900s. Although interest in the measurement of strength subsequently resumed, anthropometric measures have never regained the prominence received in the early days. Nonetheless, this type of measure still holds an important place in the physical education field in measuring growth, body composition, and body types. At the turn of the century there was considerable interest in measuring cardiorespiratory function because of the development of measures of endurance and of heart and lung tests. At that time there was also the general perception that individuals became muscle-bound by strength exercises, thus hindering athletic performance. The first test of cardiac function, the Blood Ptosis Test, was developed by C. Ward Crampton in 1905. Crampton noted changes in cardiac rate and arterial pressure on assuming the erect position from a supine position. In the 1920s more sophisticated work was published on the measurement of physical efficiency. E.C. Schneider designed a test used in aviation in World War II to determine fatigue and physical condition for flying. The relationship between pulse rate and blood pressure in the reclining position and the standing position was determined, as well as the ability to recover to normal standing values after a measured bout of exercise. In 1931 W.W. Tuttle modified a block-stepping test similar to a step test measuring endurance and general state of training called the Tuttle Pulse-Ratio Test, a forerunner of the Harvard Step Test developed in 1943. The efficiency of the circulatory system was indicated by the increase in heart rate during exercise and speed with which the heart rate returned to normal after exercise. Work in this area became increasingly sophisticated with the development of the Balke Treadmill Test in 1954 and other similar measures. The latter tests still represent the standard for measuring cardiorespiratory function in a laboratory setting. The limitation of some of these treadmill tests is that they are indirect rather than direct measures of aerobic capacity.

The earliest tests of sports skills were developed as part of athletic performance batteries. For example, in 1913 the Athletic Badge Tests were published by the Playground and Recreation Association of America. David Brace at the University of Texas first attempted to measure a group of fundamental skills for a specific sport, basketball, in 1924. He also worked on the development of tests for indoor baseball and soccer. In a 1930 measurement textbook, Bovard and Cozens noted that the area of skill testing was relatively untouched (Bovard and Cozens, 1930). They identified 1916 as the approximate year that the physical education curriculum was broadened to include game activities. Therefore, they noted, physical educators ought to be prepared to measure sports skills as well as other aspects of physical activity. Although tests were being developed during this time, many were not published. Several outstanding measurement specialists in physical education emerged during this period, including Ruth Glassow at the University of Wisconsin. Skills test development was emphasized at Wisconsin, and Glassow and Broer published a measurement book in 1938, which was almost entirely devoted to skills tests and batteries. Charles McCloy (1939) at the University of Iowa was a strong critic of subjective measures of skill in his 1939 textbook; Harrison Clarke at the University of Oregon took a similar stance in his 1945 textbook (Clarke, 1945). Subsequently Gladys Scott and her students at the University of Iowa made many contributions to the development of skills tests in the field of physical education. A number of these tests were described in the 1959 textbook by Scott and French.

After a temporary lag in the use of strength tests, interest was restored with the development of new tests in this area, such as the Strength Index and Physical Fitness Index developed by Frederick Rand Rogers in 1925. This type of measurement became much more precise with the development of the cable tensiometer tests by Harrison Clarke. Clarke's innovative thinking led to the design of equipment allowing an investigator to measure the strength of many different body parts. As more sophisticated equipment such as the dynamometers and weight-training machines became available to the exercise scientist, options for strength testing were greatly expanded.

The history of physical fitness testing is described in Chapters 16 and 17. Up to the 1950s physical fitness was typically stressed when the United States was engaged in war. In 1954 the results of administering the Kraus-Weber Test of Minimum Strength to American and English children were published. For the first time, fitness was stressed as important to the individual's health rather than solely as an indicator of readiness for combat. (Refer to Chapters 16 and 17 for details.)

Up to this point, one type of testing in the physical education field has been ignored—the measurement of general motor ability. Motor ability is an expression that was commonplace among physical educators in the early 1900s. Actually, as early as 1894 the Normal School of Gymnastics in Milwaukee and the Gymnastics Societies in Cleveland administered batteries of tests that measured ability in events such as jumping, climbing, shot-putting, lifting, and so forth. As time passed many schools began to institute testing programs, including basic events from track and field. Most of the test batteries developed then had many similarities, and none of the original batteries was based on sound test development as we know it today. In the 1930-1940 era a number of test batteries purporting to measure basic motor ability were published, based on a much stronger scientific rationale. However, the overall validity of these batteries was never firmly established. Yet the popularity of the concept of motor ability continued into the late 1950s. At that time the concept began to be questioned in light of emerging research evidence. This reexamination is described in greater detail in Chapter 21. Suffice it to say that the idea of general motor ability, while intuitively appealing, has never been verified scientifically.

In conclusion, the development of tests in physical education has occurred despite the absence of a strategy for systematically adding to various categories of tests and modifying tests when necessary. More attention has been paid to field and laboratory tests of various physiological attributes largely because of the existence of exercise physiology laboratories in departments of physical education throughout the United States. These laboratories provide a mechanism for systematic work on test development. No similar environment exists for the development of skills tests and tests of basic movement. As a result, there is a significant void in the availability of tests, in particular for preschool and elementary school children in physical education. This deficit points to the pressing need for a test service to provide the impetus for the development of tests of all aspects of motor behavior.

RECENT CHANGES IN MEASUREMENT PRACTICES

Measurement and evaluation courses have been taught for many years in physical education programs throughout the United States. Tests of sports skills, fitness, and motor ability, for example, have been advocated in these courses. Presumably, some testing has taken place in physical education programs as well as in exercise and sport programs in nonschool settings. Have measurement practices in these fields changed in recent years? Although judging the extent to which changes have taken place is difficult, events transpiring over the past two decades point to the need for certain changes. The most prominent events include modification of sports, the use of competency-based tests in the public schools, the accessibility of microcomputers, the passage of Title IX, a concern for the development of health-related physical fitness, and concern for the health and well-being of an increasing elderly population.

Modification of Sports Skills Tests

When a test of sport skill is developed, the validity of the test rests, in part, on the degree to which the test measures the skill as it is used most efficiently in the sport. For instance, it would be illogical to design a test of the basketball jump shot that requires the examinee to take the test at a distance of 30 feet from the basket, since the average student in a physical education class would not attempt a shot from that distance. On the other hand, the sport itself can be modified over the years so that tests that were previously valid are no longer appropriate. As the sport of volleyball changed to a power sport, the use of several volleyball skills also changed. Years ago, players would use an underarm serve

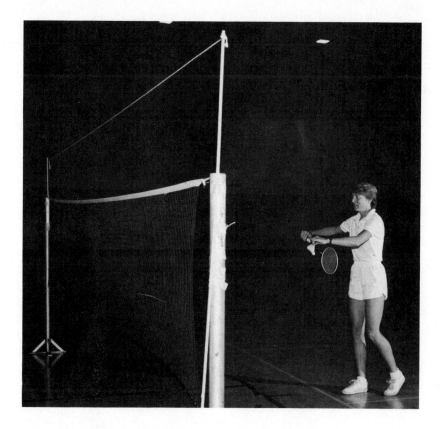

that was returned to a front-court teammate using a pass. Power volleyball incorporated an overarm serve usually returned, again to a front-court teammate, using a bump. The Liba and Stauff Volleyball Pass Test (Collins and Hodges, 1978)
was developed for the pass as it was used in an earlier version of the sport. In
the test the overhead pass was measured over a distance equivalent to executing
the pass from the backcourt to the forecourt. In power volleyball, the ball is typically hit from the backcourt to the forecourt using a bump. A pass usually follows but at a shorter distance and lower height than the dimensions required in
the earlier version of the sport. The pass as measured in the Liba and Stauff test
would not be recommended under the same conditions in power volleyball; however, the test can easily be modified to accurately measure the constraints of the
game as it is now played. Changing the constraints of a sport can invalidate a
test. This does not mean the test should be discarded but rather that the test
should be modified to fit the current version of the game. The implications of
these changes are discussed in more detail in Chapters 14 and 18.

Tests can also be modified and adapted to make them more appropriate for specific situations. For example, in a school setting, the measurement and evaluation process can match the teacher, students, and class content with its inherent methodological uniqueness.

Competency-Based Evaluation

Competency-based evaluation is based on the premise that certain competencies are identifiable for a group of examinees that ought to be mastered. A test is developed for each competency, and a test score is selected as the standard representing the criterion behavior—the behavior representing mastery of the competency. Individuals who meet or exceed the standards pass the compentency-based evaluation; all others fail. Decisions based on this type of evaluation can have a tremendous impact on the individuals involved. For example, some states have developed a competency-based program for their high school students. Students who fail to meet the standards expected for a high school graduate are sometimes denied a high school diploma. These programs are highly controversial, since the decisions about those who are competent and those who are not will never be error-free. In other words, the decisions will sometimes be wrong. The most serious consequence of an incorrect decision is the classification of a student as unsuccessful in meeting the standard, when, in reality, the student is competent. At best the student must undertake remedial work to obtain a diploma that should have been awarded in the first place. In some states competency-based evaluation is applied in the certification of teachers. A standardized test of knowledge about teaching and content areas is administered to prospective teachers. If the predetermined standard for prospective teachers in a specified area (e.g. art, physical education, or mathematics) is not met, the student will not be certified to teach in that state. As you might suspect, these programs also promote controversy because 100% accuracy is not possible when decisions are made. Criterion-referenced tests are generally used in competency-based programs, and these tests must be rigorously developed.

Microcomputers

In the early 1970s it was unusual for students in a measurement class in physical education to own minicalculators. Analyzing a set of test scores was accomplished either by hand or by using a large desk calculator, if available. Although the small hand calculators were being sold, they were expensive and capable of only a few basic arithmetic operations. By the end of that decade the cost of the minicalculator had dropped to an affordable price and the capability of the instrument had been markedly expanded, allowing many physical education majors in measurement classes to use their own minicalculators. Vast improvements in the microchip have resulted in the development of small desk-top computers called microcomputers, which have gradually become more affordable. Several brands of microcomputers are now available at a fairly modest cost. Eventually it will be commonplace for measurement students to own their own microcomputers and carry small, portable ones to class. Since the impact of microcomputers on measurement and evaluation in physical education will be significant, two chapters in this textbook are devoted to the topic. Certainly this technological advance will facilitate measurement and evaluation practices in the field.

Reassessment of Physical Performance Standards for Girls and Women

When physical education programs were first promoted in the United States, providing separate programs for boys and girls was not uncommon. Many colleges and universities even established separate physical education departments for men and women. Almost all activities were taught in separate classes for males and females. In 1975 a set of regulations known as **Title IX** of the Education Amendments of 1972 became effective. This legislation required fair and equal opportunities in all phases of education, including evaluation. It pointed to the need for greater attention to ability grouping and performance standards.

Three subparagraphs in the Title IX legislation are directed specifically to physical education.

Subparagraph 86.34 (b) provides that ability grouping in physical education classes is permissible provided that the composition of the groups is determined objectively with regard to individual performance rather than on the basis of sex. Subparagraph 86.34 (c) allows separation by sex within physical education classes during competition in wrestling, boxing, ice hockey, football, basketball, and other sports, the purpose or major activity of which involves bodily contact. Subparagraph 86.34 (d), requiring the use of standards for measuring skill or progress in physical education which do not adversely impact on members of one sex, is intended to eliminate a problem raised by many comments that, where a goal-oriented standard is used to assess skill or progress, women almost invariably score lower than men. For example, if progress is measured by determining whether an individual can perform 25 push-ups, the standard may be virtually out of reach for many more women than men because of the difference in strength between average persons of each sex. Accordingly the appropriate standard might be an individual progress chart based on the number of push-ups that might be expected of that individual (Federal Register, 1975:24132).

More research needs to be conducted on sex differences in motor performance. Some of these differences may be caused by differences in basic physiological factors; others may be culturally induced. As opportunities increase for women to participate in athletics, their physical abilities and skills are presumably also increasing. These changes should be monitored on an annual basis.

In the summer of 1981 the Illinois State Board of Education sponsored a Physical Education Ability Grouping and Performance Evaluation Symposium. The purpose of the symposium was to identify guidelines that physical education teachers could use to develop their own objective, sex-fair standards of measures for grouping and evaluating students. An outgrowth of the symposium was a useful publication including tips and techniques for the teacher (Illinois State Board of Education, 1982).

Increase in the Use of Physical Fitness Tests

Historically, Americans have been concerned about physical fitness in times of war. Many young men who were drafted during previous wars were not physically fit at the time of their induction. Thus it is not suprising that fitness received considerable emphasis when the country was involved in a war. This emphasis was also felt in the schools, especially in physical education classes. Between wars, however, the interest in fitness waned. This remained true for many years despite the stress placed on fitness by presidents such as Eisenhower and Kennedy. This pattern began to change in the 1970s when Americans became concerned about their own fitness for health-related reasons, not merely because fitness was necessary to fight in a war. The fitness explosion has led to a proliferation of fitness clubs and health spas throughout the country. Many of these organizations administer health-related fitness tests to their clients. The American Alliance for Health, Physical Education, Recreation and Dance (AAHPERD) has published a health-related physical fitness test, the Physical Best Test. In 1988 this test battery was approved as the official fitness test of the Alliance. Other tests have been sponsored by the President's Council on Physical Fitness and Sports (1987), the Institute for Aerobics Research (1987), the American Health and Fitness Foundation (1986), and the Amateur Athletic Union (1987). The development and use of tests measuring fitness have vastly increased relative to that of other types of tests in our field.

The United States Department of Health and Human Services (1985, 1987) published the results of two recent nationwide studies of youth fitness. In these studies three major questions were asked: (1) How fit are American boys and girls in grades 5 and 12? (2) What are the physical activity patterns of children and youth in these grades? (3) How do differences in physical activity patterns affect measured fitness? As a result of this investigation, a new set of fitness norms was formulated. These norms are presented in Chapter 16.

Health and Well-being of the Elderly Population

The fact that American society is aging has been widely documented and extensively discussed. The health and well-being of older adults presents a challenge to professionals in both physical education and the exercise sciences. Considerable research is already being conducted on this age group, and educational programs are being devised to meet their needs. These enterprises require a knowledge of the physiological and psychological parameters of the elderly. Many physical assessment procedures have been used to measure these parameters. Osness (1985) recommends a functional profile, which is a comprehensive evaluation of the physical functionality of the individual. This should be preceded by a thorough medical examination. "The assessment procedure must be specific to older populations and must be comprehensive enough to include all those parameters important to physical well-being" (Osness, 1985, p. 38). Assessment of the elderly has become an important activity for many professionals in our field.

SUMMARY

Measurement and evaluation represent essential aspects of most careers in physical education and exercise science. Tests are used for many purposes and can range from simple field measures to highly sophisticated laboratory measures. The more recent changes in the measurement of motor behavior have resulted from the widespread use of competency-based measurement, the availability of microcomputers, modifications of various sports, the advent of Title IX legislation, the increased interest in health-related fitness, and increasing concern for the health and well-being of the elderly. New approaches to testing motor skills and abilities have recently been proposed. Technological advances will lead to modifications of tests and testing programs, enabling physical educators and exercise scientists to measure with greater precision and accuracy.

LEARNING EXPERIENCES

1. Try to remember when tests were used in your high school physical education program. What types of tests were used? Were they administered at the end of each unit or throughout the unit? How were the test results used?
2. Familiarize yourself with one of the tests of motor skill or physical fitness included in this textbook. Think of ways in which the test could be used (a) in a school setting and (b) in a nonschool setting. Write a brief paper summarizing your thoughts.
3. Interview a physical education teacher who teaches in a public or private school in your area, or invite one to visit one of your measurement classes. Ask the teacher about the tests used in his or her classes. Ask about the major problems a physical education teacher faces in implementing a sound testing program.
4. Interview an exercise specialist who works with elderly clients. Inquire about the tests used in the exercise program. Are the clients monitored on a formative evaluation basis? How is feedback presented to them? Write a brief report on your interview.

REFERENCES

American Alliance for Health, Physical Education, Recreation and Dance. 1988. Physical Best: a physical fitness education & assessment program. Reston, Va.: AAHPERD.

American Health and Fitness Foundation. 1986. Fit Youth Today. Austin, Tex.: American Health and Fitness Foundation.

Bovard, J.F., and Cozens, F.W. 1930. Tests and measurement in physical education. Philadelphia: W.B. Saunders Co.

Chrysler Fund-Amateur Athletic Union. 1987. Physical fitness program. Bloomington, Ind.: The Chrysler Fund-Amateur Athletic Union.

Clarke, H.H. 1976. Application of measurement to health and physical education, ed. 5, Englewood Cliffs, N.J.: Prentice-Hall, Inc.

Collins, D.R., and Hodges, P.B. 1978. A comprehensive guide to sports skills tests and measurement. Springfield, Ill.: Charles C Thomas, Publisher.

Illinois State Board of Education. 1982. Tips and techniques: ability grouping and performance evaluation in physical education. Springfield, Ill.: Illinois State Board of Education.

Institute for Aerobics Research. 1987. FITNESSGRAM User's Manual. Dallas, Tex.: Institute for Aerobics Research.

McCloy, C.H. 1942. Tests and measurements in health and physical education. New York: Appleton-Century-Crofts.

Osness, W.H. 1985. Physical assessment procedures: the use of functional profiles. Journal of Physical Education, Recreation and Dance, **57**(1):22-24.

President's Council on Physical Fitness and Sports. 1987. The Presidential Award. Washington, D.C.: PCPFS.

Rogers, F.R. 1925. Physical capacity tests in the administration of physical education. New York: Teachers College Contribution to Education.

Scott, M.G., and French, E. 1959. Measurement and evaluation in physical education. Dubuque, Iowa: Wm C Brown Group.

United States Department of Health and Human Services. 1985. Summary of findings from the National Children and Youth Fitness Study. Journal of Physical Education, Recreation and Dance, **56**(1):43-90.

United States Department of Health and Human Services. 1987. Summary of findings from the National Children and Youth Fitness Study II. Journal of Physical Education, Recreation and Dance, **58**(9):49-96.

United States Department of Health, Education, and Welfare. 1975. Federal Register, **40**(108), June 4.

ANNOTATED READINGS

Daves, C.W. 1984. The uses and misuses of tests. Washington: Jossey-Bass Inc., Publishers.

Addresses several major issues associated with the use of tests: the public stake in proper test use, professional standards for proper test use, issues in test use in schools, and test use and the law; written by experts in measurement, but in readable, nontechnical language.

Disch, J.G. 1983. The measurement of basic stuff. Journal of Physical Education, Recreation, and Dance, **54**(8):17-29.

A series of articles on the measurement of the body of knowledge in physical education as presented in the Basic Stuff Series, published by the American Alliance for Health, Physical Education, Recreation and Dance; includes articles on measurement in exercise physiology, motor development, biomechanics, humanities in physical education, psychosocial aspects of physical education, and motor learning.

Perkins, M.R. 1982. Minimum competency in testing: what? why? why not? Educational Measurement, 1(4):5-9, 26.

Presents various definitions of minimum competency testing; describes the perceived benefits of this use of tests; discusses the perceived costs of minimum competency testing; valuable reading for teachers involved in competency-based testing.

Ross, J.G., and Gilbert, G.G. 1985. A summary of findings. Journal of Physical Education, Recreation, and Dance, **56**(1):45-53.

A description of the National Children and Youth Fitness Study I, which was designed to determine the fitness status and activity levels of students in grades 5 through 12; includes a brief overview of the data collection procedures, new fitness standards, and a summary of other results.

Part Two

Simplified Statistics

2 Summarizing a Set of Test Scores

It is not uncommon for the terms *measurement* and *statistics* to be used interchangeably by students. Although both disciplines deal with sets of scores, **measurement** encompasses the process of obtaining test scores and **statistics** provides the methodology for analyzing the scores. In Chapter 1 measurement was defined as the process of assigning numbers to an object or a person according to some rule. Statistics, on the other hand, is defined as a method of analyzing a set of scores to enhance its interpretation. While an extensive coverage of statistics is not necessary in a measurement textbook, a few basic concepts must be covered to provide an understanding of certain measurement practices described later in the book. The type of statistics primarily covered in this book is **descriptive statistics,** which can be used to describe a data set. Basically, statistics will be used in the following ways in this book:

1. *To describe a set of test scores.* Having obtained a set of test scores, what kind of information can be derived from these scores? The scores can be ordered in *frequency distribution* form, and a measure of the *center* and *spread* of the distribution can be calculated. (These terms are defined later in this chapter.)
2. *To standardize a test score.* Sometimes standardizing a person's score on a test is useful so that the score can be compared with those of other people. This can be accomplished by transforming scores to a different scale such as a z-score or a **percentile** scale.
3. *To estimate the validity and reliability of a test.* In measurement theory a

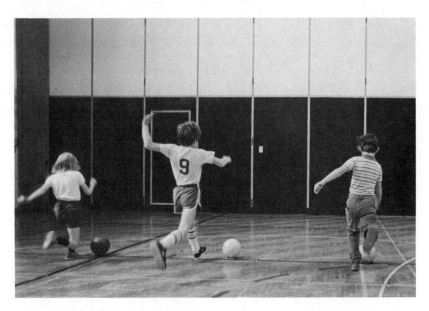

Testing elementary school children.

test has certain characteristics such as *reliability* and *validity*. These test characteristics are often estimated using a statistic known as the *correlation coefficient*.

Another branch of statistics is known as *inferential* statistics. When a data set is obtained from a sample that is assumed to be representative of the population from which the sample is drawn, it is appropriate to use inferential statistics to analyze the data. One such statistic is the t-test, which is briefly described in Chapter 3.

Numerous statistics software packages are now available for microcomputers. Some are relatively inexpensive and easy to use. Refer to Chapters 4 and 5 for more information on microcomputers.

MEASUREMENT SCALES

Whenever a measurement instrument is used, some type of score is obtained. To interpret the score, knowing the rule underlying the score is helpful. An accurate interpretation depends in part on the type of scale the score reflects. Four types of scales are commonly described: *nominal, ordinal, interval*, and *ratio*.

A nominal scale is a set of mutually exclusive categories. Each category represents one aspect of the attribute being measured. If a score can legitimately be placed in more than one category, the categories are not mutually exclusive. In a properly developed nominal scale, a score can fit one and only one category.

However, there is no meaningful order to the categorization. Classifying football players by number is an example of nominal scaling. A player who is assigned number 42 is not necessarily better than a player assigned number 12. Another example of a nominal scale is gender, that is, male or female.

An ordinal scale is determined by ranking a set of objects with regard to some specific characteristic. A basketball coach might be asked to rank the basketball teams in a league on the basis of predicted success at the end of the season. If ten teams are in the league, a rank of 1 is assigned to the team predicted to win the league title and a rank of 10 to the team expected to be at the bottom of the league. Since a rank of 1 is better than a rank of 2, the order of the numbers is important. However, the top-ranked team might be considerably better than the teams ranked 2, 3, and 4, while the latter three teams might be similar in ability. These differences are not reflected in the differences between ranks. Ordinal scales can also characterize scores that are not in the form of actual ranks. For example, when all-star teams are selected by a national press, sportswriters are asked to vote for the player of their choice. Suppose Player F receives 232 votes; Player R, 190 votes; and Player N, 93 votes. Clearly, Player F is considered outstanding by the largest number of sportswriters, but the number of votes does not disclose how much better Player F is than Player R. Because the distance between numbers does not have a meaningful interpretation, the scores represent ordinal data. Although the actual number of votes may be reported by the press, future reference to the all-star players generally centers on the ranks of the players.

In the interval scale the scores have a meaningful order, and units of measurement are an equal distance apart on the scale. On a test of motor behavior the distance between 93 and 90 represents the same range of ability as the difference between 53 and 50. If an interval scale contains a score of 0, the 0 score does not reflect total absence of the attribute being measured.

In contrast, the ratio scale uses a 0 score that represents absence of the attribute. For example, a score of 0 on a vertical jump would be interpreted as the total lack of ability to execute a jump vertically. The ordering of numbers is meaningful (larger numbers represent higher jumps), the distance between numbers is equal (the difference between 15 and 12 inches is equal to the difference between 10 and 7 inches), and the ratio of numbers is meaningful (12 inches is twice as long as 6 inches). Of course, given two examinees of equal height, 3 inches at higher heights may represent a greater performance increment than 3 inches at lower heights. Ratio scales include measures of length, weight, and time, which are frequently used in measuring motor skills.

Why is it important to understand measurement scales? Certain descriptive statistics are designed specifically for a designated scale. For example, the Spearman rank-difference (rho) correlation coefficient (described in Chapter 3) was developed to be used with ordinal data. Of greater importance is that the properties of the measurement scale should reflect the underlying characteristics of the attribute being measured. For example, if the numbers have no meaningful order and are merely used for classification purposes, the nominal scale best reflects the characteristic being measured. Scales are used in an effort to describe data as accurately as possible.

DISCRETE AND CONTINUOUS VARIABLES

A variable may be classified as either *continuous* or *discrete*. A continuous variable is one that, in theory, can be measured to continuing finer degrees. Many physical measures—such as distance, time, and weight or mass—are examples of continuous variables. A long jump, for example, can be measured to the nearest foot, the nearest inch, the nearest half-inch, and so on. Variables that are not continuous are known as discrete variables, since these variables can assume values only at distinct or discrete points on a scale. A baseball team might score 8 runs during a game, but never 8½ or 8¼ runs. Other examples of discrete variables are the number of students in a class, the number of teams in a league, and the number of books in a library.

FREQUENCY DISTRIBUTION

Suppose, as the instructor of a newly formed health and fitness class, you administer several tests to the class members before beginning instruction. These tests include body composition measures, a test of physical work capacity, and a measure of flexibility. Close examination of each data set is essential before beginning work with these individuals. A simple way of making sense of the data sets is to develop a **frequency distribution** for each set. A frequency distribution is a method of organizing data and has two basic characteristics. First, the test scores must have a meaningful order. For instance, assume that you have drawn two test scores out of one of the data sets and that each score has a different value. If the score with the higher value represents a greater amount of the attribute being measured, the scores in this set meet the criterion of having a meaningful order. Using the triceps skinfold as an example, it is obvious that a skinfold of 9 mm represents a thicker skinfold than a skinfold of 6 mm. On the surface all numbers may seem to have a meaningful order, but sometimes objects are given numerical labels merely for convenience. This is almost always the case with lockers in gymnasium dressing rooms, for example, since numbers are frequently used for identification. A locker with a higher number does not represent a better locker than one with a lower number. Thus it would be inappropriate to build a frequency distribution of locker numbers. The second characteristic is that categories in a frequency distribution must be *mutually exclusive*. Assigning a score to more than one category should not be possible. The scores in one category, then, should never overlap with those in other categories.

Frequency Distribution with Intervals of Size 1

Now let us turn to the task of actually building a frequency distribution. When the number of scores is small, the procedure is very simple. As the number of scores increases, the procedure becomes more complex, although it is certainly not difficult.

Ordered Scores Not in Frequency Distribution Form When a test is administered to a small number of people, a frequency distribution is probably not needed. However, no matter how small the data set, the test user should interpret the test scores. Administering a test and failing to use the data in any way is a waste of time for the examinee as well as the test user. Thus with a small data set the scores might simply be ordered from highest to lowest. Consider the following set of scores, representing subscapular skinfold thicknesses for 9-year-old girls:

Data set of 10 scores (in mm): 6, 9, 7, 10, 2, 4, 9, 5, 3, 6

Listing these scores from highest to lowest would yield the following order:

10-9-9-7-6-6-5-4-3-2

Such an ordering can be useful, but this is *not* a frequency distribution. If the characteristics of a frequency distribution in the previous section are reviewed, the reason this representation of the data is not a frequency distribution should be clear. The numbers have a meaningful order, but there are no mutually exclusive categories. To convert this data set into a frequency distribution, every possible score from 10 to 2 would be listed once; thus each score would form a category.

Construction of Frequency Distribution These scores are scores from a test of throwing accuracy taken by 24 elementary school children:

Data set of 24 scores (in points): 6, 1, 8, 7, 5, 5, 9, 6, 4, 10, 3, 6, 6, 5, 4, 7, 7, 8, 6, 4, 6, 5, 7, 5

The symbol for the number of test scores (or the number of people obtaining scores on a test) is N. In this example, N = 24. Note that the range is still small $(10 - 1 + 1 = 10)$; thus it would be appropriate to use intervals of size 1 to form a frequency distribution. Of course, listing each possible score in the data set, from highest to lowest, is possible; however, the data would not be in frequency-distribution form. With 24 scores, building a frequency distribution would be simpler. In addition, the description of the data would be more concise.

Score	Tally	f	cf	c%
10	x	1	24	100.0
9	x	1	23	95.8
8	xx	2	22	91.7
7	xxxx	4	20	83.3
6	xxxxxx	6	16	66.7
5	xxxxx	5	10	41.7
4	xxx	3	5	20.8
3	x	1	2	8.3
2		0	1	4.2
1	x	1	1	4.2

Note the columns in the above distribution. One is labeled **tally,** which represents the recording of a score in the appropriate interval. Each *x* designates one score in an interval. The next column, *f,* consists of the **frequency** of scores in each interval. This can be more simply expressed as the number of scores in each interval and is obtained by summing the tallies in each interval. The next column is labeled *cf,* the symbol for **cummulative frequency.** The numbers in this column are obtained by summing the frequencies from the bottom interval to the top. In the above example the *cf* for interval 6 is *16.* This indicates that 16 out of 24 people obtained scores of 6 or below on this measure. The *c%,* or **cumulative percent,** column displays the conversion of the *cf* column to percentages. Take another look at interval 6. A *cf* of 16 is converted to a *c%* of 66.7% by dividing 16 by the total number (N) of test scores, in this case, 24. The result must then be multiplied by 100. Thus, c% = cf/N × 100, or cf divided by N times 100. Referring to the interval 6, it would be appropriate to say that 66.7% of the group of 24 obtained scores of 6 or below. The percentages in this column are similar to *percentiles,* which are described later in this chapter.

With a larger range of score values, however, using intervals of size 1 would become very cumbersome. For instance, if the highest score in a data set is 80 and the lowest is 21, the range would be 60 (80 − 21 + 1). It would be tedious and very time-consuming to list 60 intervals of size 1 in forming a frequency distribution. Developing intervals greater than size 1 would be more expedient. This is sometimes referred to as a *group frequency distribution.* The major purpose of forming a frequency distribution is to summarize the data for easier interpretation. If too many intervals are used, the original purpose may be defeated. A large number of intervals often spreads the data too much to be interpretable, while a very small number of intervals can mask important trends in the data. The **range** (R) is determined by subtracting the lowest score from the highest score and adding 1 as symbolized in Formula 2-1:

$$R = (\text{Highest score} - \text{Lowest score}) + 1 \qquad \text{Formula 2-1}$$

Adding 1 to (Highest score − Lowest score) provides a more accurate indicator of the range as it reflects all possible scores in the distribution. Consider a small data set consisting of four scores: 7, 6, 5, 4. If 7 − 4 is used to calculate the range, the result is 3. Yet it is evident that there are four scores in the data set. The addition of 1 would yield a range of 4. Not all textbooks recommend adding 1 to determine the range. From a practical point of view, the difference between the two versions of the range is relatively minor.

Frequency Distribution with Intervals Greater than Size 1

When a set of test scores is distributed over a wider range, grouping the data into intervals greater than size 1 is preferred. As noted previously this is sometimes referred to as a group frequency distribution. Additional steps must be followed when the interval size exceeds 1, such as the determination of an appropriate interval size and a suitable number of intervals.

Description of Procedure Consider a data set of 22 scores on a physical fitness knowledge test, with the scores ranging from 80 to 99. The range of this set is 99 − 80 + 1 = 20. It would be more efficient and provide a better representation of the data if a frequency distribution with intervals greater than 1 were used. How many intervals should be formed? The general rule is to use *no fewer than 10 and no more than 20 intervals*. How large should the interval size be? Many interval sizes are legitimate possibilities, but the most widely used options are 2, 3, 5, 7, 10, and multiples of 5 thereafter. Since it has been determined that the range of this set of scores is 20 and that no fewer than 10 intervals should be used, the best interval size for this data set is 20/10 = 2.

Data set of 22 scores (Fitness Knowledge Test): 89, 86, 91, 82, 80, 93, 96, 87, 82, 98, 96, 99, 95, 90, 89, 91, 88, 92, 93, 87, 89, 91

$$N = 22; R = 99 - 80 + 1 = 20$$

Intervals	Tally	f	cf	c%
98-99	xx	2	22	100.0
96-97	xx	2	20	91.0
94-95	x	1	18	81.8
92-93	xxx	3	17	77.3
90-91	xxxx	4	14	63.6
88-89	xxxx	4	10	45.5
86-87	xxx	3	6	27.2
84-85		0	3	13.6
82-83	xx	2	3	13.6
80-81	x	1	1	4.5

Traditionally, frequency distributions are constructed so that the highest scores are at the top of the column and the lowest scores are at the bottom. Displaying an interval with the lowest score in the interval placed to the left of the interval and the highest score, to the right, is customary. The reason higher scores are usually placed at the top of the **interval** (i) column is that higher scores typically represent better performances. However, this is not always true in measuring motor behavior, especially when the score is recorded in time. When measuring running speed, for example, faster times (smaller scores) represent better performances. In these cases building the frequency distributions with the smaller scores at the top of the interval column would be appropriate (see example, p. 32). Keep in mind that the purpose of a frequency distribution is to present a meaningful summary of the data.

Summary of Steps The following steps are taken in constructing a frequency distribution with intervals of size 1. (Other equally effective approaches may also be used to accomplish the same purpose.)

1. Calculate the range of the set of scores (highest score − lowest score + 1). List all possible scores in the range, regardless of whether the score actually occurs in the data set. The score representing the best performance should be placed at the top of the list, and the score reflecting the poorest performance should be at the bottom of the list.
2. Tally each of the scores in the data set, using x's or 1's as tallies.
3. Develop the frequency (f) column by summing the tallies for each interval.
4. Generate the cumulative frequency (cf) column by adding the frequencies, beginning with the bottom interval.
5. Develop the cumulative percent $(c\%)$ column by dividing cf by N and multiplying by 100.

If the frequency distribution includes intervals greater than size 1, two additional steps, *1a* and *1b*, must be taken between steps *1* and *2* above.

1a. Select an appropriate number of intervals to ensure that the distribution will contain no more than 20 intervals and no fewer than 10.
1b. Select an appropriate interval size. Remember that typical interval sizes are 2, 3, 5, 7, and 10. To determine the interval size, the number of intervals can be divided into the range.

Another way to approach the development of a frequency distribution with intervals greater than size 1 is to estimate the interval size first, taking into account the range, then divide the range by the interval size to obtain the number of intervals. Let's contrast the two approaches. If the number of intervals is determined first, even a cursory examination of the frequency distribution data on p. 28 would show that the number will be relatively small. This is evident, since the range (20) itself is small. Thus a reasonable estimate of an appropriate number of intervals is 10, and 20/10 = 2. The distribution, then, would have 10 intervals with an interval size of 2. To take the other approach, determining the interval size first, simply reverse your thought process as follows. Since the range is small, the number of intervals can be maximized by keeping the interval size small. As this example deals with intervals greater than size 1, the smallest possible interval size is 2. Dividing the range (20) by 2 yields 10 intervals. This is basically a trial-and-error process. The interval size and the number of intervals are adjusted until both numbers are acceptable.

Graphing Distributions

Although the frequency distribution is a simple method of summarizing a set of scores, it may not be the most effective way of displaying the summary to others. Graphical representations are sometimes more powerful when presenting your data to principals, club managers, laboratory directors, clients, parents, and so forth. Two popular types of graphs are the **frequency polygon** and the **histogram.**

In Figure 2-1 the frequency distribution on p. 28 is shown in frequency polygon form. Since the intervals in this distribution are greater than size 1, the points used to plot the frequency polygon are the midpoints of the intervals shown on the horizontal axis. On the vertical axis of the graph, the frequency of cases (number of test scores) is depicted.

The histogram is a type of bar graph. The width of the bar represents the width of the interval displayed on the horizontal axis of the graph. As with the frequency polygon, the frequency of cases is shown on the vertical axis. Figure

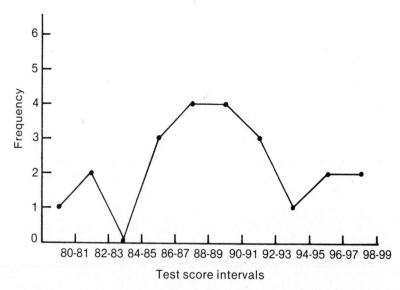

FIGURE 2-1 *Frequency polygon of scores on Physical Fitness Knowledge Test.*

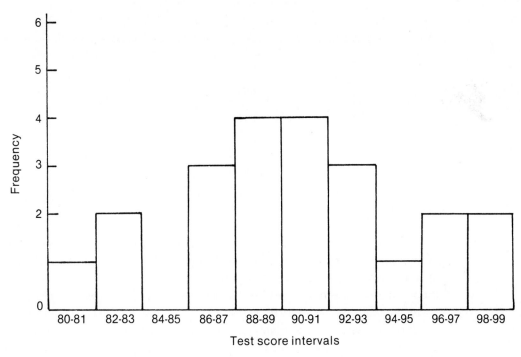

FIGURE 2-2 *Histogram of scores on Physical Fitness Knowledge Test.*

2-2 depicts the distribution on p. 28 in histogram form. The choice between using a histogram or a frequency polygon is largely a matter of personal preference.

Special Case of Frequency Distribution

In situations where lower scores represent better performances, such as golf and running events, the frequency distribution may be modified accordingly. When a frequency distribution or a graph of the distribution is of primary interest, the lowest scores can be placed at the top of the distribution. This provides a clear presentation of the set of scores, since people generally expect to see better scores at the top of a frequency distribution. The percentile and percentile rank formulas (presented later in this chapter) must be modified to be used with this type of distribution of scores. Consider the following set of time scores on a shuttle run test, where test performance is timed to the nearest tenth of a second.

Data set of 20 scores (in seconds): 9.2, 11.1, 9.7, 10.3, 10.5, 9.8, 10.9, 11.6, 11.3, 9.0, 10.0, 10.3, 10.0, 9.8, 9.8, 10.3, 9.7, 10.5, 10.0, 10.1

$$N = 20; \text{ Range} = 11.6 - 9.0 + 0.1 = 2.7 \text{ or } 27 \text{ scores recorded}$$
to the nearest tenth of a second

Interval	Tally	f
9.1-9.0	x	1
9.3-9.2	x	1
9.5-9.4		0
9.7-9.6	xx	2
9.9-9.8	xxx	3
10.1-10.0	xxxx	4
10.3-10.2	xxx	3
10.5-10.4	xx	2
10.7-10.6		0
10.9-10.8	x	1
11.1-11.0	x	1
11.3-11.2	x	1
11.5-11.4		0
11.7-11.6	x	1

Even though these scores are recorded to the nearest tenth of a second, each tenth can be considered as a score to determine the interval size. Thus the range for this set of scores is 27 (116 − 90 + 1). If an interval size of 3 were selected, the number of intervals would be 9, which would not fit the rule of thumb of 10 to 20 intervals. If an interval size of 2 were chosen, the number of intervals would be 14 (27/2 = 13.5, rounded to 14). Note that the lower scores represent better performances on the shuttle run test. Therefore these scores are placed at the top of the *interval* column. Furthermore, within each interval the lower (better) score is placed at the top of the interval (to the right) and the higher (poorer) score is placed at the bottom (to the left). If the data were presented in graph form, the scores would be plotted in the same manner, with the lower scores placed to the right of the horizontal axis and the higher values to the left. Remember, however, that the formulas described in the remaining sections of this chapter are not appropriate to use with this distribution unless they are modified.

CALCULATION OF PERCENTILES

After a test has been administered to a group of examinees and a frequency distribution has been developed using a set of scores, using the distribution to calculate one or more percentiles is often helpful. For example, the **median** is frequently of interest because it represents the center of the distribution of scores. The median is the 50th **percentile,** often expressed by the symbol $X_{.50}$. The median is the score that divides the distribution so that 50% of the scores fall above this point and 50% fall below. Of course, other percentiles also provide useful information, especially when standards of performance are needed to interpret a set of scores. In the following sections the format followed in describing the development of a frequency distribution is used. First, the calculation of percentiles for ordered scores (not in frequency distribution form) is described. Then,

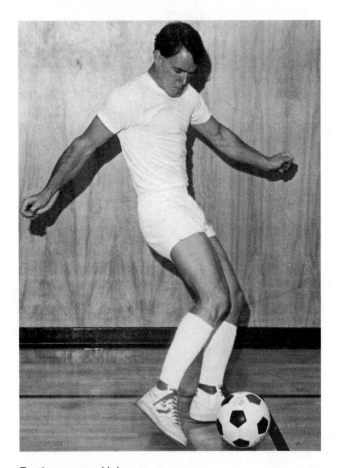

Testing soccer kick.

the procedures for calculating percentiles are presented for the simple frequency distribution (intervals of size 1) and the group frequency distribution (intervals greater than size 1).

Calculation from Ordered Scores

Using ordered scores (not in frequency distribution form), calculating the median or any other percentile is simple, especially if the number of cases is small. Consider, for example, this set representing scores on a pull-up test.

Data set of 17 scores (no. of pull-ups): 7, 4, 10, 1, 6, 6, 4, 3, 7, 10, 1, 7, 4, 10, 7, 4, 8

These scores can simply be ordered from highest to lowest, not in frequency distribution form:

10-10-10-8-7-7-7-7-6-6-4-4-4-4-3-1-1

There are 17 scores in this data set. By definition, the median will be represented by the score dividing the distribution into equal halves. The median, then, will be the ninth score, since this score divides the distribution in halves of 8 scores each. Counting up from the bottom (or down from the top), the ninth score is a score of 6. Thus the median is 6 in this example. Let's identify another percentile—the 75th percentile or $X_{.75}$. This is the score separating the top one fourth of the distribution from the bottom three fourths. Four scores fall above this point and 12 fall below; thus, the 75th percentile is 7.

Calculation from Frequency Distribution with Intervals of Size 1

This same set of 17 scores can also be displayed in simple frequency distribution form, with intervals of size 1.

Interval	Tally	f	cf
10	XXX	3	17
9		0	14
8	X	1	14
7	XXXX	4	13
6	XX	2	9
5		0	7
4	XXXX	4	7
3	X	1	3
2		0	2
1	XX	2	2

Score Limits Up to this point, the numbers used to represent intervals have been the scores an examinee might actually obtain on a test. These numbers are called the **score limits** of the interval. For example, the top two intervals in the above distribution can be displayed as follows:

$$[\underline{\hspace{2cm}}] \ [\underline{\hspace{2cm}}]$$
$$\quad 9 \qquad\qquad 10$$

Conceptually, a set of test scores is viewed as a distribution of scores. The shape of the distribution is determined by the way the scores are spread throughout the possible range of scores. If most of the scores are grouped in the center of the distribution with a smaller number of scores at each end, the distribution will resemble a normal curve. The only point to keep in mind now is that the space under the curve is the area represented by the test scores. When score limits are used to represent a data set, the representation is incomplete because a small amount of area is left out between the score limits of the intervals. Notice in the above display of score limits that all scores in the interval of 9 are considered in the middle of the interval. The same is true for the interval 10. These scores represent the score limits of the two intervals. A small amount of space is unaccounted for between the intervals. In this case the space between the two midpoints of each interval, 9 and 10, is unaccounted for. For this reason real limits must be used to calculate percentiles more precisely.

Real Limits To obtain **real limits,** first examine the score limits for any two adjacent intervals. A real limit is determined by taking half the distance between any two adjacent score limits representing the upper score limit of one interval and the lower score limit of the adjacent interval. In this case (intervals of size 1) the upper score limit and the lower score limit are the same for each interval. Look back to the two score limits in this section. The distance between the score limits is 1. By taking half of 1 and adding to and subtracting from the score limits, real limits of 8.5 to 9.5 and 9.5 to 10.5 are obtained. (Real limits are not used for purposes of tallying; only score limits are used for the placement of tallies.) Compare this representation with the one for score limits:

$$[\underline{\hspace{1.5cm}}] \ [\underline{\hspace{1.5cm}}]$$
$$\quad 8.5 \qquad 9.5 \qquad 10.5$$

When real limits are determined for every interval in a distribution, the entire area under the curve is taken into account. Real limits are also used in calculating percentiles using a group frequency distribution (intervals greater than 1) as well as in calculating percentile ranks.

Percentile Formula To use the following percentile (%ile) formula, Formula 2-2, the data must be in frequency distribution form.

$$\%ile = lrl + \frac{.x(N) - \Sigma fb}{fw}(i) \qquad\qquad \text{Formula 2-2}$$

where %ile = percentile; for example, $X_{.50}$ = 50th percentile or median
      lrl = *lower real limit* of interval containing the score representing the desired percentile
      .x = *percentile* displayed as a proportion; for example, the 50th percentile is displayed as .50
      N = total *number* of scores; total frequency in data set
      Σfb = *sum* of *frequencies* below the interval containing the score representing the desired percentile
      fw = *frequency within* this interval
      i = size (width) of the *interval*

Now Formula 2-2 is used below with the frequency distribution on p. 34 to calculate the 75th percentile.

Be certain you are working in the correct interval before you begin calculating. In this case, the correct interval is identified by determining 75%N or .75(17), which equals 12.75. This is the calculation for .x(N) in Formula 2-2. The 12.75th score is the 75th percentile in this set of scores. Checking the *cf* column of the frequency distribution, the 12.75th score is located in the interval 7, since 12.75 is larger than 9 but not greater than 13. Although the interval has now been identified, the score must still be calculated. The formula is completed as follows:

$$\text{75th \%ile} = 6.5 + \frac{12.75 - 9}{4} \tag{1}$$

$$= 7.4375$$

Calculation from Frequency Distribution with Interval Greater than Size 1

When calculating percentiles using frequency distributions with intervals greater than size 1 (group frequency distribution), Formula 2-2 *must* be used. When data are grouped in this way, information on the original data set is lost. However, the data are portrayed in a more concise form and thus are more easily interpretable. The value of the percentile calculated from a group frequency distribution will be slightly different from the value calculated from ordered data, again due to the loss of information brought about by grouping. The frequency distribution presented below is used to demonstrate this calculation. The data represent scores (in inches) on the standing long jump for a group of 14-year-old boys, where N = 60.

Interval	f	cf
80-82	1	60
77-79	3	59
74-76	5	56
71-73	6	51
68-70	9	45
65-67	12	36
62-64	9	24
59-61	6	15
56-58	5	9
53-55	3	4
50-52	1	1

Before describing the steps in this calculation, a review of the concept of real limits is appropriate, since larger (wider) intervals are being used. The score limits for the top two intervals in the above distribution can be displayed as follows:

$$\underset{77 \qquad 79}{[\underline{\qquad\qquad}]} \quad \underset{80 \qquad 82}{[\underline{\qquad\qquad}]}$$

When score limits are used to represent the data set, the distribution of the scores is not completely displayed. A small amount of area is left out between the score limits of adjacent intervals. Notice in the above display of score limits that the area between 79 and 80 is not represented. To be precise in calculating precentiles, *all* of the area must be taken into account.

In this case the lower score limit of the top interval of the above example is 80, and the upper score limit of the lower interval is 79. The distance or area between these limits is 1. Taking half of 1 and adding to and subtracting from the upper and lower score limits, real limits of 76.5 to 79.5 and 79.5 to 82.5 are obtained. The real limits are depicted as follows:

$$[\text{_____}] \, [\text{_____}]$$
$$76.5 \qquad 79.5 \qquad 82.5$$

The median and other percentiles can be calculated using Formula 2-2. Since the median is frequently of interest to a test user, let's calculate this value first.

$$X_{.50} = 64.5 + \frac{30 - 24}{12} \, (3)$$
$$= 66$$

Be certain you are working in the correct interval before you begin calculating. In this case, the correct interval is identified by determining 50%N or .5(60), which is 30. Thus, the 30th case is the median in this set of scores. Checking the *cf* column of the frequency distribution, the 30th score is located in the interval between 65 and 67 (30 is larger than 24 but less than 36). Now that the interval has been identified, the score must be calculated. Since the range of scores in the interval equals 3, the score representing the median is unknown. To determine the interval size, subtract the lower score limit from the upper score limit and add 1 to the result. For instance, if 65 were subtracted from 67, the result would equal 2. However, it is clear that the interval 65-67 contains *three* scores—65, 66, and 67. By adding 1 to the result, an interval size of 3 is obtained, which is correct. Of course, the correct size could also be obtained by subtracting the lower real limit from the upper real limit.

As another example, let's calculate the 80th percentile, or $X_{.80}$. To identify the correct interval, find 80%N or .8(60), which equals 48. Since 48 is larger than 45 in the *cf* column but not greater than 51, the interval 71–73 contains the 48th case, which in turn represents the 80th percentile. Now the percentile formula can be used to calculate the score representing the 80th percentile.

$$X_{.80} = 70.5 + \frac{48 - 45}{6} \, (3)$$
$$= 70.5 + 1.5$$
$$= 72$$

Summary of Steps

The following steps summarize the procedure for calculating percentiles:
1. Identify the interval containing the percentile by determine x%(N) or .x(N). Use the cf column to locate this number, then mark the corresponding interval.
2. Determine the lower real limit (lrl) of the interval identified in step #1.
3. Find fb, the sum of the frequencies below this interval by referring to the cf column immediately below the interval.

4. Find fw, the frequency within the interval, by noting the number of cases in the f column for this interval.
5. Determine i, the interval size, by subtracting the lower real limit from the upper real limit.
6. Use Formula 2-2 to calculate the percentile.

Calculating Percentiles When Lower Scores Represent Better Performance

On page 31 a special case of the frequency distribution was described. The special case is appropriate when lower scores represent better performance, a common occurrence in our field. The formula to calculate percentiles must be modified under these circumstances. Consider the following frequency distribution of time scores (recorded to the nearest tenth of a second) for an agility run test:

X	Tally	f	cf
10.1	x	1	20
10.2	xx	2	19
10.3	xx	2	17
10.4	xxx	3	15
10.5	xxxx	4	12
10.6	xxx	3	8
10.7	xx	2	5
10.8	xx	2	3
10.9		0	1
11.0	x	1	1

Calculate the 50th percentile:

$$\%tile = lrl + \frac{fb - .xN}{fw} (i) \qquad \text{Formula 2-3}$$

where lrl (in this case only) = X + ½ unit of measurement (½ of .1 = .05)

$$X_{.50} = 10.55 + \frac{8 - .5(20)}{4} (.1)$$

$$= 10.55 + \frac{-2}{4} (.1)$$

$$= 10.55 - .05 = 10.5$$

CALCULATION OF PERCENTILE RANKS

The answer to the question, "What is the nth **percentile?**" is always a test score. A teacher may wish to provide summary information on students' test performance for review by the principal. The manager of a fitness club may ask for information on specific percentiles for certain measures of fitness administered to clients at some point in their program. On the other hand, from the standpoint of the client or the student, the most useful information might be the percentile rank representing his or her own score. Here the known factor is the student's

score, and the unknown factor is the percentage, now called the **percentile rank.**
Now the question is, "What is the percentile rank for a score of X?" The score is
known and the percentile rank is unknown; in the previous section the percentile was known and the score was unknown. Keep in mind that percentiles and
percentile ranks are reciprocal concepts.

Calculations from Ordered Scores

You will recall that it was possible to calculate a percentile without forming a
frequency distribution at all. The scores were simply ordered from highest to
lowest, which is reasonable if the number of scores in the data set is small. Let
us use the example on p. 34 to show how percentile ranks can also be calculated
from an ordered set of scores. Consider a score of 8; what percentile rank does
this score represent? By counting from the lowest score upward, we find that the
score of 8 is the 14th score in the data set. Since N = 17, the percentile rank can
be calculated by dividing 14 by 17, which equals 82%. Therefore a score of 8
reflects a percentile rank of 82%, meaning that 82% of the examinees in this sample obtained scores of 8 or below on this test. Only 18% of the examinees scored
higher than 8; thus 8 is a very good score. Using the same set of ordered scores,
calculate the percentile rank for a score of 3. The answer you should have obtained is 18%. A score of 3 is the third score in the ordered data set, and the
percentile rank is $\frac{3}{17}$ = 18%. Percentile ranks can also be calculated from frequency distributions, either with intervals of size 1 or intervals greater than
size 1.

Calculation for Frequency Distribution with Intervals Greater than Size 1

Formula 2-4 is used to calculate more precise estimates of the percentile rank.
This formula, as well as Formula 2-2 on p. 35, has many variations that will yield
the same answer. Although the calculation will be exemplified using a frequency
distribution with intervals greater than size 1, the formula is equally applicable
when the intervals are of size 1.

$$\text{PR for X} = \frac{\left(\begin{array}{c}\text{cf in}\\\text{interval}\\\text{below}\end{array}\right) + \dfrac{X - \text{lrl}}{i}(f)}{N}(100) \qquad \text{Formula 2-4}$$

where PR = percentile rank
     X = score
   lrl = lower real limit
     i = interval size
    f = frequency

It is not necessary to perform any calculation to locate the interval, since the examinee's score is provided, which automatically locates the interval. Let's calculate the percentile rank for a score of 69, using the distribution on p. 36.

$$\text{PR for 69} = \frac{36 + \dfrac{69 - 67.5}{3}(9)}{60}(100)$$

$$= \frac{36 + \dfrac{1.5}{3}(9)}{60}(100)$$

$$= 67.5\%$$

A score of 69 has a percentile rank of 67.5.

Note that the real limits must be used in calculating this statistic. A table of percentiles and scores can easily be set up for a test, and then either the percentile or the percentile rank can be read from the table. If a test is used frequently, such a table is useful. Sample tables of percentiles are included in several chapters of this textbook. A microcomputer program for calculating a table of percentiles is included in the Appendix (see p. A-31). This program can be used when the distribution of scores forms an approximate normal curve (see Chapter 3). The mean and standard deviation of the set of scores are used to calculate percentiles. These calculations are shown in Table 2-1. Once the mean and standard deviation have been determined, this table can be set up by hand, although using a computer program is far easier.

TABLE 2-1 *Development of table of percentiles using mean and standard deviation*

PR	%	PR	%
99.9	$\bar{X} + 3.00s$	45.0	$\bar{X} - .13s$
95.0	$\bar{X} + 1.64s$	40.0	$\bar{X} - .25s$
90.0	$\bar{X} + 1.28s$	35.0	$\bar{X} - .39s$
85.0	$\bar{X} + 1.04s$	30.0	$\bar{X} - .52s$
80.0	$\bar{X} + .84s$	25.0	$\bar{X} - .67s$
75.0	$\bar{X} + .67s$	20.0	$\bar{X} - .84s$
70.0	$\bar{X} + .52s$	15.0	$\bar{X} - 1.04s$
65.0	$\bar{X} + .39s$	10.0	$\bar{X} - 1.28s$
60.0	$\bar{X} + .25s$	5.0	$\bar{X} - 1.64s$
55.0	$\bar{X} + .13s$	0.1	$\bar{X} - 3.00s$
50.0	$\bar{X} + .00s$		

Summary of Steps

The steps for calculating percentiles are summarized below:
1. Identify the interval containing the score of interest.
2. Find cf, the cumulative frequency of scores, just below the interval identified in step 1.
3. Determine lrl, the lower real limit, by subtracting half of the unit of measurement from the lowest score in the interval.
4. Find i, the interval size, and f, the frequency.
5. Calculate the percentile rank.

Calculating PR When Lower Scores Represent Better Performance

The percentile rank formula must be modified when lower scores represent better performance.

$$\text{PR for X} = \frac{\begin{array}{c}\text{cf in}\\\text{interval}\\\text{below}\end{array} + \dfrac{\text{lrl} - \text{X}}{i}(f)}{N}(100) \qquad \text{Formula 2-5}$$

The data from the frequency distribution on p. 38 will be used to exemplify this calculation:

$$\text{PR for 10.3} = \frac{15 + \dfrac{10.35 - 10.3}{.1}(2)}{20}(100)$$

$$= \frac{15 + .05/.1(2)}{20}(100)$$

$$= \frac{15 + 1}{20}(100)$$

$$= .80 \text{ or } 80\%$$

SUMMARY

Once a test has been administered to a group of examinees, a set of test scores is available to be interpreted. Several types of questions might be of interest. How are the test scores distributed for the entire group? To answer this question, a frequency distribution can be constructed and graphed for easier analysis. For example, what is the 50th percentile? For any percentile, the corresponding test score can be calculated. How good is a score of X? The percentile rank of any score in the distribution can be determined. At the very least, a frequency distribution should be formed for each set of test scores unless the number of scores is small; then a simple ordering of scores will often suffice. Test information should not be wasted. If administering the test is important enough, analyzing the scores properly is certainly worthwhile.

REFERENCES

Glass, G.V., and Stanley, J.C. 1980. Statistical methods in education and psychology. Englewood Cliffs, N.J.: Prentice-Hall, Inc.

Hopkins, K.D., and Stanley, J.C. 1981. Educational and psychological measurement and evaluation. Englewood Cliffs, N.J.: Prentice-Hall, Inc.

Mattson, D.E. 1981. Statistics: difficult concepts, understandable explanations. St. Louis: The C.V. Mosby Co.

Stahl, S.M., and Hennes, J.D. 1980. Reading and understanding applied statistics: a self-learning approach, ed. 2, St. Louis: The C.V. Mosby Co.

ANNOTATED READINGS

Gutman, A. 1984. Computerized instruction in statistics. Lavallette, N.J.: Holt, Rinehart & Winston General Book.

Consists of comprehensive courseware package; explains and illustrates the major concepts found in introductory statistics textbooks; class-tested for user friendliness and ease of operation; eight tutorial disks cover statistical concepts; interactive exercises; eight stat-paks; available for Apple II+ or IIe.

Hills, J.R. 1983. Interpreting percentile scores. Educational Measurement, 2(2):24.

Ten true-false items on the interpretation of percentile scores; provides correct answers and brief explanations for all items; useful way to review the concept of percentiles.

Spatz, C., and Johnston, J.O. 1984. Basic statistics: tales of distribution, ed. 3, Belmont, Calif.: Brooks/Cole Publishing Co.

Designed for use in a one-term introductory course; emphasizes conceptualization and interpretation of statistical results; uses distinctive pedagogical devices to stimulate interest and facilitate understanding; covers both descriptive and inferential statistics; presents problems and answers with all necessary steps and explanations.

Weinbery, S.L., and Goldberg, K.P. 1979. Basic statistics for education and the behavioral sciences. Boston: Houghton Mifflin Co.

Written for beginning students; presents case studies from education and the behavioral sciences at the end of each chapter; provides realistic examples of each concept; reviews basic mathematics in an appendix; instructor's manual includes eight sample examinations with complete solutions.

Wike, E.L. 1985. Numbers: a primer of data analysis. Columbus, Ohio: Charles E. Merrill Publishing Co.

Lays the foundation for the underlying concepts of statistics; designed for the beginning student; avoids the characteristic dryness of many statistics texts; includes a computer addendum at the end of each chapter, relating material to the MINITAB computer program; uses practical examples and problems.

PROBLEMS

1. Answer the following questions *without* forming a frequency distribution:

   Data set of 15 scores (on push-ups test):
   28, 19, 30, 15, 19, 9, 20, 28, 33, 10, 14, 32, 27, 24, 19

   a. Order the scores from highest to lowest.
   b. Calculate the median.
   c. Calculate the 66 ⅔ (round to 67th) percentile.
   d. What is the percentile rank for a score of 15?

2. Use the following data set to form a frequency distribution:

Data set of 15 scores (on sit-ups test):
62, 60, 59, 66, 60, 57, 61, 65, 58, 59, 65, 60, 64, 61, 60

    a. Form a frequency distribution with intervals of size 1. Include columns for tally, f, cf, and c%.
    b. Calculate the median.
    c. Calculate the 75th percentile.
    d. What is the percentile rank of a score of 58?

3. Use the following data set to build a frequency distribution:

Data set of 30 scores (on tennis serve test):
63, 59, 76, 60, 44, 41, 59, 68, 64, 55, 79, 65, 65, 58, 48, 65, 40, 72, 68, 70, 59, 46, 66, 51, 52, 69, 75, 46, 59, 58

    a. Form a frequency distribution with intervals of size 4. Include columns for real limits, tally, f, cf, and c%.
    b. Calculate the median.
    c. Calculate the 25th percentile.
    d. What is the percentile rank for a score of 66?

4. Use the following data to form a frequency distribution:

Data set of 20 scores (on the 50-yard dash):
7.4, 7.5, 6.8, 8.1, 8.7, 7.2, 9.1, 8.4, 7.2, 6.5, 8.2, 7.5, 8.1, 9.4, 8.0, 6.9, 7.5, 9.0, 6.7, 7.0

Form a frequency distribution with intervals of size 3 (actually .3, since the data are recorded in tenth of seconds). Remember that you are working with time scores and lower scores represent better performances. Include columns for real limits, tally, f, cf, and c%.

5. Use the following data set to form a frequency distribution:

Data set of 20 scores on 50 yard dash: (unit = seconds)
7.0, 7.8, 7.5, 7.2, 7.3, 7.4, 7.4, 7.2, 7.5, 7.6, 7.7, 8.0, 7.7, 7.5, 7.8, 7.6, 7.5, 7.7, 7.5, 7.4.

    a. Form a frequency distribution with intervals of size 0.1. Include columns for real limits, tally, f, cf, and c%.
    b. Calculate the median.
    c. Calculate the 60th percentile.
    d. What is the percentile rank of a score of 7.4 seconds?

6. Use the following data set to build a frequency distribution:

Data set of 45 scores on standing long jump: (unit = cm)
226 267 232 243 258 238 239 238 240 241 247 250 257 248 240 231 222 254 243 243 238 232 236 235 259 240 264 244 251 245 217 248 253 260 234 250 224 246 226 245 247 230 252 235 242

    a. Form a frequency distribution with intervals of size 5. Include columns for real limits, tally, f, cf, and c%.
    b. Calculate the median.
    c. Calculate the 90th percentile.

d. What is the percentile rank for a score of 248 cm?

e. What is the percentile rank for a score of 229 cm?

ANSWERS TO PROBLEMS

1. a. 33-32-30-28-28-27-24-20-19-19-19-15-14-10-9

   b. $X_{.50} = 20$

   c. $X_{.67} = 27.5$

   d. PR for score of 15 = 26.67%

2. a.

Interval	Tally	f	cf	c%
66	X	1	15	100.0
65	XX	2	14	93.3
64	X	1	12	80.0
63		0	11	73.3
62	X	1	11	73.3
61	XX	2	10	66.7
60	XXXX	4	8	53.3
59	XX	2	4	26.7
58	X	1	2	13.3
57	X	1	1	6.7

   b. $X_{.50} = 60$

   c. $X_{.75} = 64$

   d. PR for score of 58 = 13.3%

3. a.

Interval	Real limits	Tally	f	cf	c%
76-79	75.5-79.5	XX	2	30	100.0
72-75	71.5-75.5	XX	2	28	93.3
68-71	67.5-71.5	XXXX	4	26	86.7
64-67	63.5-67.5	XXXXX	5	22	73.3
60-63	59.5-63.5	XX	2	17	56.7
56-59	55.5-59.5	XXXXXX	6	15	50.0
52-55	51.5-55.5	XX	2	9	30.0
48-51	47.5-51.5	XX	2	7	23.3
44-47	43.5-47.4	XXX	3	5	16.7
40-43	39.5-43.5	XX	2	2	6.7

   b.
   $$X_{.50} = 55.5 + \frac{15 - 9}{6}(4) = 55.5 + \frac{6}{6}(4)$$
   $$= 59.5$$

   c.
   $$X_{.25} = 51.5 + \frac{7.5 - 7}{2}(4) = 51.5 + \frac{.5}{2}(4)$$
   $$= 52.5$$

   d.
   $$\text{PR for 66} = \frac{17 + \dfrac{66 - 63.5}{4}(5)}{30}(100)$$
   $$= 67.1\%$$

4.

Interval	Real limits	Tally	f	cf	c%
6.7-6.5	6.75-6.55	xx	2	20	100.0
7.0-6.8	7.05-6.75	xxx	3	18	90.0
7.3-7.1	7.35-7.05	xx	2	15	75.0
7.6-7.4	7.65-7.35	xxxx	4	13	65.0
7.9-7.7	7.95-7.65		0	9	45.0
8.2-8.0	8.25-7.95	xxxx	4	9	45.0
8.5-8.3	8.55-8.25	x	1	5	25.0
8.8-8.6	8.85-8.55	x	1	4	20.0
9.1-8.9	9.15-8.85	xx	2	3	15.0
9.4-9.2	9.45-9.15	x	1	1	5.0

5. a.

Interval	Real limits	Tally	f	cf	c%
7.0	7.05-6.95	x	1	20	100
7.1	7.15-7.05		0	19	95
7.2	7.25-7.15	xx	2	19	95
7.3	7.35-7.25	x	1	17	85
7.4	7.45-7.35	xxx	3	16	80
7.5	7.55-7.45	xxxxx	5	13	65
7.6	7.65-7.55	xx	2	8	40
7.7	7.75-7.65	xxx	3	6	30
7.8	7.85-7.75	xx	2	3	15
7.9	7.95-7.85		0	1	5
8.0	8.05-7.95	x	1	1	5

b.
$$X_{.50} = 7.55 - \frac{0.50(20) - 8}{5}(0.1)$$
$$= 7.55 - 0.04$$
$$= 7.51$$

c.
$$X_{.60} = 7.55 - \frac{0.60(20) - 8}{5}(0.1)$$
$$= 7.55 - 0.08$$
$$= 7.47$$

d.
$$\text{PR for } 7.4 = \frac{13 + \dfrac{7.45 - 7.4}{0.1}(3)}{20}(100)$$
$$= \frac{13 + 1.5}{20}(100)$$
$$= 72.5\%$$

6. a.

Interval	Real limits	Tally	f	cf	c%
263-267	262.5-267.5	xx	2	45	100.0
258-262	257.5-262.5	xxx	3	43	95.6
253-257	252.5-257.5	xxx	3	40	88.9
248-252	247.5-252.5	xxxxxx	6	37	82.2
243-247	242.5-247.5	xxxxxxxxx	9	31	68.9
238-242	237.5-242.5	xxxxxxxxx	9	22	48.9
233-237	232.5-237.5	xxxx	4	13	28.9
228-232	227.5-232.5	xxxx	4	9	20.0
223-227	222.5-227.5	xxx	3	5	11.1
218-222	217.5-222.5	x	1	2	4.4
213-217	212.5-217.5	x	1	1	2.2

b.
$$X_{.50} = 242.5 + \frac{0.50(45) - 22}{9}(5)$$
$$= 242.5 + 0.278$$
$$= 242.778$$

c.
$$X_{.90} = 257.5 + \frac{0.90(45) - 40}{3}(5)$$
$$= 257.5 + 0.833$$
$$= 258.333$$

d.
$$\text{PR for } 248 = \frac{31 + \dfrac{248 - 247.5}{5}(6)}{45}(100)$$
$$= \frac{31 + 0.6}{45}(100)$$
$$= 70.2\%$$

e.
$$\text{PR for } 229 = \frac{5 + \dfrac{229 - 227.5}{5}(4)}{45}\,100$$
$$= \frac{5 + 1.2}{45}(100)$$
$$= 13.78\%$$

3

Describing a Distribution of Test Scores

KEY WORDS   *Watch for these words as you read the following chapter:*

central tendency	median	standard scores
correlation	mode	T-scores
correlation coefficient	normal curve	variability
interpercentile range	raw score	variance
interquartile range	skewness	z-scores
mean	standard deviation	

In the previous chapter a detailed description of the process of building a frequency distribution to summarize a data set in an orderly manner was emphasized. Procedures were also set forth for calculating percentiles and percentile ranks with or without a frequency distribution. Test users and test developers frequently use two other pieces of information: a measure of **central tendency** and a measure of **variability.** The focus of the first section of this chapter is on measures of central tendency. This material is followed by a discussion of standard scores, correlation, and the use of norms. At its best, test development includes the generation of norms. Although you may not develop these norms yourself, be certain that the normative information is appropriate for the examinees.

MEASURES OF CENTRAL TENDENCY

A measure of central tendency provides information about the center of a distribution of test scores. Three measures of central tendency are commonly used to describe a set of test scores—the **mean,** the **median,** and the **mode.** Remember from Chapter 2 that the *median,* or the 50th percentile, is the score dividing the distribution into equal halves. The *mode* is the score occurring most frequently in a distribution. Consider the following set of test scores.

Data set of 12 scores: 39, 33, 31, 29, 27, 26, 26, 26, 24, 23, 23, 21

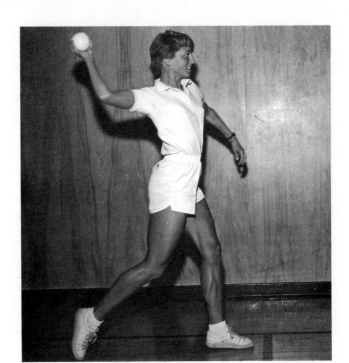

In this case, the mode is *26*, the most frequently occurring score. The *mean* is the arithmetic average of a set of scores. The mean is emphasized in this section, since the calculation of the median has already been described and the mode can be determined in a straightforward manner.

Recall that the median could be calculated for a data set that was ordered from highest to lowest scores, even when the data were not in frequency-distribution form. Neither developing a frequency distribution to compute the mean nor ordering the scores is necessary. Examine the five test scores below.

Data set of 5 scores: 20, 10, 14, 18, 15

By using elementary arithmetic a simple average can be determined by summing the scores and dividing by *N*. This is represented by Formula 3-1:

$$\overline{X} = \frac{\Sigma X}{N} \qquad \text{Formula 3-1}$$

where $\overline{X}$ = the *mean* (referred to as *X-bar*)
    Σ = *sum of*
    X = *score* for one examinee
    ΣX = *sum* of all *scores* in data set
    (20 + 10 + 14 + 18 + 15)

For the data set given on p. 48:

$$\overline{X} = \frac{77}{5} = 15.4$$

Sometimes it is more convenient to calculate the mean from a set of scores in frequency-distribution form, especially when the raw scores for the test are not available. **A raw score** is the actual score an examinee obtains on the test. Usually these scores are available; therefore only the simplest case of a frequency distribution is described here. This is the frequency distribution with interval sizes equal to 1. To keep the example simple a frequency distribution of only 6 intervals is used. (Keep in mind, however, that a proper distribution should have no fewer than 10 and no more than 20 intervals.)

X		f		fx
10		2		20
9		3		27
8		4		32
7		6		42
6		3		18
5		1		5
		N = 19		144

With the data in this form, Formula 3-1 must be modified slightly to take into account that more than one person obtained a score in most of the above intervals. If all of the scores in the X column were merely added and the sum were divided by N, the answer would be incorrect. The frequency column, as shown in Formula 3-2, must also be considered.

$$\overline{X} = \frac{\Sigma fX}{N}$$

Formula 3-2

where X = *score* in a frequency distribution
   f = *frequency* of scores in interval of frequency distribution
   fX = *frequency multiplied* by score representing interval
      [e.g., for top interval, fX = 2(10) = 20]
   ΣfX = *sum of frequency multiplied* by score for all intervals
      [2(10) + 3(9) + . . . + 1(5) = 144]

By multiplying the X column by the f column, a score for each person is included in the calculation. In this case:

$$\overline{X} = \frac{144}{19} = 7.58$$

The calculation of the mean for data sets in frequency distribution form with intervals greater than size 1 is omitted from this chapter. This calculation is not difficult, but it is cumbersome. With the ready availability of minicalculators, punching in the raw scores and computing the mean are simple transactions. A discussion of more complex procedures is unnecessary at this level; the formulas presented in this section should be adequate. Although information about the center of a distribution is useful in itself, a more accurate interpretation of the data set is possible by obtaining information on the *spread* of the scores.

MEASURES OF VARIABILITY

Suppose two friends, Jim and Paul, bowled five lines apiece and obtained the following scores:

Jim: 138 142 140 139 141
Paul: 120 140 160 100 180

Let's order these scores to compare them more easily.

Jim: 138 139 140 141 142
Paul: 100 120 140 160 180

Which score represents the center of Jim's set of scores? Which represents Paul's set of scores? In this example both the mean and the median of each set of scores equal 140. Does the fact that these measures of central tendency are the same for both boys suggest that they have similar levels of ability in bowling?

If only the means and medians were available, this conclusion might be drawn. Since all five scores are available for each boy, let's look at them more closely in their ordered form. Jim's raw scores are similar, but Paul's vary to a great degree. One might say Paul is a more erratic bowler than Jim. Thus even though the sets of scores have one characteristic in common—their centrality—they are quite different in another way—their variability.

Range and Interpercentile Range

Three measures of variability are described in this section. The first is the **range** (highest score − lowest score + 1). The second measure is the **interpercentile range,** which provides an indication of how scores vary around the median, the 50th percentile. The most frequently used interpercentile range is the absolute value of $X_{.75} - X_{.25}$, known as the **interquartile range.** The method for obtaining interpercentile ranges involves removing a small percentage of scores from both ends of the distribution. As a result the most extreme scores are not allowed to affect the indicators of variability. If $X_{.75} = 50$ and $X_{.25} = 27$, the interquartile range is $50 - 27 = 23$. The number 23 is expressed in raw score units. Smaller numbers represent smaller ranges, with more scores clustering around the center of the distribution. Many other interpercentile ranges may be used, such as $X_{.90} - X_{.10}$ or $X_{.85} - X_{.15}$, as long as equal portions of the distribution are deleted from both ends.

Standard Deviation

When the mean is used as the measure of the center of the distribution, variability is estimated using the **standard deviation.** This statistic provides information about the extent to which scores deviate from the mean. In statistics Greek lowercase sigma, σ, is sometimes used to represent the standard deviation of a population of examinees, and s is used to represent the standard deviation of a sample of examinees drawn from the population. For convenience and simplicity the symbol s is used in this chapter.

Conceptual Formula Earlier in this chapter, Formula 3-1 was used to calculate the mean of 15.4 for a set of five scores. The same set of five scores is listed below, this time from highest to lowest.

X	X − X̄	(X − X̄)²
20	4.6	21.16
18	2.6	6.76
15	−.4	.16
14	−1.4	1.96
10	−5.4	29.16
	0	59.20
	$[\Sigma(X-\overline{X})]$	$[\Sigma(X-\overline{X})^2]$

Since the standard deviation reflects the deviation of scores from the mean, it seems logical to calculate this statistic by subtracting the mean from each score and summing the deviations. This calculation is demonstrated in the second column in the above example. Note the result of obtaining the deviations and summing them. The answer of 0 would be obtained regardless of the data set used. Look back and examine the individual deviations from the mean. Although an answer of 0 indicates no variability in the data set, this is obviously not true for this set of scores. An answer of 0 would only *accurately* reflect no variability in a data set if all scores were identical. Thus, to obtain a deviation score that provides an accurate indication of the deviation of scores from the mean, these deviations are squared. The squared deviations are shown in the third column of the above example. The sum of these deviations is 59.20.

Now that we are working with *squared* deviations, the statistic being calculated is s^2, which is known as the **variance.** Once the variance is known, the standard deviation can be calculated by taking the square root of the variance. Formula 3-3 for the variance follows:

$$s^2 = \frac{\Sigma(X - \overline{X})^2}{N} \qquad \text{Formula 3-3}$$

The sum of the squared deviations is divided by N to determine the average of the deviations. The numerator of this formula has already been determined for the set of 5 scores and, of course, $N = 5$. Thus,

$$s^2 = \frac{59.20}{5} = 11.84$$

Although calculating the variance to obtain the standard deviation is necessary, the numerical value for the variance is not as easily interpreted as the standard deviation. The variance is not expressed in the original raw score units of the test. The square root of this value, the standard deviation, is more useful in describing a set of test scores, since it is expressed in the actual score units of the test. Formula 3-4 for calculating the standard deviation follows:

$$s = \sqrt{\frac{\Sigma(X - \overline{X})^2}{N}} \qquad \text{Formula 3-4}$$

A variance of 11.84 yields a standard deviation of 3.44. To summarize for the set of five scores, the mean is 15.4 and the standard deviation is 3.44. Assume that the five scores were obtained by administering an agility test to five students. The scores are expressed in seconds. A small standard deviation means that the scores tend to cluster around the mean. In this case the standard deviation indicates that the scores are spread out on both sides of the mean rather than clustered. Since the time scores are for a test of short duration, a deviation of 3 seconds or greater is considerable. In a measure of much longer duration, such as a long-distance run, a deviation of 3 seconds would carry much less significance. The standard deviation must be interpreted in light of the actual score units of the test. In the previous example the examinees would not have similar abilities on the attribute being measured. If the standard deviation were smaller (e.g., 1.1 seconds), the scores would be clustered much more closely around the mean. In this case the ability levels of the examinees would be similar. Formula 3-4 is known as a conceptual formula rather than a computational formula. In other words, it depicts in a clear-cut manner the meaning and derivation of the standard deviation. (Do not use Formula 3-4 in the actual calculation of the standard deviation.)

If you have previously taken an elementary statistics course, you might have used a formula for the standard deviation with $N - 1$ in the denominator rather than N, as shown in Formulas 3-4 and 3-5. When $N - 1$ is used, the test user wishes to use a set of test scores to estimate the standard deviation of a population of individuals like those in the group being tested. For example, a teacher might administer a standing long jump test to a group of fourth-grade girls randomly selected from the entire school district. The mean and standard deviation calculated for the set of test scores could be interpreted as representative of all fourth-grade girls in the district. Under these circumstances the standard deviation formula should be used with $N - 1$ in the denominator so that the estimate of the standard deviation will be unbiased. In contrast, the more typical situation encountered in test administration is the use of a test with a specific group. Of greatest interest is the mean and standard deviation for this specific group. Generalizing to a population of individuals may not be important or, more often, may not be feasible. In this case the standard deviation formula with N in the denominator is appropriate. Thus, throughout this text, any version of the standard deviation formula will include N in the denominator. If you use a minicalculator that is programmed to calculate the standard deviation, determine which term is used in the denominator. Many minicalculators provide two estimates of s, one calculated using N in the denominator and the other using N − 1 in the denominator.

Computational Formula   The standard deviation can be easily calculated from a set of raw scores by using many of the inexpensive minicalculators now on the market. In some cases after the scores have been entered, the standard deviation can be calculated with the push of a button. In others the sum of squares needed in the computational formula is automatically calculated. The computational formula for the standard deviation used in this textbook is Formula 3-5. (A number of equivalent formulas that are equally appropriate may be used.)

$$s = \sqrt{\frac{N\Sigma X^2 - (\Sigma X)^2}{N(N)}} \qquad \text{Formula 3-5}$$

where ΣX^2 = the *sum* of each *number squared;* for the data set of 5 scores.
This would be $20^2 + 18^2 + \ldots + 10^2$
$(\Sigma X)^2$ = the *square* of the *sum* of all *scores;* in this example
$(20 + 18 + \ldots + 10)^2$

Let's apply Formula 3-5 to the small data set on p. 48.

$$s = \sqrt{\frac{5(1245) - (77)^2}{5(5)}}$$
$$= \sqrt{\frac{6225 - 5929}{25}}$$
$$= \sqrt{11.84}$$
$$= 3.44$$

To summarize, the standard deviation is the square root of the variance. The variance must be calculated first because the sum of the deviations of scores from the mean is *always* 0. However, the standard deviation is the statistic of greater interest, since it is expressed in raw score units. Now both the mean and standard deviation of this small set of five scores have been calculated. Interpreting these values is easier if the normal curve and its characteristics are clarified.

SCORE DISTRIBUTIONS

When data obtained from a test administration are graphed in the form of a curve, the shape of the curve will depend on the way in which the scores are distributed. The most common types of curves represented in data sets at this level are the normal curve and the skewed curve.

Normal Curve

In the previous chapter test scores were graphed in frequency polygon or histogram form. If it were possible to administer a test to a large number of examinees, perhaps several thousand, and the test scores were graphed, the resultant curve would approach the **normal curve** for most physical performance tests.

The normal curve (Fig. 3-1) has several characteristics that can be of assistance in interpreting a set of scores. First, the curve is symmetrical. If the curve were lifted at one tail and folded over on top of the other side, the two halves of the curve would match precisely. In this case the mean, median, and mode would be identical. Second, the area under the curve represents 100%. It is possible to calculate the area for any portion of the curve. On the baseline of the curve, a mark is placed in the center to represent the center of the distribution. In addition, three marks are placed equidistant from each other above the center (in this context, the mean), and three marks are placed below the mean. These marks, representing 3 standard deviations both above and below the mean, divide the normal curve into six portions. The percentage of area between these points is calculated and provides useful information for test users and developers. These portions and the percentage of area in each are displayed in Figure 3-2. Note that the tails of the curve do not touch the baseline. Obtaining scores representing 4 or more standard deviations above or below the mean is possible. For example, a genius might have an IQ that is greater than 5 or 6 standard deviations above the mean of the distribution of IQ scores. However, the likelihood of obtaining extreme scores is remote; thus the normal curve is usually described as being characterized by ±3 standard deviations.

FIGURE 3-1 Normal curve.

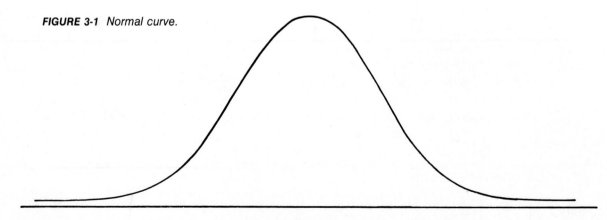

What kind of information can be obtained from Figure 3-2? Look at the point designated as +1*s*, or 1 standard deviation above the mean. If an examinee's score falls at exactly this point, approximately 84% of the group taking the test scored below this point. The 84% was approximated by adding the percentages in each section to the left of +1*s*. A distribution of scores for a sit-ups test is depicted in Figure 3-3. The mean for this set of scores is 40, and the standard deviation is 7. One standard deviation above the mean is a score of 47 (40 + 7).

FIGURE 3-2 *Areas under normal curve.*
From Test Service Notebook 148.

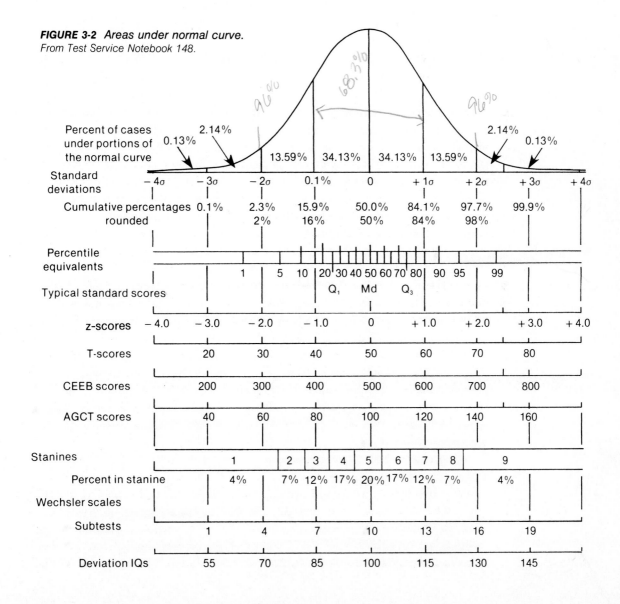

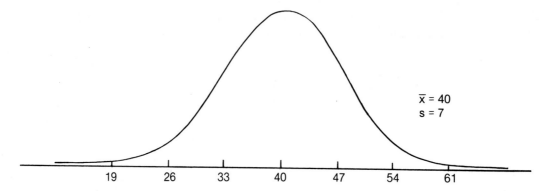

FIGURE 3-3 *Normal curve with standard deviations expressed in score units (number of sit-ups).*

One standard deviation below the mean is a score of 33 (40 − 7). Thus 84% of the group of examinees received scores at or below 47, while scores for approximately 16% of the group were at or below a score of 33. Of course, many scores fall between standard deviations expressed as whole numbers (e.g., +2, −1). For example, how should a score of 35 be interpreted? Certainly this score is below average, falling between the mean and 1 standard deviation below the mean. However, the score cannot be interpreted with precision unless it is converted to standard score form.

Skewed Distributions

The bell shape typically associated with the normal curve shows that most of the examinees obtained scores in the middle of the distribution, with a few people scoring at each end. The two ends of the distribution are referred to as *tails* of the distribution. In short, the majority of the examinees represented under the normal curve obtained scores surrounding the average, while a smaller number received high and low scores. However, in real-life testing situations the test scores do not always approximate the normal curve. Sometimes most of the examinees will do well on a test, or sometimes most will perform poorly. Then these scores form **skewed** distributions, with most of the area clustered at one end of the distribution.

When most of the examinees receive low scores on the test, the distribution is positively skewed. As shown in Figure 3-4, the majority of scores fall in the lower portion of the distribution, with a small number of high scores occurring in the long tail stretching out to the right. The *skewed* end of the distribution is the one with the long tail. If the skewness is located to the right, as in Figure 3-4, the distribution is labeled positively skewed. If the skewed end is located to the left, the distribution is labeled negatively skewed, as depicted in Figure 3-5. In

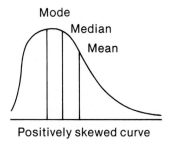

FIGURE 3-4 *Positively skewed distribution.*

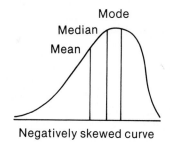

FIGURE 3-5 *Negatively skewed distribution.*

this case a large portion of the examinees received high scores on the test, and only a few scored at the lower end of the distribution. When mastery tests are used, a negatively skewed distribution is often a desirable result. If most individuals master the material, they will do well on the test.

Consider the best way to describe these distributions. Should the mean and standard deviation be used as measure of central tendency and variability, or should the median be used? How is this decision made? First, a set of test scores should be summarized in frequency distribution form and graphed as a frequency polygon. Next, the graph (frequency polygon) should be examined. If the distribution of scores appears to approximate the normal curve, the mean and standard deviation should be used, since these values have stronger mathematical properties than the median and interpercentile range. If the distribution of scores is skewed, the mean will be closer to the skewed tail of the distribution than the median because the mean is affected by the extreme scores in the tail. Therefore, the median is a better representation of the center of the distribution when it is skewed. Since the median is a percentile, the corresponding measure of variability is one of the interpercentile ranges.

STANDARD SCORES

In Chapter 2 you learned how to convert test scores to percentile ranks. Two rules of thumb apply when transforming scores to standard scores. First, the median and the interpercentile range are used together. If these statistics are used to describe the center and spread of the distribution, percentile ranks should be used to convert scores. Second, the mean and the standard deviation are used together. When these statistics are used to describe a data set, a standard score transformation should be used.

The z-Score Transformation

Standard scores may take many forms, but all are based on the **z-score transformation,** which is the basic standard score transformation. Another term for this unit of transformation is the *standard deviation unit*. Formula 3-6 converts test scores to z-scores.

$$\text{z-score} = \frac{X - \overline{X}}{s}$$

Formula 3-6

All the symbols in Formula 3-6 should look familiar. Refer back to the data from the sit-ups test. The mean of 40, the standard deviation of 7, and the precise interpretation of a score of 35 were of interest. The z-score transformation is one way of providing greater precision. Let's apply the data to Formula 3-6 and calculate the z-score for a score of 35.

$$\text{z-score} = \frac{35 - 40}{7} = -.71$$

The z-scores form a distribution with fixed parameters—a mean of 0 and a standard deviation of 1. Examine the z-score distribution in Figure 3-6. The mean of the distribution is 0, and 1 standard deviation above the mean is +1. One standard deviation below the mean is −1. The z-score values above the mean are all positive; those below the mean are all negative. Whatever the metric of the test score, the z-score formula converts it to the standard z-score metric. In other words, across a wide variety of distributions the mean of each distribution is converted to a z-score mean of 0. One of these tests might be scored in feet and inches, and another may be scored in minutes and seconds; yet the z-score means of the two tests will both be 0. The standard deviations are standardized in the same way.

Certain raw scores can be easily determined without the use of Formula 3-6, if the score is equal to 1 or more standard deviations above or below the mean. In the previous example it is apparent that a z-score of +1 equals 47 and a z-score of −1 equals 33. Both a z-score of +1 and a raw score of 47 equal 1 stan-

FIGURE 3-6 *Graph of z-score distribution.*

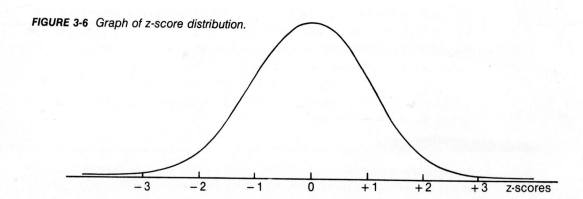

dard deviation above the mean. A z-score of −1 and a raw score of 33 both equal 1 standard deviation below the mean.

Refer to the interpretations of a score of 35 on the sit-ups test; the z-score for this score is −.71. The negative sign indicates that the score falls below the mean, and the size of the z-score (.71) indicates that almost three quarters of a standard deviation is represented. Thus a score of 35 is approximately three quarters of 1 standard deviation below the mean.

When interpreting only a few test scores from a single data set, it is possible to interpret the scores without converting them to z-scores if the mean and standard deviation of the data set are known. However, in the physical education field several tests are often administered to a group of examinees during a single testing session. Each of the tests may be scored in different units. For example, a set of tests might include a test of skinfold thickness, a 1-mile run, and a sit-and-reach test of flexibility. The first measure is scored in millimeters; the second, in minutes and seconds; and the third, in centimeters (cm). How can an examinee's score on these three tests be compared? For this purpose the z-score transformation is a very useful tool. Assume that the examinee who performed 35 sit-ups in the previous example also took the sit-and-reach test and obtained a score of 25 cm. The mean and standard deviation of the group on the test was 23 cm and 2 cm, respectively. It is rather cumbersome to graph a distribution and mark the mean and standard deviations for the sit-ups test and sit-and-reach test so that the two test scores could be compared. If the score transformations of many examinees are needed, then the graphing approach is totally inefficient. What is the z-score for a sit-and-reach score of 25 cm?

$$\text{z-score} = \frac{25 - 23}{2} = +1$$

Now the score on the sit-ups test can be compared with the score on the sit-and-reach test. The score of 35 on the sit-ups test is represented by a z-score of −.71 and the sit-and-reach score of 25 by a z-score of +1. Referring to any other information about either of the two data sets is not necessary when comparing the two z-scores. This particular examinee is below average in abdominal strength and above average in low-back flexibility. This same procedure could be used to compare the scores of two or more individuals on the same test.

The T-Score Transformation

A practical reason for converting test scores to standard scores is to inform others of the examinee's performance on a test. For instance, a comparison of scores on different tests is information that is often requested by parents of a child in a physical education class, by the principal of a school, or by the manager of a fitness club. While z-scores provide a logical means of comparison, the z-score scale itself is not the easiest standard score to explain. This difficulty is primarily because the negative scores occur below the mean and the scores with decimal points can be found both above and below the mean. Most test developers resolve this problem by transforming the z-scores to another standard score that is easier for the layman to interpret. Generally these transformations remove the negative sign and the decimal point from the z-scores. All these transformations, however, are based on the z-score distribution.

The **T-score distribution** is a popular conversion with developers of sport skills and basic motor abilities tests. The T-score distribution has a mean of 50 and a standard deviation of 10. To convert z-scores to T-scores, Formula 3-7 is used.

$$\text{T-score} = 10z + 50 \qquad \qquad \text{Formula 3-7}$$

Since two T-scores were calculated in the previous section, let's use these to calculate T-scores.

$$\text{T-score (for sit-ups score)} = 10(-.71) + 50 = 42.9$$
$$\text{T-score (for sit-and-reach score)} = 10(1) + 50 = 60$$

Compare these scores using the T-score distribution presented in Figure 3-7. Note that no transformed score begins with a negative sign or a decimal. At the same time the information obtained from the T-score calculations does not conceal anything previously secured from the z-scores themselves. However, T-scores have a few inherent qualities that allow this distribution to be explained more easily to the public. In general, the scores range between 0 and 100. Al-

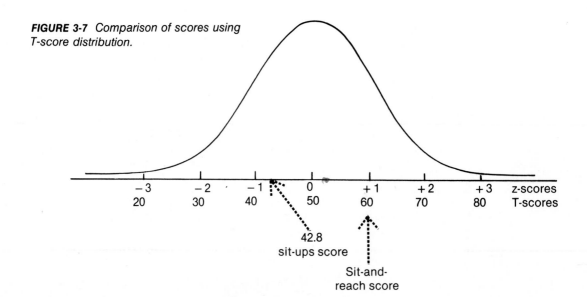

FIGURE 3-7 *Comparison of scores using T-score distribution.*

though scores exceeding a −3 or +3 standard deviation (exceeding T-scores of 20 or 80) are rare, a range of scores from 0 to 100 seems plausible. Furthermore, the mean of the T-score distribution is 50, which seems like a reasonable average for a test to many people.

Constant-Value Method Frequently a test user is more interested in determining the T-scores for an entire set of test scores than in calculating individual T-scores. If so, the *constant-value method* can be used to contruct a T-score table for the data set. This table can be used to convert raw scores to T-scores, not only for this year's examinees but also for those who take the test in future years. Of course, these types of tables must be recalculated periodically so that they remain updated. The following steps are used in the constant-value method.

1. Calculate the mean and standard deviation for a set of test scores. For the sit-ups test the mean was 40 and the standard deviation was 7.
2. Calculate $s/10$. In our example, $7/10 = .7$. This is the constant used to add and subtract from the mean.
3. List each possible T-score from 20 to 80.
4. Add the constant to the mean (40) to obtain the raw score for a T-score of 51. In this case, $40 + .7 = 40.7$. Proceed in the same manner for T-scores 52-80. Note that the addition is cumulative. For example, to calculate the raw score for a T-score of 52, add the constant (.7) to the raw score for a T-score of 51 (40.7). The raw score for a T-score of 52 is 41.4.
5. For all T-scores below the mean, subtract the constant. For a T-score of 49, subtract the constant (.7) from the mean (40) to obtain an equivalent raw score. The raw score for a T-score of 49 is 39.3. Proceed in the same manner for T-scores of 48 down to 20.
6. Round off the raw scores to correspond with the actual test scores. In this case the actual test scores are in whole numbers (number of sit-ups); therefore, the raw scores should be rounded to the nearest whole number.

As an example, the use of the constant-value method is exemplified for T-scores of 45 to 55.

T-score	Corresponding raw score	Rounded raw score
55	43.5	44
54	42.8	43
53	42.1	42
52	41.4	41
51	40.7	41
50	40.0	40
49	39.3	39
48	38.6	39
47	37.9	38
46	37.2	37
45	36.5	37

To complete the table of T-scores, raw score values must be calculated for all T-scores from 20 to 80. Note that several T-score values have the same raw score values. This is not unusual, especially when the standard deviation is a small number. Once the completed T-score table has been developed, it can be used to convert all scores in a data set, assuming the test examinees are similar to those whose scores were used to prepare the table. This method is much simpler than calculating T-scores for each raw score in a set of test scores.

Lower Scores/Better Performances   For certain measures of motor behavior, higher scores reflect poorer performance. If the data set consists of scores on a shuttle run test, lower times are faster times and thus reflect better performance. When a z-score is calculated for a time score that is actually better than the mean in a performance context but lower than the mean in a numerical context, the result may be confusing. As an example, the mean of a set of shuttle run test scores is 11.2 seconds and the standard deviation is 0.4 second. What is the z-score for a raw score of 11.8? Use Formula 3-6 to solve this problem.

$$\text{z-score} = \frac{11.8 - 11.2}{4} = +1.5$$

The result is a +1.5 z-score, which indicates that the score is above the mean. This, of course, implies above-average performance. Yet in a performance context this is not true. A shuttle run score of 11.8 is slower than the average score for the group; it is a below-average score. The formula for calculating z-scores, as with any other statistical formulas, only deals with numbers and not with their interpretations. Therefore whenever lower scores equal better performances, change the sign of the z-score to the opposite; the result will then represent the correct *interpretation* of the score. Instead of obtaining a +1.5 z-score for a shuttle run score of 11.8, the answer would be −1.5. When the z-score is transformed to a T-score, it will also be correct in an interpretive sense. A z-score of −1.5 is equal to a T-score of 35, a below-average score.

When lower scores represent better performances, an easier method of calculating the z-score is to use a variation of Formula 3-6 shown in Formula 3-8.

$$\text{z-score} = \frac{\overline{X} - X}{s} \qquad\qquad \text{Formula 3-8}$$

This formula is a special case of the usual z-score formula.

When using Formula 3-8, the resulting answer corresponds with the interpretation of the score in a performance context. In other words, a time score larger than the mean actually represents poorer performance; thus, the negative z-score provides the correct interpretation.

CORRELATION

To be able to analyze a test, a basic understanding of test reliability and validity is necessary. To estimate these two test characteristics, a statistic known as the **correlation coefficient** is often used. The term **correlation** refers to the *relationship between two variables, X and Y*. The symbol X already represents a score on a test; now Y will be used to represent a score on another test. Is the ability to perform one skill related to the ability to perform a second skill? To gain insight into this type of question, a correlation coefficient can be calculated.

Pearson Product-Moment Correlation Coefficient

The *Pearson product-moment correlation coefficient,* the most commonly used correlation coefficient, is symbolized as r_{xy}. Correlation coefficients can range from $+1.00$ to -1.00. These extremes are depicted in the data sets below.

	Data set A		Data set B	
	Leg strength	Standing long jump	Leg strength	Arm strength
A	42	7 ft, 5 in	42	8
B	40	7 ft, 0 in	40	10
C	38	6 ft, 5 in	38	12
D	36	6 ft, 0 in	36	14
E	34	5 ft, 5 in	34	16

In both data sets the leg strength measure (X) is an indicator of leg extensor strength measured in foot-pounds. In Data set A the second variable (Y) is the standing long jump, and in Data set B arm strength is measured by a test of pull-ups. All these data sets are formed hypothetically to demonstrate the extreme range of correlation coefficients, $r_{xy} = +1.00$ and $r_{xy} = -1.00$. In Data set A the first examinee, A, has the highest scores on both tests, and the fifth examinee, E, has the lowest scores. This pattern can be observed across all examinees. Thus it is intuitively obvious that a high relationship exists between leg strength and the ability to perform the standing long jump (i.e., those with greater leg strength are able to jump longer distances). If r_{xy}, the Pearson product-moment correlation coefficient, were calculated for this data set, it would equal $+1.00$. A correlation coefficient of $+1.00$ represents a *perfect positive correlation*.

Now examine the two sets of scores in Data set B. Note that precisely the reverse trend is evident in the arm strength and leg strength scores. As the leg strength scores decrease, the arm strength scores increase. The correlation between these two sets of scores is negative. In fact, in this example, the correlation coefficient is -1.00, a perfect negative correlation. Normally, it is not appropriate to calculate the correlation coefficients for such small data sets. With only five examinees the resultant coefficients may not be an accurate indicator of the relationship between two variables, since the idiosyncrasies of one person could drastically affect the coefficient. Even in the next example, the number of cases is too small; 30 or more examinees would be desirable. However, a small data set is convenient for demonstrating the calculation of the correlation coefficient. In this example the correlation coefficient for scores of eight examinees on two variables, pull-ups and push-ups, will be determined.

Examinee	Pull-ups(X)	Push-ups(Y)	X²	Y²	XY
A	10	15	100	225	150
B	2	5	4	25	10
C	5	11	25	121	55
D	6	10	36	100	60
E	7	14	49	196	98
F	1	3	1	9	3
G	9	16	81	256	144
H	5	8	25	64	40
	45	82	321	996	560

The Pearson product-moment correlation coefficient, r_{xy}, is calculated using Formula 3-9.

$$r_{xy} = \frac{N\Sigma XY - (\Sigma X)(\Sigma Y)}{\sqrt{[N\Sigma X^2 - (\Sigma X)^2][N\Sigma Y^2 - (\Sigma Y)^2]}} \qquad \text{Formula 3-9}$$

where ΣXY = the *sum* of the products of XY for each examinee;
    in this example, $(10)(15)+(2)(5)+ \ldots +(5)(8) = 560$
$(\Sigma X)(\Sigma Y)$ = the *product* of the *sum* of the X scores and the *sum* of the Y scores;
    in this example, $(45)(82) = 3690$
ΣX^2 = the *sum* of each X value *squared;* in this example,
    $(10^2 + \ldots + 5^2) = 321$; use the same concept for Y^2
$(\Sigma X)^2$ = the *square* of the *sum* of all X values; in this example,
    $(10 + 2 + \ldots + 5)^2 = 2025$; use the same concept for $(\Sigma Y)^2$

Now Formula 3-9 will be used with the pull-ups and push-ups data.

$$r_{xy} = \frac{8(560) - (45)(82)}{\sqrt{[8(321) - (45)^2][8(996) - (82)^2]}} = 0.96$$

A coefficient of 0.96 represents a high positive relationship between push-ups and pull-ups, suggesting that performance of each measure is dependent to a large extent on a similar type of arm and shoulder girdle strength.

Rank Difference Correlation Coefficient

Ranking the scores in each data set on p. 64 is also possible. The highest scores in each data set would be given ranks of 1, and so forth. In the pull-ups data set, Examinees C and H received the same score of 5. The scores represent two rank positions, yet the ranks for the two scores should be identical. These ranks are calculated by *averaging* the two rank positions, in this case 5 and 6, and assigning the average rank of 5.5 to each score of 5. Without performing any type of calculation on the ranks, it is possible to obtain a general feeling about the degree of relationship between two variables from a visual examination of the ranks. For example, Examinee A would be assigned ranks of 1 on pull-ups and 2 on push-ups; Examinee F would be assigned ranks of 8 and 8, respectively. Although the ranks are not identical for each person, they are similar; this points to a substantial relationship between the two variables. Of course it is known that the relationship is high, since r_{xy} has already been calculated using the raw scores. Calculating a correlation coefficient using ranks only is also possible, it requires a different statistic known as the **rank difference correlation coefficient** (ρ). Formula 3-10 is used to calculate rho, ρ.

$$\rho = 1 - \frac{6(\Sigma D^2)}{N(N^2 - 1)} \qquad \text{Formula 3-10}$$

where D = the *difference* between the two ranks for each subject
  D^2 = *square* of the *difference* between ranks for an examinee
  ΣD^2 = *sum* of D^2 for all examinees

The push-ups and pull-ups data will be used again, and for purposes of convenience the raw scores will be reproduced as well as ranked. Note that D equals 0. This is always true, regardless of the data set. This calculation is a convenient way to check the numbers in the *D* column.

X	Rank(X)	Y	Rank(Y)	D	D^2
10	1	15	2	−1	1
2	7	5	7	0	0
5	5.5	11	4	1.5	2.25
6	4	10	5	−1	1
7	3	14	3	0	0
1	8	3	8	0	0
9	2	16	1	1	1
5	5.5	8	6	−0.5	0.25
					5.50
					(ΣD^2)

$$\rho = 1 - \frac{6(5.50)}{8(8^2 - 1)} = 0.935$$

Note that the result of the rank difference method is not the same as the result obtained using r_{xy}, although the values are similar. This is expected, since the process of converting raw scores to ranks leads to a loss of information about the original data sets.

To summarize, when two sets of scores are available for the same set of examinees, the relationship between the two variables can be estimated using a correlation coefficient. When the raw scores are continuous or discrete data (not initially in rank form), the Pearson product-moment correlation coefficient (r_{xy}) is appropriate under most circumstances. When the scores are converted to ranks, or obtained as ranks initially, the rank difference correlation coefficient (ρ) may be used. The rank difference formula is easier to use, but its result is not as accurate as r_{xy}. For all practical purposes, however, the discrepancy between estimates is not serious.

Graph of Relationship Between Two Variables

Correlational information is often presented in graphic form by plotting the *coordinates* of the X and Y scores, with the Y scores represented on the *vertical* axis and the X scores represented on the *horizontal* axis. Lower or poorer scores are located on the lower portion of the Y axis and higher or better scores on the upper portion. On the X axis lower or poorer scores are placed to the left; higher or better scores are to the right. A coordinate is a point on the graph representing the paired X and Y scores for each examinee. The push-ups and pull-ups scores for 8 examinees are presented in graph form in Figure 3-8.

Each point on the graph represents two scores for an examinee. If the X and Y scores increase proportionally, that is, as the X scores increase the Y scores also increase by the same proportion, the coordinates will fall on or close to a straight line that slants from the lower left corner of the graph to the upper right corner. While the increase in X and Y scores is not precisely proportional in Figure 3-8 the tendency can be observed. This is an example of a high positive correlation represented in graph form. Examples of other sizes and signs of correlation coefficients are displayed in graph form in Figure 3-9.

Interpretation of Correlation Coefficients

Opinions vary about how the size of a correlation coefficient should be interpreted. How high should a coefficient be to be classified as high? Moderate? Low? A general rule of thumb is presented below, but under certain circumstances the interpretation may vary even from this general rule.

± .80-1.00	High
± .60-0.79	Moderately high
± .40-0.59	Moderate
± .20-0.39	Low
± .00-0.19	No relationship

Another way of interpreting the coefficient is to square it. This statistic, r_{xy}^2, is known as the *coefficient of determination*. As an example, assume the correlation between two measures of arm strength is 0.80. The square of the correlation is an indication of the *shared variance between two variables*. In other words, this is the variance the two variables share. For the two measures of arm

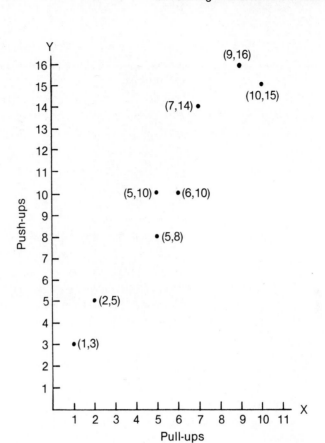

FIGURE 3-8 *Graph of relationship between push-up and pull-up scores.*

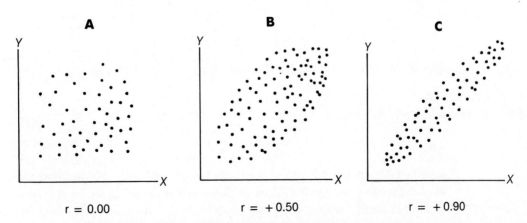

FIGURE 3-9 *Graph of various sizes of correlation coefficients.* **A,** *No relationship between X and Y.* **B,** *Moderate relationship.* **C,** *High relationship.*

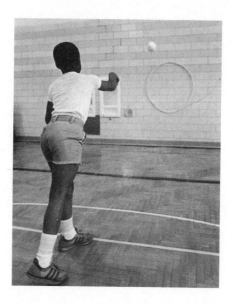

strength, the shared variance is 0.64. This means that 64% of the variance between these two measures taps a common element, which can be assumed to be
arm strength. With higher correlation coefficients the shared variance is substantial. However, with correlation coefficients of moderate and small sizes, the coefficient of determination is affected to a greater extent. For example, if $r_{xy} =$
0.50, the square of the coefficient equals 0.25. Another advantage of using the
squared correlation coefficient in interpreting r_{xy} is that squared coefficients can
be compared as ratios, unlike the regular correlation coefficient. For example, a
coefficient of 0.90 does not represent twice as much of a relationship as a coefficient of 0.45. However, when r_{xy} is squared, coefficients can legitimately be
compared in this manner. For example, a coefficient of determination of 0.50
represents twice as much variance as a coefficient of 0.25.

USE OF NORMS
Raw Scores and Derived Scores

A raw score is the score an individual obtains on a test. If the only information
available about an examinee's test performance is the raw score, interpreting it
meaningfully can be difficult. For instance, if Mary runs the 50-yard dash in 7.8
seconds, is the score good? To answer this question the score can be transformed
to another scale, yielding a *derived score*. In Chapters 2 and 3 procedures are
described for developing both percentile and standard score norms. Even better
the raw scores can be compared to a table in which derived scores have already
been calculated for the raw scores.

Types of Norms

Norms are derived scores determined from the raw scores obtained by a specific group on a specific test. Whenever percentile norms are determined for a group of examinees, half will score above the middle of the distribution and half will score below. No inherent value is attached to any given norm score. The norm describes an examinee in relation to a large sample of people who have taken the test. Any judgment made about the norm is made by the test user. Several types of norms might be used, including grade norms, age norms, percentiles, and standard scores.

Grade Norms *Grade norms* are calculated by determining the average of the raw scores for a grade and using the grade equivalent in place of that average. For example, if the average distance that a class of fifth-grade boys could throw a softball were 96 feet, a score of 96 feet would represent a grade norm of 5. However, scores on measures of physical performance are rarely transformed to grade norms because each grade includes children of different ages; the older children, more advanced in physical growth and development, have a natural advantage in many motor skills.

The use of grade norms has several other limitations. The units from one grade to another are not equal over different parts of the scale. Thus achievement from grade 2 to grade 3 may be greater or less than achievement from grade 8 to grade 9. Performance on physical fitness items, for instance, usually increases consistently from grade to grade for elementary school girls. However, this performance increment may level off before entrance into high school. Thus the significance of a grade norm of 11 for a ninth-grade student is not nearly as great as a grade norm of 4 for a second-grade student.

Furthermore, grade units may be unequal from test to test. A seventh-grade student with grade norms of 11 on the distance run and 9 on the sit-and-reach test would appear to have more cardiorespiratory endurance than flexibility. However, there may be a greater range of distance run scores than flexibility scores for the sixth grade, and the student might actually have high percentile ranks on both tests.

Grade norms are useful for reporting growth in basic skills at the elementary school level. Since this type of norm can be misinterpreted so easily, other types are often preferred.

Age Norms *Age norms* are determined by calculating the average score for a given age. A raw score is then interpreted in terms of an age equivalent. If the average performance by 17-year-old boys on the standing long jump is 7 feet 2 inches, then a raw score of 7 feet 2 inches is used to represent an age norm of 17. Although this type of norm has been used with tests of physical performance, in reality skeletal maturation may play a more significant role than age. In growth and development scales a form of age norms is sometimes used to describe sequences of motor behavior.

Percentile Rank Norms The standardized tests published by AAHPERD include tables of norms based on percentile ranks. These include the Health-Related Physical Fitness Test (1980), the Youth Fitness Test (1976), the Cooperative Physical Education Tests (1970), and the Sports Skills Tests (1967). Both fitness test manuals present norms by age and gender. Grouping by age or grade should not be confused with age norms and grade norms. In the latter case ages or grades represent the norms; in the former case percentiles represent the norms.

In Chapter 2 you learned how to calculate percentile ranks. The *percentile rank norm* is based on the position of the person's score relative to others in the group. Whatever the range of raw scores, the percentiles can only range from 1 to 99. Percentiles divide a distribution of scores into 100 groups of equal size. Although a set of raw scores often forms a bell-like distribution, percentiles form a rectangular one, as shown in Figure 3-10. Percentiles are not equally spaced throughout the distribution because more people are clustered at the middle of

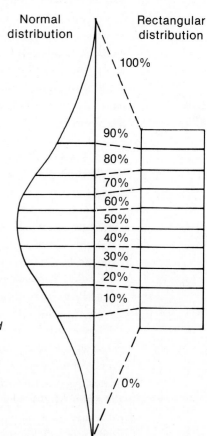

FIGURE 3-10 *Relationship between normal and rectangular distributions.*

the distribution than at the extremes. Only if the same number of examinees obtains each score are the percentiles equally spaced. However, such a distribution is not likely. Therefore, although percentiles seem simple to interpret, it is easy to overemphasize differences near the median and underemphasize differences near the extremes.

Sometimes averaging percentile ranks for several tests is desirable. To do so, the percentiles must first be converted to z-scores. This conversion can be made using tables that are available in most statistics textbooks. The z-scores are then averaged, and this average is converted back to a percentile rank using the same table. The raw score distribution is assumed to be normal for each set of raw scores. Also, the same norm group should be used to generate the percentiles.

Standard Score Norms *Standard score norms*, like percentile norms, are widely used for measures of physical performance, although they have typically not been used to determine national norms in the physical education field. Figure 3-2 represents the relationship between percentiles and standard scores. All standard scores are based on the z-score distribution, which was described earlier in this chapter. Most test users prefer to use a transformation of the z-score because this score is expressed in decimal places and, in some instances, is a negative number. The most widely used transformation in the field is the T-score, also described earlier in this chapter.

T-scores are sometimes confused with T-scaled scores, which are also standard scores, or percentiles, because all three use similar ranges of numbers. However, the T-score reflects the raw score distribution; the T-scaled score alters (normalizes) the raw score distribution unless it is normal to begin with. If the raw score distribution is normal, the T-scores and T-scaled scores will be identical. To obtain a T-scaled score, first convert the raw score to percentiles.

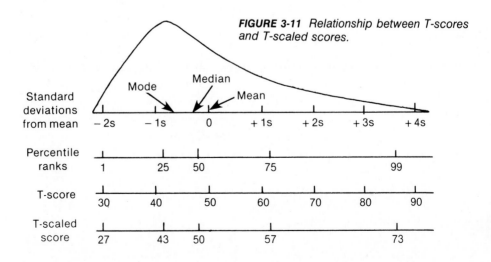

FIGURE 3-11 *Relationship between T-scores and T-scaled scores.*

Then the median of the percentile distribution is set at a z-score of 0 (or a T-score of 50, now referred to as a T-scaled score of 50), and the standard score values are set for other points on the distribution. The T-scaled distribution, like the T-score distribution, has a mean of 50 and a standard deviation of 10. Figure 3-11 shows the relationship of the T-scaled score to T-scores and percentiles.

Local and National Norms

National norms, if properly developed, can be useful for certain purposes. A physical education teacher may wish to compare students' test scores with a national sample as partial evidence of a successful program. If the test scores match high norms, the program is obviously achieving satisfactory results in the area tested. If the norms are low, perhaps certain aspects of the program need to be improved. National norms are also useful for comparisons among distinct sub-populations within an area. For example, in a large metropolitan area comparisons of performance level of "inner city," "fringe-area," and suburban students with national norms could yield interesting results.

On the other hand, national norms are limited in the type of information they can provide. In a school with a good physical education program, all the students may score above the middle of the distribution using a table of national norms. Although this information may be useful in justifying a physical education program, the individual student receives little feedback on personal performance relative to other students in the same school. *Local norms* would provide more useful information in this case. A student who is above average using national norms may be average or even below average compared with local norms. Teachers within a school district can develop local norms by collecting test scores over a period of several years to obtain adequate data; these norms should also be revised periodically so that they remain up-to-date.

CALCULATION OF T-TEST

The purpose of the t-test is to statistically determine if there is a significant difference between two groups that represent independent samples.

A physical educator may want to compare two groups who received different training methods, a trained group versus an untrained one, or male achievement versus female achievement at the end of a semester. This is a test of the hypothesis that $\mu_1 - \mu_2 = 0$. The test is based on the difference in the sample means, $\bar{X}_1 - \bar{X}_2$ that is based on *random* samples of n_1 and n_2 observations drawn from two independent populations.

The following assumptions, besides the randomization and independence mentioned before, must be met for the test to be valid.

1. Populations are normally distributed.
2. Homogeneity of variance: Both populations have the same variance
   $\sigma_1^2 = \sigma_2^2 = \sigma^2.$

Violating the assumption of equal variance is not serious if the two samples are of equal size. The t-test should be used whenever the sample size is smaller than 30. The t-distribution for a given test depends on the degrees of freedom of the samples (n_1, n_2). A table of percentile points of the t-distribution (see appendix) gives the value of t that is to be used as the critical value (to locate the rejection region) to determine whether the groups are statistically different from each other.

The degrees of freedom are determined by adding the two sample sizes and subtracting 2 (df = $n_1 + n_2 - 2$).

The t-test for comparing two means is performed as shown below:

$$t = \frac{\overline{X}_1 - \overline{X}_2}{\sqrt{\dfrac{S_1^2}{n_1} + \dfrac{S_2^2}{n_2}}}$$
Formula 3-11

where $\overline{X}_1$ = mean of group 1
$\overline{X}_2$ = mean of group 2
S_1 = the standard deviation of group 1
S_2 = the standard deviation of group 2
n_1 = number of subjects in group 1
n_2 = number of subjects in group 2

The rejection region or the t critical value for the t-test is identified as follows:

For a two-tailed test with $\alpha = 0.05$, look up the t-value corresponding to $\alpha = 0.05/2 = 0.025$ and degrees of freedom, df = $n_1 + n_2 - 2$. If the obtained t value (formula above) is greater than the positive value or less than the negative value found in the table, reject the hypothesis that the two means are equal and conclude with an $\alpha = 0.05$ (Type I error) that the difference between the two samples is statistically significant. If the obtained t-value does not fall within the critical region, do not reject H_o and conclude that there is no evidence that the samples differ significantly from each other.

Examples

1. Suppose a physical education teacher administers a basketball skill test to two groups of physical education students. One group received instruction for 2 months, and the other did not. Test the mean difference for significance at the 0.05 level using the following data:

	Trained	Untrained
	9	3
	15	6
	4	2
	11	3
	5	6
	7	5
	5	2
	8	4
	10	9
	8	2

Answer

$$\Sigma X \qquad 82 \qquad 42$$
$$\Sigma X^2 \qquad 770 \qquad 224$$

$$\overline{X}_1 = 82/10 = 8.2 \quad \overline{X}_2 = 42/10 = 4.2$$

$$S_1 = \sqrt{\frac{10(770) - (82)^2}{10(10)}} = 3.124 \quad S_2 = \sqrt{\frac{10(224) - (42)^2}{10(10)}} = 2.182$$

$$t = \frac{8.2 - 4.2}{\sqrt{\dfrac{3.124^2}{10} + \dfrac{2.182^2}{10}}} = \frac{4}{\sqrt{1.4520}} = \frac{4}{1.2050} = 3.320$$

The critical value for $\alpha = 0.05$ and 18 degrees of freedom $(10+10-2)$ is ± 2.101 (from t-table). For a more precise estimate of S, use $N(N - 1)$ in the demonstration.

Since the computed value is 3.320 and is greater than $+2.101$, we conclude that there is a significant difference between the trained and untrained group. The trained group displayed superior performance.

2. A physical education teacher gave a bowling test on the last day of class. There were 20 boys and 20 girls in the class. The teacher wished to find out if boys differ from girls in their performance. The number of pins knocked down when the first ball was bowled for each of 10 frames was recorded. A trial performance standard of 8 was used to classify students as master or nonmaster.

Based on the following data that are the number of times that each student was classified as master (in 10 trials), test whether the boys' performance is different from the girls' performance.

	Boys		Girls	
1 - 4	11 - 8	1 - 2	11 - 6
2 - 3	12 - 4	2 - 4	12 - 5
3 - 6	13 - 5	3 - 6	13 - 4
4 - 7	14 - 9	4 - 5	14 - 5
5 - 3	15 - 3	5 - 6	15 - 4
6 - 6	16 - 1	6 - 3	16 - 5
7 - 4	17 - 7	7 - 3	17 - 3
8 - 6	18 - 6	8 - 3	18 - 5
9 - 3	19 - 6	9 - 4	19 - 5
10 - 10	20 - 8	10 - 4	20 - 7

Answer

$$\Sigma X_{boys} = 109 \qquad \Sigma X_{girls} = 89$$
$$\overline{X}_{boys} = 109/20 = 5.45 \qquad \overline{X}_{girls} = 89/20 = 4.45$$
$$\Sigma X^2_{boys} = 697 \qquad \Sigma X^2_{girls} = 427$$

$$S_{boys} = \sqrt{\frac{20(697) - (109)^2}{20(20)}} = 2.27 \quad S_{girls} = \sqrt{\frac{20(427) - (89)^2}{20(20)}} = 1.24$$

$$t = \frac{5.45 - 4.45}{\sqrt{\dfrac{2.27^2}{20} + \dfrac{1.24^2}{20}}} = \frac{1}{\sqrt{0.3345}} = \frac{1}{0.5784} = 1.729$$

The critical value for $\alpha = 0.05$ and 38 degrees of freedom is ± 2.03.

Since the obtained t-value, 1.729, is not greater than $+2.03$ and not smaller than -2.03, there is no evidence to suggest that the performance of girls is significantly different from the performance of boys in this particular class.

SUMMARY

Measures of central tendency and variability provide essential information for a concise interpretation of a set of test scores. If the test scores are distributed so that they approximate the normal curve, the mean and standard deviation are preferred measures. When the distribution is skewed, the median is a more accurate representation of the center of the distribution. In this case the interpercentile range would be used as the measure of variability. Because tests of motor skill and physical fitness are scored in different metrics, scores are frequently transformed to a common scale using percentiles, z-score transformations, or T-score transformations. In this way scores recorded in minutes and seconds can be compared with scores recorded in feet and inches.

Sometimes it is of interest to know whether two variables bear a relationship to each other. This can be examined by calculating a correlation coefficient using the two variables. The Pearson product-moment procedure can be used to calculate this statistic; if the scores are ranked, the rank difference method can be used. These coefficients may be interpreted on both practical and statistical grounds.

The scores of normative groups should be taken into account in interpreting scores on tests of motor behavior. Information on local and national norms is useful in obtaining an overall perspective of the ability of individual examinees in relation to others.

LEARNING EXPERIENCES

1. Ten students were given the long jump test and the 50-yard-dash test. Their scores were:

Student	Long jump (inches) (Test A)	50-Yard dash (sec. tenths) (Test B)
1	72	8.0
2	69	8.0
3	51	9.7
4	69	7.6
5	63	8.3
6	81	7.3
7	66	8.2
8	78	7.5
9	72	7.4
10	75	7.8

a. Calculate the mean, median, and mode for Test A and Test B.
b. Calculate the range and interquartile range for Test A and Test B.
c. Calculate the standard deviation for Test A and Test B.
d. Calculate z-scores and T-scores for each score on Test A.
e. Calculate z-scores and T-scores for each score on Test B.
f. Calculate the correlation coefficient between Test A and Test B using the Pearson product-moment method. Interpret the correlation coefficient.
g. Calculate the percentage of variance that Test A and Test B share.
h. Rank the Test A scores.
i. Rank the Test B scores.
j. Calculate the rank-difference correlation coefficient.

REFERENCES

American Association for Health, Physical Education and Recreation. 1967. AAHPER sports skills tests. Washington, D.C.: AAHPER.

American Association for Health, Physical Education and Recreation. 1976. Youth Fitness Test manual. Washington, D.C.: AAHPER.

American Alliance for Health, Physical Education, Recreation and Dance. 1980. Health-Related Physical Fitness Test manual. Reston, Va.: AAHPERD.

American Psychological Association. 1985. Standards for educational and psychological tests. Washington, D.C.: APA.

Downing, D., and Clark, J. 1983. Statistics the easy way. Woodbury, N.Y.: Barron's Educational Series, Inc.

Lyman, H.B. 1978. Test scores and what they mean, ed. 3, Englewood Cliffs, N.J.: Prentice-Hall, Inc.

Mosteller, F., Fienberg, S.E., and Rourke, R.E.K. 1983. Beginning statistics with data analysis. Reading, Mass.: Addison-Wesley Publishing Co.

Rothstein, A.L. 1985. Research design and statistics for physical education. Englewood Cliffs, N.J.: Prentice-Hall, Inc.

Sprinthall, R.C. 1982. Basic statistical analysis. Reading, Mass.: Addison-Wesley Publishing Co.

ANNOTATED READINGS

Glasnapp, D.R., and Popglo, J.P. 1985. Essentials of statistical analysis for the behavioral sciences. Columbus, Ohio: Charles E. Merrill Publishing Co.

Introductory statistics text tailored to students with little math background and no experience studying statistics; focuses on applied statistics; problems use data reflecting children in actual situations—the "Sesame Street" data base; includes enough theory to lay a firm foundation and enough application to be genuinely practical; emphasizes key concepts.

Hinkle, D.E., Wiersma, W., and Jurs, S.G. 1979. Applied statistics for the behavioral sciences. Boston: Houghton Mifflin Co.

Emphasizes conceptual understanding of basic statistical procedures; helps students achieve computational skills needed for statistical procedures in practical settings; examples taken from actual settings (40% from education); begins with elementary descriptive statistics and progresses to more sophisticated procedures.

Jaeger, R. 1983. Statistics: a spectator sport. Beverly Hills, Calif.: Sage Publications, Inc.

Designed to help anyone who wants to understand statistics; includes clear explanations that enable readers to learn what statistics are, what they mean, and how they are used and interpreted; does not include any equations; applications to a wide range of research and evaluation problems, giving particular attention to studies in the computerized files of Educational Resources Information Center (ERIC).

Kirk, R.E. 1984. Elementary statistics, ed. 2, Florence, Ky.: Brooks/Cole Publishing Co.

Introduction to statistics for students in education and behavioral sciences; emphasizes verbal rather than mathematical problems; includes in-depth treatments of individual concepts and their interrelationships; develops the underpinnings of statistics through the use of high school mathematics; a concise review of elementary math in an appendix; incorporates real-life examples in the review exercises; provides interesting introduction to the history of statistics, as well as extensive references on important topics.

Witte, R.S. 1984. Statistics, ed. 2. Lavallette, N.J.: Holt, Rinehart & Winston General Book.

Emphasizes concepts rather than just computations; covers wide range of topics in descriptive and inferential statistics without overwhelming students with mathematics; includes extensive problem sets in each chapter, ranging from simple computational tasks to questions of interpretation, with step-by-step progressions to problem solving.

PROBLEMS

1. Use the data set below to calculate the mean and the standard deviation.

   Data set of 30 max $\dot{V}o_2$ scores:
   54, 49, 53, 56, 55, 50, 47, 60, 53, 41, 58, 53, 48, 37, 55, 62, 54, 51, 39, 54, 53, 47, 57, 55, 42, 57, 54, 45, 49, 53

2. a. Use the above data set of 30 max $\dot{V}_{O_2}$ scores to form a frequency distribution with intervals of size 2. Include columns for tally, f, cf, and c%.
    b. Calculate the interquartile range for this distribution, using the frequency distribution in a.

3. The mean of a set of basketball scores is 32 and the standard deviation is 3. Calculate z-scores and T-scores for the following test scores: 31, 39, 29, 27, 33, 25.

4. Using the Pearson product-moment method, calculate the correlation coefficient for the scores on the first (X) and second (Y) examinations given in an undergraduate course on measurement in physical education.

Student	Test 1 (X)	Test 2 (Y)	x^2	y^2
1	47	33		
2	54	49		
3	48	40		
4	47	44		
5	50	48		
6	45	36		
7	50	35		
8	56	50		
9	54	46		
10	48	37		
11	53	40		
12	47	39		
13	38	32		
14	47	42		
15	48	39		
16	49	37		
17	53	42		
18	53	40		
19	49	40		
20	52	47		

988   816   49,118

a. Draw a graph of the relationship between X and Y. Plot the coordinates and record their numerical values at each point, as in Figure 3-8.

5. Thought question: Interpret the relationship between the scores on the two measurement exams that were correlated in 4. Consider both the size and sign of the correlation coefficient. What does this mean in terms of the students' abilities on the two tests?

6. Use the data set below to calculate the mean and standard deviation.

    Data set of nine 100-meter dash scores: (unit = second) 12.9, 13.1, 13.5, 13.8, 14.0, 14.2, 14.5, 14.7, 15.4

7. The mean of a set of 400-meter run scores is 70.5 seconds and the standard deviation is 6.0 seconds. Calculate z-scores and T-scores for the following scores:

    58.7, 64.5, 70.5, 76.5, 88.0

8. The mean of a set of standing long jump scores is 100.5 inches and the standard deviation is 4.47 inches. Calculate z-scores and T-scores for the following test scores:

    89, 92, 100.5, 105, 112.

9. a. Using the Pearson product-moment method, calculate the correlation coefficient for the scores on 100-meter dash (X) scores and the average length of steps in dash (Y) collected from 12 male athletes in competition.

Athlete no.	100-Meter time X (sec)	Average length of steps Y (m)
1	9.98	2.23
2	9.90	2.13
3	10.22	2.15
4	10.11	2.13
5	10.25	2.11
6	10.41	2.29
7	10.00	2.00
8	10.30	2.04
9	10.30	2.00
10	10.30	1.95
11	10.30	2.04
12	10.70	1.98

b. Draw a graph of the relationship between X and Y. Plot the coordinates and record their numerical values at each point, as in Figure 3-8.

10. The data set below is the scoring rate of spikes (X) and the winning order (Y) of the first eight winning teams in a volleyball competition.

Team no.	Scoring rate of spikes X (%)	Winning order Y
1	44.0	1
2	40.3	2
3	40.6	3
4	46.1	4
5	37.4	5
6	43.5	6
7	37.4	7
8	38.9	8

Calculate the rank difference correlation coefficient for the scoring rate of spikes (X) and the winning order (Y) of the volleyball teams.

11. Two groups of students were trained on their vertical jump ability. After same period of training, the increasing values of the vertical jump test of both groups are as follows:

Group 1: $\bar{X}_1 = 7.6$ $S_1 = 3.90$ $n_1 = 17$
Group 2: $\bar{X}_2 = 4.8$ $S_2 = 3.29$ $n_2 = 15$

Test the significance of the mean difference between two groups at 0.05 level. (Assume the increasing value of vertical jump is normally distributed.)

12. The data below represent the heart rate of male and female athletes measured from a maximum exercise test between the 60th and 70th second.

Male: $\bar{X}_1 = 27.52$ beats/10 sec. $S_1 = 2.87$ beats/10 sec. $n_1 = 32$
Female: $\bar{X}_2 = 28.78$ beats/10 sec. $S_2 = 2.42$ beats/10 sec. $n_2 = 28$

Test the significance of the difference between the mean heart rate of male and female athletes at the 0.05 level. (Assume the distribution of heart rate during maximum exercise is normal.)

13. Assume you have two samples from two normal population. Your sample values are as follows:

$$\text{Sample 1:} \quad \bar{X}_1 = 36 \quad S_1 = 4.00 \quad n_1 = 15$$
$$\text{Sample 2:} \quad \bar{X}_2 = 30 \quad S_2 = 6.00 \quad n_2 = 16$$

Test the significance of the mean difference between two samples at 0.05 level.

14. Ten hypertensive patients participated in a physical therapy program. The diastolic blood pressure values of the patients measured before and after the program are given below. Test the significance of the mean difference between the pre and post-test blood pressure values.

Patient	Pretest	Posttest
1	100	94
2	113	98
3	134	118
4	95	84
5	122	116
6	117	119
7	92	85
8	120	96
9	114	104
10	138	120

15. Repeat problem 14 by using t-test considering the pretest and posttest as two independent samples. Compare and explain the results of problem 14 and problem 15.

ANSWERS TO PROBLEMS

1. $\bar{X} = \dfrac{1541}{30} = 51.37; \ s = \sqrt{\dfrac{(30)(80211) - (1541)^2}{(30)(30)}} = 5.93$

2. a.

Intervals	Tally	f	cf	c%
61-62	X	1	30	100.0
59-60	X	1	29	96.7
57-58	XXX	3	28	93.3
55-56	XXXX	4	25	83.3
53-54	XXXXXXXXX	9	21	70.0
51-52	X	1	12	40.0
49-50	XXX	3	11	36.7
47-48	XXX	3	8	26.7
45-46	X	1	5	16.7
43-44		0	4	13.3
41-42	XX	2	4	13.3
39-40	X	1	2	6.7
37-38	X	1	1	3.3

b. $X_{.75} = 55.25; \ X_{.25} = 48.17$
Interquartile range $= 55.25 - 48.17 = 7.08$

3.

Score	z-Score	T-score
31	−.33	46.7
39	2.33	73.3
29	−1.00	40.0
27	−1.67	33.3
33	.33	53.3
25	−2.33	26.7

4. a. 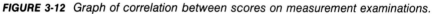 $r_{xy} = \dfrac{20(40593) - 988(816)}{\sqrt{[20(49118) - 976144][20(33808) - 665856)]}} = 0.706$

b. Answer is depicted in Fig. 3-12, as shown on p. 81.

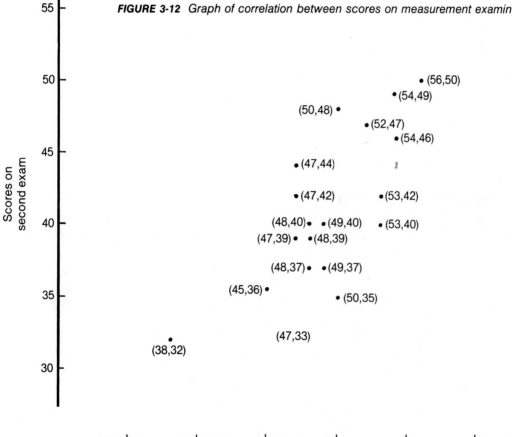

FIGURE 3-12 *Graph of correlation between scores on measurement examinations.*

6. $\bar{X} = \dfrac{\Sigma X}{N} = \dfrac{126.1}{9} = 14.01$

$$S = \sqrt{\dfrac{N\Sigma X^2 - (\Sigma X)^2}{N(N)}}$$

$$= \sqrt{\dfrac{9(1771.85) - (126.1)^2}{9(9)}}$$

$$= \sqrt{\dfrac{45.44}{81}}$$

$$= \sqrt{0.561}$$

$$= 0.75$$

7.

Raw score	z-Score	T-score
58.7	1.97	69.7
64.5	1.00	60.0
70.5	0.00	50.0
76.5	−1.00	40.0
88.0	−2.92	20.8

8.

Raw score	z-Score	T-score
112	2.57	75.7
105	1.01	60.1
100.5	0.00	50.0
92	−1.90	30.9
89	−2.57	24.3

9. a. $r_{xy} = \dfrac{12(256.2111) - (122.77)(25.05)}{\sqrt{[12(1256.5515) - (122.77)^2][12(52.4115) - (25.05)^2]}}$

$$= \dfrac{-0.8553}{2.9701}$$

$$= -0.288$$

10.

Team no.	X	Rank(X)	Y	Rank (Y)	D	D²
1	44.0	2	1	1	1	1
2	40.3	5	2	2	3	9
3	40.6	4	3	3	1	1
4	46.1	1	4	4	−3	9
5	37.4	7.5	5	5	2.5	6.25
6	43.5	3	6	6	−3	9
7	37.4	7.5	7	7	0.5	0.25
8	38.9	6	8	8	−2	4

$$\Sigma D^2 = \overline{39.5}$$

$$P = 1 - \dfrac{6(39.5)}{8(8 - 1)}$$

$$= 1 - 0.47$$

$$= 0.53$$

11. $t = \dfrac{|7.6 - 4.8|}{\sqrt{\dfrac{3.90^2}{17} + \dfrac{3.29^2}{15}}} = \dfrac{2.8}{\sqrt{1.6163}} = \dfrac{2.8}{1.2713} = 2.2025$

df $= 17 + 15 - 2 = 30 \qquad t_{.05(30)} = 2.042$

$t = 2.2025 > t_{.05(30)} = 2.042$. Therefore, there is a significant difference between two means (p < 0.05).

12. $t = \dfrac{|28.78 - 27.52|}{\sqrt{\dfrac{2.87^2}{32} + \dfrac{2.42^2}{28}}} = \dfrac{1.26}{\sqrt{.4666}} = \dfrac{1.26}{0.6831} = 1.8445$

df $= 32 + 28 - 2 = 58 \qquad t_{.05(58)} = 2.000.$

$t = 1.8445 < t_{.05(58)} = 2.000$. Therefore, there is no significant difference between two means (p > 0.05).

13. $t = \dfrac{|30 - 36|}{\sqrt{\dfrac{4^2}{15} + \dfrac{6^2}{16}}} = \dfrac{6}{\sqrt{3.3167}} = \dfrac{6}{1.8212} = 3.2945$

df $= 15 + 16 - 2 = 29 \qquad t_{.05(29)} = 2.045$

$t = 3.2945 > t_{.05(29)} = 2.045$. Therefore, there is a significant difference between two means (p < 0.05).

14.

Patient	Pretest	Postest	d	d²
1	100	94	6	36
2	113	98	15	225
3	134	118	16	256
4	95	84	11	121
5	122	116	6	36
6	117	119	−2	4
7	92	85	7	49
8	120	96	24	576
9	114	104	10	100
10	138	120	18	324

$\Sigma d = 111 \qquad \Sigma d^2 = 1727 \qquad \bar{d} = 11.1 \qquad S_d = 7.0349 \qquad N = 10$

$t = \dfrac{\bar{d}}{S_d/\sqrt{N}} = \dfrac{11.1}{7.0349/\sqrt{10}} = \dfrac{11.1}{2.3450} = 4.7335$

df $= 10 - 1 = 9 \qquad t_{.05(9)} = 2.262$

$t = 4.7335 > t_{.05(9)} = 2.262$. Therefore, there is a significant difference between the blood pressure values of pretest and posttest (p < 0.05).

15. $t = \dfrac{|103.4 - 114.5|}{\sqrt{\dfrac{14.5757^2}{10} + \dfrac{13.3357^2}{10}}} = \dfrac{11.1}{\sqrt{39.0292}}$

$= \dfrac{11.1}{6.2473}$

$= 1.7768$

df $= 10 + 10 - 2 = 18 \qquad t_{.05(18)} = 2.101$

$t = 1.7768 < t_{.05(18)} = 2.101$. Therefore, there is no significant difference between two means (p > 0.05).

Part Three

The Use of Microcomputers in Measuring Motor Behavior

4

Conceptual Overview of a Microcomputer

KEY WORDS *Watch for these words as you read the following chapter:*

bit	display	monitor
booting	gates	peripheral
Central Processing Unit (CPU)	hardware	Random Access Memory (RAM)
byte	keyboard	Read Only Memory (ROM)
computer literacy	kilobyte (k)	software
disk drive	microchip	
Disk Operating System (DOS)	modem	

The use of microcomputers in measurement and evaluation has unlimited potential. They can be used to administer, score, and develop tests; summarize, analyze, and transform scores; and compare scores with norms. Data banks consisting of tests scores can be established and expanded using the microcomputer. The objective of this chapter is to familiarize the novice with the microcomputer. For the student with some expertise with a microcomputer, this chapter serves as a cursory overview. For the student who is a rank beginner, even this chapter may seem overwhelming at first. Learning to use a microcomputer requires a considerable amount of patience. Rereading various sections of this chapter now and returning to review this chapter after completing Chapter 5, which covers some applications in the field, will help the material to fall into place.

Keep in mind, however, that entire books have been written on using microcomputers, even a specific microcomputer brand, and other texts are devoted entirely to a programming language. Although covering a great amount of information in a textbook on measurement and evaluation is not feasible, a general overview is essential. Microcomputers are here to stay. They will be a part of your life, both personally and professionally. If you plan to teach, your students will probably be receiving a constant exposure to microcomputers. A general understanding of these machines is therefore essential for every teacher in the public schools, even those who do not teach microcomputer skills. For those who intend to be exercise specialists, a knowledge of computers is valuable for more

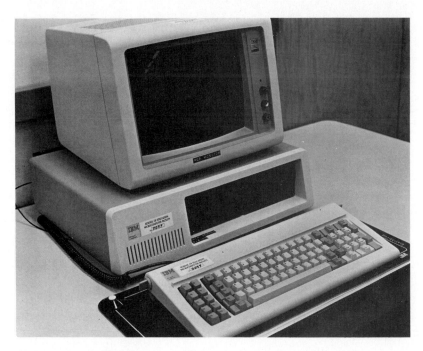

IBM-PC microcomputer.

efficient recordkeeping as well as a means of providing information to clients on their health and fitness status. In some corporate fitness centers a bank of microcomputers is installed in a central location. As employees enter the center, they slip an identification card into the slot in one of the microcomputers and data on their exercise prescription and physiological state are printed on the screen. On completion of the exercise period the employee enters information on the type, duration, and intensity of the exercise, along with his or her exercise heart rate. This information is added to the employee's records on the computer and is used to modify, if necessary, the exercise prescription. Since all employees participating in the fitness program use a microcomputer to record their fitness data, a summary of these data may be obtained for the total corporation to use in evaluating the program.

A BRIEF HISTORY

The first large-scale electronic computer was built at the University of Pennsylvania in 1946. This huge machine required a room 30 feet by 50 feet for its storage. It used 18,000 vacuum tubes and miles of wiring to operate. In the 1960s the **microchip,** a silicon board the size of a fingernail, was developed, resulting in a tremendous impact on our society. By 1981 the equivalent of 750,000 microchips could be etched on a single microchip.

A microchip contains many microscopic switches known as **gates.** An electrical charge opens some gates and closes others, creating a pattern simulating human logic. The chips in a microcomputer contain thousands of electronic circuits. One kind of microchip executes instructions; the other stores information in memory. The development of the microchip made manufacturing small desktop computers at affordable prices possible. In the 1970s the microcomputer boom became so widespread that it was inconceivable that anyone in our society would be unaware of its existence.

How did our society respond to this technology? Astronomical numbers of microcomputers were sold every month. Sales are continuing at an astonishing pace. How microcomputers are being used is another matter. Many schools have microcomputer laboratories. What kind of instruction takes place in these labs? Issues of this type are being hotly debated across the country, often under the label of **computer literacy.** An unresolved question among educators and scientists is how computer literacy should be defined. Some believe it should reflect a knowledge of programming and programming skills. Others describe it as a knowledge of computer systems and what they can do. A loose definition of computer literacy is "a threshold of knowledge that qualifies an individual for participation in the computer age" (Benderson, 1983). The Educational Testing Service (1985, p. 10) prepared a more precise definition: "Computer literacy may be defined as whatever a person needs to know and do with computers to function competently in our information based society. It involves three kinds of competence—the ability to use and instruct computers to aid in learning, solving problems, and managing information; the knowledge of functions, applications, capabilities, limitations, and social implications of computers and related technology; and the understanding needed to learn and evaluate new applications and social issues as they arise." Although a limited discussion of the BASIC (Beginners All-Purpose Symbolic Instruction Code) programming language is presented in Chapter 5, the primary objective of these two chapters is to help you to develop a small amount of computer literacy.

THE MAKEUP OF A MICROCOMPUTER

In the past, microcomputers have been referred to as personal computers, which indicates that only one person can use the computer at a time. These single-user computers process information more slowly than the larger versions and are generally affordable to the average person. Microcomputers are sometimes used exclusively for entertainment. Two other types of computers, minicomputers and mainframe computers, have been available for many years. A minicomputer can process information faster than a microcomputer and accommodate several users at once. Of course, it is also costlier than the microcomputer. The grandfather of all computers, the mainframe computer, is a large multiuser machine, which is faster and more expensive than the minicomputer.

In the 1990s the conception of the types of computers described in the above paragraph will change. The computer age can be divided into two eras. The first, occurring from 1945 to 1980, was characterized by linear processing, which solved problems one step at a time. Since 1980, the focus has been on parallel processing, which assigns portions of a problem to several microprocessors working at the same time. As a result, the problem is solved in significantly less time. Clearly, the next computer revolution is underway. Desktop supercomputers as fast and powerful as today's multimillion-dollar mainframe supercomputers will become commonplace in the late 1990s. A superchip with the equivalent of a supercomputer's computation power is already available. Experts predict that in a few years, scientists will link several such chips in a parallel supersystem. Not many physical educators or exercise scientists will need this much computing power, however. There will still be a need for simpler and cheaper desktop computers, or microcomputers as they are currently known.

If you went to a computer store today and asked about purchasing a microcomputer, you would be shown a bewildering array of equipment. The physical components of the computer and its peripherals are referred to as **hardware.** A **peripheral** is a device that can send information to the computer as well as receive information from it. At the very least the hardware you would probably need includes the computer itself (a case housing the central processing unit), a keyboard, a monitor, and a disk drive or a tape recorder. The **keyboard** is similar to the keyboard on a typewriter and is used to transmit information to the computer. **A monitor** is like a television set; in fact, a television set can easily be

Dual disk drive.

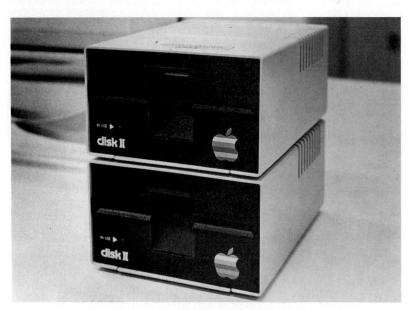

used for this purpose. A monitor purchased specifically to use with a computer consists of a screen and a cathode ray tube (CRT). A **display** appears on the screen, either in color or monochrome. A **disk drive** is a storage device that can store data and retrieve it. A dual disk drive is shown in the photograph.

The basic features are shown in the following photograph of the Apple IIe microcomputer. This brand of microcomputer is used to exemplify microcomputers and their operation in both this chapter and Chapter 5. The Apple IIe was chosen for two reasons: it is inexpensive, and many are available in the public schools. However, this does not mean that the Apple is the best microcomputer.

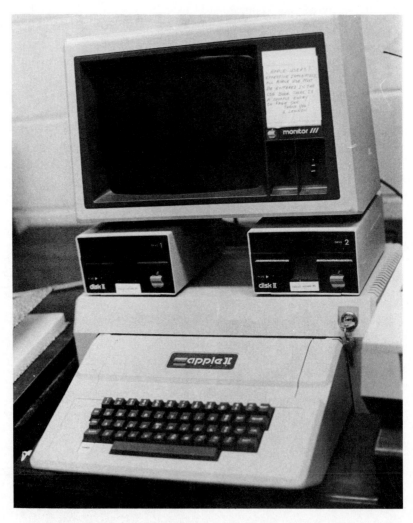

Apple IIe microcomputer, keyboard, monitor, two disk drives.

Many other fine brands have been manufactured, such as the IBM-PC (the photograph at the beginning of the chapter), Commodore (the photograph at the end of this chapter), Corona, TRS (Radio Shack), Zenith, Atari, Compaq, and Epson. Many models that were popular 10 years ago, including the Apple IIe, are no longer being manufactured. However, many of these computers are still being used. Furthermore, most programs written for them can be run on the newer computers manufactured by the same company.

Computer Memory

Computer hardware must use a machine language that is compatible with the **central processing unit** (CPU). The CPU of a microcomputer may be a single microchip or a portion of a microchip. This unit controls peripherals and memory. Remember that there are two kinds of microchips, one to execute commands and one to store information. Some of the microchips contain information stored permanently in the computer. These form the **Read Only Memory,** or ROM, section of the computer. ROM is the control system for the whole computer, including the program that allows the use of BASIC, a machine language. It is impossible to put any information into ROM. Recall that electric charges open and close gates on a microchip. In ROM the gates are permanently fixed in either the open or closed position. Other microchips can read and store information temporarily. This section of the computer is called **Random Access Memory,** or RAM. When you turn on a computer and begin using it, you are working in the RAM section. When you turn the computer off, you lose all the information in RAM.

Data Storage

Even though information can be stored temporarily in RAM, this information is lost once the computer is turned off. Thus a more permanent means of storage is needed. Information can be stored on tape cassettes, hard disks, floppy disks (see photograph), and video disks. The use of the floppy disk (also known as a

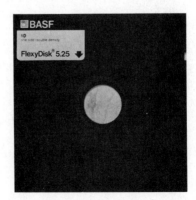

Floppy disk.

diskette) is described here, although hard disk usage is becoming much more commonplace. A hard disk alleviates the need to constantly use diskettes when operating the computer. It also stores far more data than a diskette. Many computers use 5¼ inch floppy disks. However, the Apple Macintosh computer and, more recently, the IBM PS/2 series use 3½ inch disks. The smaller disks are encased in a hard cover and cannot be damaged as easily as the larger ones. A peripheral device can be purchased to transfer the data from a 5¼ inch disk to a 3½ inch disk.

To use the disk, insert it into the disk drive, or storage device. There must be a means of communicating between the disk in the disk drive and the central processor. The **Disk Operating System** (DOS) is a program written to establish this communication. The program must be loaded into the computer's memory (RAM) from a disk. The process is often referred to as **booting** a disk.

Computer Languages

Computer languages use the two-digit system of binary mathematics. It is based on a Boolean algebra, a system of logic devised in the nineteenth century for solving complex problems through a series of binary (yes or no) choices. A discussion of how it works using a language such as BASIC follows. Each letter, number, and punctuation mark is represented by a **byte.** Each byte contains eight **bits** (or two nibbles), which are the yes-no choices represented by open and closed gates. Each byte, then, has eight gates. There are also 16-bit processors such as the IBM Personal Computer (IBM-PC). This simply means that each byte in the IBM contains 16 bits and is approximately twice as fast as the 8-bit processors such as the Apple. The IBM PC-AT uses a 32-bit processor and is four times as fast as the microcomputers with the 8-bit processors.

The amount of memory in a computer is determined by the number of bytes in a system. For convenience, computer memory is usually reported in **kilobytes,** or k, with 1k equal to 1024 bytes. If an advertisement indicates that a microcomputer has 48k memory, it usually means there is a 48k memory capacity in RAM.

Software

Previously, DOS was described as a program; thus it is not hardware. A computer program is referred to as software. Specifically, **software** refers to a set of instructions that makes the computer function in some desired way, such as word processing or statistical calculations. Many programs can be purchased through computer stores or companies advertising in computer magazines. It is not necessary to have any programming skills to use these programs. However, the software must be compatible with your computer. Furthermore, your computer must have the memory capacity required to use the program.

Peripherals

Other hardware may also be added to the basic components described above. A printer is useful for obtaining a paper copy of a computer program, the data you entered into the computer, and the results of running a program. When the information is printed on paper, this is referred to as a hard copy.

To communicate with other microcomputers, mainframe computers, and information services, a **modem** is needed. A modem is a device allowing a computer to communicate over telephone lines and other communication media. The term is actually a contraction of modulator-demodulator. Modems transmit information at different speeds, measured in a unit called a baud. A 1200 baud modem will send or receive about 120 characters a second. There are two types of modems—acoustic and direct-connect. The acoustic modem consists of two cups in which the telephone's handset fits. To use this modem the telephone number of another computer is dialed, and the handset is placed in the modem's cups to allow communication. A direct-connect modem clips into a jack attached to your telephone line.

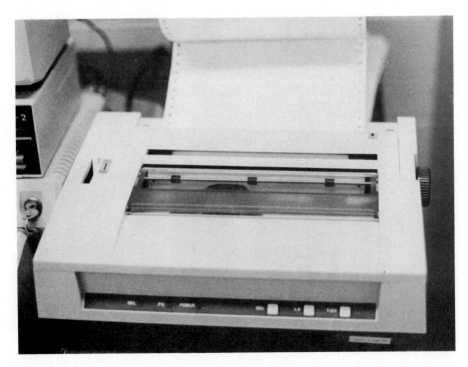

Printer.

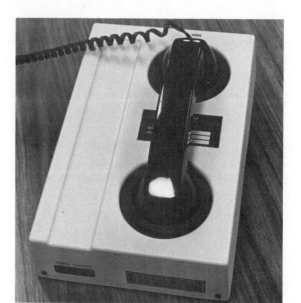

Modem.

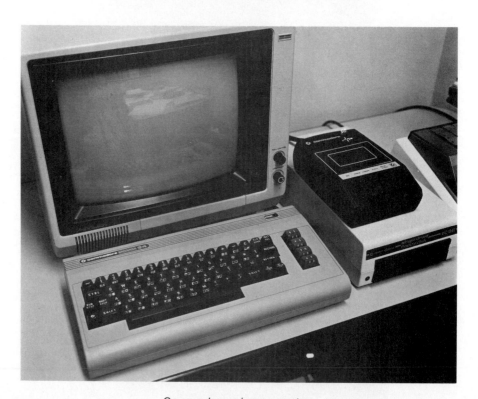

Commodore microcomputer.

SUMMARY

The refinement of computer technology has been nothing short of phenomenal. The invention of the microchip has made relatively efficient desktop computers available to the masses. Both teachers of physical education and exercise specialists in nonschool settings will find many uses for these machines, not only to handle sets of test scores but also to provide computer-aided instruction. Imagine using the computer to teach students the rules of a sport or to instruct clients on nutritional factors related to physical fitness. Once basic computing skills have been mastered, the possibilities for applications in physical education and exercise science are unlimited.

LEARNING EXPERIENCES

1. Visit the computer center or one of the microcomputer laboratories on your campus and try a demonstration disk that describes ways in which a microcomputer can be used. Select the type of computer available to you on your campus and ask for the demonstration disk for this type. Try it on a microcomputer in the laboratory. Do not hesitate to ask the staff members questions.
2. Visit a computer store and ask the salesman to demonstrate a commercially developed program dealing with statistical analyses. Actually try a portion of the demonstration disk that comes with the program, using one of the microcomputers on display in the store.

REFERENCES

Benderson, A. 1983. Computer literacy. Focus, **11**:1-32.
Educational Testing Service. 1985. A unique effort to create a computer literacy pool. Examiner. Princeton, N.J.: Educational Testing Service.

ANNOTATED READINGS

Bork, A. 1985. Personal computers for education. New York: Harper & Row, Publishers, Inc.
Discusses the use of computers in education and the profound effects they will have in the future; focuses on computer literacy and programming; examines the computer as an intellectual tool and as an instructional device; surveys the role of the computer in the management of learning; proves to be a practical book for teachers, parents, and administrators.
Farrell, P. 1984. Computer literacy: what does it mean? Journal of Physical Education, Recreation and Dance, **55**(4):54-55.
Advocates the use of computers at all levels of learning; defines and discusses computer literacy.
Hiscox, M.D. 1985. Computer-based testing systems. Educational Measurement, 4(1):27-28.
Discusses the use of computers in item banking and test construction; analyzes the problems faced in attempting to develop a new micro-based testing system to be used on a widespread basis; suggests that the method of developing the system is more important than the product.

Kanter, H.M. 1985. Computer applications of educational measurement concepts. New York: Macmillan Publishing Co.

Provides a brief, hands-on introduction to the microcomputer system and descriptive statistical concepts; incorporates computer literacy into coursework; contains a variety of examples and illustrations in each unit.

Poole, L. 1983. Apple II user's guide. Berkeley, Calif.: Osborne/McGraw-Hill, Inc.

First three chapters are especially useful to the first-time computer user; describes hardware and software; explains how to use the computer system; describes disk commands needed to run existing programs.

5 *Microcomputer Applications*

KEY WORDS *Watch for these words as you read the following chapter:*

BASIC language	enter key	LOAD (program)
CATALOG	formatting a disk	NEW
compatibles	HOME	RUN (program)
DELETE (program)	initializing a disk	SAVE (program)
disk (floppy)	LIST	

The technology explosion elicited by the microcomputer has already influenced society a great deal and will continue to do so in the future, just as the Sputnik flight influenced curricular offerings in the public school systems by increasing the emphasis on sciences. The widespread availability of microcomputers has already spawned studies of users and potential users. Some of these studies have shown that many people suffer from computer phobia, a general anxiety or apprehension about using computers. Although the computer user actually controls the computer, this sometimes does not appear to be true. It helps to remember that microcomputers are virtually indestructable during the normal course of operating them. Children often play aimlessly with a home computer, and no damage is done. Of course, programs can be accidentally erased, but it is extremely unlikely that the hardware would be damaged.

Microcomputers are being used in many aspects of physical education and exercise science. At least one test-writing program has been developed by a physical educator and is being sold commercially (Cicciarella, 1983).* This program produces equivalent-form examinations of 100 questions or less on any topic from a pool of questions the user has originated. A microcomputer can control cardiovascular fitness testing. In one laboratory a microcomputer controls the speed and the grade of the treadmill according to any protocol, turns on an electrocardiograph (ECG) at any predetermined time or on demand, converts the ECG signal for computer storage, and generates data, summaries, and individualized

---

*For more information on this program, known as Test Writer, write to Persimmon Software, 1901 Gemway Drive, Charlotte, N.C. 28216.

programs based on test results (Donnelly, 1983). At the University of Delaware, computer-aided instruction is provided in fitness, sports such as volleyball and racquetball, biomechanics, nutrition, basic mathematics, and social dance (Barlow and Bayalis, 1983). A microcomputer can be used for data management (Mayhew and Rankin, 1983) and dance notation (Sealy, 1983).

According to Kelly (1987), computer-assisted instruction (CAI) programs can be classified in three broad categories: drill and practice, tutorial, and simulation programs. In drill and practice programs the user reads information on a topic and responds to questions presented on the computer screen. Tutorials are similar types of programs; however, they typically allow the user more options (e.g., to return to information section). Simulation programs are more sophisticated versions of CAI. The user reviews an event, then responds to questions that require problem solving. Different paths can be taken, depending on the responses of the user. The user may ask for information or review tutorials. "CAI programs allow a learner to progress at an individual rate, keep the learner actively involved, provide immediate feedback and reinforcement, and maximize success and minimize failure" (Kelly, 1987, p. 75).

In Chapter 4 microcomputers are described in a general context; this chapter provides a few practical experiences with a microcomputer. Anytime a set of test scores is obtained, certain summary information should be calculated. If the appropriate program has been written for the microcomputer, this information can be obtained in minutes. However, the process should not be oversimplified. Learning to use a microcomputer takes time and patience, even if you are using software rather than writing your own programs. However, your efforts will be well rewarded, both by making your job easier and by enhancing your understanding of a significant phenomenon in our society.

VARIATIONS IN MICROCOMPUTERS

Even though you may not have shopped for a microcomputer of your own, you are undoubtedly aware of the wide array of machines available on the market. In fact, because of the extensive advertising campaigns by certain companies, names such as Apple, IBM, Commodore, Radio Shack, and Texas Instruments are probably very familiar. Each of these machines has a different operating system. If you bought a program written for the Apple, it could not be used on the IBM unless an interpreter program was used to translate the Apple program. Many features of the computer differ across brands. For example, even keys on the keyboard are dissimilar in number, type, and layout. Of course, the prices can be notably different for various brands of microcomputers.

Richards and Engelhorn (1983) prepared a brief overview of microcomputer systems. Even though this type of information is rapidly outdated, many of the precautions they noted remain timely. A rank beginner in desktop computing

B.C. **by johnny hart**

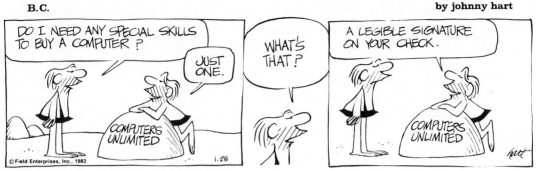

By permission of Johnny Hart and Field Enterprises, Inc.

would be wise to become familiar with one type of computer and to use it exclusively. Experienced users having some programming background will find it relatively easy to switch back and forth between certain brands of microcomputers once they are aware of the computers' basic differences. One final point—when a microcomputer appears on the market and becomes a best seller, other companies try to build a machine that is referred to as **compatible** with the first one. If the machine is truly compatible, it can use software for the well-known microcomputer, and vice versa. However, the primary feature of the compatibles is usually that they are less expensive than the best seller and yet can perform most, if not all, of the same operations.

COMPUTER LANGUAGES

To communicate with a computer a special language must be used. Language options can range from the straightforward BASIC, the *Beginners All-Purpose Symbolic Instruction Code*, to more structured languages such as COBOL, FORTRAN, PASCAL, and C. Most microcomputers are set up to use BASIC. To use other languages with these computers a special board must be inserted in a slot in the computer's central processing unit, or a disk containing the program must be inserted into the disk drive and stored in RAM. The BASIC language is used in the examples in this text. Generally, microcomputer manufacturers install BASIC in the machine at the factory; then if you use a disk drive, a disk operating system must also be used. This may include a version of BASIC that is compatible with the operating system. Many brands use a version of Microsoft BASIC to achieve this compatibility. Although versions of Microsoft BASIC differ across brands, they are quite similar. This means that programming in BASIC is markedly similar, no matter what machine is used. Even so, these versions are not identical. For purposes of simplicity, Microsoft BASIC for the Apple computer is used in the examples in this textbook. Not only are Apple computers widely available in the public schools, but many colleges and universities also have microcomputer laboratories that include a number of Apple computers. These programs will usually work on other brands, but they sometimes require minor revisions. In most cases the commands differ across machines, but the actual program does not differ. In fact, the programs included in this chapter were written on an IBM microcomputer and then were modified for the Apple. The modifications consisted of making a few minor program alterations and changing some of the commands.

PREPARING THE DISK

This section should be covered only if you wish to store your work on file using a disk. You can go through every example in this chapter using the screen on your monitor, but you will lose the results of running the program when you turn off the machine. If you do not want to type a program on the screen each time you wish to try it, you will want to file the program on a disk.

With the Apple computer, you will need a **floppy disk,** a round sheet of plastic coated with iron oxide and inserted in a protective black jacket. The disk should never be removed from its jacket. A disk 5¼ inches in diameter will be needed. However, remember that the size of the disk depends on the computer you will be using. Both single-sided and double-sided disks are available. You might start with a single-sided, single-density disk, which holds about 125,000 letters and numbers. Before a new disk can be used, it must be prepared in a special way known as **formatting.** Formatting magnetically imprints tracks, sectors, and other information onto the disk exactly where the computer's memory system needs them. Once the disk has been formatted, it is ready to store files.

On the Apple the process of formatting the disk is referred to as **initializing** the disk. First, the new disk is inserted in the disk drive. The program for initializing can be called any term, but it is usually referred to as the HELLO program. Follow these steps to initialize a disk:

1. Load the DOS. (This system is on a disk that comes with the Apple. If you are working in a microcomputer laboratory, your instructor will provide the disk with the operating system.)
2. Insert the new disk in the disk drive.
3. Press the Caps Lock key to the down position.
4. Use the keyboard to type the following information:

```
NEW
10 TEXT:HOME:?"MY FIRST DISK"
RUN
INIT HELLO
```

Now the new disk is initialized and ready to use. To check, shut off the machine, then turn it back on again. The words MY FIRST DISK should be on the screen.

ELEMENTARY COMPUTER COMMANDS

Before discussing a few simple computer programs usable with a set of test scores, a review of several commands used in the operation of the Apple is provided. Although an occasional point is made about programming in BASIC, keep in mind that the purpose of this chapter is not to teach you to program in BASIC but rather to illustrate how a simple program operates.

Commercial Software

An enormous amount of commercial software is available through computer stores, magazines, and catalogs. For example, a number of word processing programs have been developed for a wide variety of computers. Screenwriter and Applewriter are popular programs written for the Apple; Volkswriter and Wordperfect have been well received by IBM users. Statistical program packages are also available, allowing the user to calculate both descriptive and inferential statistics with ease. Some examples of these are SPSS^X, BMDP, SAS, and Systat. One of the best-selling pieces of software has been Visicalc, a spreadsheet for accounting. Many other versions of spreadsheets are also available. Another category of software packages includes the database programs, such as the Database series. These programs handle filing and data management problems. A good software program is written so that it can be used by the computer novice. Any computer commands that are needed should be presented to the user within the program itself. A tutorial, a file that helps the user learn to use the program, is included. A well-developed software program can be most valuable to the user; however, these programs can be expensive, so be certain your purchase is worthwhile. Do not buy a program until you have used the demonstration disk. Keep in mind that a lot of poor software is on the market too.

Very little commercial software is available in physical education and exercise science. Wendt and Morrow (1986) describe some of this software, which can be used to describe sport performance, evaluate physiological parameters, summarize scouting statistics, plan strategies, and schedule tournaments.

User-Developed Software

Perhaps your instructor has several programs that have been written for the Apple for use in your class. A few simple programs written in BASIC are provided in the next section. Although these programs are quite easy to use, they are not as "user friendly" as commercial programs. In other words, you will need to know how to use a few simple commands on the Apple to use these programs. Let's review a few of these commands before trying out the programs. Note that each of these commands must be **entered** by pressing the Return key on the right side of the keyboard before the computer will respond to them.

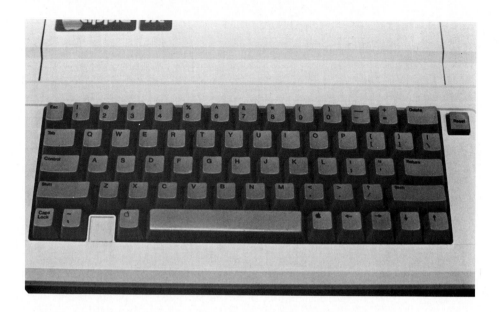

NEW: The NEW command erases everything stored in random access memory (RAM), although it does not erase the screen. You were asked to type NEW when you initialized your disk to tell the computer that a new program was being initiated and that it should not confuse this program with anything else previously stored in RAM; therefore the NEW command instructs the computer to erase any information in RAM. Remember to press the Return key after you have typed NEW.

HOME: The HOME command clears the screen, but it does not tamper with any information now in RAM. As long as you do not turn off your machine, nothing currently in RAM memory is destroyed.

CATALOG: If you have a disk in your disk drive, the CATALOG command lets you know what is on the disk. The computer will list the files on the disk. If you initialized a disk according to the instructions in the previous section, put this disk in the disk drive and type CATALOG. You should see the HELLO file listed. If nothing happens, it may be because you put the disk in after the computer had been turned on. The computer should not be turned on until after the disk is in the disk drive. Turn the computer off, put the disk in, and turn the computer back on. Since the disk has been initialized, it contains the disk operating system, which must be loaded before the disk can be used.

RUN (program): The command RUN in capital letters and another word (program) in small letters and in parentheses means that you should type in the RUN command and the name of the program or file you wish to run. You must use capital letters for all your entries, including the name you gave to the program.

Let's say you are interested in calculating the mean of a set of scores, and a program named MEAN is on the disk in a disk drive. You should type RUN MEAN and press the return key. The computer will load the program from the disk to RAM and run it. If you are not using a disk, you can type a program directly on the screen and instruct the computer to run it. Then you do not have to type in the program name since the program is already in RAM memory. (Although it is redundant to use the term *memory* after RAM, this is done on occasion to remind you of the various memories associated with a microcomputer.) Thus the computer knows which program you are referring to when you type RUN. Sometimes you might wish to do something with the program before you run it. If so, the program can be loaded (see the next command description) into RAM initially. If you load the program, only RUN is needed to operate it. Again, once the program is in RAM memory, the computer does not have to be given the program name.

LOAD (**program**): The LOAD (**program**) command instructs the computer to take a program, for which you have provided the name, and put it into RAM. Remember that the program is automatically loaded if you type RUN and then the program name. On the other hand, once you have loaded the program, only the RUN command is necessary to execute it. Typing in the program name is not necessary.

LIST: The LIST command instructs the computer to list each line of the program. One reason the LIST command is used is to enable the user to see how the program is listed. A programmer may list a program to revise it in some way. All but one of the programs in this chapter are short and can be seen in their entirety on the fixed screen. Many programs are longer than the screen length; the command LIST causes the computer to scroll the lines of the program. The listing begins at the top of the screen. When the screen is filled, the top lines begin "scrolling" off the top of the screen, and new lines appear at the bottom.

SAVE (**program**): The SAVE (**program**) command takes the program out of RAM and puts it onto the disk. If the program is a new one, you must give it a name. If it is already on your disk with a specified name and you wish to continue using this name, do so. If the program was revised while in RAM, the revised form will take the place of the previous version on the disk.

DELETE (**program**): The DELETE (**program**) command is used to erase a program from a disk. Be sure you will no longer need the program before deleting it. These commands should enable you to use the following simple programs.

EXAMPLES OF PROGRAMS

Four simple programs are included in this section to illustrate calculation of the mean, z-scores, T-scores, and grades. All the programs are written in BASIC. Each line is preceded by a line number. Without these line numbers the computer would carry out the operations immediately, and the program lines would not be stored. The lines allow storage of the program and its operations until the RUN command is given. Be sure the Caps Lock key is down.

Program MEAN

Program MEAN was written to calculate the mean of a set of scores. To familiarize yourself with the program, enter it in your computer's memory using the keyboard. If you plan to save the program on a disk, be sure that the disk has been initialized. (The disk should have been inserted in the disk drive before the computer was turned on.) The program is so short that typing it on the screen whenever you want to use it will not be difficult. On the other hand, disk storage saves time and prevents errors that can occur when retyping.

Enter the commands and program as presented below. Do not forget to enter each line after you have typed it by pressing the Return key.

```
NEW
10 INPUT "How many scores are in the data set? ";N
20 FOR S=1 TO N
30 INPUT "SCORE ";X
40 SUM = SUM + X
50 NEXT S
60 MEAN = SUM/N
70 PRINT "MEAN = ";MEAN
80 END
```

The number at the beginning of each line is used to identify the line. The first line is 10; the next line is 20. Using 11 rather than 20 is permissible; however, if the program required an addition between lines 10 and 11, it would have to be renumbered. Renumbering would not be a problem if the addition were made between lines 10 and 20, because a new line, given a number from 11 to 19, could be entered. The program is now in RAM. Try using a few computer commands. Enter HOME. Notice that the screen has been cleared but the program has not been lost. To take another look at the program, enter LIST. Now run the program using the following data:

$$N = 5$$
$$\text{Scores} = 30, 48, 37, 52, 29$$

Enter RUN. The computer will ask you how many scores are in the data set. Type 5 and press the Return key. The computer will then ask you to enter each score. Remember to press the Return key after typing each score. Since the computer knows that five scores are in the data set, it will not ask you for any more scores after the fifth one. In this case the mean equals 39.2.

Clear the screen by typing HOME, then list the program by entering LIST. Since this is such a short, simple program, following instructions given to the computer in BASIC is easy. Spend a few minutes studying the program. Of course, you can also study the printed version in this book. If your computer is hooked up to a printer, you could also print a copy of the program. Let's assume you do not have a printer available, but you would like to save the MEAN program on your disk. Enter SAVE MEAN. Now check to see if the program has been filed on the disk by entering CATALOG. If your disk only included the HELLO program before, the list should now show both the HELLO and MEAN programs. Experiment with this program using several other data sets.

Program Z-SCORE

Program Z-SCORE was written to convert raw scores to z-scores. (See Chapter 3.) Assume you have administered a test and obtained a set of scores. You would like to compare these scores with the scores on another test. Unless the two tests have the same score range, mean, and standard deviation, the raw scores cannot be directly compared. However, by converting the raw scores to z-scores, even different score units can be compared.

Type the z-score program onto the screen. Remember to press the Return key after each program line.

```
NEW
10 INPUT "How many scores do you want to convert to z-scores? ";N
20 INPUT "What is the mean? ";M
30 INPUT "What is the standard deviation? ";S
40 FOR A = 1 TO N
50 INPUT "What is the score? ";X
60 PRINT
70 PRINT "The z-score equals   ";(X-M)/S
80 PRINT
90 NEXT A
100 END
```

You can now type HOME, clear the screen, and run the program by typing RUN, or you can run the program without clearing the screen. Notice that this program asks for the mean and standard deviation before the test scores are input. However, this information needs to be provided only once for each data set. The program moves to a "loop" where a score is input and its z-score calculated. The next score is input, and so on, until N scores have been input; the program then ends. Use the following data to run the program:

$$\overline{X} = 50$$
$$s = 2$$
Scores: 56, 51, 48, 49, 45, 50
$$N = 6$$

The z-scores for the above raw scores are 3, 0.5, −1, −0.5, −2.5, and 0. After you have typed in the sixth score, the program should end. The program is still in RAM and can be used repeatedly as long as you do not turn off the machine or accidentally erase it (by typing NEW, for example). If you want to keep the program on a disk, be sure your disk is in the disk drive. Then type SAVE Z-SCORE. As soon as the whirring sound has stopped, type CATALOG. Don't forget to press the Return key after each of these commands. The list of programs on your disk should now be on the screen. It should include HELLO, MEAN, and Z-SCORE, if you saved the MEAN program. Now you can turn off your machine or type NEW and go on to another program.

Since this program is short and simple, review the program line by line and see if it makes sense to you. If program Z-SCORE is no longer in RAM but was stored on a disk, reload it into your machine memory by typing LOAD Z-SCORE. Then type LIST. Now examine the program closely. The calculation is straightforward, since the mean and standard deviation are provided as input. A more complex program could be written in which the mean and standard deviation are calculated as part of the program. In line 50 the computer is instructed to print a statement "The z-score equals " and then print the results of the calculation $(X-M)/S$. Several spaces were inserted after the word "equals" purely for cosmetic purposes to separate the answer from the statement and make it easier to read. When you have completed your examination of the program, type SAVE Z-SCORE if you wish to save the program on your disk.

Program T-SCORE

When test scores are transformed, the z-score transformation is often used. However, because z-scores can be negative and represented as decimals, it is not uncommon to transform these scores so they can be more easily interpreted. A transformation commonly used in measures of motor performance is the T-score. In the next program, T-scores are calculated. The required input consists of the mean and standard deviation of the set of scores, along with the raw scores. In this program the z-score is also calculated, but it is not printed since the T-score is of primary interest. First, type in the program as it is listed below. (An asterisk [*] is the multiplication symbol, and a slash [/] is the division symbol.)

```
NEW
10 INPUT "How many scores do you want to convert to T-scores? ";N
20 INPUT "What is the mean? ";M
30 INPUT "What is the standard deviation? ";S
40 FOR A = 1 TO N
50 INPUT "What is the score? ";X
60 PRINT
70 PRINT "The T-score equals "50 + ( (X−M)/S)*10
```

```
80 PRINT
90 NEXT A
100 END
```

As an example, use the six test scores given in the previous section on Program z-score. Type RUN and then go through the program. The correct answers for the T-score calculations are 80, 55, 40, 45, 25, and 50.

Now list the program and examine it. Find the line in which the z-score is calculated, and note how the z-score is modified to obtain the T-score. You should be looking at line 70 now. If you would like to keep this program, save it on your disk.

A more elaborate T-score program is included in Appendix E. This program accepts a larger number of test scores and provides an option for printing a hard copy of the results.

Program GRADES

The following program can be used to determine the final grades for students in physical education classes. Although it is a little longer than the previous ones, it runs just as easily. The input needed to operate this program includes individual test grades for each student and the weight given to each test by the teacher. Since the same weights apply to all grades, they need only be input once. If one skill test is twice as important as another, you might assign it a weight of 2 and the second test, a weight of 1.

First enter the program into RAM memory.

```
10 HOME
20 INPUT "How many students? ";S
30 INPUT "How many grades for each student   ";N
40 PRINT
100 DIM GD(N,3), GD$(N)
120 FOR X = 1 TO N
130 INPUT "WEIGHT? ";GD(X,2)
135 ADD = ADD + GD(X,2)
140 NEXT X
150 FOR Y = 1 TO S
155 PRINT
200 FOR X = 1 TO N
210 INPUT "GRADE? ";GD$(X)
211 IF GD$(X) = "A+" THEN GD(X,1) = 12
212 IF GD$(X) = "A" THEN GD(X,1) = 11
213 IF GD$(X) = "A−" THEN GD(X,1) = 10
214 IF GD$(X) = "B+" THEN GD(X,1) = 9
215 IF GD$(X) = "B" THEN GD(X,1) = 8
216 IF GD$(X) = "B−" THEN GD(X,1) = 7
```

```
217 IF GD$(X) = "C+" THEN GD(X,1) = 6
218 IF GD$(X) = "C" THEN GD(X,1) = 5
219 IF GD$(X) = "C−" THEN GD(X,1) = 4
220 IF GD$(X) = "D+" THEN GD(X,1) = 3
221 IF GD$(X) = "D" THEN GD(X,1) = 2
222 IF GD$(X) = "D−" THEN GD(X,1) = 1
223 IF GD$(X) = "F" THEN GD(X,1) = 0
310 GD(X,3) = GD(X,1)*GD(X,2)
320 NEXT X
330 LET SUM = 0
340 FOR X = 1 TO N
350 SUM = SUM + GD(X,3)
360 NEXT X
370 PRINT
375 T = SUM/ADD
380 PRINT "AVERAGE GRADE = ";T
381 IF T < 12.1 THEN T$ = "A+"
382 IF T < 11.5 THEN T$ = "A"
383 IF T < 10.5 THEN T$ = "A−"
384 IF T < 9.5 THEN T$ = "B+"
385 IF T < 8.5 THEN T$ = "B"
386 IF T < 7.5 THEN T$ = "B−"
387 IF T < 6.5 THEN T$ = "C+"
388 IF T < 5.5 THEN T$ = "C"
389 IF T < 4.5 THEN T$ = "C−"
390 IF T < 3.5 THEN T$ = "D+"
391 IF T < 2.5 THEN T$ = "D"
392 IF T < 1.5 THEN T$ = "D−"
393 IF T < 0.5 THEN T$ = "F"
398 PRINT "AVERAGE LETTER GRADE = ";T$
399 PRINT
400 PRINT
410 NEXT Y
420 END
```

Now that you have typed in the program, perhaps you should check it line by line. If you enter LIST, you will find that this program is too long to be displayed on the screen in its entirety. The computer will execute your command, but the first lines will scroll off the screen fairly quickly. You can instruct the computer to list specific lines you wish to see. If you are interested in the first 150 lines, enter LIST 1-150. If you have checked each line for accuracy, try to run the program.

For purposes of simplicity in an example the final grades for two students will be calculated. Three tests were administered to each student during the unit of instruction. The computer will ask for the following information for the entire class: the number of students in class, the number of grades for each student, and the weights for each grade. Once this information has been entered, the program is completed by entering the numerical value of the grades for each student. Let's use the following information in our example:

> Number of students = 2
> Number of grades per student = 3
> Weights for the three grades = 1.5, 3.0, 2.5
> Grades for the first student = C, B+, C+
> Grades for the second student = A, B, C

When this program is run, the screen will automatically clear and the following question will appear: How many students? The output from the program will be displayed on your screen as follows, as long as you enter the appropriate information at the correct time. (The notes are used to clarify the example and will not appear on the screen.)

How many students? 2
How many grades for each student? 3
Weight? 1.5
Weight? 3
Weight? 2.5

Note: This information is input only once for each group of students, since the weights are the same for all students.

Grade? C
Grade? B+
Grade? C+

Note: The program now asks you to input the grades for each student, beginning with the first one on your roster.

AVERAGE GRADE = 7.071429
AVERAGE LETTER GRADE = B−

Note: The computer provides both the numerical average and the average letter grade. The grade should be recorded for each student whenever it appears on the screen.
Note: Now the program asks for the grades of the next student.

Grade? A
Grade? B
Grade? C
AVERAGE GRADE = 7.571429
AVERAGE LETTER GRADE = B

The previous program will automatically terminate at this point since we had indicated previously that grades for only two students would be input. This program can calculate a small number of final grades in a short period. The teacher's only task is to enter each student's grades and record the final grade once the information for the entire class (number of students, number of grades per student, and the weights for the grades) has been entered. An expanded version of this program is listed in Appendix E. It can handle grades for a large number of students and provides the option for obtaining a hard copy of the student's names and grades.

List the program again and examine the program lines closely. In the first 130 lines, data for the entire class are entered. In the remainder of the program, four loops are included—one to add the weights, one to average the grades numerically, one to convert the numerical average to a letter grade, and one to repeat the process for each student until the number of students (S) has been reached. Now run the program again, either using hypothetical data or data provided by your instructor. If you want to save the program, enter SAVE GRADES.

SUMMARY

Some of the mystique of the computer is eliminated once you have completed a few simple, practical tasks. The programs included in this chapter provide a few examples of how computers can be used to facilitate measurement and evaluation, yet these examples only scratch the surface of their innumerable possibilities. New programs for physical educators and exercise scientists will become available every year, and these programs should be increasingly easy to use.

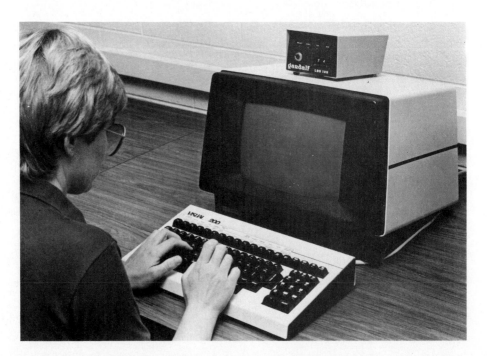

LEARNING EXPERIENCES

1. Read the article by Mayhew and Rankin (1983) included in the References. Try out at least one of the simple programs listed in the article. Your instructor may have a data set you can use. If not, make up a few numbers and use them to execute the program.
2. Use the Z-SCORE and T-SCORE programs to solve Problem 3 at the end of Chapter 3.

SOURCES FOR PHYSICAL EDUCATION SOFTWARE

1. CompTech Systems Design
   P.O. Box 516
   Hastings, MN 55033
   (612)437-1350
2. Directory of Computer Software with Application to Sport Science, Health and Dance
   AAHPERD
   American Alliance Publications
   P.O. Box 704
   Waldorf, MD 20601
   (703)476-3481
3. Human Factors Software
   755 University Avenue, Suite S
   Sacramento, CA 95825
   (916)454-6389
4. Minnesota Education Computer Consortium (MECC)
   2520 Broadway Drive
   St. Paul, MN 55113
   (612)376-1101
5. Project React
   66 Malcolm Avenue, S.E.
   Minneapolis, MN 55414
   (612)379-0428

REFERENCES

Barlow, D.A., and Bayalis, P.A. 1983. Computer facilitated learning. Journal of Physical Education, Recreation and Dance, **54**(9):27-29.

Cicciarella, C.F. 1983. The computer in physical education. Journal of Physical Education, Recreation and Dance, **54**(9):18, 32.

Donnelly, J.E. 1983. Physiology and fitness testing. Journal of Physical Education, Recreation and Dance, **54**(9):24-26.

Kelly, L. 1987. Computer assisted instruction—applications for physical education. Journal of Physical Education, Recreation and Dance, **58**(4):74-79.

Mayhew, J.L., and Rankin, B.A. 1983. Data management. Journal of Physical Education, Recreation and Dance, **54**(9):22-23.

Richards, J.G., and Engelhorn, R. 1983. Selecting a microcomputer. Journal of Physical Education, Recreation and Dance, **54**(9):19-21.

Sealy, D. 1983. Computer programs for dance notation. Journal of Physical Education and Dance, **54**(9):36-37.

Wendt, J.C., and Morrow, J.R., Jr. 1986. Microcomputer software: practical applications for coaches and teachers. Journal of Physical Education, Recreation and Dance, **57**(6):54-57.

ANNOTATED READINGS

Baun, M. and Baun, W.B. 1984. A corporate health and fitness program: motivation and management by computers. Journal of Physical Education, Recreation and Dance, **55**(4):42-45.

Describes the computer system used in Tenneco's health and fitness program in Houston, Texas; incorporates a unique exercise logging function; produces feedback to participants and health and fitness staff.

Brownell, B.A. 1985. Using microcomputers; a guidebook for writers, teachers, and researchers. Beverly Hills, Calif.: Sage Publications, Inc.

Written for people who have limited understanding of the many ways in which microcomputers enhance their professional lives; includes specific illustrations of computer applications, such as the creation and maintenance of bibliographies and references and the production of instructional materials; describes the most popular microcomputers and their operating systems; examines a variety of software.

Graham, G.P., and Woolridge, W. 1983. Computer measurements of skinfolds. Journal of Physical Education, Recreation and Dance, **54**(7):68-69.

Presents a microcomputer program for the Apple II to estimate the percentage of body fat for men (using chest, abdomen, and thigh) and women (using triceps and suprailiac) from skinfold measurements.

Kelly, L.E. 1986. Physical Education Management System. Northbrook, Ill: Hubbard. (Computer Program and Manual)

A computer database program used as a management system for physical education; the Physical Education Management System (PEMS); allows students to be managed on up to 15 objectives defined by the teacher; provides teachers with summative feedback on the achievement levels of their students; provides option for statistical analysis of data.

Marley, W.P. 1972. The computer in measurement and evaluation class. Journal of Health, Physical Education, and Recreation, **43**:39.

Demonstrates the usefulness of computers in testing and evaluation in physical education; stresses the practical applications that are possible; emphasizes developing an understanding of the ways a computer can be used; deemphasizes the need for teachers to learn programming skills.

Mood, D.P. 1978. The undergraduate physical education major and the computer. Journal of Physical Education and Recreation, **49**:66-67.

Provides rationale for using computers for statistics, calculating velocities and limb length, and movement analysis; also valuable for individualized instruction; enhances recordkeeping procedures in physical education courses; provides examples of ways computers can be used in physical education.

Vockell, E.L., and Rivers, R.H. 1984. Instructional computing for today's teachers. New York: Macmillan Publishing Co.

Assumes user has no prior knowledge of computers; gives an overview of Computer Aided Instruction (CAI); provides guidelines for the selection of microcomputers and software; teaches readers to program using BASIC by modifying existing instructional programs; contains program modules for improving user friendliness, information on the use of sequential data files, and a comprehensive list of software.

Part Four

Characteristics of a Good Test

6

Validity and Reliability of Norm-Referenced Tests

KEY WORDS *Watch for these words as you read the following chapter:*

concurrent validity

construct validity

content validity

contingency table

criterion

criterion-related validity

intraclass correlation coefficient

logical validity

objective test

objectivity

predictors

predictive validity

reliability

split-half reliability estimate

standard error of measurement

subjective test

test-retest reliability

validity

validity coefficient

In Chapter 1 the concept of *norm-referenced* measurement was introduced. This type of test, in which the *score* is interpreted by comparing it to a *norm*, is used when both the test user and the examinee want to know who has the most ability, who has the least, and so forth. Before placing any faith in the test results, one must be certain that the test is a good one: the test should measure what it is

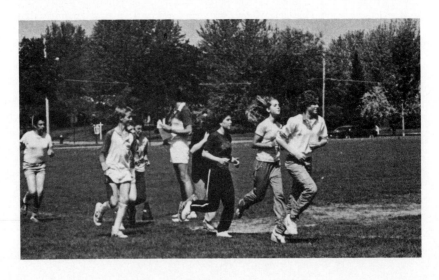

supposed to measure (**validity**) with consistency (**reliability**), using an accurate scoring system (**objectivity**). (For a discussion of these characteristics in a criterion-referenced measurement framework, see Chapter 7.) A more comprehensive view of validity is that it encompasses two components: relevance and reliability. Reliability and objectivity are therefore subsumed under validity. In this chapter the concept of relevance is covered first, because a test can be reliable but not necessarily relevant. Validity is the most important element of test theory. More practical attributes of a test—such as cost, ease of administration, and appropriateness—are discussed in other chapters.

VALIDITY

Assume you are a student who has just completed a basketball unit. Mr. Miller, your teacher, announces that he will give a written test on skill execution, game strategy, and rules—the content he taught during the unit. You carefully study all three areas and feel well prepared to take the test. When the test is administered, you skim through it quickly and find that all the items deal with rules. No questions on skill execution and game strategy are included. After completing the test, you might comment to the teacher or a classmate that this was not a good test because it did not measure what it was supposed to measure. In other words, the test lacked *validity*.

A valid test can be loosely defined as a measure that is sound in terms of the purpose of the test and that meets satisfactory criteria for test construction. More broadly, validity is the soundness of the interpretation of the test. It is the closeness of agreement between what the test measures and the behavior it is intended to measure. Furthermore, to be valid a test must also have acceptable reliability, or consistency of measure, which is discussed more thoroughly later in this chapter.

How does one evaluate the validity of a test? First, it is important to recognize that a test can have many validities. Therefore to describe a test as "valid" is really not accurate; rather, a test should be designated as "valid for a given purpose." For example, a test might be valid for 5-year-old girls but not 25-year-old women. It might be valid for measuring an individual skill but not game-playing ability. The first step in interpreting test validity is to think through how you plan to use the test. Then the *type* of validity of greatest interest must be determined. The most common types of validity are *content, criterion-related,* and *construct.* In the physical education field, logical validity, a special case of content validity, is frequently used (see Figure 6-1).

Types of Validity

Because many definitions of validity have been proposed, the concept can be confusing to the test user. In an effort to alleviate this confusion several national

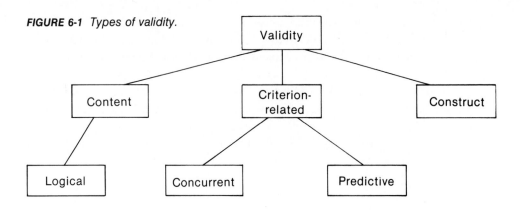

FIGURE 6-1 *Types of validity.*

measurement organizations have developed a set of standards for educational and psychological tests. These standards include the categorization of validity into three types of evidence—**content-related, criterion-related,** and **construct-related** (American Psychological Association, 1985). The most important point to keep in mind is that validity, no matter what type, is the single most important concept in evaluating a test.

   Content-Related Evidence of Validity The content validity of a test is "the degree to which the sample of items, tasks, or questions on a test are representative of some defined universe or 'domain' of content" (American Psychological Association, 1985). More simply stated, when a test developer demonstrates that the items in a test adequately represent all important areas of content, the test has content validity. This type of validity is appropriate for written tests. How is the content-related evidence of validity of a test evaluated? This process can be demonstrated by analyzing the AAHPER Cooperative Physical Education Test (Cooperative Tests and Services, 1970), one of the few standardized written tests published for physical education students in public schools. This test was developed according to a table of specifications, sometimes referred to as a *test blueprint*. Table 6-1 shows the specifications for grades 10 through 12. The content areas are listed on the left side of the table and represent the content judged to be important for students in physical education classes. Across the top of the table are levels of cognitive behavior, which will be described in Chapter 8. The cells under the heading reflecting cognitive behaviors contain one or more numbers. These numbers represent the actual test question numbers. For example, 11 represents item 11 on the test. For each cell in the table, the test developer writes a predetermined number of test items. The number of items is determined by the educational importance attached to each category of content and cognitive behavior. Refer to the column labeled "Numbers of items" at the top. The number in each cell in this column represents the number of items written

TABLE 6-1 *Item classification, Forms 2A and 2B, AAHPER Cooperative Physical Education Tests*

Content	Form 2A				Form 2B			
	Knowledge	Under-standing	Thinking	Numbers of items	Knowledge	Under-standing	Thinking	Numbers of items
I. *Activity performance* Basic sports skills	45, 55			2		57		1
Concepts fundamental to movement skills in strategy and activities patterns	23, 59	10	24	4	9	40, 46	15	4
Body mechanics, rules and procedures, and protective requirements		4, 11, 37	15, 26	5		14, 23, 24, 48	47	5
II. *Effects of activities* Immediate	1, 2, 12, 16, 25, 47, 52	6, 9, 13, 17, 27, 28, 36, 44, 46	48	17	20, 22, 30, 34, 35, 50, 55	6, 7, 11, 13, 32, 37, 38, 39, 58	8, 12, 59	19
Long-term health and appearance	18, 21, 42	5, 29, 30, 50	54	8	2, 25, 31	21, 29, 53, 56	19, 45	9
Capacity for effort	7, 56, 57, 58	3, 31, 32, 40	39	9	4, 10, 18, 60	26, 33, 49, 52		8
III. *Factors modifying participation in activities and their efforts*	8, 20, 41, 51	14, 19, 22, 35, 38, 43, 53	33, 34, 49, 60	15	17, 28, 44	1, 16, 27, 36, 41, 42, 54	3, 5, 43, 51	14
Number of items	20	30	10	60	18	31	11	60

From Handbook for AAHPER Cooperative Physical Education Tests.

for each area of content. The largest number of items for a content area in Form 2A is 17. This suggests that the test developers viewed the immediate effects of physical activity as the most important content area. Now look at the same label "Numbers of items" at the bottom of the page. The largest number of items for an area of cognitive behavior in Form 2A is 30, placing the greatest weight on understanding the content.

Begin analyzing the test itself by evaluating its content validity. Copies of the test and the table of specifications are needed. First, take the test just as a student would be required to do. Then arbitrarily select several items from the test and find them in the table of specifications. Answer the following question about each item: Does the item properly fit the cell designated by the test publisher? Suppose one of the items in Table 6-1 you have chosen to analyze is *42* in Form 2A. This item is written as follows:

Item 42. Which of the following represents specificity of training?
A. Training to run distance events also improves sprinting.
B. Practice in tennis skills improves badminton skills.
C. Training in one sport skill limits performance in other sports.
D. Training for one event is directed to that event alone.

According to its placement, Item *42* is a measure of knowledge about the long-term effects of physical activity. The knowledge is factual and could be learned by memorization, a low level of cognitive behavior. Reread the test item. Does it measure what it is supposed to measure? If so, the item contributes to the content validity of the test. If not, it is not a valid item. Obviously this is a demanding job, but a test user is obligated to at least spot-check the test developer's decisions.

Another important aspect of content validity is whether the content areas are important in terms of the test user's educational goals. Should an area be emphasized more, deemphasized, added, or eliminated? These are judgments the test user must make. In the preceding paragraph a substantial number of items measuring the acute effects of physical activity were noted. One might question whether the degree of emphasis on this content area is warranted. The relative importance of various areas of content might differ markedly across school districts, depending on the curricular objectives of the particular physical education program. Including a substantial number of test items on the short-term and long-term effects of physical activity might be desirable in a program where physical fitness is an important part of the curriculum. In a program where skill development is stressed in the curricular objectives, a strong emphasis on exercise physiology might be unacceptable. Is it appropriate to use a standardized test to judge the outcomes of a physical education program, when the content taught in the curriculum receives a different emphasis from that provided in the test? The test may not be useful for judging program outcomes, but it can still provide valuable information to the physical education staff in a school system. For example, the test might be administered to determine the status of student knowledge in three content areas, without making a judgment on the quality of their physical education program. The test results might then be used to reexamine the current physical education curriculum. Standardized tests of this type should never be used to determine grades. They can be used appropriately as a part of program evaluation or simply to determine how well students can perform on a nationally standardized test.

To summarize, the following steps are recommended for reviewing a published test to determine its content validity:

1. Answer the test items and score your responses. This step should be standard procedure for *any* teacher with *any* test. If this step is taken seriously, detecting weaknesses in a test, including one's own test, is much easier.
2. Review the publisher's statement on content validity.
3. Examine the table of specifications.
4. Assess the appropriateness of the placement of items in the content/behavior categories.
5. Examine the universe (content and behavior categories) and respond to the following four questions:
    a. Are important elements of a content area omitted from the universe?
    b. Are unimportant elements of the content area erroneously included?
    c. Are any categories included in the content and behavior areas weighted improperly? (Weighting is reflected in the number of items included in a category.)
    d. Are all elements of the content and behavior areas educationally important?

Now that the procedure for evaluating the content validity of a published test has been described, let's examine the approach to be used when planning to develop your own test. Perhaps you are interested in developing a test of basketball rules. Obviously, including questions on all the rules in the rule book is not possible; therefore a representative sample of rules must be selected. The rules should be categorized in a table of specifications. Two of the categories might be offensive and defensive rules. If there are more offensive rules than defensive, the proportions of test items should reflect this difference. Levels of cognitive behavior can also be considered. When students are first learning the rules, the test might primarily measure a low level of cognitive behavior. If the rules test is intended for experienced players, you may be more interested in the degree to which students can apply the rules and thus design items measuring higher levels of cognitive behavior. Many tests include items reflecting several levels of cognitive behavior. Whatever the case, the identification of items should follow a systematic plan.

To summarize, the following steps should be taken to demonstrate content validity when you have developed the test yourself:

1. Develop a table of specifications for the test. Determine the number of items that should be written for each cell of the table. Write the appropriate number of items for each cell.
2. Prepare the test items in the format you plan to use with your students.
3. Take the test and score your responses. This step should be taken even if the test is your own!
4. Select 25% of the test items and reexamine the appropriateness of their placement in the content/behavior categories of the table of specifications. Revise the items if necessary. If more than 5% (of the 25% selected) of the items are inappropriately placed, reexamine the placement of the remaining 75% of the items.
5. Determine whether the content/behavior categories should be altered in any way. Additions? Deletions? Increased emphasis? Decreased emphasis?

Often a test is developed by writing down item after item as each one comes to mind, until enough items have been written to fill the testing period. Such an approach may lead to haphazard results. The test may be heavily weighted with items in one or two categories and slighted in others. It behooves the teacher to begin by preparing a table of specifications, deciding in advance on the number of items for each category based on its relative importance. When the item-writing process is begun, it becomes a more purposeful activity. In addition, the test developer can have greater confidence that the test will be valid.

Logical Validity Although written tests are used frequently in physical education and the exercise sciences, the most predominantly used tests are those measuring physical skills and abilities. The concept of content validity does not make much sense for tests of motor performance. Instead of using clusters of items to measure various content areas, the test may consist of a single item or a repetition of the same item, usually referred to as *trials* of the test. However, the initial validation of these types of tests follows a set of rules similar in concept to content validity—**logical validity.** Logical validity is defined as the extent to which a test measures the most important components of skill necessary to perform a motor task adequately.

A test of motor skill is used to demonstrate how logical validity is evaluated. If the test incorporates and directly measures the important components of the skill being evaluated, logical validity can be claimed. The concept of logical validity was proposed by Ruth B. Glassow and Marie R. Liba at the University of Wisconsin. Both were interested in developing skills tests that measured the most important aspects of skills. They had observed that many of the tests in physical education measured only accuracy in performing a skill. While accuracy is undeniably important in the execution of many skills, it is not the only important factor. Glassow and Liba reasoned that these limitations were occurring because tests were not being developed according to some logical plan, similar to the development of a good written test. Thus the idea of logical validity came into being. The general procedure to be followed in constructing a skills test is to define good performance in executing the skill, construct a test that measures the important components of skill in the definition, and score the test so that the best score represents a performance that approximates the definition of good performance.

Consider, for example, a test of the tennis forehand drive. Ms. Spencer, a physical education teacher, describes a good forehand drive as a ball hit so that it travels low over the net and deep into the backcourt. She decides to test her students on this skill using a test in which a target is placed in the backcourt. The target is sectioned so that the areas with the higher scores are closer to the baseline of the tennis court. Is this a valid test? The test measures whether the ball is hit deep into the backcourt by giving more points to the ball landing close to the baseline, but it does not measure the height of the ball's flight over the net. Thus the evidence of logical validity is insufficient, and the test is not valid. Test validity could be increased by placing extensions on the standards holding the tennis nets and by stretching a rope across the middle of the court above the net. Then the examinee would attempt to hit the ball so that it passed between the rope and the top of the net.

Because logical validity is the degree to which the components of skill measured by a test correspond with those required to perform the skill adequately, the identification of important components of a skill is important. The previous section on logical validity dealt primarily with a single skills test. Although it is appropriate to measure specific skills when students are learning a sport, skills tests should not mistakenly be thought to measure playing ability. To measure playing ability, a battery of tests is often used. One of the first steps in validating a test battery of this type is to use logical validity. Logical validity in this context involves the definition of the important skills constituting playing ability. Tests are then selected to measure each of the skills identified as most important. Of course, each individual test must have logical validity as well.

Four major steps can be identified in assessing the logical validity of a skills test:

1. Review the test developer's statement on the purpose of the test and the components of skill the test is designed to measure. These components should be clearly stated in the test description. Make a list of these components.

2. Examine the test. List the components *actually* measured in the test.
3. Compare the two lists. Are the components identified and defined by the test developer actually measured by the test?
4. Examine the educational importance of the test:
   a. Are unimportant components of skill measured by the test?
   b. Are important components of skill omitted from the test?
   c. Do certain components of the skill receive inappropriate emphasis in the text?

Published tests of sports skills and playing ability frequently lack a statement identifying the important components of skill. In these cases, the test must be examined and the components being measured must be listed. Then the educational importance of the test must be analyzed. If developing your own test is necessary, start with a list of the important components of skill, which will provide the basis for the design of the test.

Criterion-Related Evidence of Validity Criterion-related evidence of validity is demonstrated by comparing test scores with one or more external variables that are considered direct measures of the characteristic or behavior in question (known as the *criterion*). Two of the most common types of **criterion-related validity** are concurrent validity, which involves the comparison of a test with a criterion measure, and predictive validity, dealing with prediction of a behavior on a criterion test. Criterion-related evidence of validity is determined by statistical methods, although content and logical validity may play a part in the initial stages of constructing the test.

Concurrent validity is used when a test is proposed as a substitute for another test that is known to be valid. The latter test is called the **criterion** test, with criterion defined as a standard of behavior. More precisely, concurrent validity is defined as the degree to which a test correlates with (is related to) a criterion test, which has already been established as a valid test of the attribute of interest. Why would one search for a substitute test when a valid test is already available? Although the criterion test's validity has been established, it may be impractical. For example, administration of the test may require an excessive amount of time, trained personnel, or expensive equipment. Laboratory tests administered on a one-to-one basis are usually impractical in a school setting. Consider the wide variety of measures of cardiorespiratory (CR) function. It is well known that testing an examinee on the treadmill provides more valid indicators of CR function than a field test; however, trained physiologists, expensive laboratory equipment, and one-to-one testing are required. Therefore field tests are used most frequently in fitness clubs and physical education classes. Yet how is the adequacy of the field test determined? Usually a **validity coefficient** is reported for the test. This coefficient represents the correlation between scores on the field test (X) and the laboratory test (Y). This is the same correlation coefficient (r_{xy}) that was studied in Chapter 3, only now it is being used as an estimate of test validity. The higher the estimate, the stronger the relationship between the field test and the laboratory (criterion) test.

Three steps should be followed in evaluating the concurrent validity of a published test. To exemplify each step the 12-Minute Run Test is used as the field test of interest, and the maximal stress test on the treadmill is used as the laboratory (criterion) test.

1. *Identify and examine the criterion test. Is it a logically valid measure of the attribute of interest?*

Although there are other valid indicators of CR function, the measure of max $\dot{V}O_2$ obtained from maximal stress testing on the treadmill is generally accepted as a valid criterion measure. (See Chapter 16 for additional information.)

2. *Evaluate the correlation (validity coefficient) between the criterion test and the test you are interested in using. Is the correlation high enough to justify substituting the test you wish to use for the criterion test?*

The validity coefficient for the 12-Minute Run Test when compared with max $\dot{V}O_2$ is reported as 0.897 in one of Cooper's first published reports (Cooper, 1968). Thus, people who run longer distances tend to have higher max $\dot{V}O_2$ values, and vice versa. The validity coefficient is high enough to justify substituting the 12-Minute Run Test for the treadmill test. If you are developing the test yourself, you must calculate the validity coefficient. Use Formula 3-9 for calculating the Pearson product-moment correlation coefficient (r_{xy}).

3. *If the criterion test is valid and the validity coefficient is 0.80 or above, use the test. If not, look for another test.*

In general the Cooper test appears to be an excellent field test. However, several factors should be considered before using the test. Cooper's test group consisted of adult males who were well trained and highly motivated. The test user should consider the examinee's sex, age, body fatness, and ability to pace properly and run efficiently during the test. (These elements are considered in more detail in Chapter 16.)

Predictive validity is defined as the degree to which a criterion behavior can be predicted using a score from a predictor test. Two uses of predictive validity are commonly observed in physical education and exercise science: as a *description* of the current status of an individual on the criterion behavior and as a *predictor* of the future behavior on the criterion. (The criterion again refers to the standard against which the usefulness of the test is judged.) The **predictors** are tests or variables that predict criterion behavior.

Predictive validity used to describe the current status of an individual is essentially an extension of the concept of concurrent validity. Usually the test user is interested in estimating performance on an often complex criterion variable by obtaining a score on a simple predictor variable. To be reasonably accurate in the prediction, a relationship must exist between the predictor and criterion variables. In other words, the correlation between the two variables should be substantial. Consider a prediction study by Getchell and associates (1977) in which scores on the 1.5-mile run were used to predict CR function, specifically max $\dot{V}O_2$ as measured in a treadmill test. The relationship between the two measures was determined to be -0.915. Since shorter times are associated with higher max $\dot{V}O_2$ values, the validity coefficient is expected to be negative. In this case the predictor measure, the 1.5-mile run, had high validity. This is essentially an estimate of *concurrent* validity.

Multiple Correlation In many cases the use of only one predictor is not reasonable. In assessing body fatness using skinfold measures, for example, the use of more than one skinfold site is often recommended. When two or more predictors are used with one criterion measure (underwater weighing, for instance, in this example), multiple correlation procedures are used.

Regression In addition to knowing that the 1.5-mile run test can be substituted for the treadmill test, one may also wish to predict or estimate the examinee's max $\dot{V}O_2$ value from his or her score on the 1.5-mile run. This can be done if a *regression equation* has been developed. The simple linear regression equation takes the following form:

$$Y' = a + bX \qquad\qquad \text{Formula 6-1}$$

where Y' = predicted max $\dot{V}O_2$ value
    a = intercept of the regression line
    b = slope of the regression line
    X = score on the 1.5-mile run expressed as a decimal per minute

The *a* and *b* values are presented by the test developer but can be calculated using simple formulas found in elementary statistics textbooks. The value for X, the examinee's score on the 1.5-mile run, is inserted in Formula 6-1, and Y', the estimated max $\dot{V}O_2$, is then calculated. In the Getchell et al. (1977) report, the following regression equation was presented for college women:

$$Y' = 98.3 - 4.182X \qquad\qquad \text{Formula 6-2}$$

Suppose that a woman in a college conditioning course ran the 1.5-mile run in 12 minutes. Using Formula 6-2,

$$Y' = 98.3 - (4.182)(12)$$
$$= 48.1 \text{ (estimated max } \dot{V}O_2)$$

How much faith can be placed in this estimated value? This depends on the care with which the test developer carried out the study. Factors such as sample size, standard error of estimate, and cross-validation must be considered.

The steps for conducting a predictive validity study are relatively straightforward:

1. Draw a random sample of approximately 200 subjects. Randomization is sometimes not possible; using the entire population is equally acceptable. If neither alternative is possible, the size of the sample should still be substantial.
2. Administer the predictor and criterion tests.
3. Correlate the predictor and criterion tests. If the validity coefficient is sizable, proceed with the next step.
4. Randomly divide the sample into two groups of equal size (100 in each group). Randomization is an essential process. Using group 1, calculate the intercept (a) and the slope (b) for the regression equation. These formulas are not included in this textbook but can be easily obtained in an elementary statistics book. Using the scores from group 2, apply the unknowns (*a* and *b*) from the first groups's equation and estimate the Y values for group 2 (even though in reality these values are already known).
5. Since criterion test scores are available for group 2, these scores can be compared with the *estimated* criterion scores obtained in step 4. This process is known as *cross-validation*. The closer the two values, the more accurate is the estimate. The use of a statistic known as the *standard error of estimate* provides a means of evaluating the accuracy of the estimate. The standard error of estimate can be calculated using Formula 6-3.

$$s_{y-x} = s_y \sqrt{1 - r_{xy}^2} \qquad \text{Formula 6-3}$$

where s_{y-x} = standard error of estimate
s_y = standard deviation of the group on the criterion test
r_{xy}^2 = square of the correlation coefficient between the predictor and the criterion test

If the standard error of estimate is sufficiently small, the estimate of the criterion score can be viewed as accurate.

The application of predictive validity in *predicting future behavior* uses one or more predictor variables to predict criterion behavior at some future point. Within this context, scores on the predictor and criterion variables are not obtained at the same time. Although this may initially seem strange, it actually is the only logical way to proceed. When future behavior is being predicted, the interest focuses on the person's future performance instead of present performance. For instance, one may wish to predict the degree of success an athlete might have if selected for a team. The prediction would have to be made before the team members are selected; yet the success of the individual would be unknown until the end of the season. Thus this is a more difficult type of predictive validity to determine. Fortunately a test developer will handle the difficult part. The concern here is how well the predictor works.

Let's look at an example of predicting future behavior from the sports psychology literature. A number of studies have centered on the psychological factors that can be used to predict success in sport. For example, Morgan and Johnson (1978) studied the psychological characteristics of highly skilled oarsmen. For many years all entering freshmen at the University of Wisconsin were required to take the Minnesota Multiphasic Personality Inventory. Using the scores on this inventory, Morgan and Johnson evaluated the psychological profiles of successful and unsuccessful oarsmen on the University of Wisconsin teams. Successful oarsmen tended to be less anxious, depressed, angry, fatigued, confused, and neurotic and more vigorous and extroverted. In 1974 at a training camp for potential Olympic oarsmen, the investigators administered a similar battery of psychological scales to all 57 candidates at the camp. No one, not even the investigators themselves, knew of the results of the psychological tests until the end of the training camp session. (Not until after the Olympic team members had been selected did Morgan and Johnson prepare the psychological profiles of the total group of candidates, since knowledge of these results might have influenced the coaches' decisions in making selections.)

After the team members had been selected, the psychological profiles were compared with the profiles of successful and unsuccessful oarsmen identified in Morgan and Johnson's earlier work. Based on these comparisons, each member of the group at the training camp was classified as successful (likely to be chosen for the Olympic team) or unsuccessful (unlikely to be chosen). Of course, at that point they knew who the actual team members were. Therefore Morgan and Johnson were able to compare their predictions with the actual results, as shown in Table 6-2. This is known as a **contingency table.**

Of the 57 candidates, 10 were accurately predicted for the Success category and 31 for the Fail category. The profiles accurately predicted 62% (10/16 = .62) of the oarsmen selected for the team and 76% (31/41 = .76) of those rejected. Thus psychological variables alone cannot be used to predict team membership, although knowledge of these variables can contribute to the accuracy of prediction.

Before proceeding to the next example, be sure you understand how to read a contingency table, since they are discussed in the next chapter. Do you under-

---

TABLE 6-2 *Evaluation of the clinical (a priori) prediction model's accuracy*

Actual category	Predicted category		Total
	Success	Fail	
Success	10	6	16
Fail	10	31	41
TOTAL	20	37	57

From Morgan, W.P., and Johnson R.W.

stand how the 62% success rate in predicting team membership was determined? The 76% success rate in rejection?

In a more recent study, Morgan and Raven (1985) evaluated the effectiveness of trait anxiety in predicting respiratory distress during heavy physical work performed by subjects wearing an industrial respirator. The predictor test, the Spielberger State-Trait Anxiety Inventory, was administered to all subjects on the first day of the experiment. The criterion measure was a seven-point perceived exertion scale designed to assess respiratory distress. The subjects performed three submaximal exercise tests at light, moderate, and heavy work intensities. Of the 45 subjects, 6 were predicted to manifest respiratory distress and 5 actually did. (See Table 6-3.) This represented a hit rate of 83% (5 of 6). Thirty-nine subjects were expected not to display respiratory distress, and 38 did not. The hit rate for this prediction was 97% (38 of 39). Thus this predictive validity study demonstrated that it is possible to identify individuals who are likely to experience respiratory distress when performing heavy work and wearing an industrial respirator.

Construct-Related Evidence of Validity   The last type of validity to be examined in this textbook is construct-related evidence of validity. **Construct validity** can be defined as the degree to which a test measures an attribute or trait that cannot be directly measured. Think about an attribute like athletic ability. Everyone assumes such an attribute exists, but it cannot be measured directly. Of course, certain aspects of athletic ability can be measured, but as a whole it defies precise measurement. Athletic ability can be thought of as a *construct*, a trait that cannot be directly measured.

Another example of a construct is anxiety, often an attribute of concern in athletics. Measuring the sweatiness of palms, administering an anxiety inventory, and checking heart rate or blood pressure are ways to determine if a person is anxious. However, these are merely *indicators* of anxiety. Anxiety cannot really be measured directly. Although a construct cannot be measured precisely,

TABLE 6-3 *Prediction of distress for individuals wearing industrial respirators*

Actual respiratory distress	Predicted respiratory distress		
	Yes	No	Total
Yes	5	1	6
No	1	38	39
TOTAL	6	39	45

From Morgan, W.P., and Raven, P.B.

indicators of the construct behavior are often measured. How is this type of test validated, since no criterion test is available?

Although there are many ways of determining construct validity, only one will be discussed in this textbook—the *group differences method*. Let's use Kenyon's Attitude Toward Physical Activity Inventory (Kenyon, 1968) as an example. One of the scales in the Kenyon Inventory is labeled "Vertigo." Essentially this scale is a measure of the risk-taking capacity of an individual in situations involving vigorous physical activity. How should this scale be validated? Logically, persons who participate in forms of vigorous physical activity involving risk taking would be more likely to obtain high scores on the scale than sedentary individuals. For example, a group of mountain climbers should score significantly higher on the scale than a group of sedentary office workers. If not, the validity of the scale is questionable. Comparing two groups' scores, which are expected to differ, is one way of providing evidence of construct validity. This can be accomplished using a t-test, which was described in Chapter 3. The group difference method alone does not establish construct validity; many pieces of evidence are required for this purpose.

Another example of the use of the group-difference approach is to compare groups on scores on the Health and Fitness scale of the Kenyon Inventory. Individuals who are known to be highly fit should score higher than those who are not (e.g., sedentary office workers). If those with a high level of CR function do not score higher than those with low CR function, the construct validity of the scale would be open to question.

Interpretation of the Validity Coefficient

When selecting a test, one of the factors to be evaluated is the size of the validity coefficient. How high should the coefficient be to be acceptable? If the test is being used as a substitute for a more sophisticated but impractical test, the validity coefficient should be high. Generally, coefficients of 0.90 and above are desirable, but those exceeding 0.80 are acceptable. Squaring the correlation coefficient demonstrates the amount of variance common to both tests, that is, the extent to which the two tests are measuring the same attribute. Thus a lower coefficient would not be acceptable. For a validity coefficient of 0.50, only 25% of the variance of the test and of the criterion measure overlap. For the most part these tests are measuring different qualities.

When a test is constructed for predictive purposes, a lower validity coefficient may sometimes be acceptable. Even tests with validity estimates of 0.50 or 0.60 may be retained. The key question is whether the test does a better job of predicting than any other method; that is, is the test superior to another test or a subjective method of making the prediction? The accuracy of the prediction increases as the size of the validity coefficient increases.

RELIABILITY

One of the most confusing points in measurement to the beginning student is the definition of test reliability. The reliability of a test refers to the dependability of scores, their relative freedom from error. Reliability is popularly defined as the consistency of an individual in performing a test. Suppose an examinee took a test once and then was able to go back in time as if the test had never been taken. Then suppose the same test was administered again. We would expect the scores on the two tests to be quite similar. If not, the test would be unreliable. If a test is administered at the end of a unit of instruction, we assume the scores will represent a stable level of achievement. In other words, if the test were administered again the next day, the test scores would be similiar to those obtained on the first day.

The definition of reliability as consistency is both meaningful and appropriate; however, when reliability is estimated within a norm-referenced framework, a more complex definition is implied. The term **reliability** reflects the ability of the test to detect reliable differences *between* examinees; that is, given that the test was administered on two occasions to the same students, the *same differences* between students would be detected. Remember that a norm-referenced test is designed to reflect individual differences; thus this interpretation of reliability makes sense.

A test can be reliable without being valid, but a valid test has to be reliable. Reliability, then, refers to the consistency, not the general worthiness, or the validity, of the test. For example, suppose a physical education teacher administers a test of the football place-kick from the 20-yard line. An assistant holds the ball in place on the tee, and the student taking the test kicks the ball 10 times to complete the test. The test may be highly reliable, but its validity might be questioned, especially if the examinees have had previous experience playing football. One way of improving the validity is to snap the ball to an assistant, who must place the ball on the tee before the kick. There is a trade-off, however, in that the increased complexity of the test would probably reduce its reliability. The fewer the extraneous factors associated with the parameters of the test, the more reliable the test.

The same point can be exemplified using another test. A popular test in volleyball classes is the wall volley test, designed to measure volleying skill. Generally the test score is the number of times the ball hits the wall, with certain distance and height restrictions. A student might be able to perform the test reliably, yet use poor form, executing the skill poorly and perhaps illegally by game rules. Reliability does not ensure validity.

Types of Reliability

Most developers of motor performance tests do not provide much information about test reliability. Often a reliability coefficient is presented with little expla-

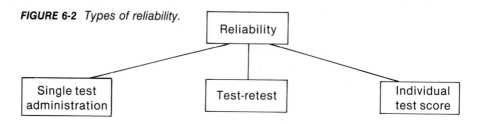

FIGURE 6-2 Types of reliability.

nation. The coefficient will usually be symbolized by either $r_{xx'}$, the interclass correlation (or Pearson product-moment correlation) coefficient, or $R_{xx'}$, intraclass correlation coefficient. Both of these symbols represent correlation coefficients, but the second represents a more informative estimate. Both reflect the ratio of true scores to obtained scores. A *true score* is the score an individual would obtain on a test if there were no measurement error. An *obtained score* is the sum of true score plus error score. A true score is unknown but can be estimated by determining measurement error and subtracting it from the obtained score. The two reliability estimates mentioned represent the ratio of the true score to the obtained score.

The types of reliability described in the next sections are those most likely seen in the physical education field. These types, shown in Figure 6-2, are single test administration, test-retest reliability, and precision of an individual test score.

Single Test Administration The reliability of a test can be estimated from a single administration of the test on any one occasion. The resultant **interclass** reliability coefficient estimates the reliability of the test at one point. There is no guarantee that an examinee's score on the test would be similar if the test were administered again the next day. However, sometimes this does not matter. For instance, sport competition anxiety can be measured using an inventory developed by Martens (1977). Test users would not use this inventory unless it measured with consistency the anxiety level of an athlete before a game. However, the athlete would not be expected to obtain the same score the next day (even if another game was being played) or even after the game ended. Anxiety levels usually fluctuate, depending on the situation.

If a student is repeatedly tested during the time a skill is being learned, one might not expect his or her scores to be consistent from one day to the next. The student has been taught more about the skill before the second testing period. One point should be clarified before proceeding. Whenever test developers administer a test more than once to establish reliability, it does not mean that all test users are expected to give the test twice. However, this information is important to know when selecting a test. If test reliability was established based on one administration of the test on a single occasion, the test is expected to elicit reliable performance only for that occasion. If test reliability was established based on two administrations of the test, each one on a different occasion, the test is expected to be reliable for that general period of time. If a test is used in a different situation than that proposed by the test developer, test reliability must be re-established.

Now, how is the reliability of a test established when the test is administered on one occasion only? Either of two procedures for estimating reliability can be used. One is the *Pearson product-moment correlation coefficient* ($r_{xx'}$) (see Formula 3-9). The test must consist of at least two trials. If more than two trials are used, the trials must be reduced (usually by averaging) to two sets. You will recall that the correlation coefficient estimates the relationship between two sets of scores. In Chapter 3 the two sets of scores represented different variables, similar to the validity coefficients in this chapter. The reliability coefficient, however, represents two sets of scores on the *same* variable.

The second method is the **intraclass correlation coefficient,** known as $R_{xx'}$. This coefficient is estimated by calculating an analysis of variance. Generally, $r_{xx'}$ and $R_{xx'}$ are interpreted similarly. However, $R_{xx'}$ is a more accurate estimate of reliability for two reasons. First, it is not necessary to reduce the trials to two sets to calculate $R_{xx'}$. This is important because many tests of motor skill consist of more than two trials. A major portion of the test error could occur among trials, but this would not be detected when $r_{xx'}$ is used. Second, if trial scores increase or decrease systematically, this should lower the reliability of the test. Yet these changes do not affect $r_{xx'}$. This fact can be verified by examining the scores in Table 6-4. Note that the scores on trial 2 are much higher than the trial 1 scores. However, $r_{xx'}$ equals +1.00, reflecting perfect reliability. It is obvious that the examinees' performances were not consistent. Detailed information on

TABLE 6-4 *Systematic increase in scores from day 1 to day 2*

Student	Test 1, day 1	Test 1, day 2
A	2	20
B	4	40
C	6	60
D	8	80
E	10	100
	30	300
	$\bar{X} = 6$	$\bar{X} = 60$
	$s = 3.16$	$s = 31.62$

the calculation of the intraclass correlation coefficient can be found in the Instructor's Manual accompanying this textbook.

Another way of estimating reliability on the basis of a single test administration is to divide the test into halves and correlate the two half-tests. This is referred to as a **split-half reliability estimate.** This procedure was originally devised for written tests but was subsequently used with tests in the exercise sciences. For example, the reliability of a 10-trial test of a sports skill could be determined by correlating the average of one set of five trial scores with the average of the scores on the remaining five trials. There are several ways the trials could be split. Two possibilities are a first half-second half split, where the two halves consist of trials 1 to 5 and trials 6 to 10, or an odd-even split, where the two halves consist of trials 1, 3, 5, 7, and 9 and trials 2, 4, 6, 8, and 10.

The odd-even split is used most frequently in tests of motor skill to guard against the possibility of fatigue or lack of motivation affecting performance on the last few trials of the test. To exemplify this point, let's use an extreme example. Suppose we were interested in the reliability of a 10-trial shuttle run test. If the division into halves was accomplished using a first half-second half split, the average of the first five trials is likely to be lower (better performance) than the average of the last five trials. This would result in a lower reliability estimate. If an odd-even split were used, the average of the odd-numbered trials would probably be similar to the average of the even-numbered trials. This comparison is demonstrated in Figure 6-3.

If a first half-second half split is used, the average of the second five trials (11.44 seconds) clearly differs from the average of the first five trials (10.96 seconds), as shown in Figure 6-3. This is probably caused by the effect of fatigue.

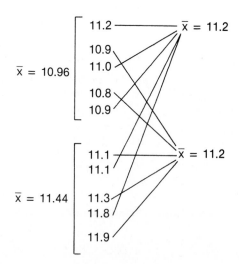

FIGURE 6-3 *Comparison of odd-even split with first half-second half split using 10 shuttle run test scores (seconds).*

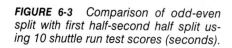

An odd-even split, on the other hand, yields identical averages for the odd-numbered and the even-numbered trials.

Once a test is split in halves and the averages of the halves determined, these scores can be correlated to yield $r_{xx'}$. However, since only half the test has been correlated with the other half, the resultant reliability coefficient represents an estimate for a 5-trial test. We, of course, would like to know how reliable a 10-trial test would be. The formula used to estimate the reliability of the full length (in this case, 10-trial) test, called the *Spearman-Brown prophecy formula,* is shown in Formula 6-4.

$$r^*_{xx'} = \frac{nr_{xx'}}{1 + (n - 1)r_{xx'}} \qquad \text{Formula 6-4}$$

where n = number of times test length is increased
$r_{xx'}$ = reliability of half of the test length
$r^*_{xx'}$ = estimated reliability for the full test length

If the correlation between half-tests of a 10-trial test is 0.60, the estimated reliability of the full-length test would be 0.75. In this case, $n = 2$. Longer tests are expected to be more reliable than shorter ones.

The Spearman-Brown prophecy formula generally provides an overestimate of the actual reliability of the full-length test. Intraclass correlation procedures can also be used to estimate the reliability of a shortened or lengthened test.

Test-Retest Reliability If a test is used to assess achievement on a skill at the end of a unit of instruction, obtaining a test score that reflects the examinee's skill level with precision would be desirable. The assessment would be inaccurate if some examinees who obtained high scores on the day testing took place would have received low scores if the test had been administered on a second day. To avoid this possibility the test user should look for a test with an acceptable reliability coefficient that has been established on a test-retest context.

Either of the two correlational procedures described in the previous section would be appropriate for estimating the reliability in a test-retest context. The split-half procedure, however, is not appropriate in this setting. See Instructor's Manual for details on calculating $R_{xx'}$.

Precision of an Individual Test Score Thus far reliability estimates that are determined for groups have been discussed. In other words, reliability is estimated by using the test scores obtained from administering the test to a group of examinees. Sometimes it is of greater interest to evaluate the reliability of an individual examinee's score. This can be done using the **standard error of measurement.** Let's assume we could administer a test to an examinee 1000 times, with each administration completely independent of the others. We would plot a distribution of these 1000 scores as described in Chapter 2. The standard deviation of this distribution of scores is the *standard error of measurement* for the examinee. As the examinee's scores become more similar, the standard error of measurement becomes smaller. Thus a smaller standard error of measurement is associated with a more precise score. This differs from other types of reliability discussed previously, where higher values of $r_{xx'}$ and $R_{xx'}$ represent greater consistency.

Since a test cannot be administered repeatedly to an individual, the standard error of measurement is estimated using Formula 6-5.

$$SE_m = s\sqrt{1 - r_{xx'}} \qquad \text{Formula 6-5}$$

where SE_m = *standard error of measurement*
s = *standard* deviation of a group of examinees
$r_{xx'}$ = *reliability coefficient*

Suppose, for example, that the standard deviation of a set of shuttle run test scores is 2 seconds and the test reliability is 0.84.

$$SE_m = 2\sqrt{1 - 0.84} = 0.80 \text{ seconds}$$

How is an SE_m of 0.80 interpreted? First, it represents seconds, in this case. In other words, the SE_m for the shuttle run test is 0.80 seconds. The standard error of measurement is always presented in the actual score units of the test. Now, suppose Mary obtained a score of 9.8 seconds on the shuttle run test. How precise is her score? The SE_m can be used to form a band around the examinee's score. The smaller the band, the more precise the score. Remember that the SE_m is actually a standard deviation. Thus if a ± 1 SE_m band around Mary's score is used, it would be expected to span her true score 68% of the time. The SE_m is subtracted from Mary's score to obtain the lower bound of the band and added to obtain the upper bound. In this example Mary's band is 9.0–10.6 seconds. If Mary repeatedly took the shuttle run test, we would not necessarily expect her scores to be close to the original 9.8 seconds, since the standard error of measurement band is relatively large. As the band decreases in size, we can have more faith in the precision of Mary's score.

To summarize, the standard error of measurement provides an indicator of the precision of an individual's test score. The smaller the SE_m, the greater the reliability of the score.

Factors Influencing the Reliability of a Test

Numerous factors influence the reliability of a test. Many of the factors are more important to test developers than test users, but knowledge of a few of these factors helps in selecting a test with acceptable reliability. See Figure 6-4 for an overview of the factors to be described in the next sections.

Type of Test To expect the reliability of all tests in our field to be 0.90 or above is not reasonable. The type of test must be taken into account when interpreting the reliability of a test. If performance on the test requires a maximum

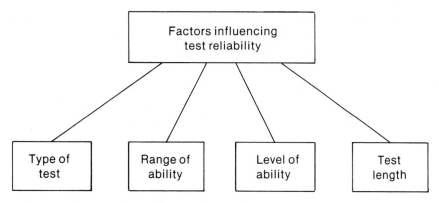

FIGURE 6-4 *Factors influencing test reliability.*

expenditure of effort, it is reasonable to expect reliabilities of around 0.85 or higher. For example, a grip strength test is taken by squeezing a hand dynamometer as hard as possible. This requires all-out physical effort. Performance on this test ought to be highly reliable. This is also true for measures of the long jump, vertical jump, dashes, distance throw, and other similar abilities. The greater the force requirements (throw as hard as possible, jump as far as possible, squeeze the hand dynamometer as hard as possible), the higher the reliability coefficient should be.

As the accuracy demands of a test increase, reliability decreases. To expect reliability coefficients to be 0.85 or higher in most instances is not reasonable. In fact, a test primarily measuring accuracy, such as a test of the chip shot in golf or the short serve in badminton, might be acceptable with a reliability estimate of 0.70, assuming satisfactory validity. At the same time estimates below 0.70 are rarely acceptable, regardless of the type of test, even though reliability estimates theoretically range from .00 to 1.00. Negative reliability coefficients are uninterpretable. A test can be reliable or it can have little or no reliability.

Range of Ability When reliability is estimated using test scores from a group with a wide range of ability, the estimate is artificially inflated. For example, assume a test of the softball throw for distance was given to a group of children in grades 2 through 6. In this case, reliability is almost guaranteed to be high. The children in sixth grade will throw the ball farther than the second graders, primarily because sixth graders are bigger and stronger than second graders. This would be true as often as the test is repeated. In a relative sense the test is highly reliable. On the other hand, it is more informative to know whether the test is reliable for sixth graders—or second graders—and this suggests that reliability must be estimated for each grade separately. Although the scores will still fluctuate within each grade, the reliability estimate for each grade will not be an artifact of a wide range of ability. In short, when planning to test sixth graders, select a test with acceptable reliability for sixth-grade children.

Level of Ability Closely related to range of ability is level of ability and its effect on reliability. In physical education there has been a tendency to expect skilled individuals to perform with more consistency than beginners. Therefore a specific skills test might be more reliable when administered to a highly skilled player. Interestingly enough, research in motor development has not totally verified this assumption. When a number of basic movement patterns are measured, poorly skilled individuals—presumably beginners in learning the pattern—tend to display highly reliable performances. They may not be very good, but they are consistent in their performance! As individuals learn more about the movement pattern—presumably moving up to intermediate level—their performances become less reliable. This may seem incongruous, but an intermediate-level performer is refining the movement pattern. At the advanced level these individuals become more consistent, with highly reliable performance. At this level the performer has begun to have control over the potential error and can perform with relative consistency.

Test Length The reliability of a test can be increased by making it longer. This is a well-established fact. When measuring sports skills, increasing the number of trials will lead to a higher reliability estimate. Adding more items to a written test will have the same effect.

OBJECTIVITY OF SCORING

The degree of accuracy in scoring a test is often referred to as the **objectivity** of the test. If a test is labeled highly objective, this means there will be little error in scoring the test. Many individuals could score the test and obtain the same result. A **subjective** test might be scored quite differently, depending upon the scorer. Variability among scorers increases when the scorer is required to make judgments that are more subjective, as in rating playing ability in a sport.

When a target is used to score a test or when a distance is measured, the test can be scored at a high level of objectivity. The objectivity is so obvious that an estimate of objectivity is rarely calculated. As the subjectivity of the test increases, the test developer is obligated to report an objectivity estimate. There are two types of objectivity as depicted in Figure 6-5.

FIGURE 6-5 *Types of objectivity.*

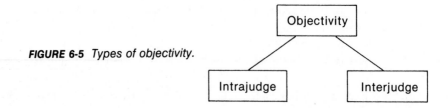

Intrajudge objectivity, the first type of objectivity, is the consistency in scoring when a test user scores the same test two or more times. If a written test is being considered, intrajudge objectivity can easily be determined. A set of tests can be graded once, put aside until a later date, and then graded again by the same person. Comparison of the two sets of scores would reflect the consistency of the individual in scoring the test. In testing motor skills, estimates of intrajudge objectivity are more difficult to obtain because the same performance must be viewed twice. This is usually facilitated by recording the performance on film or videotape.

The second type of objectivity is *interjudge objectivity*, which is the consistency between two or more independent judgments of the same performance. Interjudge objectivity is an important part of rating events in gymnastics, diving, and figure skating, where several judges rate each performance.

Both types of objectivity can be estimated using correlational procedures similar to estimating reliability. The estimates are expected to be relatively high (0.80 or above), since lower values suggest that the judges are weighting the various components of skill differently.

A method has been proposed to objectify judging of springboard diving (McCormick, Subbaiah, and Arnold, 1982). For example, a videotape recording can be made of the front half-twist dive, and clear plastic grids are placed over the video monitor to measure various components of the dive, such as deviation of twist from 180 degrees. A total of four measures can be used to predict judges' scores—height of the diver above the board (see Figure 6-6), distance out from board, twist, and one or two angle measurements.

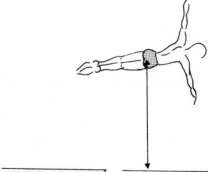

FIGURE 6-6   *Measurement of maximum height of diver in front half-twist dive.*

Efforts to identify the sources of biasing factors in judging motor performance have been numerous. Although knowing whether judges agree in their ratings is useful, knowing *why* they differ is more important. The possibility of reducing the bias and increasing the objectivity of ratings then exists.

SUMMARY

The characteristics of a test should be carefully evaluated before its administration to a group of examinees. Test validity, reliability, and objectivity are of major importance. Validity is the soundness of the interpretation of the test. It can be established on logical and/or statistical grounds. Through a logical analysis evidence of content validity can be demonstrated for a written test, and evidence of logical validity can be demonstrated for a test of motor performance. Statistical evidence is used to determine criterion-related validity, and both logical and statistical information are needed to establish construct validity. Reliability is the consistency of performance on a test. Test reliability can be established for a single occasion or a general period of time. Either $r_{xx'}$ or $R_{xx'}$ can be used as reliability coefficients, although $R_{xx'}$ is generally viewed as the superior estimate. Objectivity is the accuracy of scoring a test. Statistical evidence of this characteristic should be provided when the scoring is subjective, as in gymnastics and diving. A good test will possess high levels of all three of these elements.

LEARNING EXPERIENCES

1. Select a test you might consider using in the future. (Examples of a wide variety of tests can be found in Chapters 18 to 21.) Carefully evaluate its evidence of validity, reliability, and objectivity. Suggest ways in which each of these test characteristics might be improved for the test you selected.
2. Develop a simple rating scale for a skill in a sport such as basketball (See Chapter 14 for information on developing rating scales.) Attend a game with a friend who is also in your measurement and evaluation course, and use the scale to rate the skill. Do not try to rate more than one player. Each of you should independently rate the same person. Periodically compare ratings; if they are discrepant, discuss ways of improving the use of the scale or the scale itself.
3. Six trials of a basketball shooting test were administered to each of five students. Using this data set, answer the three questions below.

Student	Trial 1	Trial 2	Trial 3	Trial 4	Trial 5	Trial 6
A	10	11	11	12	11	12
B	14	13	14	14	15	14
C	12	12	12	13	12	13
D	9	8	8	9	9	8
E	7	9	8	8	9	9

   a. Calculate the split-half reliability coefficient for this six-trial test. Use an odd-even split.

   b. Use the Spearman-Brown formula to estimate the reliability coefficient for six trials.

   c. Briefly interpret this coefficient.

ANSWERS TO LEARNING EXPERIENCES

3a. The mean of the odd trials and the mean of the even trials should be determined for each person.

Student	Odd (X)	Even (X')	XX'
A	10.67	11.67	124.52
B	14.33	13.67	195.89
C	12.00	12.67	152.04
D	8.67	8.33	72.22
E	8.00	8.67	69.36

Use the Pearson product-moment correlation coefficient formula to determine the correlation between the odd (X) and even (X^1) means (Formula 3-9). The following values are needed for the formula:

$$\Sigma X = 53.67$$
$$\Sigma X' = 55.01$$
$$\Sigma XX' = 614.03$$
$$\Sigma X^2 = 602.37$$
$$\Sigma (X')^2 = 628.14$$
$$(\Sigma X)^2 = 2880.47$$
$$(\Sigma X')^2 = 3026.10$$

$$r_{xx'} = \frac{5(614.03) - 2952.39}{\sqrt{[5(602.37) - 2880.47][5(628.16) - 3026.10]}}$$
$$= \frac{117.76}{122.76} = 0.959$$

3b. The answer to 3a is the reliability for a three-trial test, since the six-trial test was split into three halves to obtain the reliability coefficient. The reliability of the six-trial test must now be estimated using the Spearman-Brown prophecy formula (Formula 6-4).

$$r^*_{xx'} = \frac{2(.959)}{1 + (2 - 1)(.959)}$$
$$= \frac{117.76}{122.70} = 0.979$$

3c. The estimated reliability of the six-trial test (0.979) is quite high, indicating that the basketball test is a reliable measure of performance. Since the three-trial test reliability (0.959) is also high, this suggests that administering the full-length six-trial test to measure performance adequately is not necessary. A three-trial test would be adequate.

REFERENCES

American Psychological Association. 1985. Joint standards for educational and psychological tests. Washington, D.C.: APA.

Cooper, K.H. 1968. A means of assessing maximal oxygen intake. Journal of the American Medical Association, **203**:201-204.

Cooperative Tests and Services. 1970. AAHPERD Cooperative Physical Education Tests. Princeton, N.J.: Educational Testing Service.

Getchell, L.H., Kirkendall, D., and Robbins, G. 1977. Prediction of maximal oxygen uptake in young adult women joggers. Research Quarterly, **48**:61-67.

Kenyon, G.S. 1968. Six scales for assessing attitude toward physical activity. Research Quarterly, **39**:566-574.

Martens, R. 1977. Sport Competition Anxiety Test. Champaign, Ill.: Human Kinetics Publishers, Inc.

McCormick, J.H., Subbaiah, P., and Arnold, H.J. 1982. A method for identification of some components of judging springboard diving. Research Quarterly for Exercise and Sport, **53**(4):313-322.

Morgan, W.P., and Johnson, R.W. 1978. Personality characteristics of successful and unsuccessful oarsmen. International Journal of Sport Psychology, **9**:119-133.

Morgan, W.P., and Raven, P.B. 1985. Prediction of distress for individuals wearing industrial respirators. American Industrial Hygiene Association Journal, **46**(7):363-368.

ANNOTATED READINGS

Brown, F.G. 1983. Principles of educational and psychological testing, ed. 3. Lavallette, N.J.: Holt, Rinehart & Winston.

Thorough coverage of both theory and techniques of educational and psychological testing: presents basic concepts in testing—validity, reliability, and types of scores—and illustrates how to apply those principles in test construction, use, evaluation, and interpretation; explores rationale underlying educational and psychological testing.

Gronlund, N.E. 1985. Measurement and evaluation in teaching, ed. 5. New York: Macmillan Publishing Co.

Emphasizes principles and procedures of testing and evaluation important to elementary and secondary teachers; assumes no prior knowledge of measurement or statistics; illustrates both norm-referenced and criterion-referenced test specifications.

Mehrens, W.A., and Lehmann, I.J. 1984. Measurement and evaluation in education and psychology, ed. 3. Lavallette, N.J.: Holt, Rinehart & Winston.

Introduction to the construction, evaluation, interpretation, and uses of tests; offers a contemporary look at testing and some of its practical applications; includes updated discussion of criterion-referenced measurement; contains detailed information on the practical uses of assessment data; covers current issues in testing.

Noll, V.H., Scannell, D.P., and Craig, R.C. 1979. Introduction to educational measurement, ed. 4. Boston: Houghton Mifflin Co.

Nontechnical orientation to educational measurement; includes thorough coverage of criterion-referenced tests and national and state assessment programs.

7
Validity and Reliability of Criterion-Referenced Tests

KEY WORDS *Watch for these words as you read the following chapter:*

contingency coefficient	domain	kappa coefficient
contrasting groups method	domain-referenced validity	mastery learning
criterion-referenced test	instructed/uninstructed approach	proportion of agreement
decision validity		reliability

Although most published tests in physical education and exercise science are norm-referenced, a great deal of informal testing goes on in the field that is more similar to the criterion-referenced approach to testing (Safrit, 1981). A physical education teacher, for example, may set a standard that students are expected to achieve on a test. Those whose test scores equal or surpass the test standard are classified as masters on the test; those with scores falling below the standard are labeled nonmasters (or some similar term). In a fitness laboratory clients are often placed in a category reflecting their level of fitness based on the results of a test. In a situation where there are no constraints on who can be classified as masters, a criterion-referenced test is appropriate. When only the top four or five examinees will be selected for a given purpose, a norm-referenced approach is more useful. A **criterion-referenced test** is defined as *a test with a predetermined standard of performance that is tied to a specified domain of behavior.* There is more to a criterion-referenced test than setting a standard, although this is an important part of this type of measure. The standard must be referenced to a criterion behavior. Suppose an exercise specialist administers a battery of fitness tests to all new clients joining a fitness club. One of these tests is modified sit-ups measure of abdominal strength. A woman who is a new member of the club is classified "average" in abdominal strength based on the test results. The exercise specialist suggests a series of exercises to increase abdominal strength and sets a goal of 45 sit-ups (in 1 minute) for her. How was this standard set? What does it mean? If this is a legitimate criterion-referenced test, the standard should have meaning in terms of a criterion behavior. This means that 45 sit-ups (standard) should reflect adequate abdominal strength for a woman in this fitness category. Of course, there is no way of knowing this is true. A standard could be set for any test, but it might not be clearly interpretable in light of the criterion behavior.

Even though there are problems in developing this type of test, it has certain advantages over a norm-referenced test. A norm-referenced test measures the status of the normative group, that is, "what is" rather than "what should be." For example, consider a measure of body fatness, the sum of a set of skinfold measures. Perhaps these measures are obtained from a large group of adult female examinees and used to estimate their percent body fat. The average percent fat for this group is 36%. Does this reflect a desirable standard for women to attain? This is legitimate normative data. However, it is well known that adult women tend to be overweight; therefore, normative data do not represent the most desirable standards in this case.

Furthermore, norm-referenced tests rarely provide extensive diagnostic feedback to the examinee. Think about the many tests you have taken in past years. How often did you receive meaningful feedback on your test score? In physical education few tests provide specific feedback. All over the United States students are tested on the basketball free throw by taking a predetermined number of shots at the basket. The student who makes most of these shots gets feedback on his or her skill level. The shooting technique of this individual is assumed to be good enough to be successful. However, the student who misses the shot receives little systematic feedback. If a criterion-referenced test is tied to a criterion behavior, it will provide needed feedback to the examinee. An excellent overview of the criterion-referenced approach to measurement can be found in Popham (1978, 1981).

MASTERY LEARNING

The normal distribution, as described in Chapter 3, is used in determining norm-referenced grades. Regardless of the ability levels of students, some will receive A's, B's, and so forth, according to a predetermined set of percentages. In a **mastery learning** setting (Nitko, 1984) an individual is expected to be a nonmaster before instruction or a training program. At this point when tests are administered to the nonmasters, the distribution of scores will be skewed in a positive direction, since most examinees would receive low scores and only a small percentage would receive high scores. At the end of the unit of instruction or a training program, the majority in the group is expected to master the objective. In this case, test scores will be skewed negatively, since only a few people received low scores.

Criterion-referenced testing, then, is closely associated with the mastery model of instruction. Frequently, teachers care little about individual differences. If many students can master the test, so much the better. (Is not the objective of education for all or most students to learn?) Many educators feel it re-

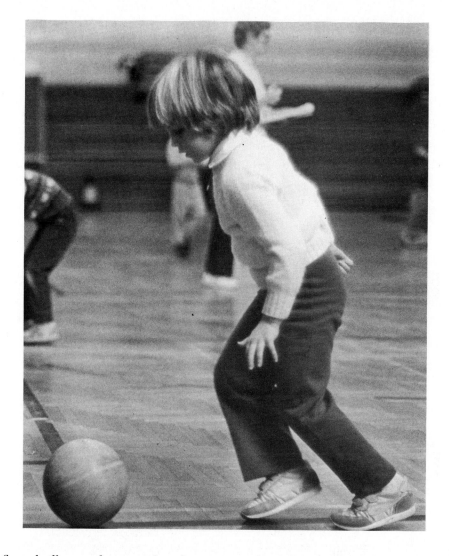

flects badly on education if students are taught skills, yet conclude the unit by being normally distributed on their abilities. Should not a large percentage of the students have at least minimal success in a unit? If this mode of instruction is adopted, the norm-referenced approach to testing is not quite appropriate. The criterion-referenced test is better suited to this instructional model.

USES OF A CRITERION-REFERENCED TEST

Criterion-referenced tests have a variety of uses. Sometimes we seek information on a person's capabilities, even though we have no interest in comparing the test score to a standard. For example, an exercise specialist might be interested in determining the strength of a client by administering a strength test at various parts of the body. Yet the individual is not classified according to some predetermined standard. In the physical education field, however, the most widespread use of criterion-referenced tests is to assign people to mastery states by administering *mastery tests.*

Several of the national physical fitness tests use criterion-referenced standards instead of providing tables of norms in the test manual. In these tests, desirable levels of fitness are promoted rather than normative assessments. The Physical Best Program, FITNESSGRAM, and Youth Fit Today are prominent examples of these tests. All three tests are described in Chapter 16.

VALIDITY

The techniques for validating a criterion-referenced test are unique, although there are similarities conceptually to norm-referenced test validity methodology. Generally, the definition of validity for a norm-referenced test applies to a criterion-referenced test; that is, validity is the soundness of the interpretation of the test. However, more precise definitions must be used that are unique to the criterion-referenced test. These definitions vary according to the type of validity of interest.

Types of Validity

Validity can be determined logically through domain-referenced validity or statistically, using decision validity methods. The focus here is on the mastery test, where examinees are classified as masters or nonmasters on the basis of their test score.

Domain-Referenced Validity Remember that a criterion-referenced test has been defined as a measure of performance referenced to a criterion behavior. To develop a test of this type, the criterion behavior must be defined. Then the test is logically validated by showing that the tasks sampled by the test adequately represent the criterion behavior. This is called **domain-referenced validity,** with the term **domain** used to represent the criterion behavior. This has many parallels with both content and logical validity, which were described in Chapter 6. However, the focus of a criterion-referenced test is much narrower than its norm-referenced counterpart. A criterion-referenced test is usually designed to measure a single objective and is frequently used as formative evaluation.

How might domain-referenced validity be established for a test of a sports skill? Let's use a test of the basketball jump shot as an example. The first steps in developing the test would be to analyze the skill, identify its most important elements, and devise a test to measure these elements. This is precisely how logical validity is determined, and it is equally appropriate in criterion-referenced testing. Suppose the test specifies that the student take 10 jump shots from a restraining line 15 feet away from the basket. In a physical education class of high school boys, a standard of 7 out of 10 successful jump shots might be set. This is a typical approach to testing in the physical education field. How is the placement of the restraining line for the test chosen? Usually it is arbitrary, although the distance from the basket would be expected to be realistic. Yet any one of a number of realistic locations might be selected. Would it not be a better test of the boy's jump-shooting ability if he could make successful shots from several points on the court? In the context of domain-referenced validity, this would be desirable. Of course, testing from every possible spot would be impossible. A procedure needs to be developed for systematically identifying several spots on the court from which the jump shot may be taken. One way of doing this would be to divide the basketball half-court into sections, as shown in Figure 7-1.

Thinking of each of the sections in Figure 7-1 as test items may be helpful. How many sections should be selected? For the sake of simplicity and practicality, let's use four sections. How should these sections be selected? Drawing a random sample from the entire set does not seem appropriate, since a player is much less likely to attempt a jump shot from certain sections of the court than others. Areas O through S represent sections seldom used for jump shots; therefore, the sections to be sampled might reasonably be limited to A through N. These letters were converted to numbers from 1 to 14, and four numbers were randomly drawn from the set. Their corresponding letters—E, I, K, and M— are circled in Figure 7-1.

The number of trials to be taken from each area should also be determined.

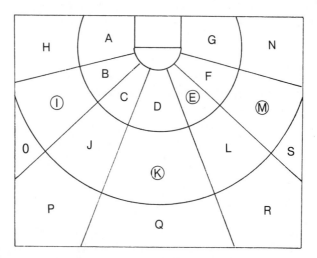

FIGURE 7-1 *Sampling of basketball court areas to test jump shot.*

Actual test scores are necessary for this purpose. Certainly more than one trial would be taken from each of the areas to have a reliable test.

Would this be a practical test to administer in a physical education class? Possibly not, in many school settings, but tests are not developed solely for use in classes. The jump shot test, with several trials taken from four spots on the court, might be useful for a basketball camp or an all-school testing program. Actually, it is not as cumbersome as it might seem for use in a physical education class. If the students are divided into four groups, they could rotate from one testing station to the other. In this way more students would be active than if only one restraining line location were used.

Domain-referenced validity, then, requires a careful description of the criterion behavior, or domain, along with evidence that the test adequately represents this domain. Although this is a logical rather than a statistical analysis, it should not be viewed as an arbitrary process.

Decision Validity   In addition to evidence of the adequacy of the test as a measure of the criterion behavior, the *accuracy of classification* as masters and nonmasters must be determined. This is done using **decision validity** procedures, which typically require the use of statistical procedures. Does the test classify people accurately? Two approaches—empirical methods and judgmental-empirical methods—are described in the next section.

As the name implies, *empirical methods* require a data base, and statistical procedures are used to estimate validity. One example of empirical procedures is a method that can be used by physical education teachers to select a valid cutoff point for a mastery test. This is usually referred to as the **instructed/uninstructed approach.** It assumes that an objective has been written, a test has been identified to measure the objective, but no performance standard has been set. The test is administered to two groups of students—one that has received no instruction on the objective and one that has received previous instruction. Then the two distributions of test scores are compared, as shown in Figure 7-2. A degree of overlap is expected between the distributions. The best students in the uninstructed group should have scores similar to the poorest in the instructed group.

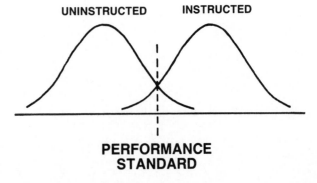

FIGURE 7-2 Setting standards using the instructed/uninstructed group approach.

The point at which the two distributions overlap represents the cutoff score, which can be used to classify future students as masters or nonmasters.

This is a viable approach *if* the uninstructed group really is uninstructed. A unit may represent the first formal instruction the students have had in school, but many students will have learned a few skills in other settings. In the Measurement Laboratory at the University of Wisconsin the difficulty in finding a true uninstructed group has been demonstrated in several activities. Because the uninstructed group does not consist only of nonmasters, the curves overlap too much; no meaningful cutoff point can be identified. This approach is probably most appropriate in units where more unusual activities are taught, such as self-defense or fencing, or when all students could be tested and the lower third of the distribution could be used to represent the uninstructed and the upper third, the instructed.

The second type of decision validity is *judgmental-empirical* methods. These methods require judgment on the part of the test user as well as a data base. One type of judgmental-empirical method is known as the **contrasting groups method.** Although it can be used outside a school setting, the following example is relevant for physical education teachers in a school. To use the system properly, more than one physical education teacher must be knowledgeable about the physical capabilities of the students who will be tested. Assume again that an education objective has been set and ways of evaluating the objective have been determined, but no standard has been set. The only information the teacher needs is a list of names of the students involved. Based on his or her knowledge of the students, the teacher classifies each one as either a master or a nonmaster on the objective in question. Then the entire group of students is evaluated on the objective using the predetermined procedure. A distribution of scores is formed for those students who are expected to master the objective and one for those not expected to master it. These distributions are then compared for overlap, as shown in Figure 7-3. As in the previous approach, the point of overlap is the best estimate of the cutoff score.

FIGURE 7-3 Setting standards using the contrasting groups approach.

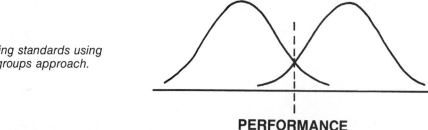

NONMASTERY EXPECTED

MASTERY EXPECTED

PERFORMANCE STANDARD

Notice that both of the above methods use the comparison of distributions of scores to validate a cutoff score. An easier way to estimate test validity using these approaches is to set up a *contingency table*. An example of displaying the results of the instructed/uninstructed approach in a contingency table can be found in Figure 7-4. The examinees in the instructed and uninstructed groups have already been identified. The only factor that can be varied is the cutoff score used to identify masters and nonmasters. The master/nonmaster classifications are shown on the left of the table.

The teacher's job is to select a cutoff score that seems reasonable. Then the examinees' scores are tallied in the table. For example, a student in the instructed group who is identified as a master by the test would be placed in the upper left cell (A) of the table. A student in the uninstructed group who is classified as a master would be tallied in the upper right cell (B) of the table. When all students have been tallied, the sum of the tallies in each cell is converted to a proportion. Each proportion is calculated by dividing the number of students within a cell by N, the total number of students. For example, in cell D the proportion of students is 75/190 or 0.39. The *validity coefficient* is calculated by summing the proportions in the upper left cell (A) and the lower right cell (D). The symbol for this coefficient is C, representing the **contingency coefficient.** Don't confuse this symbol with the letter C used to identify one of the cells in the contingency table in Figure 7-4. Different sizes of the coefficient C can be examined by changing the cutoff score. The highest C value will represent the most valid cutoff score.

Review the numerical example in Figure 7-4. Note that the whole numbers in the cells of the table represent the number of examinees; the numbers in pa-

FIGURE 7-4 *Procedure for estimating test validity using the contingency coefficient (C).*

	Criterion groups	
	Instructed	Uninstructed
Master	A 80[a] (.42)[b]	B 20 (.11)
Nonmaster	C 15 (.08)	D 75 (.39)

Test classification

$C = 0.81$

[a]Number of students
[b]Proportion of students

rentheses represent the proportion of examinees. Adding the proportion of examinees correctly classified (A + D) yields C, the contingency coefficient. In this case, C equals (0.42 + 0.39) or 0.81. If a higher validity coefficient were desired, the test developer would set a different cutoff point and develop a new contingency table. In this way the cutoff score that maximizes the differences between groups is determined.

In summary, a criterion-referenced test, like a norm-referenced test, can be validated both logically and statistically. If a mastery test is to be used in an informal setting, logical validation of the test would probably suffice. If the test is used to make major decisions about examinees, both logical and statistical validity should be established. Since the test is used to classify students as masters or nonmasters, the accuracy of these classifications should be evident.

Interpretation of the Validity Coefficient

Since C, the validity coefficient, is the sum of two proportions, a high coefficient is desirable. In fact, if $C = 0.50$, this suggests that the classification may be no better than chance. Therefore when $C = 0.50$, the validity is essentially zero. The interpretable range of C values is 0.50 to 1.00. Although no hard rule has been set for evaluating the size of the validity coefficient, certainly values of 0.80 or above would be desirable.

RELIABILITY

Criterion-referenced **reliability** is defined differently from norm-referenced reliability. In the criterion-referenced context, reliability is defined as *consistency of classification.* In other words, if the examinees were classified as masters or nonmasters on one occasion, would they be classified the same way on a second occasion?

Procedures for Estimating Reliability

The simplest way to estimate reliability is to administer a mastery test on 2 days and tally the scores in a contingency table. The general layout of this contingency table is shown in Figure 7-5. To the left of the table, M (mastery) and NM (nonmastery) classifications for the first day (Day 1) of testing are displayed. Across the top of the table, M and NM classifications are identified for the second day of testing. If a student is classified as a master on both days, a tally is placed in the upper left cell of the table. If a student is classified as a master on Day 1 and a nonmaster on Day 2, the tally is placed in the upper right cell. Locate the appropriate cell for the examinee who is a nonmaster on Day 1 and a master on Day 2. This is the lower left cell of the table. Once the scores have been tallied, the tallies in each cell are summed and converted to proportions.

Proportion of Agreement The most popular method for estimating reliability from a contingency table is to use P, which is the symbol for **proportion of**

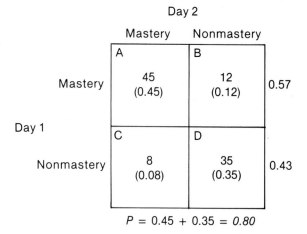

FIGURE 7-5 *Procedure for calculating P, the proportion of agreement.*

$$P = 0.45 + 0.35 = 0.80$$

agreement. The coefficient P is calculated by summing the proportions in cell A and D. This should sound familiar because it is the same procedure used to estimate C, the validity coefficient. Of course, the two coefficients have different interpretations because the contingency tables are set up differently, but the calculation is identical. Look at the data in Figure 7-5. Of the 100 examinees taking this test, 45 were classified as masters on both days, and 35 were classified as nonmasters. There were errors in classification as well, with 12 examinees labeled masters on the first day and nonmasters on the second, while the remaining 8 students received the reverse classifications. Since N equals 100 in this case, the proportions will be the same numerical value as the number of students within cells preceded by a decimal point. In cell A, for example, the proportion is 45/100 or 0.45. The proportion of agreement P is $(0.45 + 0.35)$ or 0.80.

Kappa Coefficient The coefficient P fails to take into account that some correct categorizations will be made purely by chance. If we tested a group of examinees and randomly placed their scores into the four cells of a contingency table, .25 of the sample would be placed in each cell purely by chance. A P of .50 could be obtained merely by chance. It would be of interest to know what degree of agreement has been obtained beyond the expectation of chance? One approach to this problem is to use k, **kappa coefficient,** to estimate reliability (Swaminathan, Hambleton, and Algina, 1974). Formula 7-1 is used to calculate k.

$$k = \frac{P_o - P_c}{1 - P_c}$$ Formula 7-1

where P_o = *proportion of agreement*
$\quad P_c$ = *proportion of agreement* expected by *chance*

OR

$\quad P_c = \Sigma \ (P_i) \ (P_i)$
where P_i = *marginal proportion*

To calculate P_c, follow this rule of thumb. Determine the marginal proportions by adding the proportions for each column and row of the contingency table. For example, in the first row of the table, the proportions for cells A and B are summed $(0.45 + 0.12)$ to equal the marginal proportion for this row (0.57). Multiply the marginal proportions of the outermost row and column of the table $[(0.57) (0.53)$, in this case] and add to the product of the marginal proportions of the innermost row and column $[(0.43) (0.47)$, in this case]. The outermost row and column represent the first row and column of the contingency table, while the innermost row and column represent the second row and column. In the example in Figure 7-5, $P_c = (0.57) (0.53) + (0.43) (0.47) = 0.3021 + 0.2021 = 0.5042$.

$$k = \frac{0.80 - 0.5042}{1 - 0.5042} = \frac{0.2958}{0.4958} = 0.597$$

Not surprisingly, when chance is taken into account, the size of the proportion of agreement decreases.

Interpretation of the Reliability Coefficient

Since the proportion of agreement, P, can be affected by chance allocations, values of P below 0.50 are unacceptable. Thus the *interpretable range* of P is 0.50 to 1.00. In other words, a P of 0.50 is interpreted as a P of 0.00. Although values of k can range from -1.00 to $+1.00$, the interpretable range of k is 0.00 to 1.00. Negative values of k have no meaning in the context of reliability, since test information either contributes positively to the consistency of classification or it does not.

When the group being tested consists of a large proportion of masters or nonmasters, P tends to be high. This is an expected characteristic of P, since it will be easier to classify people when they display low or high skill levels because their scores will be far below or above the cutoff point. Examinees who fall in between are more difficult to classify. When the test group consists primarily of this category of examinees, P typically drops, reflecting the difficulty of classifying people consistently as their scores approach the cutoff score.

SUMMARY

The criterion-referenced test offers an excellent option to norm-referenced testing when the identification of masters and nonmasters based on test performance is of interest. On the other hand, the concept of criterion-referenced measurement is often not fully understood, leading to oversimplified tests of mastery. Although a cutoff score can be determined with relative ease if set arbitrarily, this score, and thus the test, lacks validity unless the score can be interpreted in light of a criterion behavior. The validity and reliability of criterion-referenced tests

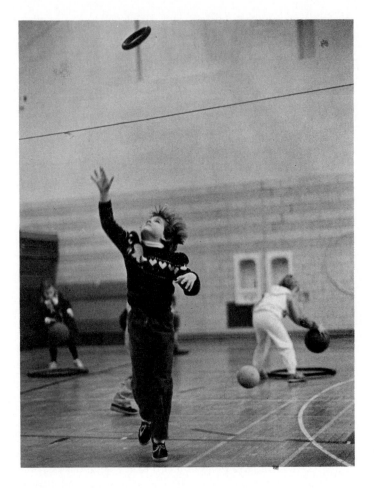

are defined differently from the definitions of these concepts in a norm-referenced context. The validity of a mastery test is defined as the accuracy of classifications; reliability is the consistency of classifications.

LEARNING EXPERIENCES

1. This exercise is designed to give you some practical experience with criterion-referenced testing. Collect 15 pennies and a plastic container. Ask 10 people to try to toss the pennies in the container one at a time. Tell them that mastery on this task is successfully tossing 10 of the 15 pennies into the container. (Try it first yourself, so that the distance of the toss is realistic.) Record the number of successes out of 15 trials. Then ask each person to repeat the test, beginning again with all 15 pennies. After recording these successes, calculate P, the proportion of agreement. How reliable is this data set? Evaluate the size of this coefficient and indicate ways it might be increased.

2. An exercise specialist wishes to check the validity of a sit-ups test as a measure of abdominal strength. He compares the sit-ups test activity with a criterion test, electromyographic (EMG) readings of the abdominal muscles. Both tests are used in a crite-

rion-referenced framework. On the EMG test a cutoff score of 27 or above reflects substantial activity in the abdominal muscles. The exercise specialist decides to try using a cutoff score of 55 or above on the sit-ups test to check the criterion-referenced test validity. He obtains the following test scores.

Subject	Sit-ups test	EMG test
1	73	32
2	42	20
3	51	19
4	63	25
5	59	27
6	39	18
7	57	33
8	70	36
9	65	29
10	69	28
11	46	19
12	51	21
13	52	30
14	56	31
15	64	27
16	71	17
17	42	19
18	50	25
19	50	23
20	60	29

a. Develop a contingency table for these scores.
b. Calculate C, the validity coefficient.
c. Is the sit-ups test valid? Explain.

ANSWERS TO LEARNING EXPERIENCES

2a. Hint: To develop the contingency table, each of the scores must be converted to a 0 or 1 score. See Figure 7-6 for the answer to this problem.

EMG test

		M(1)	NM(0)
Sit-ups test	M(1)	(9)* .45†	(2) .10
	NM(0)	(1) .05	(8) .40

FIGURE 7-6 *Contingency table; answer to Learning Experience 2a.*

*Number of people

†Proportion of people (number in cell divided by total number; in this case, N = 20)

b. $C = 0.45 + 0.40 = 0.85$

c. A C of 0.85 indicates a high degree of accuracy of classification; thus the validity of the sit-ups test is acceptable.

REFERENCES

Nitko, A.J. 1984. Defining "criterion-referenced test." In R.A. Berk, editor. A guide to criterion-referenced test construction. Baltimore: The Johns Hopkins University Press.

Popham, W.J. 1978. Criterion-referenced measurement. Englewood Cliffs, N.J.: Prentice-Hall, Inc.

Popham, W.J. 1981. Modern educational measurement. Englewood Cliffs, N.J.: Prentice-Hall, Inc.

Safrit, M.J. 1981. Evaluation in physical education. Englewood Cliffs, N.J.: Prentice-Hall, Inc.

Swaminathan, H., Hambleton, R.K., and Algina, J.A. 1974. Reliability of criterion-referenced tests: a decision-theoretic formulation. Journal of Educational Measurement, **11**:263-268.

ANNOTATED READINGS

Educational Testing Service. 1982. Passing scores. Princeton. N.J.: Educational Testing Service.

Focuses on setting standards of performance on test; describes in clear, nontechnical language various methods of making decisions related to passing scores; provides advice for making fair and impartial decisions.

Glass, G.V. 1978. Standards and criteria. Journal of Educational Measurement, **15**:237-271.

An excellent treatise of the current procedures used to set standards along with a critique of their shortcomings; suggests that the arbitrariness of standard-setting is predominant, and other alternatives to determining mastery may be more viable.

Guskey, T.R. 1985. Implementing mastery learning. Belmont, Calif.: Wadsworth Publishing Co.

Written specifically for teachers; describes the system of mastery learning and how to implement it in the schools; includes examples of teacher-made lesson plans based on mastery learning; demonstrates and explains formative and summative evaluation.

Linn, R.L. 1982. Two weak spots in the practice of criterion-referenced measurement. Educational Measurement, **1**(1):12-13, 25.

Discusses the terminology associated with criterion-referenced measurement; describes several of the problems associated with setting standards.

Nitko, A.J. 1984. Defining "criterion-referenced test." In R.A. Berk, editor. A guide to criterion-referenced test construction. Baltimore: The Johns Hopkins University Press.

Differentiates between norm-referenced and criterion-referenced tests; reviews various definitions of criterion-referenced tests; proposes two categories for classifying criterion-referenced tests; provides guidelines for practitioners.

Safrit, M.J., Baumgartner, T.A., Jackson, A.S., and Stamm, C.L. 1980. Issues in setting motor performance standards. Quest, **32**(2):152-162.

Discusses issues in setting standards in physical education; a brief review of procedures for standard-setting; an examination of gender differences in motor performance and the impact of these differences on standard setting.

Part Five

Measurement in a School Setting

8 Tests and Testing

KEY WORDS *Watch for these words as you read the following chapter:*

accountability	curriculum objectives	needs assessment
affective domain	evaluation objectives	psychomotor domain
behavioral objectives	immediate objectives	standard of performance
cognitive domain	long-range goals	taxonomy

If you plan to teach physical education in the schools, you will be expected to evaluate your students' performance on a variety of tasks. Most schools use several testing programs that have varying degrees of formality. The most formal program encompasses the administration of standardized achievement tests, although these will not comprise a sizable part of the testing because not many standardized tests are available in the physical education field. Several organizations have published standardized tests of physical fitness for school children, described in Chapters 16 and 17. A series of test manuals for several sports can also be obtained through the American Alliance for Health, Physical Education, Recreation and Dance (AAHPERD). Certain types of standardized tests have been developed for special populations. Of the tests mentioned thus far, all are measures of motor behavior. Only one standardized knowledge test has been published in the field. In 1970 the Cooperative Knowledge Test was made available as a measure of the knowledge students in grades 4 through 12 have about physical education. However, the content of a knowledge test ought to be revised periodically, and this test has not been updated since its original development. This more formal part of the testing program is often the basis for informing people outside the school of the physical education program's effectiveness. Reports of test results and comparisons with national norms are prepared for parents, other schools in the district, the school board, and all tax-paying citizens in the community.

Testing also occurs at a less formal level in the schools. At this level the teacher selects or develops tests to be used in his or her classes. This differs from school-wide testing in which all students at a given grade level are administered the same standardized test. For example, Mr. Moore, a physical education

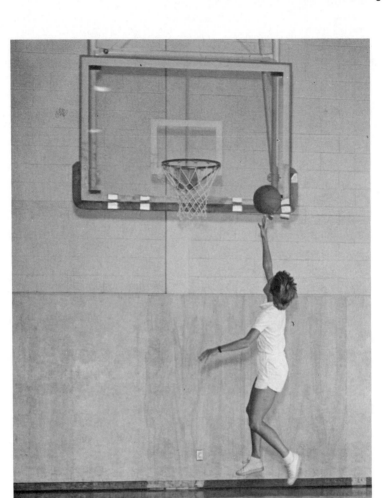

teacher, might use a specific health-related physical fitness test to measure the fitness of his students because it is a requirement in all physical education classes in the system. On the other hand, it might be Mr. Moore's responsibility to select additional tests to be administered to his students throughout a unit or at the end of a unit. These tests may or may not be used by any of the other physical education teachers in his school or school system. The fact that this level of testing is less formal is not meant to suggest that the tests are handled more casually. *Less formal* in this context means that the decision to use certain tests is made individually rather than on a school-wide basis. One of the positive features of our society is that schools operate in various ways to achieve the goals of education. For instance, in some schools the entire staff of physical education teachers may decide that a certain series of tests will be used in all classes in the school. In others, each teacher makes these decisions; although this may result in different tests being used by each teacher, the objectives of the physical education program may be the same for all.

In this chapter some of the most basic decision-making processes in teaching will be reviewed. How do you decide what to test in your physical education classes? This decision can be made in a systematic manner if behavioral objectives have been properly prepared. This process is reviewed in the forthcoming sections after a discussion of the current status of testing in physical education.

DO PHYSICAL EDUCATION TEACHERS USE TESTS?

When you accept your first teaching position, what sort of expectations should you have about the testing program? The program may be excellent or virtually nonexistent. Probably most programs fall somewhere in between these extremes.

In the 1958 edition of a measurement textbook by Mathews, he referred to an informal survey of 50 student teachers on the grading practices in their cooperating schools. In 80% of the systems, the student's mark was based solely on being present and in uniform daily. In 1974 Cousins gave a keynote speech at a measurement symposium at Indiana University. He cited a number of incidents reflecting the misuse of tests in our field and suggested that the greatest misuse of tests was the lack of use by physical education teachers. In 1978 Morrow conducted a survey on the use of evaluation techniques and concluded that tests were simply not being used in the schools he sampled. Assessment of students was made on the basis of dress and participation. All these reports were published before 1980; surely the situation has improved. A 1982 survey of Florida physical education teachers (Imwold, Rider, and Johnson, 1982) suggests this is not true, however. A portion of their survey appears in the boxed material. These results were substantiated in a 1986 survey of physical education teachers in Iowa, Wyoming, Kansas, and Georgia (Hensley and others, 1988).

According to the results of the Florida survey, skills tests were used by only 54% of the teachers; fewer than 40% used knowledge tests. Skills tests were administered more frequently by female teachers, junior high teachers, and those with 4 or more years' experience. In general, norm-referenced tests were selected more frequently than criterion-referenced tests, with the latter being used primarily by senior high school teachers with 4 or more years' experience. Few teachers graded on the curve. The most popular method of grading was a performance scale; however, this was used by less than 50% of the teachers. This survey clearly demonstrates that many teachers still use a subjective assessment of effort, sportsmanship, class attendance, and assessment of behavior to determine grades. The subjective approach was most frequently used by elementary physical education teachers, the group most likely to use no tests at all. (However,

---

Use of evaluation in Florida public school physical education programs

---

Use of tests

Skills tests	54%
Written tests	Less than 40%
Measurement model	Predominantly norm-referenced
Major users	Women teachers
	Junior high teachers
	Teachers with more experience
	Teachers with coaching responsibilities
Least frequent users	Elementary physical education teachers

Determination of grades

Bases for grading	Performance scale (less than 50%)
	Subjective assessment
Type of grade	Letter (high school)
	P-F (elementary school)

Modified from Imwold, C.H., Rider, R.A., and Johnson, D.J.

---

elementary physical education classes often meet infrequently and for short durations.) Although it has been suggested that some coaches are too involved in athletics to be conscientious about their teaching, the Florida survey showed that teachers with coaching responsibilities used more skills tests than those without these responsibilities. The evidence points to an irrefutable conclusion: A sound testing program is not a strong feature of physical education programs in the United States.

Where should the blame for this dilemma be placed? The likely culprit may appear to be the physical education teachers in the public schools. Perhaps some teachers are to blame, yet there are teachers who do use tests and use them very effectively. Before the total blame is placed hastily on teachers, the situation should be looked at from a broader perspective. King (1983) suggested that the tests available to physical education teachers are not being used because they are not appropriate for a school setting. He was not enthusiastic about these tests because most of them are norm-referenced, require too much time to administer, and often have an overly elaborate test set-up. His solution to the problem is, at least in part, to develop new types of criterion-referenced tests that have satisfactory validity and reliability and yet are practical enough to be used in schools. While there is considerable merit in King's criticisms, tests are available that are appropriate for the school setting and feasible from an administrative standpoint. However, many of these tests require the use of a special test set-up, such as a target. Taking a reasonable amount of time to prepare for testing should not be viewed as a burden but simply as a part of good teaching. Certainly teachers will come across tests that require expensive equipment their schools cannot afford. If a version of the equipment cannot be constructed or purchased by school personnel, then the test cannot be used. Also, some tests require so much time to set up that they may not be reasonable options. Yet this does not mean that all tests requiring set-up time should not be used. A test requires preplanning, organization, and preparation time.

Of course, evaluating students by observing and rating their performance is always possible. This may be an effective approach if the rating scale is well defined and can be demonstrated to be valid. Unfortunately, this approach is all too often used in the worst possible way—by merely looking at the student and jotting down a score, with no breakdown of the component of skill being rated and no assurance that the teacher is rating objectively. This is a form of *subjective evaluation* that is discussed more thoroughly later in this book.

What is the best way to begin planning your testing program once you arrive at your new school? First, review the objectives that have been agreed upon for the *total* school as well as the physical education program. Always keep in mind that you are a part of a total school system and that the physical education program should contribute to the objectives of the school. The physical education objectives may be written for the program as a whole. Then you may be expected to prepare the objectives specifically for your classes. After all, how will you know what to evaluate, if you do not know what your objectives are?

REVIEW OF DOMAINS OF BEHAVIOR

Students enrolled in a measurement and evaluation course are expected to have had experience in preparing educational objectives. This book will not attempt to replicate this process; however, a brief review of the most pertinent information about behavioral objectives is appropriate.

In a school setting, the curriculum typically includes cognitive, affective, and psychomotor objectives. Each type of objective represents a domain of behavior.

Cognitive Domain

The classification of educational objectives for the **cognitive domain** is a result of the work of Bloom and his associates (1956). These were presented in the form of a **taxonomy,** which is defined as a *classification scheme*. The taxonomy represents levels of intellectual behavior ranging from a low level (memorization of facts) to a higher level (application of these facts). The levels of the taxonomy are hierarchical, with each one building on the other(s). It is assumed that mastery of a designated level of cognitive behavior must be preceded by mastery of all lower levels. For example, to apply facts, one must be able to recall them.

This taxonomy can be used in a physical education setting to develop knowledge tests. The teacher must decide on the levels of cognitive behavior that should be mastered by the class; then objectives can be written for each level.

Affective Domain

A taxonomy for the affective domain was developed by Krathwohl and associates (1964). An *affect* is defined as an emotional behavior. The **affective domain** encompasses levels of emotional behavior, including interests, attitudes, and personality characteristics. At a low level of affective behavior, an individual may display acceptable behavior because an authority figure (e.g., teacher or parent) is present. At higher levels of affective behavior, the individual's actions are based on personal beliefs about the value of a certain response. This belief is often strongly influenced by societal standards of affective behavior. In a sports setting players are expected to maintain acceptable levels of sportsmanship. If sportsmanlike behavior occurs only when an official is nearby, the player is operating at a low level of affective behavior. If the desired behaviors are displayed consistently, regardless of the situation, a higher level has been incorporated by the player.

Psychomotor Domain

The **psychomotor domain** is of greatest interest to the readers of this textbook. Several classification schemes for motor behavior have been proposed for physical education. An excellent example of one of these schemes is a taxonomy developed by Jewett (Nixon and Jewett, 1980). Jewett's taxonomy more closely parallels the cognitive and affective schemes than any other taxonomy of motor behavior. Her categories are hierarchical and deal with process rather than content.

At low levels of psychomotor behavior, the individual perceives the components of the movement and attempts to pattern the movement based on recall or observation of a demonstration of the movement. At higher levels, emphasis is placed on creating movement designed to fit a specific situation in sport, dance, or other forms of physical activity.

Although criticisms of behavioral objectives have been numerous, emphasis on their tie to taxonomies has brought about a reexamination of teaching and learning in the classroom. As the motor domain is developed in a useful way for physical educators, a similar reexamination of what is being taught in the gymnasium should take place. This reexamination may show that a teacher spent an entire unit patterning basic skills, emphasizing a low level of motor behavior despite the fact that a number of students in class should actually be working at higher levels. If the objectives for this class were written in behavioral terms, it would be clear that either instruction ought to be modified so that all students were learning patterning skills or that objectives ought to be written to reflect actual student behavior. This type of information, when carefully analyzed, can lead to improved instruction.

PREPARING EDUCATIONAL OBJECTIVES

The process of preparing educational objectives is the first step in implementing the concept of **accountability,** that is, holding teachers in a school accountable for the results of their program. An educational objective can be defined as a statement of proposed change in the learner (Mager, 1962). This change will presumably take place as the result of planned learning experiences. When an objective is stated in terms of the performance or behavior that the student will exhibit upon successful attainment of the objective, it is referred to as a **behavioral objective.** Note that the objective refers to the behavior of the *student*. Objectives can be written in two ways: a description of the expected behavior of the teacher and a description of the expected behavior of the student. The latter type is of interest in a behavioral objective because the primary interest in education is the student's achievement. The assumption is that educators will teach in such a way that the desired results will be attained. Thus the following is the first rule of thumb in writing behavioral objectives: Incorporate the behavior the student is expected to display when the objective has been successfully met. By stating objectives in terms of student response rather than teaching material, both the student and the teacher will know precisely what to expect. Also, stating objectives in behavioral terms helps to establish evaluation procedures that relate to student performance as it has been described.

In a school setting both long-range and immediate objectives are usually identified. Long-range goals specify the behavior of a fully educated person and are by nature general. Typically these goals are first established within the school system. To learn whether students are moving toward the long-range goals, **immediate objectives** are determined that provide guidance for the selection of activities to be incorporated into a unit of instruction. These objectives can be attained in a relatively short period.

Many terms have been used to describe different types of behavioral objectives. In this book the terms *long-range goals, curriculum objectives*, and *evaluation objectives* will be used to specify three levels of objectives that establish a link between long-range goals and immediate objectives. The relationship among these levels is shown in Figure 8-1.

The first level, **long-range goals,** represents the long-term general goals of education that describe the final product of a complete education. These goals

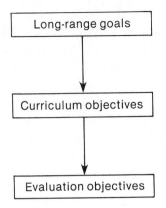

FIGURE 8-1 *Relationship among levels of objectives.*

might be a part of the overall objectives of the school or even the school system. New teachers' orientation will probably include a review of these long-range goals.

Once the long-range goals have been established, curriculum objectives are derived from these goals. This second level, **curriculum objectives,** is the reduction of the general goals into precise behaviors that reflect the terminal performance of students successfully completing an instructional unit during a course or following an entire course. Instead of stating expectations in general terms, curriculum objectives are written for specific courses or groups of courses. These objectives represent examples of ways in which the broad-based goals can be met.

At the third level **evaluation objectives** are used to describe at the unit or course level of specificity a step-by-step hierarchy, each step representing a behavior more sophisticated than the previous one. Evaluation objectives are derived from the curriculum objectives and specify the **standards of performance** that students are expected to meet after the objectives have been implemented. An essential part is the specification of a standard of performance. Usually the curriculum and evaluation objectives will have been written by the physical education staff. However, you may be responsible for writing the evaluation objectives. Notice that the evaluation objectives may not specify exactly how the skills should be measured. This may be determined either by the physical education staff as a whole or by the individual teacher. In a large high school it is not unusual for the physical education teachers to work cooperatively to develop a testing program. In an elementary school where the physical education teacher often works on a part-time basis, the testing program is usually developed by the individual teacher. Behavioral objectives become increasingly specific and require different levels of decision making.

Selection of Objectives

Covering all aspects of the physical education program within a school program is impossible; therefore, choices must be made before writing objectives. Before beginning, ask two important questions: What are the bases for the choices? Are the choices sound?

Curriculum developers often use the following information as a basis for making choices:

1. Data regarding the students themselves, their pretest abilities, knowledges, skills, interests, attitudes, and needs.
2. Data regarding the demands society is making on the graduates, opportunities and defects of contemporary society that have significance for education, and similar data.
3. Suggestions of specialists in various fields regarding the contribution they think their subjects can make to the education of students (Tyler, 1951, p. 50).

You may find these suggestions useful in writing objectives for your classes. Of course, considering this information could still lead to an excessive number of objectives, but the final choice should be based on a sound philosophy of physical education, the school's philosophy, and principles derived from motor learning. If other physical education teachers are members of the teaching staff in your school, a mutually agreeable approach to the formulation of objectives should be reached.

Decision making based on the previous information may take place at the district level, but a number of choices are still left as the daily instructional program is planned. Certainly these choices will be influenced by personal interests and values. In a soccer unit, for example, an educator must decide which skills to teach, how much time to devote to learning skills, how much time to devote to playing the game, and so on. Most teachers and coaches would agree that several soccer skills are essential to the game. Beyond these, the teacher makes choices based on personal values, interests, knowledge of course content, and level of students, as considered in the perspective of the expectations of the physical education staff within a school and the school district as a whole.

Writing one's own objectives is not always necessary. Another teacher or a staff of teachers may have written behavioral objectives for specific units of instruction in physical education, and these objectives may be suitable for you, especially as a new teacher. However, you may wish to individualize those objectives, which requires writing your own. Even if you initially use someone else's objectives, you will probably want to modify these objectives after you become a more experienced teacher. Of course, this assumes that objectives have not been predetermined for physical education within your school.

CONDUCTING A NEEDS ASSESSMENT

Once your objectives have been written in behavioral form, your expectations of students are clearly defined by the standards of performance. Setting standards is, at best, an arbitrary procedure. What if your standards are inappropriate for your students? How will you know? If the standards have been used in the school for a number of years, the other teachers have probably established that they are reasonable for the students. If not, data can be collected to assist in the preparation of objectives. It might be wise to consider conducting a *needs assessment* before writing a set of objectives. This is a process for determining the appropriateness of the objectives for the targeted group of students. Each objective has a built-in evaluation procedure. In a needs assessment, students are evaluated on each objective at the beginning of the school year. This determines their *actual* status on each objective. These results are compared with the standards already specified in the objectives, referred to as their *desired* status. If the actual status is equal to or better than the desired status, the objective should be rewritten. In other words, students should be expected to improve beyond their actual states from the beginning of the year to the end. The definition of a **needs assessment,** then, is a comparison of actual and desired states. See Figure 8-2 for a flow chart of this process.

IMPORTANCE OF ACCOUNTABILITY

If you become a physical educator, you can expect to hear a great deal about accountability in the schools. Although emphasis may be placed on the so-called basic skills of reading, writing, and so forth, the physical educator is expected to be equally accountable for the learning outcomes of his or her students. Teaching students new skill and knowledge about physical activity is not enough; you must be able to demonstrate that your students have actually accomplished these abilities at the expected level. Perhaps physical fitness is one of your major goals, and you have stressed its importance throughout the year. The important question concerns your success in emphasizing this concept by changing student behavior. Remember—it's not what *you* do but what *your students* are able to do after instruction is completed. Thus to be accountable you must show how your students have changed behavior. To do so, a testing program must be implemented. Of course, the tests you select must be feasible for a school setting. In the context of your fitness goal, although you realize a maximal stress test of cardiorespiratory function (shown in the illustration) is the most valid measure you could use, it is not realistic to consider using this test in a school. Instead, a battery of physical fitness tests might be administered at the end of the year so that changes in performance could be plotted. This information provides you with evidence that you are accountable for your work with students in their physical ed-

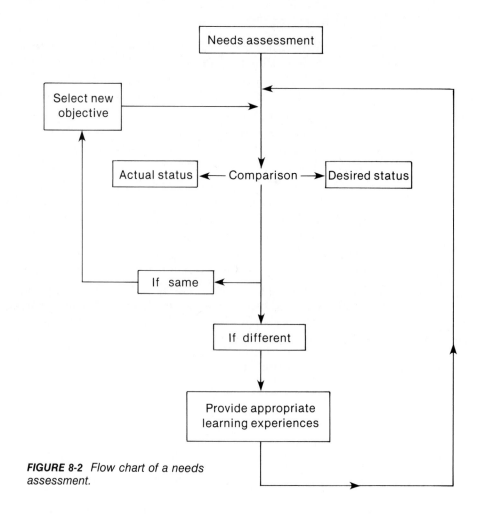

FIGURE 8-2 *Flow chart of a needs assessment.*

ucation classes. The accountability concept is not going to disappear, so expect to deal with it throughout your teaching career. Make it work for you rather than against you by planning ahead. It is difficult to demonstrate that you are accountable for your teaching when you do not think about it until the end of the year. Accountability is a sound educational concept and a reasonable job expectation. Even if communities did not demand accountability in school systems, good teachers and schools would still hold themselves accountable for their teaching.

SUMMARY

New teachers of physical education face a formidable task in planning for their classes. This includes the formulation of behavioral objectives along with evaluation procedures for each objective. Even if a set of objectives has already been

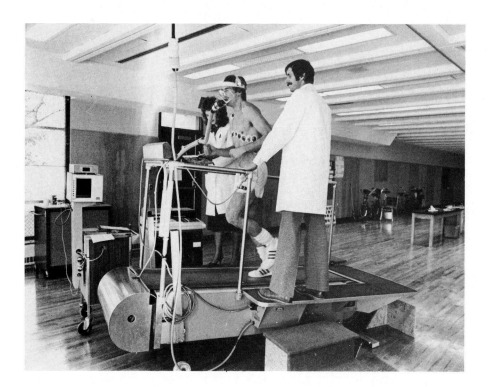

written for the physical education teachers in a school, writing more specific objectives for classes may be necessary. Of course, these must be in line with the broader objectives of physical education. A new set of objectives should be tested on students by first conducting a needs assessment. Objectives also serve as evidence of the accountability of a physical education teacher. Taxonomies of cognitive, affective, and psychomotor behavior can provide a firm basis for enhancing measurement practices as teaching experience is gained.

LEARNING EXPERIENCES

1. Choose one of your favorite sports. Select a skill and write a behavioral objective at a low level of motor behavior. Don't hesitate to use detailed descriptions. Most people are much too brief when they first begin writing behavioral objectives.
2. Form small groups in your class. Review the evaluation portion of the objectives written by members of your group. As changes are suggested, revise the objectives. Then pass your objective to someone else in another group and take someone else's objective. As a homework assignment carefully assess the evaluation portion of the objective you received from someone else. Write suggestions for improving the objective, as well as good points about it. Return the objective to the instructor at the beginning of the next class period.

3. Using the sport skill you selected in *1*, write an objective for a group of individuals operating at a high level of motor behavior. Be specific, especially in your description of the performance standard. Compare the standard with the one you described in *1*. Be sure both testing situations are clearly explained. On what basis did you determine the more difficult standard? How do you know it will not be too difficult? In other words, justify the standards you identified.

REFERENCES

Bloom, B., and others. 1956. Taxonomy of educational objectives: Handbook I: the cognitive domain. New York: David McKay Co., Inc.

Hensley, L.D., Lambert, L.T., Baumgartner, T.A., and Stillwell, J.L. 1988. Is evaluation worth the effort? Journal of Physical Education, Recreation and Dance, **59**(1):59-62.

Imwold, C.H., Rider, R.A., and Johnson, D.J. 1982. The use of evaluation in public school physical education programs. Journal of Teaching in Physical Education, **2**: 13-18.

King, H.A. 1983. Measurement and evaluation as an area of study: a plea for new perspectives. In Tipton, C.H., and Hay, J.G., editors, Specialization in physical education: the Alley legacy. Iowa City: University of Iowa.

Krathwohl, D.R., and others. 1964. Taxonomy of educational objectives: Handbook II: the affective domain. New York: David McKay Co., Inc.

Mager, R.F. 1962. Preparing instructional objectives. Palo Alto, Calif.: Fearon Publishers.

Nixon, J.E., and Jewett, A.E. 1980. An introduction to physical education, ed. 9. Philadelphia: W.B. Saunders Co.

Popham, W.J., and Baker, E.L. 1970. Establishing instructional goals. Englewood Cliffs, N.J.: Prentice-Hall, Inc.

Tyler, R.W. 1951. The functions of measurement in improving instruction. In Lindquist, E.L., editor, Educational measurement. Washington, D.C.: American Council on Education.

ANNOTATED READINGS

Bain, L.L. 1980. Program evaluation. Journal of Physical Education and Recreation **51**(2): 67-69.

Proposes a framework for program evaluation that includes both an internal and external perspective; emphasizes criterion-referenced measurement for internal evaluation and either normative or criterion-referenced measurement for external evaluation; includes an excellent summary of the total framework in chart form; discusses how to use the results to revise a physical education program.

Bayless, J.G. 1978. Conflicts and confusion over evaluation. Journal of Physical Education and Recreation, **49**(7): 54-55.

Describes a study of the evaluation of physical education programs in Oklahoma and the success of the evaluation; shows that students and physical education teachers had different perspectives of the types of evaluation taking place in class; discusses the overemphasis on dress for class, attitude, and participation in determining grades; points to the need for tests appropriate for school-age children.

Dunham, P., Jr. 1986. Evaluation for excellence: a systematic approach. Journal of Physical Education, Recreation and Dance, **57**(6): 34-36, 60.

Discusses evaluation as an integral aspect of the educational process; describes evaluation as the basis for determining the appropriateness of the curriculum, effectiveness of instructional strategies, and magnitude of student achievement; presents strategy for planning, evaluating, and implementing aspects of physical education instruction.

Gronlund, N.E. 1985. Stating objectives for classroom instruction, ed. 3. New York: Macmillan Publishing Co.

Provides a practical guide for stating instructional objectives as intended learning outcomes, then defining the objectives by student performance; presents sample objectives for all three taxonomy domains — cognitive, affective, and psychomotor; includes sample specifications for computer banking of objectives.

Jewett, A.E., and Bain, L.L. 1985. The curriculum process in physical education. Dubuque, Iowa: Wm C Brown Group.

Presents an updated version of the Jewett Purpose-Process Curriculum Framework, which encompasses the Jewett taxonomy of motor behavior; includes examples of behavioral objectives written for various levels of framework.

McCormick, J. 1988. A field experience: enhancing instruction in measurement and evaluation. Journal of Physical Education, Recreation and Dance, **59**: 27-29.

Discusses the relevance of measurement and evaluation courses in professional preparation programs in physical education; points to the need to bridge the gap between theory and practice in measurement; notes ways in which measurement and evaluation material can be made more acceptable to the practicing physical education teacher; describes a learning experience in which measurement and evaluation students administer a test battery to elementary school students.

Pflug, J. 1980. Evaluating high school coaches. Journal of Physical Education and Recreation, **51**(4): 76-77.

Describes a comprehensive, objective coaching evaluation program; provides a self appraisal by the coach, evaluation by the head coach (if an assistant coach is present) and the building athletic administrator, and a conference with the building coordinator and the district athletic director; program encompasses evaluation in five areas: administration, skills, relationships, performance, and self-improvement.

Vargas, J.S. 1982. Writing worthwhile behavioral objectives. New York: Harper & Row, Publishers Inc.

Self-instructional text; teaches students to recognize and classify behavioral objectives and to write quality objectives; presents fundamentals of writing behavioral objectives; includes examples from different subject areas and grade levels.

9 Grading

If you plan to teach physical education, you must be prepared to establish some sort of grading system as soon as you assume your first teaching position. This is not an easy task. In fact, even seasoned teachers often express dissatisfaction with the grading system they use. A **grade** is a permanent record of a student's achievement. It remains on record during and even after the lifetime of a student. Thus it is reasonable to expect teachers to think carefully about their approach to grading, making every effort to use the fairest and most objective system possible. Most prospective teachers would welcome straightforward recommendations from experienced teachers, administrators, and measurement specialists on the best grading system to use. Unfortunately, with all the advances in education, no one has developed a foolproof system of grading.

In this chapter several approaches to grading are examined, but no specific system is recommended. Each system has advantages and disadvantages that must be taken into account. Sometimes a teacher's choice of a grading system depends on his or her general philosophy about how students learn. It would be

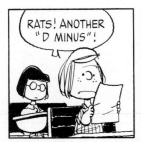
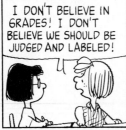
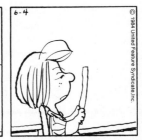
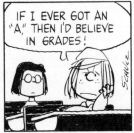

© 1984 United Feature Syndicate, Inc.

ideal if every teacher developed a grading system in this manner, but all too often an armchair approach (i.e., teacher sits in chair and determines grades subjectively) is taken in grading.

Why does grading present such a problem? Averaging a set of unit grades to calculate a final grade certainly is not difficult. It is the decision-making aspect of grading that presents the problem. What does the grade mean? Does it reflect achievement? Improvement? Attitude? How is a letter grade assigned? Is a normative approach to grading used or an approach involving mastery of a set of standards? If these questions are not carefully analyzed, inappropriate grading systems often result. Grades can vary from class to class and teacher to teacher; for example, an A in one course may be the equivalent of a C in another course of the same type. Furthermore, the grades may not be based on objective evidence. The halo effect often operates in the determination of grades. Good grades may be used as a reward and poor grades as a punishment. Teachers are human beings and can succumb to a tendency to allow a student's personality to influence his or her grade. However, this is less likely to happen if the system is formulated as objectively as possible.

An unfortunate tie has been made between grades and testing. Testing is often perceived to take place for the sole purpose of determining grades. This is one of the reasons for testing but certainly not the only one. In several other chapters measurement as an integral part of learning is discussed. Even if there were no grades, testing would be worthwhile as a means of improving performance.

The student should be informed at the beginning of a unit how the unit grade is to be determined. For older students a handout describing the grading system is helpful. If some tests are to be weighted more heavily than others, this should be noted. At the end of a unit the student should receive no surprises regarding the prearranged grading system.

One final point should be emphasized: Grades should always reflect the objectives of the course. Physical education teachers should be aware of the relationship between the initial objectives of a unit and the degree to which these objectives have been met in determining the grade. Otherwise, the basis for determining grades might be quite arbitrary. This is one of the most important concepts to remember about grading. In fact, it is one of the basic tenets of good teaching.

USE OF GRADES

Grades have many uses in the school system. They are used to inform the student of his or her status; inform parents, teachers, and administrators of the student's status; provide information for the student's permanent record; and motivate students. Even though many people dislike grades, they are a part of the

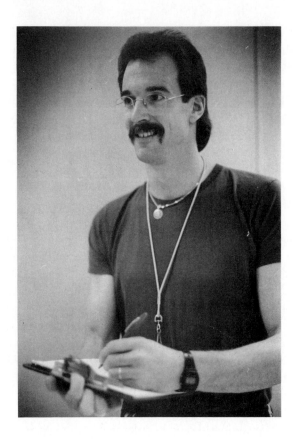

American school system. Grading, although an imperfect aspect of education, can be acceptable if the system is carefully developed and refined.

Inform Students of Status

In a physical education class where the teaching/learning process is operating efficiently, students will continually receive feedback on performance. However, at the end of a unit most students would probably benefit from some type of summary information of their achievement. A unit grade can provide this kind of information.

Inform Parents of Student's Status

Although a student may receive feedback from day to day in a physical education class, the student's grade is the major method of communication between the school and the parents. As much information as possible should be given along with the grade. For example, the major objectives of the unit might be listed along with an indication of the student's progress toward meeting them. An excellent example of a well-developed procedure for informing students of their children's fitness state is the FITNESSGRAM program. The FITNESSGRAM, described in Chapter 16, includes a student's fitness test scores and the corresponding norms, along with a brief exercise prescription for areas needing improvement. This information is printed on a computer and mailed to the child's parents.

Inform Teachers of Student's Status

Although all good teachers have a fairly concise view of the level of ability of each student, an overview of the ability of all students in the class may not be as clear. The class grades can be useful for providing this overview. They can be used to aid in the evaluation of teaching effectiveness, course content, and curriculum. A most valuable outcome of grading is to help the teacher gain a better overall understanding of the students' achievement. Information on grades can be valuable in providing future instruction to each individual in the class as well as the class as a whole.

When a teacher begins a new year with a group of new students, grades from the previous year can be used in classifying the students into groups. Previous grades can also be used in planning units of instruction. However, teachers should avoid placing total reliance on previous grades, since there will always be a margin for error in grading.

Inform Administrators of Student's Status

The student's grades are used in many ways within a school system. They provide evidence that students are either meeting or not meeting stated objectives. Grades are also used for purposes of promotion, graduation, honors, athletic eligibility, and college entrance.

Add to a Student's Permanent Record

Grades are routinely added to a student's permanent record in the administrative office and retained indefinitely, often beyond a student's lifetime. This suggests that each grade has considerable importance to the student. Teachers must understand that a casually determined grade is not only unfair to the student at the time it is given, but that it can also have a long-term negative impact.

Motivate Students

Grades are a motivational device for most students. Whether teachers like it or not, students' motivation is often to do whatever is needed to receive a satisfactory grade. If the process of grading improves learning in the desired direction, deriving motivation from grades is not necessarily bad. In this context, working for a grade may not be undesirable.

DETERMINING A FINAL UNIT GRADE

Measurement specialists in physical education agree that one important basis for determining a grade is achievement in one or more aspects of motor performance. These can include sports skills, playing ability, and physical fitness. Specialists also generally agree that the achievement of cognitive skills (including knowledge and understanding of the principles and mechanics of movement, safety, conditioning, history, and so forth) should be graded, although perhaps to a lesser extent. The predominant area of disagreement is whether a physical education grade should be based, in part, on the student's affective behavior (including social behaviors such as effort, attitude, sportsmanship, and citizenship). Whether all three areas—motor, cognitive, and affective—should be considered in determining a grade is largely a matter of philosophy. Whether all three areas can be measured with sufficient objectivity to justify contributing to the determination of a grade is another matter.

Achievement in Motor Skills as a Basis for Grading

Many physical educators believe that the achievement of skill and ability in physical education should receive the greatest emphasis in grading. The type of achievement expected depends on the objectives of the unit. In a beginning class, emphasis may be placed on skill development, whereas in an intermediate class, skill development and playing ability may be equally stressed.

One objective of many physical education programs is the development of physical fitness. Assessment of the level of fitness of students in these programs should be incorporated into their final grade. It might be informative to separate the fitness grade from the unit grades that are given throughout the year. Hanson (1967) suggests using several criteria rather than a single standard of fitness because there are individual differences in body build. These differences may be partially taken into account by using tables of norms adjusted for body weight, particularly for measures of muscular strength and endurance.

Another objective is the development of sports skills. An A in tennis should mean the student can play tennis well, considering the level of ability of the students in the course.

Improvement in Motor Skills as a Basis for Grading

When a student's performance improves over a given period of time, we assume that learning has taken place, although performance and learning are not synonymous. Intuitively, it seems highly desirable to use improvement as one means of determining a student's grade. After all, a teacher may reason, isn't the fact that improvement took place more important than the final level of achievement? This seems plausible to many physical education teachers. Obviously stu-

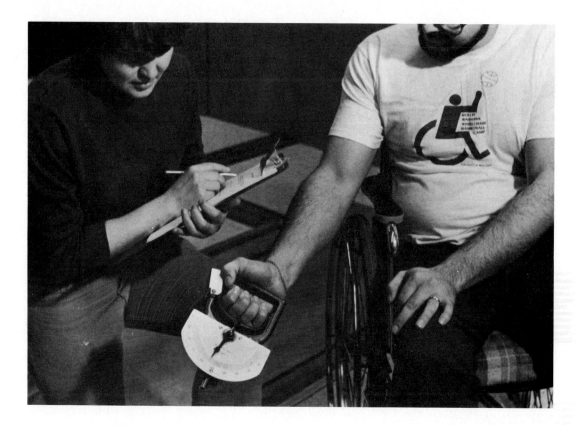

dents hope to improve, and teachers want them to do so. The difficulty lies in attempting to use improvement as a basis for grading. Several problems are associated with the measurement of improvement—unreliability of improvement scores, inequality of scale units, and difficulty in motivating students during the first testing session.

In the first place, how is improvement usually determined? Usually a test is administered at the beginning and at the end of a unit. The pretest score is subtracted from the posttest score to yield an improvement score. Unfortunately, an improvement score calculated this way has been shown to be notably unreliable. This is a well established fact. There is a degree of unreliability associated with both the pretest and posttest scores. The measurement error associated with each of these tests is compounded in the improvement score.

Furthermore, the amount of improvement a student can attain depends on his or her initial level of skill. This is referred to as inequality of scale units. The highly skilled person cannot be expected to improve as much as the poorly skilled because there is less room for improvement at higher levels of performance. For example, an improvement of 4 seconds on the 1-mile run has a different meaning for a world-class runner than it does for a novice runner, even though the numerical value of the improvement score (4 seconds) is the same for each performer. If the world-class runner's time improved from 4:11 to 4:07, it would represent a significant improvement. On the other hand, a change in the novice runner's time from 8:11 to 8:07 might have little or no practical significance. Decreasing one's running time by 4 seconds is easy if the time is initially slow. In addition, a child's performance on a test of physical performance may improve simply because he or she has grown older and become more mature physically during the time period between the pretest and the posttest. For example, as a child grows taller and heavier, throwing a ball farther or jumping a longer distance is possible as a result of the maturation factor. In other words, little or no actual improvement due to learning might have taken place.

One procedure developed for measuring improvement in physical education shows promise. Hale and Hale (1972) used a mathematical procedure to transform test scores so that improvement at a low level of performance is not weighted as heavily as the same amount of improvement at a higher level of performance. This procedure, in its simplest form, requires the standardization of initial and final test scores by converting them to T-scores. In some cases, tables of T-scores are published for skills tests; otherwise, the teacher can easily develop such a table, as described in Chapter 3. Once the raw scores have been transformed to T-scores, a conversion table (see Table 9-1) is used to determine each student's progression score. The progression score representing the initial score is subtracted from the progression score for the final test score.

As an example, consider the pretest and the posttest scores of two students in a bowling class, as shown in Table 9-2. Student A bowled an average of 90 during the testing period at the beginning of the unit and an average of 120 during the posttest period. These scores were converted to T-scores of 30 and 50, respectively. Using these T-scores and referring to the conversion table in Table 9-1, subtract the progression score for a T-score of 30 (3.99) from the progression score for a T-score of 50 (10.05). The improvement score for Student A was 6.06. Note that the raw gain was 30 points, the T-score gain was 20 units, and the actual improvement score was 6.06.

Student B, on the other hand, bowled an average of 170 during initial testing and 180 during final testing. In this case the raw gain was 10 points and the T-score gain (70-75) was 5 units. If these students had been graded on their raw gain scores, Student A would have received a higher grade than Student B; yet, in terms of actual performance, B's improvement may be equal to or better than A's. When the conversion table was used to calculate B's improvement score, the score was 6.57, slightly higher than A's score.

Even though the application of this procedure yields more valid improvement scores, there are problems with this approach. The exponential equations

TABLE 9-1 *Conversion of T-scores to progression scores*

T-score	Progression score	T-score	Progression score	T-score	Progression score
20	2.52	40	6.34	60	15.94
21	2.64	41	6.65	61	16.70
22	2.76	42	6.95	62	17.48
23	2.89	43	7.27	63	18.31
24	3.03	44	7.62	64	19.16
25	3.17	45	7.98	65	20.09
26	3.32	46	8.35	66	21.03
27	3.48	47	8.75	67	22.02
28	3.64	48	9.16	68	23.07
29	3.81	49	9.60	69	24.14
30	3.99	50	10.05	70	25.29
31	4.18	51	10.52	71	26.46
32	4.38	52	11.03	72	27.72
33	4.59	53	11.54	73	29.09
34	4.80	54	12.09	74	30.42
35	5.03	55	12.66	75	31.86
36	5.26	56	13.25	76	33.37
37	5.51	57	13.87	77	34.92
38	5.77	58	14.53	78	36.58
39	6.05	59	15.23	79	38.31
				80	40.13

From Hale, P.W., and Hale, R.M.

TABLE 9-2 *Example of Hale and Hale (1972) method*

Student	Pretest score	T-score	Posttest score	T-score	Progression score
A	90	30	120	50	6.06
B	170	70	180	75	6.57

used to convert scores to progression scores are not necessarily an accurate reflection of actual changes in performance. Although the transformation represents a rough adjustment of scores that appear to be conceptually sound, there is no scientific evidence supporting this particular exponential equation over others. For a more detailed analysis of the problems in measuring change, refer to

Schutz (1989). PROGRAM CHANGE, a refinement of the Hale and Hale procedure, was programmed for the Apple IIe by East (1985) and is included in Appendix E.

Another problem associated with grading on improvement is commonly known as *sandbagging*. If it is common knowledge that final grades are to be based on improvement, some students may deliberately perform at a low level of skill on the pretest when they are capable of obtaining higher test scores. By obtaining a low pretest score, greater improvement will be reflected in the pretest-posttest score comparison at the end of the unit.

Hanson (1967) noted that if improvement is to occur, adequate time must be allowed for it. Some students need to practice over long periods to improve. Instructional units in physical education are often scheduled for 6 weeks or less; therefore there may not be adequate time for improvement. For example, expecting students to hit 8 out of 10 free throws successfully after only a 6-week basketball unit may be unrealistic.

Finally, emphasizing the student's improvement score does not conceal the true achievement level. If a student's performance is poor compared to others in class, it will be obvious. Grading on improvement, although desirable, should probably be minimized until more appropriate ways are developed to handle improvement scores.

Development of Cognitive Skills as a Basis for Grading

There is general agreement that knowledge of the course content of the instructional unit in physical education should be part of the final grade. Understanding the principles and mechanics of movement, along with the application of these principles to specific activities, are among the most important cognitive skills. Lower-level cognitive skills such as knowledge of rules and strategies of a sport can also be used in determining grades. Other cognitive skills that might be measured are safety factors, history of the sport, and principles of conditioning.

Development of Affective Skills as a Basis for Grading

Grades based on affective skills are determined by factors such as attitude, attendance, sportsmanship, effort, dress, and, in some instances, whether a student showers after participating in a physical education class. Unfortunately, these factors constitute the major part of the grade in some physical education classes, even though their assessment is generally unreliable and frequently punitive. They are often considered a reflection of attitude; that is, if a student's attitude is good, he or she will attend class, be a good sport, try hard, wear the proper clothes, and shower after class. The measurement of some of these factors is highly subjective, often bringing into play the halo effect. Moreover, an overemphasis on affective behavior often leads to neglect of cognitive and motor skills. Furthermore, the presence of the desired affective skills in no way guarantees achievement in motor skills or understanding movement. On the other hand, we must recognize that some physical education teachers use these factors in determining grades in an attempt to deal with student apathy or disciplinary problems. Although these are genuine concerns and must be dealt with in some way, grades may not be the best or most appropriate alternative. Of greater importance is that grades based only on these factors are not valid. Let's examine more closely a few of the affective skills that are often used in determining a grade.

Attendance According to a report by Mathews (1958), in 80% of the schools to which 50 student teachers were assigned, grades were based solely on students being present and in uniform daily. Since that time, the observation by Mathews has been verified in a number of surveys. Generally, the factors on which a grade is based depend on the course objectives. Is regular attendance a course objective, or is it a matter of school policy? Attendance is usually governed by school policy, and deviant behavior related to attendance is dealt with by the principal or other designated authorities.

The practice of grading has sometimes been justified by the view that a student cannot learn when not in class. If, however, the student is able to meet the course objectives satisfactorily, his or her grade should not be reduced because of poor attendance. Certainly disciplinary action should be taken against a student who is in school but does not attend class. Whether this action comes from the principal or the teacher, however, punishment should never take the form of reducing a grade.

As Cotten and Cotten (1985) aptly noted, grades should never be used as a weapon for dealing with behaviors and attitudes. Grades should be based on objectives. Does an A in history mean the student displayed a good attitude in the history class? Obviously, the answer is *no*.

Effort Effort is extremely difficult to evaluate. Does a student who performs well with seemingly little effort work less than the student with less skill who obviously works hard? Can a teacher judge the amount of effort displayed by an individual based on facial expression or how tired he or she looks? If part of the grade is based on effort, it must be evaluated with a reasonable degree of objectivity. A physical education teacher may genuinely feel effort can be judged adequately using subjective judgment, but personal values will probably interfere. Usually we assume that effort is reflected in achievement. However, if the achievement level is unchanged, is the effort meaningful? If effort is so important that it is part of the course objective, a procedure should be developed to objectively and systematically measure this affective skill.

Dress and Showers The need for gym clothes appropriate for physical education classes is obvious; however, the practice of grading on uniforms is questionable. In fact, few schools in the United States now require uniforms for physical education. However, most students are expected to change into clothing suitable for participation in physical activity. If the student has dirty gym clothes, or no gym clothes at all, a penalty is appropriate, although not in the form of lowering an achievement grade.

No longer do a majority of physical education programs require students to take a shower at the end of class. In settings where this is still a practice, the requirement should be controlled by departmental policy. What represents a satisfactory shower? A wet body? Wetness on some part of the body? Some teachers think that showering is an important enough health habit to be graded. Some believe that it reflects a positive attitude. Explaining the importance of showers to students and encouraging them to take showers regularly is not unreasonable, yet grading the student on showers is no assurance that the value will become ingrained. Whether showers are mandatory or not, grades should not be based on them.

Sportsmanship Every physical education teacher hopes to implant in students values associated with good sportsmanship. The development and encouragement of habits reflecting good sportsmanship are basic to all physical education programs, yet this is a difficult affective trait to measure. The measurement of good sportsmanship is often haphazard and unreliable. If this affective skill is to be graded, the teacher should systematically record incidents of behavior for each student that reflect varying degrees of sportsmanship in a class situation. Although this process may be unrealistic because of the time involved, this is the only way to reduce the effect of the teacher's personal values on such judgments. (For more details, see Chapter 22).

Comments In a 1982 survey of the use of evaluation by physical education teachers, many teachers still used a subjective assessment of effort, sportsmanship, class attendance, and assessment of behavior to determine grades (Imwold, Rider, and Johnson, 1982). The subjective approach was used most frequently by elementary physical education teachers, the group most likely to use no tests at all. While it might be desirable to include information on the child's behavior on the report form, an assessment of achievement should not be ignored. In fact, achievement of skills and abilities should be the primary focus of a report form. "If the teacher . . . has used the grade as a disciplinary tool, to enforce class policies, or to reflect anything other than final achievement in the course, the grade will be deceptive and misleading" (Cotten and Cotten, 1985, p. 53).

NORM-REFERENCED APPROACH TO GRADING

In general, a norm-referenced test (see Chapter 1) is used to detect individual differences among examinees. Grades can also be determined in a norm-referenced context by considering a student's performance relative to others in class. This system is based on the normal probability curve. If letter grades of A, B, C,

D, and F are used, the curve is divided into five sections with each section representing a letter grade. As you know from reading the statistics chapters in this book, the entire area under the curve equals 100%. If the curve is divided into sections, the area in each section represents a certain percentage of the whole, and the sum of the percentages across all sections would equal 100%. When you use a norm-referenced system of grading, your primary task is to identify the areas under the curve that will represent each grade and their corresponding percentages.

In the following section, two methods of norm-referenced grading are described—the **standard deviation method** and the **percentage method.** Although all the examples use five grade categories (representing A, B, C, D, and F), any number of grade categories could be used in the same way. Note that this type of grading is sometimes referred to as *grading on the curve* and criticized as being unfair to students. The criticism need not be true if the grade categories are properly determined. They should, for example, be based on a large number of students, not merely on one or two classes. This issue is examined in the next section.

Standard Deviation Method

You have just given a test to a group of students, and now you wish to assign a grade to each test score. The standard deviation method is based on the standard deviation of the distribution of scores. Thus the first step is to calculate the mean and the standard deviation of the test scores, then divide the distribution into five sections using the standard deviation values. For example, in Table 9-3, note the area of the curve that is 1.5 standard deviations above the mean or higher. All scores falling in this area would receive a grade of A. Let's assume a test has a mean of 60 and a standard deviation of 8. Using Table 9-3, a score of 72 (mean plus 1.5 standard deviations = 60 + 12 = 72) or higher would receive an A. Scores ranging from 71 to 64 (mean plus 0.5 standard deviation = 60 + 4 = 64) would receive a B, and so forth.

TABLE 9-3 *Example of the standard deviation method of grading*

Grade	Standard(s) deviation range	Percent
A	1.5s or more above mean	7
B	Between +0.5s and +1.5s	24
C	Between +0.5s and −0.5s	38
D	Between −0.5s and −1.5s	24
F	1.5s or more below the mean	7

The score ranges for each grade are given below:

A	72 and above
B	64 – 71
C	56 – 63
D	48 – 55
F	47 and below

Go through the calculations for the C, D, and F grade ranges to verify these figures.

The following steps summarize this approach to grading:

1. Calculate the mean and standard deviation of the set of test scores. Assume these values are obtained: $\overline{X} = 64$ and $s = 8$.
2. Using Table 9-3, determine the range for a grade of A. Using the mean +1.5 standard deviations:

$$64 + 1.5(8) = 76$$

A student scoring 76 or above would receive an A on the test.

3. Determine the range for a grade of B. To obtain the upper score in the range, subtract 1 from the lower score in the A range (76), $76 - 1 = 75$. For the lower score in the B range, calculate the mean +.5 standard deviation:

$$64 + .5(8) = 68$$

Students scoring from 68 to 75 would receive a grade of B.

4. Determine the range for a grade of C. For the upper score in the range, subtract 1 from the lower score in the range for B (68), $68 - 1 = 67$. For the lower end of the C range, calculate the mean −.5 standard deviation:

$$64 - .5(8) = 60$$

The range for a grade of C is 60 to 67.

5. For a grade of D, calculate the scores for −.5s to −1.5s. For the upper score in the range, subtract 1 from the lower score in the C range(60), $60 - 1 = 59$. For the lower score, calculate the mean −1.5 standard deviations.

$$64 - 1.5(8) = 52$$

The range for a grade of D is 52 – 59.

6. A grade of F can be determined by subtracting 1 from the lower score in the D range (52), $52 - 1 = 51$. A student scoring 51 or below would receive an F on the test.

7. Lay out the entire scale for convenient usage:

A = 76 and above
B = 68 − 75
C = 60 − 67
D = 52 − 59
F = 51 and below

Note that we calculated the mean and standard deviation for a group of students in the above example. However, the group might consist of only 30 or 40 people. Because the number is so small, the distribution of scores might be badly distorted. Thus it is best to accumulate scores from several classes, even if it takes a year or more to do so. The grade categories can be determined from this larger data set, since we have more faith in categories based on a distribution of this size. In subsequent classes, you only need convert scores to letter grades using the grade ranges calculated from the large distribution of scores. Don't be concerned if the percentage of students in each category differs from the percentages in the Table 9-3. Remember that the table is meant to be applied to a large sample. Your small sample may fluctuate because of the small numbers, but nothing at all is wrong with this.

This method is similar to the **standard score method.** In this approach, the raw score is converted to a standard score; otherwise, the procedure is identical to the one described in this section. Actually, the example in Table 9-3 can be viewed as the standard score method. Consider the grade of A, for example. The number 1.5 preceding a score can be referred to as a z-score.

An advantage of this system is that scores for all tests are transformed to a common scale. For example, assume two tests are administered in a basketball unit. One test measures dribbling skill and is scored in seconds. The other is a shooting test, scored according to the number of successful shots in a given time period. By using standard score units, the same grading standard can be used for each test even though their actual score units are different. For each test a score falling at or above +1.5 standard deviation would receive an A, following the example shown in Table 9-3. In this way scores can be directly compared from test to test, then the grades can be averaged to determine a final grade.

A disadvantage of the system is that students set the standard. Not all classes are typical, yet some students in each class will receive As and some will receive Fs. This problem is reduced by using a large data set to determine the scale. This is the most reliable of any grading system. The standard deviation method can be used in physical education classes for grading cognitive skills (Weber and Paul, 1971), as well as sports skills and other forms of physical activity (Barrow and McGee, 1980; Broer, 1959).

TABLE 9-4 *Examples of the percentage method of grading*

Grade	Example 1	Example 2	Example 3
A	7	10	15
B	24	20	20
C	38	40	30
D	24	20	20
F	7	10	15

When this approach to grading is used, the test with the greatest variability will automatically be weighted most heavily. For example, a test that is twice as variable as another is weighted twice as much. The variability of each test, then, must be taken into account when developing a system of weights.

Percentage Method

In the percentage method of grading, grade categories are assigned by designating the percentage of students who are to receive each grade. For instance, a teacher might decide to give As to the top 10% of the students, as shown in Example 2 in Table 9-4. If the percentages in this table are based on a large sample of students, this method is no different from the standard deviation method. The percentages in Example 1 will divide distributions of test scores at the same (or very close to) standard deviation points (z-scores), as shown in Table 9-3. If the method is used with sets of test scores from one small class, comparing the grades of different tests may not be feasible because of fluctuations that can occur with small samples. Only three varieties of the percentage method of grading are presented in Table 9-4, although many other varieties are possible.

The following steps summarize the use of the percentage method of grading:

1. Determine the percentage of students who should receive each grade on a test. For example, consider the following grades and percentages:

A	10%
B	20%
C	40%
D	20%
E	10%

2. Rank the raw scores on a test from highest to lowest. Note the sample data set in Table 9-5.
3. Determine the number of students receiving each grade:

TABLE 9-5 *Modified pull-ups scores*

Student	No. of pull-ups	Grade
1	25	A
2	24	
3	23	B
4	23	
5	22	
6	22	
7	22	C
8	21	
9	21	
10	20	
11	17	
12	16	
13	15	
14	15	
15	14	D
16	13	
17	13	
18	12	
19	9	F
20	3	

A	10% of 20 = 2
B	20% of 20 = 4
C	40% of 20 = 8
D	20% of 20 = 4
F	10% of 20 = 2

4. Assign grades to ranked scores, as shown in the right side of the table.

Which Method to Use?

Which method of norm-referenced grading is preferred—the standard deviation method or the percentage method? If the grade categories are determined using a large sample of students, either approach will lead to similar results. They merely approach the same problem from different directions. When the categories are used with small classes, the percentages of students in each category are not necessarily identical to those in Tables 9-3 or 9-4. This is not a problem as we expect it to occur with small sample fluctuations. The major decision to be made is whether to use a norm-referenced or criterion-referenced approach to grading. Sometimes this is a policy dictated by the school, rather than a decision to be made by individual teachers.

CRITERION-REFERENCED APPROACH TO GRADING

How is a criterion-referenced approach to grading applied? First of all, recall that a criterion-referenced measure is a type of measure in which a standard of performance is identified that is referenced to a criterion behavior. This is a seemingly simple definition but defines a decidedly complex process. Once the performance standard is set, students scoring at or above the standard are given a grade (for instance, Pass) and those scoring below the standard are given another grade (Fail). However, as discussed earlier, school systems use a five-point grading scale. Using the criterion-referenced approach, this means that we have to identify four cutoff points or performance standards to obtain five grade categories.

Percentage-Correct Method

In the section on norm-referenced grading, the determination of grade categories based on the percentage of students in a given category is discussed. Here we will review a method where the percentage of items or trials successfully completed (**percentage-correct method**) is used to determine grade categories. (See Table 9-6). To receive an A on a test, the student would have to successfully complete 90% of the trials. In other words, for a 10-trial test, 9 out of 10 trials (or 18 out of 20 for a 20-trial test) must be properly executed. For a 100-item written test, 90 out of 100 items would have to be answered correctly.

It may be necessary to use a point system rather than percentages to designate grade categories, especially when there is no maximum score. For example, in a softball throw for distance, the maximum score for a given age group is unknown. In this case, a distance of x feet or greater could be set for the category for a grade of A. However, grades cannot be directly compared across tests,

---

TABLE 9-6 *Example of percentage-correct method of grading*

Grade	Percentage-correct score
A	90-100
B	80-89
C	70-79
D	60-69
F	Below 60

since the level of difficulty of each test will vary. This is readily apparent in testing muscular endurance, where different levels of endurance may be observed across muscle groups.

Setting Performance Standards for Grading

How are performance standards set? Let's go back to the definition of criterion-referenced measurement. It specifies that the performance standard must be referenced to a criterion behavior. In Chapter 7, the cutoff score of 42 sit-ups for 14 to 15-year-old girls was discussed in terms of a criterion behavior. Does the ability to perform 42 sit-ups mean that a 14- or 15-year-old girl has adequate abdominal strength? Of course there is no evidence to support such a statement. We know that only 25% of the girls in this age group can perform more than 42 sit-ups in 1 minute, but this is a norm-referenced rather than a criterion-referenced statement. As you can see, proper standard setting is very difficult.

With this seemingly insoluble problem in determining a cutoff score, why discuss the criterion-referenced approach to grading? Primarily because teachers who use the mastery learning model of instruction feel it is a more appropriate method for establishing grades than the norm-referenced approach. In the mastery learning model, there are no constraints on the number of students who can satisfactorily meet an objective. Thus there are no limits on the number of students who receive A's, B's, and so forth. This means the grade distribution for a class is not determined in advance. This is not true when the normal distribution is used in determining norm-referenced grades. Regardless of the ability level of the students, some will receive A's, B's, and so forth, according to a predetermined categorization of the distribution. Of course, as noted on p. 183, the grade distribution in an ordinary class is not necessarily the same as the distribution for a large sample used to determine the categories. Nonetheless, this approach is designed to reflect individual differences in ability, and it should be expected that the entire grade range will be represented in any class.

In a mastery learning setting, the teacher typically expects his or her class to consist of nonmasters at the beginning of the year. When students are measured on an objective at this point, the distribution of scores should be skewed in a positive direction, since most of the students should receive low scores and only a small percentage should receive high scores. At the end of the unit of instruction, the majority of the students are expected to master the skill. Now the students' scores on this objective are distributed negatively, since only a few students receive low scores. It is possible that many students would receive A's and B's. Once a letter grade has been determined for each test administered during the unit, the unit grade is calculated in the usual manner. Each letter grade is converted to a numerical value, weighted according to its importance, and the weighted grades are then averaged to yield a unit grade.

TABLE 9-7 *Table for converting letter grades to numbers*

Grade	Number	Grade	Number
A+	12	C	5
A	11	C−	4
A−	10	D+	3
B+	9	D	2
B	8	D−	1
B−	7	F	0
C+	6		

Another advantage of the criterion-referenced approach to grading is that repeated testing of the student in a formative evaluation context is encouraged. The disadvantages of criterion-referenced grading are associated with setting standards. First of all, it is an arbitrary process. However, this does not sanction careless standard setting. Every effort must be made to reduce the degree of subjectivity in setting standards. Several solutions to this problem were discussed in Chapter 7. The second disadvantage of criterion-referenced grading is the problem of misclassifications. In classifying students in different grade categories, it is evident that sometimes we will be wrong. Sometimes a student will be given a C and should have been given a B, and vice versa. This is a measurement problem that may never be fully resolved, yet the probability of misclassifications can be reduced as the validity of the cutoff score is increased. (See Chapter 7 for more information on procedures for determining validity.)

CALCULATING FINAL GRADES

Once letter grades have been assigned to each test, they must be converted to numbers to calculate the final grade. The conversion table given in Table 9-7 exemplifies the finest breakdown a teacher could possibly need for grade conversion. If desired, the scale can easily be reduced to a smaller size. Some teachers prefer to use a point system whereby test scores are not assigned to a letter grade. The total points for each test are accumulated and weighted accordingly; grade categories are then developed and a letter grade assigned to each. To use this approach, the test scales must be compatible. For example, it would be inappropriate to add time scores (in seconds) and distance scores (in inches). This is a valid way to determine a final grade and does not require a series of conversions from test score to letter grade to letter grade conversion, and so forth. Furthermore, averaging letter grades may result in a loss of precision compared with averaging raw test scores. On the other hand, raw scores often must be converted to standard scores, as test scales are frequently not compatible.

TABLE 9-8 *Use of weights in determining grades*

Badminton unit for beginners			
Test	Weight	Grade	Total

Skill development
    Short serve
    Long serve
    Overhead clear
	3	B−	3 × 7 = 21

Development of knowledges
    Knowledge of rules
    Knowledge of principles
	2	C	2 × 5 = 10

Playing ability	1 — 6	B+	1 × 9 = 9 40

Grade = 40/6 = 6.67 = B−

AVERAGING LETTER GRADES

Averaging letter grades is a simple way to determine a final grade. Some tests will be of greater importance than others in a given unit, therefore many teachers use a system of *weighting* the tests. If the scores of each test are averaged using a transformation and the tests are similar in difficulty level, each test automatically receives the same weight. A teacher assigns higher weights to tests of greater importance. If one test is twice as important as another, a 2:1 ratio of weights might be used, as shown in Table 9-8. The knowledge test is given a weight of 2, while the test of playing ability is weighted 1. Note that skill development in badminton is weighted more heavily than any other ability. This is appropriate if skill development received the greatest emphasis in the instructional unit.

Three letter grades are shown in Table 9-8. Using the conversion Table 9-7, we can determine the numerical value for each letter grade. For example, the numerical value for the skills grade of B− is 7. The weight for skill development (3) is multiplied by the numerical value for B− (7), yielding a total of 21. Follow this procedure for each component to be used in determining the final grade, then add the total points for the components (40) and divide by the sum of the weights (6). In this case, the average numerical grade is 6.67, which should be rounded off to a 7. Referring to Table 9-7, notice that the letter grade for a numerical grade of 7 is B−. (It is merely coincidental that the final grade is the same as the grade for the skill development test.)

AVERAGING T-SCORES

Test scores can also be converted to standard scores (e.g., T-scores) and averaged to determine final grades. This provides a finer distinction among students in calculating grades, as two students who receive the same grade on a test will not necessarily receive the same standard score. The standard scores can be weighted in the same way letter grades are weighted.

The following steps summarize the use of T-scores to determine a final grade:

1. Convert the raw scores on each test to T-scores. Tables can be developed to make these conversions, as described in Chapter 3. An even simpler method is the use of the T-score microcomputer program presented in the appendix.

2. Establish a grading scale for the averaged T-score values. For example:

A	65 and above
B	55-64
C	45-54
D	35-44
F	34 and below

3. At the end of the grading period, sum the T-scores for each student and average them. Weights may be used, as shown below:

Test	T-score	Weight	Total
1	55	2	110
2	70	1	70
3	40	2	80
4	47	3	141
5	62	1	62
6	50	1	50
		10	513

Grade = 513/10 = 51.3 or C

USING THE MICROCOMPUTER TO CALCULATE FINAL GRADES

A program to calculate final grades, either using letter grades or total points, has been written for the Apple IIe computer; however, it can easily be modified for other brands of microcomputers. This program is described in Chapter 5 and included in its entirety in Appendix E (2). It can be used with or without a printer, although the availability of a printer allows a printed copy of each student's name, individual grades, and final grade to be obtained.

OTHER SYSTEMS OF GRADING

Educators have used many other systems of grading, including pass-fail grading and a checklist of objectives.

Pass-Fail Method

Physical educators sometimes prefer the use of a two-grade category, such as **pass-fail** or mastery-nonmastery, so that the students' attempts to achieve for the sake of a grade will be reduced. In addition, this method is thought to reduce the error that occurs when attempting to classify students into a five-grade category. According to the literature, two-grade categories are less reliable than their five-grade category counterparts. This may be true if a norm-referenced approach is used to estimate reliability. However, when a criterion-referenced reliability estimate is computed, a two-category grade system can be quite reliable. On the other hand, the larger the number of grade categories, the more information is available about the students in a class. A two-category system is simply not as discriminatory as a more elaborate system, although a more elaborate system will yield a larger number of misclassifications. When a misclassification occurs, it is more serious in the two-category case. In other words, giving a student a grade of C when the grade should have been a B is a serious matter, but not nearly as severe as giving the student a Fail when he or she should have received a Pass.

Checklist of Objectives

A grading system commonly used at the elementary school level is a system of symbols that can be used with a list of major objectives of the program (**checklist of objectives**). The following symbols might be used to rate each objective:

O (Outstanding)
S (Satisfactory)
N (Needs improvement)

The appropriate symbol is placed next to each objective in the list. This system of marking is exemplified in Table 9-9.

The student's report card will probably not have adequate space to list the major objectives for each class; therefore, the physical education teacher may wish to send a letter containing more detailed information to the parents of each child or develop a special report card for physical education. An example of a complete report card used in elementary physical education in Madison, Wisconsin, is shown in Figure 9-1. This report includes an evaluation of specific objectives as well as an overall assessment of the child's performance.

An excellent way of reporting the student's fitness status is the use of the FITNESSGRAM, depicted in Chapter 16. A report can be prepared for children and youth 5 through 17+ years of age.

TABLE 9-9 *Sample checklist of objectives for elementary school physical education*

Symbol	Objective
S	Ability to move at different speeds, using different levels.
S	Ability to handle various sizes of balls in a variety of ways.
N	Ability to use a variety of locomotor patterns.

MADISON METROPOLITAN SCHOOL DISTRICT

PUPIL _____

TEACHER _____

SCHOOL _____

GRADE LEVEL _____

Physical Education

Semester
1   2

Achievement: [ ]   [ ]

EXPLANATION OF SYMBOLS

ACHIEVEMENT

E – EXCELLENT

V – VERY GOOD

S – SATISFACTORY

N – NEEDS IMPROVEMENT

PROGRESS

1 Consistent

2 Improving

3 Inconsistent

4 Having difficulty

X Does not apply at this time

MOVEMENT UNDERSTANDINGS
Progress

Semester
1 2

• Understands effects of exercise
• Understands simple strategies applied to game settings
• Understands basic movement concepts

Additional Information as needed:

WORK HABITS
Progress

Semester
1 2

• Listens and follows directions
• Works well independently
• Works well with others
• Participates readily (effort, enthusiasm)
• Respects rights and feelings of others
• Stays on task
• Makes appropriate decisions and choices
• Dresses appropriately for activity

Additional Information as needed:

NOTE TO PARENTS: Each skill listed can be performed at different levels of difficulty and with varying degrees of quality. Your child's progress is evaluated through skills and learning experiences considered developmentally appropriate at grade level.

MOVEMENT SKILLS
Progress

Semester
1 2

• Performs all types of foot locomotion (walk, hop, skip, etc.)
• Controls application of force in throwing, striking, kicking
• Controls absorption of force in catching and fielding
• Uses space effectively
• Maintains balance and control in quick starts and stops
• Uses a variety of body parts to support, hold or transfer own body weight
• Maintains a steady even rhythm
• Responds to rhythmic patterns with appropriate body movements
• Uses movement to express ideas and feelings
• Creates combinations of movements and repeats them in order
• Shows control and flow in combining movements
• Sustains prolonged physical activity (endurance)
• Demonstrates muscle strength appropriate to movement task
• Demonstrates joint flexibility appropriate to movement task

Additional Information as needed:

FIGURE 9-1 Sample report form for elementary physical education.

USE OF INSTITUTIONAL GRADES

Measurement specialists unanimously recommend the use of a common grading system throughout a school. When a common grading system is used, the grades will form a similar distribution, regardless of the area of instruction. In addition the reliability of the grading system is somewhat increased. The same kind of information is provided for students in all areas of the curriculum. Special areas, such as physical education, should use grades to discriminate to the same degree as other parts of the curriculum so that excellence in performance is recognized in all areas.

REPORTING MULTIPLE GRADES

A procedure for reporting more than one grade for each curricular area is often recommended so that one of the grades can be based purely on achievement. Frequently a second grade is classified as a "citizenship" grade. In physical education, separating motor skill grades from cognitive and affective grades would also provide useful information for all concerned. Although such a separation is somewhat artificial, the use of multiple grades will have more meaning than a single grade.

SUMMARY

Grades in physical education should represent the degree to which students have attained the objectives of the curricular units. These often include the development of motor, cognitive, and affective skills within the physical education program. There is general agreement that the achievement of sports skills and other forms of physical activity should be given major emphasis in determining a physical education grade. Cognitive skills may be given less weight but nonetheless represent an important component of the grade. Although grading the affective behavior of students is intuitively appealing, it is difficult to measure these skills objectively and systematically.

Two systems of grading for physical education students are the norm-referenced method and the criterion-referenced method. The normal distribution is the basis for determining grade categories in the norm-referenced approach. Of primary interest is the student's performance relative to others in class. The criterion-referenced method of grading designates grade categories based on predetermined performance standards. This method is tied to the mastery learning instructional method, where many students are expected to meet minimal standards at the end of a unit. Either system can be used effectively in a school setting. The choice of a grading system is dependent on the philosophy of teaching and learning adopted by the instructional staff.

LEARNING EXPERIENCES

1. A test was administered to five beginning badminton classes. The mean for the set of test scores is 32 and the standard deviation is 4. Using Table 9-3, develop a table showing the range of test scores for each grade category. Then calculate the grades for the following five students:

Student	Test score
A	40
B	30
C	25
D	33
E	36

Using the information given below, calculate the final grades for five students.

Test	Weight
No. 1	1
No. 2	2
No. 3	1.5
No. 4	2.5

Student	Test No. 1	Test No. 2	Test No. 3	Test No. 4
A	A	C	B	D+
B	C	B	B−	C+
C	B	A	A−	A
D	B	D	C+	B+
E	B−	C	D	C

REFERENCES

Baumgartner, T.A., and Jackson, A.S. 1987. Measurement for evaluation in physical education and exercise science. Dubuque, IA: Wm. C. Brown Publishers.

Barrow, H.M., and McGee, R. 1980. A practical approach to measurement in physical education, ed. 3. Philadelphia: Lea & Febiger.

Broer, M.R. 1959. Are physical education grades fair? Journal of Health, Physical Education, and Recreation, **20**:27, 83.

Cotten, D.J., and Cotten, M.B. 1985. Grading: the ultimate weapon? Journal of Physical Education, Recreation and Dance, **56**(2):52-53.

Hanson, D.L. 1967. Grading in physical education. Journal of Health, Physical Education, and Recreation, **38**:34-39.

Imwold, C.H., Rider, R.A., and Johnson, D.J. 1982. The use of evaluation in public school physical education. Journal of Teaching in Physical Education, **2**:13-18.

Mathews, D.K. 1958. Measurement in physical education. Philadelphia: W.B. Saunders Co.

Schutz, R.W. 1989. Analyzing change. Chapter 10 in M.J. Safrit and T.M. Wood (Eds.), Measurement Concepts in Physical Education and Exercise Science. Champaign, IL: Human Kinetics Publishers, Inc.

Shea, J.B. 1971. The pass-fail option in physical education. Journal of Health, Physical Education, and Recreation, **42**:19-20.

Weber, L.J., and Paul, T.L. 1971. Approaches to grading in physical education. The Physical Educator, **28**:59-62.

ANNOTATED READINGS

Cotten, D.J., and Cotten, M.B. 1985. Grading: the ultimate weapon? Journal of Physical Education, Recreation and Dance, **56**(2):52-53.

Emphasizes the importance of basing grades on objectives; identifies issues that should be considered when formulating a grading strategy; discusses the grading of group assignments.

Davis, M.W. 1983. Let's talk about Johnny's 'C' in P.E.! In Hensley, L., and East, W., editors. Measurement and evaluation symposium proceedings. Cedar Falls, IA: University of Northern Iowa.

Discusses the need for meaningful and effective evaluation in physical education; proposes a sports skill and physical fitness profile as the most desirable approach to an individualized evaluation summary; describes and illustrates the phases of profile development.

Hensley, L.D., and East, W.B. 1989. Testing and grading in the psychomotor domain. In M.J. Safrit and T.M. Wood (Eds.), Measurement Concepts in Physical Education and Exercise Science. Champaign, IL: Human Kinetics Publishers, Inc.

An up-to-date treatise of literature dealing with testing in the psychomotor domain and evaluating student achievement in physical education; provides an interesting philosophical perspective of grading.

Shea, J.B. 1971. The pass-fail option and physical education. Journal of Health, Physical Education, and Recreation, **42**:19-20.

Recommends the pass-fail option as the most practical approach to grading in physical education, since it does not require changes in the basic requirements in physical education; lists advantages of the pass-fail option; provides suggested guidelines for structuring a pass-fail grading system.

Turner, E.T. 1975. A creative evaluation experiment. Journal of Physical Education and Recreation, **46**:24-25.

Points to increased effort to reform grading practices; discusses a recently adopted practice by many schools to use a pass-fail system of grading; this system has led to lack of incentive among students; believes that pass-fail systems provide little information about the student's capabilities and achievement; describes student evaluation profile as a more viable approach to grading.

ANSWERS TO LEARNING EXPERIENCES

1. The following table was developed showing the range of test scores for each grade category by using Table 9-3.

Grade	Range of test scores
A	38 and above
B	34-37
C	30-33
D	26-29
F	25 and below

A grade was determined for each of the students listed below:

Student	Test score	Grade
A	40	A
B	30	C
C	25	F
D	33	C
E	36	B

Table 9-7 was used to convert letter grades to numbers. The individual test grades (now numbers) were multiplied by the weighting for the respective test. These values were summed across all four tests and are shown below in column 2:

Student	Sum of grade by weight	Average of column 2	Grade
A	40.5	5.78	C+
B	46.5	6.64	B−
C	72.5	10.36	A−
D	43.5	6.21	C+
E	32.5	4.64	C

In the third column, the sums in the second column were divided by the sum of the weights for the four tests, in this case, 7. Then, Table 9-7 was used to convert the numerical value in column 3 to a composite letter grade, shown in the fourth column.

10

Measuring Motor Performance in Children

KEY WORDS *Watch for these words as you read the following chapter:*

basic movement pattern	face validity	motor ability
component model of intratask development	intratask analysis	

Several surveys in recent years have verified that less testing in physical education occurs at the elementary school level than at any other level. Why is this true? One reason advanced by some is that the limited number of days and short class hours scheduled for physical education in most elementary schools is prohibitive for testing as well as teaching. Furthermore, physical education classes in the elementary schools are not always taught by trained specialists in physical education. In many schools, the regular classroom teacher may not be as knowledgeable about testing motor behavior as he or she is about testing cognitive skills. Another reason for the infrequent use of tests is that test development for this age group has been limited. The existing tests may not be the most useful ones in the elementary school setting. For instance, the teacher may be interested in the measurement of basic movement patterns, such as running, throwing, and jumping. Some may stress the outcome of the movement—how fast the child can run, how far the child can throw the ball, and so forth. Others may emphasize the execution of the movement—the form displayed in running, jumping, or batting, for example, as shown in Figure 10-1. Regardless of the approach used, the measuring instruments available to the teacher are limited. Thus teachers often resort to subjective evaluation of performance based on a cursory judgment of the child's skills.

A third reason for not using tests is the notion that testing must be formal, with time set aside from instruction for this purpose. This point of view, discussed in Chapter 1, suggests that testing automatically takes time away from instruction. Implicit in this way of thinking is the assumption that testing is not desirable because it interferes with teaching. This, of course, does not have to be true. Rather than considering testing and teaching as separate activities, testing should be viewed as an integral part of teaching. In this context, testing is an

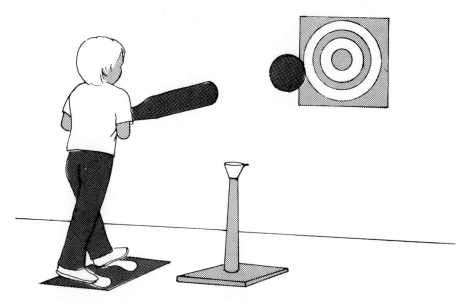

FIGURE 10-1 *Child taking batting test.*

ongoing activity. This is the concept of formative evaluation, previously described in Chapter 1. When this approach is used, children can take some responsibility for their own learning. They can keep records of their performance using charts posted on bulletin boards in the gymnasium. They can work independently on a task and then check with the teacher when ready to be evaluated. In other words, self-assessment can become an important part of the learning process.

In this chapter, examples of the types of tests that can be used in an elementary physical education program are discussed. This assumes that a well-rounded physical education program is implemented, including the following aspects of motor behavior: basic movement patterns, basic skills and games, physical fitness, perceptual motor behavior, and athletic competition. Affective tests for children are described in Chapter 22, and cognitive test development is discussed in Chapter 15.

ASSESSING BASIC MOVEMENT PATTERNS

The area of motor development in the physical education field has encompassed the study of the development of basic movement patterns in children. **Basic movement patterns** are types of movement that emerge developmentally, usually at a young age, such as running, jumping, and throwing. In general, two theories have been espoused to describe motor development in children. Seefeldt, Reuschlein, and Vogel (1972) advocate one approach; Roberton (Roberton and Halverson, 1984), the other. The assessment of movement patterns usually involves the use of a checklist. It must be carefully validated and have satisfactory reliability and objectivity just like any other test. Objectivity is extremely important when developing a checklist, since a highly valid instrument might be too complex for an observer to use. All too often, the development of a checklist is handled in a casual, offhand manner. This criticism also applies to the development of rating scales, perhaps because these measures seem to be so easy to compile. The checklist may be short and easy to use, but it should also include all appropriate test characteristics.

No matter how valid a checklist has been shown to be, it can easily be misused if the user does not have the ability to observe movement competently. Both Allison (1985) and Barrett (1983) have described the components of observational competence. The observer must have the ability to pick out the critical features of the movement designated in the checklist.

Intratask Analysis

The **intratask analysis** of a basic movement pattern is based on the identification of stages of the development of a task from the time it is first attempted to the time it is performed at a mature or adult level. Seefeldt and associates (1972) identify the stages of development of a number of motor tasks, based on the work of Wild (1938). An example of their description of stages is shown in the boxed material on p. 200. The task is the overarm throw, and five developmental stages have been identified. The child is observed throwing a ball and is then placed in one of the five categories.

The throwing pattern should be observed several times on one or more days. On a given day, observing more than one stage in a child's performance is possible. If this happens, the stage represented most frequently should be used to classify the child. Also, the type of throw should be standardized for all children. Force should be emphasized, with accuracy viewed as secondary. If the child throws at a target, with the only force requirement being to project the ball to the target, a different movement pattern is elicited. Once the child is throwing at the level of Stage 5, skills tests can be used to measure the force and accuracy.

Components of Intratask Development

The **component model of intratask development** is based on the identification of developmental characteristics of body parts within a task. This approach evolved from the work of Roberton (Roberton and Halverson, 1984), whose innovative thinking about motor development led to the idea that changes in one body part in executing a task are not always associated with specified changes in another body part. For example, one child may display the trunk action of one stage and

Stages in overarm throwing

Stage 1

The throwing motion is essentially posterior-anterior in direction. The feet usually remain stationary during the throw.

There is little or no trunk rotation in the most rudimentary pattern at this stage, but those at the point of transition between Stages 1 and 2 may evoke a slight trunk rotation in preparation for the throw and extensive hip and trunk rotation in the follow-through.

The force of projection of the ball comes primarily from hip flexion, shoulder protraction, and elbow extension.

Stage 2

The distinctive feature of this stage is the rotation of the body about an imaginary vertical axis, with the hips, spine, and shoulders rotating as one unit. The performer may step forward with either an ipsilateral or contralateral pattern, but the arm is brought forward in transverse plane.

The motion may resemble a sling rather than a throw because of the extended arm position during the course of the throw.

Stage 3

The distinctive characteristic is the ipsilateral arm-leg action. The ball is placed into a throwing position above the shoulder by a vertical and posterior motion of the arm at the time the ipsilateral leg is moving forward. There is little or no rotation of the spine and hips in preparation for the throw.

The follow-through phase includes flexion at the hip joint and some trunk rotation toward the side opposite the throwing hand.

Stage 4

The movement is contralateral, with the leg opposite the throwing arm striding forward as the throwing arm is moved in a vertical and posterior direction during the "wind-up phase." Thus, the motion of the trunk and arm closely resembles those of Stages 1 and 3.

The stride forward with the contralateral leg provides for a wide base of support and greater stability during the force production phase.

Stage 5

The shift of weight is entirely to the rear leg, as it pivots in response to the rotating joints above it.

The throwing hand moves in a downward arc and then backward as the opposite leg moves forward.

Concurrently, the hip and spine rotate into position for forceful derotation.

As the contralateral foot strikes the surface, the hips, spine, and shoulder begin to derotate in sequence.

The contralateral leg begins to extend at the knee as the shoulder protracts, the humerus rotates, and the elbow extends, thus providing an equal and opposite reaction to the throwing arm.

The opposite arm also moves forcefully toward the body to assist in the equal and opposite reaction to the throwing arm.

From Seefeldt, V., and Haulenstricker, J.

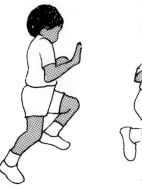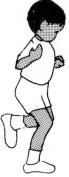

FIGURE 10-2 *Hopping: Leg action, Step 3; Arm action, Step 5.*
Redrawn from Roberton, M.A., and Halverson, L.E.

the arm action of another. Thus Roberton proposed analyzing the development of body parts as separate components. Her model can be used to generate checklists, as exemplified in the boxed material on p. 202. This checklist was developed to assess the child's level of ability in hopping.

Note that two different movement components have been identified for hopping—leg action and arm action. Under leg action four steps (somewhat like stages within a component) were delineated. In the example, the child being observed was placed in Step 3 of the leg action. As the body projection was initiated, the swing leg (left leg in this case) was used to assist the movement. However, he was classified in Step 5 of the arm action, which includes 5 steps altogether. The opposing arm was used to assist the movement. The movement profile recorded on the checklist is illustrated in Figure 10-2. Two other pieces of information are recorded—movement situation, which includes whether the child or teacher selected the movement to be observed, and the observation type, which determines whether the child was observed directly or on film or videotape. The hopping components and their associated steps have been partially validated, and the checklist is reliable and objective. For information on checklists to be used with other movement patterns, refer to Roberton and Halverson (1984).

TESTS OF SPORTS SKILLS

Few tests of sports skills have been developed specifically for children, especially in recent years. Although a great deal of informal skills testing may take place in the elementary schools, much of this work has not been published. Examples of tests of sports skills in this chapter are limited to those with published evidence of reliability and validity. Although they were developed many years ago, they represent the small number of sports skills tests for elementary school children that are available. The reliability and validity of these tests are not always acceptable; however, this information is the basis on which a test user makes a decision

Observation checklist for hopping

Child: *Jones, Randy*   Classroom: *S. Johnson*
Motor task: *Hopping*

	Level observed		
Movement component: *leg action*	Jan. 4		
Step 1. Momentary flight			
Step 2: Fall and catch; swing leg inactive			
Step 3: Projected takeoff; swing leg assists	√		
Step 4. Projection delay; swing leg leads			
Movement component: *arm action*			
Step 1. Bilateral inactive			
Step 2. Bilateral reactive			
Step 3. Bilateral assist			
Step 4. Semiopposition			
Step 5. Opposing assist	√		
Overall movement profile Legs	3		
Arms	5		
Movement situation Teacher selected			
Child selected	√		
Observation type Direct	√		
Videotape			.
Film			
Comments:			

From Roberton, M.A., and Halverson, L.E.

on whether or not to use a test. Although portions of some of these tests may be outdated, they serve as a useful framework for revising the tests in light of the skills as they are used today.

Basketball Wall Pass Test (Latchaw, 1954)

Test Objective To measure passing skills of fourth-, fifth-, and sixth-grade students.

Description The test layout is shown in Figure 10-3. The student stands behind the restraining line. On the signal Ready, Go! the ball is thrown at the target as many times as possible in 15 seconds. If a student loses control of the ball, he or she is responsible for recovering it. A 10-second practice period is allowed, followed by two 15-second trials.

Test Area Floor area 8 feet by 4 feet; wall area 7 feet by 8 feet.

Equipment Stopwatch, regulation basketballs, tape measure, floor tape, and scorecards.

Scoring The trial score is the number of correct hits in the 15-second period. The test score is the best of the two trials. Balls touching the target line do not count. If a student steps on or over the restraining line, the pass does not count.

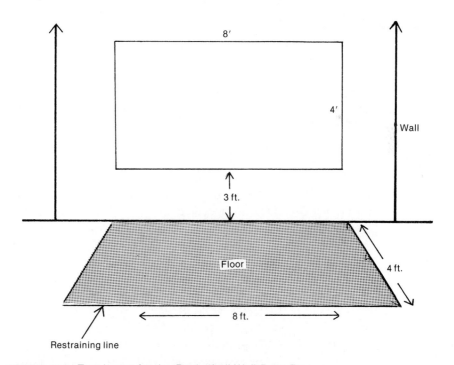

FIGURE 10-3 *Test layout for the Basketball Wall Pass Test.*
Reprinted by permission of the American Alliance for Health, Physical Education, Recreation, and Dance.

TABLE 10-1 *Achievement scales: Basketball Wall Pass Test*

T-Score	Girls Grade IV	Grade V	Grade VI	Boys Grade IV	Grade V	Grade VI	Percentile
77				24	27		99
76	19						99
75			22	23	26	30	99
74					25		99
73		20		22	24		98
72	18				23	29	98
71				21	22	28	98
70						27	97
69						26	97
68	17		21		21	25	96
67		19				24	95
66				20			94
65						23	93
64		18	20				92
63	16	17		19	20		90
62						22	88
61				18			86
60	15		19		19		84
59		16		17			81
58						21	78
57			18		18		75
56	14	15		16			72
55							69
54			17			20	65
53					17		61

From Scott, M.G., and French, E.

Validity **Face validity.** (A test with face validity is one that appears to be valid but has not been formally validated.)

Reliability Boys $r_{xx'} = 0.91$ 4th grade

$r_{xx'} = 0.84$ 5th grade

$r_{xx'} = 0.78$ 6th grade

Girls $r_{xx'} = 0.94$ 4th grade

$r_{xx'} = 0.89$ 5th grade

$r_{xx'} = 0.83$ 6th grade

Norms Norms are presented in Table 10-1.

Comments Use two assistants at each testing station, if possible. One should count the hits and the other, the faults. The ball must land inside the target, not on the line, to score a point.

TABLE 10-1 *Achievement scales: Basketball Wall Pass Test—cont'd*

T-Score	Girls			Boys			Percentile
	Grade IV	Grade V	Grade VI	Grade IV	Grade V	Grade VI	
52	13	14					57
51			16			19	53
50	12				16		50
49						18	46
48			15	14			42
47	11	13			15		38
46						17	34
45	10		14				30
44		12		13	14		27
43	9						24
42			13			16	21
41		11		12	13		18
40	8						15
39		10			12	15	13
38			12				11
37				11	11		9
36	7	9				14	8
35			11				6
34		8		10	10		5
33			10				4
32	6	7				13	3
31				9	9		3
30			9				2
29					8		2
28		6			7		2
27				8			1
26	5						1
25			8		6	12	1

Volleyball Wall Test (Latchaw, 1954)

Test Objective To measure the ability of fourth-, fifth-, and sixth-grade students to strike objects.

Description Use the test setup for the Basketball Wall Pass Test, shown in Figure 10-3. The student stands behind the restraining line. On the signal Ready, Go!, the ball is thrown against the wall. As it bounces off the wall, the student attempts to hit the ball repeatedly against the target. Any type of hit may be used. Allow one 10-second practice trial and four 15-second test trials.

Test Area Same as the Basketball Wall Pass Test.

Equipment Volleyballs, stopwatch, tape measure, floor tape, and scorecards.

Scoring The trial score is the number of correct hits in the 15-second period.

The test score is the best of four trials. The initial throw against the wall is not scored. Only balls that are hit count. If a student throws or carries the ball, it is not scored. If control of the ball is lost, it is the responsibility of the student to recover it. The ball must again be put into play with a throw against the target.

Validity Face validity.

Reliability Boys $r_{xx'} = 0.89$ 4th grade

$$r_{xx'} = 0.89 \text{ 5th grade}$$
$$r_{xx'} = 0.89 \text{ 6th grade}$$

Girls $r_{xx'} = 0.84$ 4th grade

$$r_{xx'} = 0.85 \text{ 5th grade}$$
$$r_{xx'} = 0.79 \text{ 6th grade}$$

TABLE 10-2 *Achievement scales: Volleyball Wall Volley Test*

T-Score	Girls Grade IV	Girls Grade V	Girls Grade VI	Boys Grade IV	Boys Grade V	Boys Grade VI	Percentile
77			21			29	99
76		18					99
75						28	99
74	13	17				27	99
73		15	20	20		26	98
72	12	14			20		98
71	11	13	19	18		25	98
70				16		24	97
69	10		18	15			97
68		12		14	19		96
67			17	13		23	95
66	9			12	18	22	94
65		11		11	17	21	93
64			16		16		92
63	8	10	15		15	20	90
62			14	10		19	88
61		9			14	18	86
60			13				84
59	7					17	81
58		8	12		13		78
57			11		12	16	75
56	6	7		8	11		72
55			10				69
54					10	15	65
53	5		9	7			61
52		6			9	14	57
51							53

From Scott, M.G., and French, E.

Norms Norms are presented in Table 10-2.

Comments Balls must land inside the target, not touching the line, to be scored.

Soccer Wall Volley Test (Latchaw, 1954)

Test Objective To measure the ability of fourth-, fifth-, and sixth-grade students to kick the ball.

Description Use the target layout shown in Figure 10-4. The student stands behind the restraining line. Place the ball anywhere in back of the line. On the signal Ready, Go! the student attempts to kick the ball into the target area of the wall as many times as possible in 15 seconds. If the student loses control of the ball, he or she must recover it. If the ball is within the 4 feet by 2½ feet floor area, the hands cannot be used for retrieval. If the ball is outside this area, the

TABLE 10-2 *Achievement scales: Volleyball Wall Volley Test—cont'd*

T-Score	Girls Grade IV	Girls Grade V	Girls Grade VI	Boys Grade IV	Boys Grade V	Boys Grade VI	Percentile
50	4		8	6	8	13	50
49							46
48		5			7	12	42
47						11	38
46	3		7	5			34
45						10	30
44					6		27
43		4				9	24
42			6	4		8	21
41					5		18
40	2						15
39		3				7	13
38							11
37				3			9
36			5		4	6	8
35						5	6
34		2		2			5
33							4
32	1				3	4	3
31							3
30			3			3	2
29		1					2
28							2
27				1		2	1
26							1
25							1
24					2	1	1
23			2				0

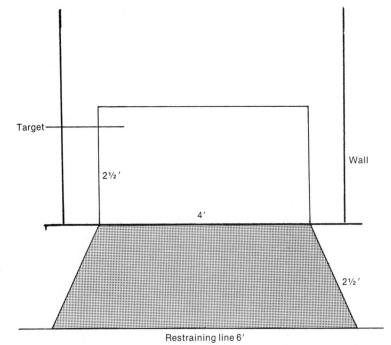

FIGURE 10-4
Test layout for the Soccer Wall Volley Test.
Reprinted by permission of the American Alliance for Health, Physical Education, Recreation, and Dance.

hands may be used. Allow one 15-second practice period and four test trials.

Test Area Wall area 4 feet by 2½ feet; floor area 4 feet by 2½ feet, with a 6-foot restraining line.

Equipment Soccer balls, stopwatch, tape measure, floor tape, and score-cards.

Scoring The trial score is the number of correct hits in 15 seconds. The test score is the best of four trials. Deduct a 1-point penalty whenever the ball is touched with the hands within the rectangular floor area.

Validity Face validity.

Reliability Boys $r_{xx'} = 0.82$ 4th grade

$r_{xx'} = 0.89$ 5th grade

$r_{xx'} = 0.88$ 6th grade

Girls $r_{xx'} = 0.77$ 4th grade

$r_{xx'} = 0.83$ 5th grade

$r_{xx'} = 0.77$ 6th grade

Norms Norms are presented in Table 10-3.

Comments The ball can be kicked from within the rectangular area, but the kick is not scored; however, this can be followed by a kick from behind the re-straining line, which is legal.

TABLE 10-3 *Achievement scales: Soccer Wall Volley Test*

T-Score	Girls Grade IV	Girls Grade V	Girls Grade VI	Boys Grade IV	Boys Grade V	Boys Grade VI	Percentile
76		15		14	16		99
74	13					18	99
73		14			15		98
71				13		17	98
70		13	13				97
69	12					16	97
68					14		96
67						15	95
66	11	12	12				94
65				12			93
64		11			13	14	92
63	10						90
61			11		12		86
60		10		11		13	84
59	9						81
57			10		11		75
56		9		10		12	72
54	8						65
53			9	9	10	11	61
52		8					57
49	7					10	46
48			8	8	9		42
46		7				9	34
44	6						27
43			7	7	8		24
40		6				8	15
39					7		13
38			6	6			11
37	5						9
35						7	6
34		5					5
32			5				3
29	4					6	2
27		4		4			1
26			4				1
24			3	3	5	5	0

From Scott, M.G., and French, E.

Softball Repeated Throws Test (Latchaw, 1954)

Test Objective To measure the ball-throwing ability of fourth-, fifth-, and sixth-grade students.

Description The layout for this test is shown in Figure 10-5. The student stands anywhere within the 5½ -foot square throwing area. On the signal Ready,

FIGURE 10-5 *Test layout for the Softball Repeated Throws Test.*
Reprinted by permission of the American Alliance for Health, Physical Education, Recreation, and Dance.

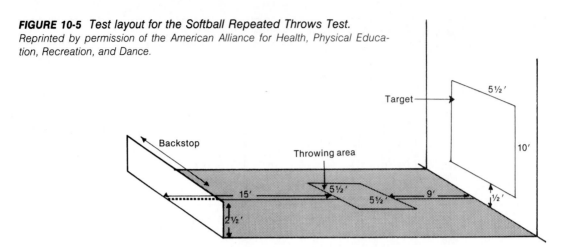

Go!, the ball is thrown at the target using an overarm throw. The rebound is caught, either in the air or on the bounce, and the student continues throwing as many times as possible in 15 seconds. A 10-second practice trial is allowed, followed by two 15-second test trials.

Test Area Floor area 6 feet by 30 feet; wall area 5½ feet by 10½ feet.

Equipment Softballs, stopwatch, tape measure, floor tape, and scorecards.

Scoring The trial is the number of correct hits in 15 seconds. The test score is the best of two trials. A hit is not scored if the examinee steps on or over any one of the lines of the throwing area or the ball lands on or outside one of the target lines.

Validity Face validity.

Reliability Boys $r_{xx'}$ = 0.82 4th grade
$r_{xx'}$ = 0.81 5th grade
$r_{xx'}$ = 0.85 6th grade
Girls $r_{xx'}$ = 0.80 4th grade
$r_{xx'}$ = 0.82 5th grade
$r_{xx'}$ = 0.85 6th grade

Norms Norms are presented in Table 10-4.

Comments If the student loses control of the ball, he or she is responsible for retrieving it. It is desirable to have on hand a dozen or more balls, since the impact of the ball hitting the wall may affect the shape of the ball. If construction of a backstop is not feasible a rolled mat may be used.

Kicking Test (Johnson, 1962)

Test Objective To measure the kicking skills (accuracy) of children in grades 1 through 6.

Description Use the test setup depicted in Figure 10-6. Begin the test by

TABLE 10-4 *Achievement scales: Softball Repeated Throws Test*

T-Score	Girls Grade IV	Girls Grade V	Girls Grade VI	Boys Grade IV	Boys Grade V	Boys Grade VI	Percentile
78	9	10					99
76				12			99
74			12			15	99
73				11	14		98
72	8	9					98
68					13	14	96
66			11				94
65				10			93
64					12		92
63	7					13	90
61			10				86
60					11		84
58				9		12	78
55		8	9		10		69
54						11	65
51				8	9		53
49			8			10	46
48		7					42
47	6						38
46					8		34
45			7	7			30
44						9	27
41	5						18
40		6			7		15
39				6		8	13
38			6				11
35	4						6
33				5		7	4
32		5			6		3
29			5				2
28	3	4				6	2
27				4			1
24		3	4		5	5	1

From Scott, M.G., and French, E.

placing a soccer ball behind the 10-foot line. The student kicks the ball against the wall, trying to hit the center of the target. Two practice kicks and three trials are taken. The same procedure is followed from behind the 20-foot and 30-foot lines.

Test Area Wall area 5 feet by 10 feet; floor area 30 feet by 10 feet.

Equipment Soccer balls, floor and wall tape, tape measure, and scorecards.

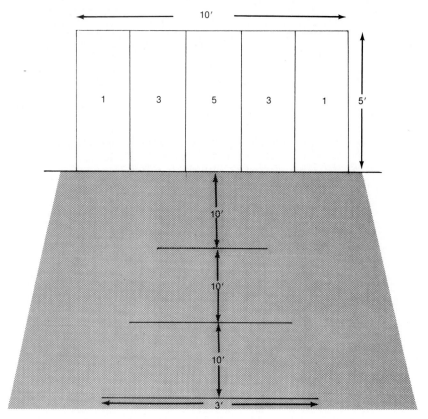

FIGURE 10-6 *Test layout for the Kicking Test.*
From the American Alliance for Health, Physical Education, Recreation, and Dance.

Scoring The score for each kick is the number of the target area the ball hits. Add the total of the nine trials to obtain the total test score. A ball landing on a line between two target areas receives the higher point value of the two areas.

Validity Concurrent validity, using a criterion measure of teachers' ratings of kicking performance.

Grade	Boys*	Girls*
1	0.29	0.41
2	0.66	0.43
3	0.34	0.13
4	0.38	0.51
5	0.04	0.12
6	0.17	0.49

*Correlation coefficients.

TABLE 10-5 *Percentiles for Kicking Test (points)*

	Grades											
	1		2		3		4		5		6	
Percentile	B†	G‡	B	G	B	G	B	G	B	G	B	G
100	34	30	36	35	40	36	42	39	43	40	44	42
95	28	27	33	33	37	34	38	37	40	38	41	40
90	27	26	31	31	36	32	37	35	39	36	40	38
85	26	25	30	30	34	31	36	34	38	35	39	36
80			28	29	33	30	35	33	37	34	37	35
75	25	24		28				32	36	33		34
70			27	27	32	29	34	31	35		36	
65	24	23		26	31	28				32	35	33
60		22	26		30	27	33	30	34	31		
55	23			25		26						32
50			25	24	29	25	32	29	33		34	
45						24	31			30		31
40	22	21	24	23	28				32		33	
35			23	22	27	23	30	28		29	32	30
30	21		21	20		22	29	27	31	28		
25		19	20		26	21		26		27	31	29
20	19	18	19	19	25	20	28	25	30	26	30	28
15	18	16	18	18	23	19	27	24	29	25	29	27
10	17	14	17	16	22	18	25	22	28	23	28	25
5	14	10	14	14	20	17	23	20	26	20	26	20
0	12	8	10	12	16	16	19	16	23	14	23	15

From Johnson, R.D.
†Boys.
‡Girls.

Reliability Test-retest coefficients.

Grade	Boys*	Girls*
1	0.38	0.82
2	0.86	0.88
3	0.83	0.80
4	0.78	0.78
5	0.49	0.67
6	0.84	0.82

*Correlation coefficients.

Norms A table of percentiles is presented in Table 10-5.

Comments If the examinee steps on or over the restraining line, the trial is retaken.

Throw-and-Catch Test (Johnson, 1962)

Test Objective To measure the ability of first- through sixth-grade students to throw and catch.

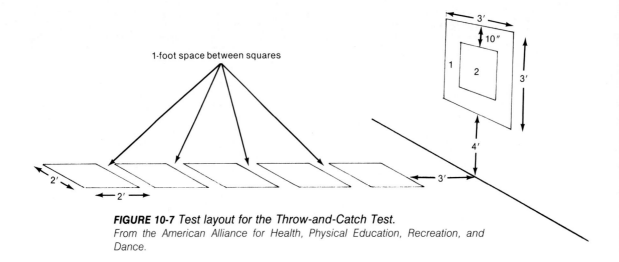

FIGURE 10-7 *Test layout for the Throw-and-Catch Test.*
From the American Alliance for Health, Physical Education, Recreation, and Dance.

Description Use the test setup shown in Figure 10-7. To begin the test the student stands in the first square and throws the ball at the wall target, using an underhand throw. Two practice trials are taken. The same sequence is repeated from each of the remaining four squares.

Test Area Wall area 7 feet by 4 feet; floor area 20 feet by 3 feet.

Equipment Playground balls (8½ inches in diameter) for the first through third grades; volleyballs for fourth through sixth grades.

Scoring The total test score is the sum of 15 trials. The following scoring system is used:

1. Score 2 points for hitting the inner wall target.
2. Score 2 points for catching the rebound in the air while standing in the proper floor square.
3. Score 1 point for hitting the outer section of the wall target.
4. Score 1 point for catching the rebound in the air while standing on the line or outside the proper floor square.

Validity Concurrent validity, using a criterion measure of teachers' ratings of throwing and catching performance.

Grade	Girls*	Boys*
1	0.54	0.47
2	0.33	0.54
3	0.33	0.54
4	0.50	0.45
5	0.15	0.38
6	0.30	0.47

*Correlation coefficients.

TABLE 10-6 *Percentiles for Throw-and-Catch Test (points)*

	Grades											
	1		2		3		4		5		6	
Percentile	B†	G‡	B	G	B	G	B	G	B	G	B	G
100	34	29	39	35	41	38	50	43	57	53	59	55
95	26	23	38	31	40	34	47	40	54	50	56	51
90	24	21	34	28	39	33	45	39	52	45	54	49
85	23	20	32	27	38	32	43	38	50	44	53	47
80	22	19	31	26	37	30	42	37	48	43	52	46
75	21	18	30	25	36	29	41	36	47	42	51	45
70	20	17	29	24	35	28	40	35	46	41	50	44
65	19		28	23	34			34	45	40	49	43
60	18	16	27	22	33	27	39		44		48	
55		15	26	21		26	38	33		39	47	42
50	17		25		32	25		32	43	38	46	41
45		14	24	20	31		37		42	37		40
40	16	13		19	30	24	36		41		45	
35	15	12	23	18		23	35	30	40	36	44	39
30	14	11	22	17	29	22	34	29	39	35	43	38
25	13	10	21	16		21	33	28	38	34	42	37
20	12		20	15	28	20	32	27	37	33	41	36
15	11	9	19	14	27	19	31	26	36	32	40	35
10	10	8	17	12	25	18	30	24	34	31	39	33
5	9	5	13	10	21	16	27	21	33	29	37	31
0	6	3	8	7	17	13	23	16	29	24	34	28

From Johnson, R.D.
†Boys.
‡Girls.

Reliability Test-retest coefficients.

Grade	Girls*	Boys*
1	0.94	0.89
2	0.79	0.92
3	0.90	0.84
4	0.78	0.81
5	0.65	0.84
6	0.93	0.91

*Correlation coefficients.

Norms A table of percentiles is presented in Table 10-6.

Comments The trial is retaken if the student steps out of the square while throwing.

TESTS OF PHYSICAL FITNESS AND MOTOR ABILITY

Tests focusing on other aspects of physical education for the elementary school child can be found in the testing literature. Two of these aspects are physical fitness and motor ability.

Physical Fitness

A well-rounded curriculum for elementary school physical education should include physical fitness. Two types of fitness might be emphasized: One is the type needed for athletic performance; the other is tied to the individual's health state, focusing on the relationship between physical activity and a positive health state. Standardized tests available for each type of fitness are described in the following section.

AAHPERD Youth Fitness Test The AAHPERD Youth Fitness Test (1976), described in detail in Chapter 17, includes six items—Pull-ups Test (or Flexed Arm Hang), Sit-ups Test, Standing Long Jump, 50-yard dash, Shuttle Run Test, and 600-yard Run. Recommended for use with examinees ages 9 through 17 and those of college age, this test measures primarily the type of fitness needed for athletic performance.

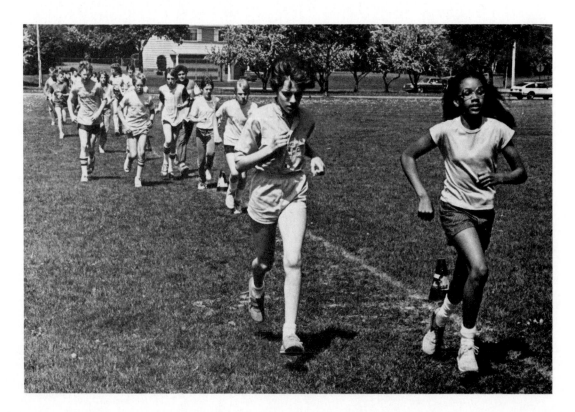

AAHPERD Physical Best Test The AAHPERD Physical Best Test (1988) is described in detail in Chapter 16. Five items are included in this test—Distance Run, Sit-ups Test, Sit-and-Reach Test, Skinfold Measures, and Pull-ups Test. Each item measures a component of health-related physical fitness that is affected by vigorous physical activity. This test is appropriate for any school-age child, including ages 5 through 17 and those of college age. Norms for children are presented in Chapter 16.

Several other national physical fitness test batteries are recommended for children of elementary school age. These include FITNESSGRAM, Fit Youth Today, Chrysler/AAU, and the President's Council on Physical Fitness and Sports. All these tests are described in Chapter 16.

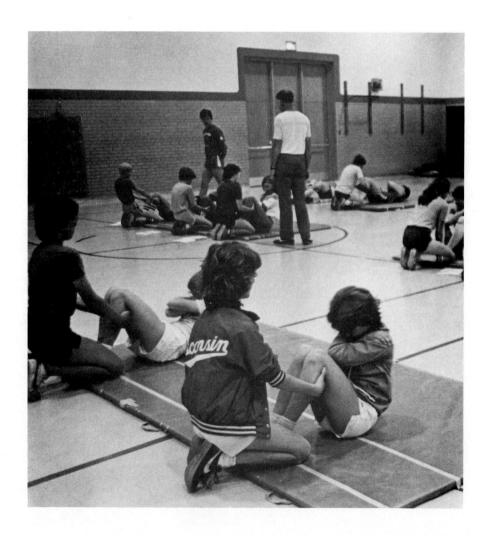

Motor Ability

The difficulties in defining and measuring something called motor ability are discussed in detail in Chapter 21. Research evidence has shown that general motor ability may not exist; rather, a number of abilities, each specific to a given task, can be identified. However, efforts have been made to develop test batteries measuring some sort of general ability in children, although not in recent years. Two of these batteries, which include sports skill–related items, are briefly described here.

Latchaw Motor Achievement Test The Latchaw Motor Achievement Test (1954) was designed to measure general motor achievement in fourth-, fifth-, and sixth-grade students. The Basketball Wall Pass Test, Volleyball Wall Volley Test, Soccer Wall Volley Test, and Softball Repeated Throws Test, all described earlier in this chapter, are four tests designed to measure basic sports skills (or basic movement patterns, as some might interpret it). Three other tests are part of the battery—Vertical Jump (Chapter 17), Standing Broad Jump (Chapter 19), and Shuttle Run. The Shuttle Run Test is similar to the Youth Fitness Test version in Chapter 17, except that no blocks are used. Instead, the examinee merely has to touch the lines with his or her foot. Although T-score tables for each test are presented in Scott and French (1959), they should be updated.

Johnson Test of Achievement in Fundamental Skills The Johnson Test of Achievement in Fundamental Skills (1962) was developed to measure the achievement of elementary school children (grades 1 through 6) in selected fun-

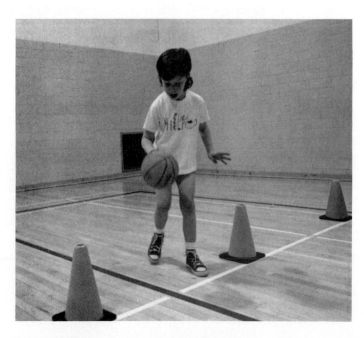

Dribbling task.
Courtesy of Dale A. Ulrich.

damental skills. Five tests are included in this battery—Throw and Catch Test, Jump and Reach Test, Zigzag Run Test, Kicking Test, and Batting Test. The Throw and Catch Test and Kicking Test are described in detail as measures of sports skills on pp. 210-215. The Batting Test is not described, since it requires a special batting kit that must be ordered from a distributor. The Jump and Reach Test is similar to the Vertical Jump, described in Chapter 19, and the Zig-Zag Run Test is fairly typical of the agility tests used in the physical education field. It uses four chairs placed 6 feet apart between a starting line and an "X" placed on the gymnasium wall. As usual, the run is timed to the nearest tenth of a second. Percentile tables are included in the original source, but these should be updated.

TESTS OF PERCEPTUAL MOTOR BEHAVIOR

Educators and clinicians working with preschool and early elementary age children are frequently interested in their perceptual motor behavior. Perceptual motor domains include spatial orientation, body image and differentiation, ocular control, form perception, perception of position in space, perceptual constancy, tactile discrimination, visual closure, and memory (Auxter and Pyfer, 1985). A number of well-known tests of this type are described in Chapter 11. Most of these tests are appropriate for children with or without handicaps, although many are used to screen children to identify those with perceptual motor deficiencies.

EXAMPLES OF GROWTH CHARTS

A number of procedures may be used to monitor the physical growth and development of children, but two of the most widely used growth charts are available from the American Medical Association (AMA) (discussed below) and Ross Laboratories (see Figures 10-8 and 10-9).

AMA Growth Charts (AMA, 1978)

Test Objective To plot the growth curves of children 4 to 18 years of age.

Description Two charts are available, one for boys and one for girls. The most recent version of the charts (AMA, 1978) was developed by H.V. Meredith and J.H. Spurgeon for the Joint Committee on Health Problems in Education of the National Education Association (NEA) and the AMA. To ensure accuracy in assessing students' weight, students should remove their shoes and wear minimal or lightweight clothing. Record weight to the nearest ½ pound and height to the nearest ¼ inch. Then find the age of the child on the appropriate chart. Plot and record the height and weight measurements in the respective portions of the chart. Repeat the assessment on an annual basis and connect the points within each portion (height and weight) of the chart. Both portions contain channels representing tall, heavy (upper 10%), average (next 20% and middle 40%), and

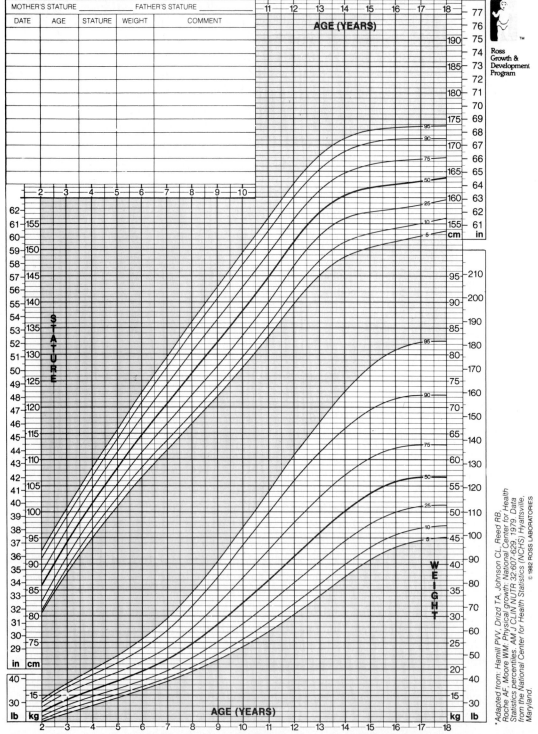

FIGURE 10-8 *Physical Growth NCHS Percentile Chart for Girls.*

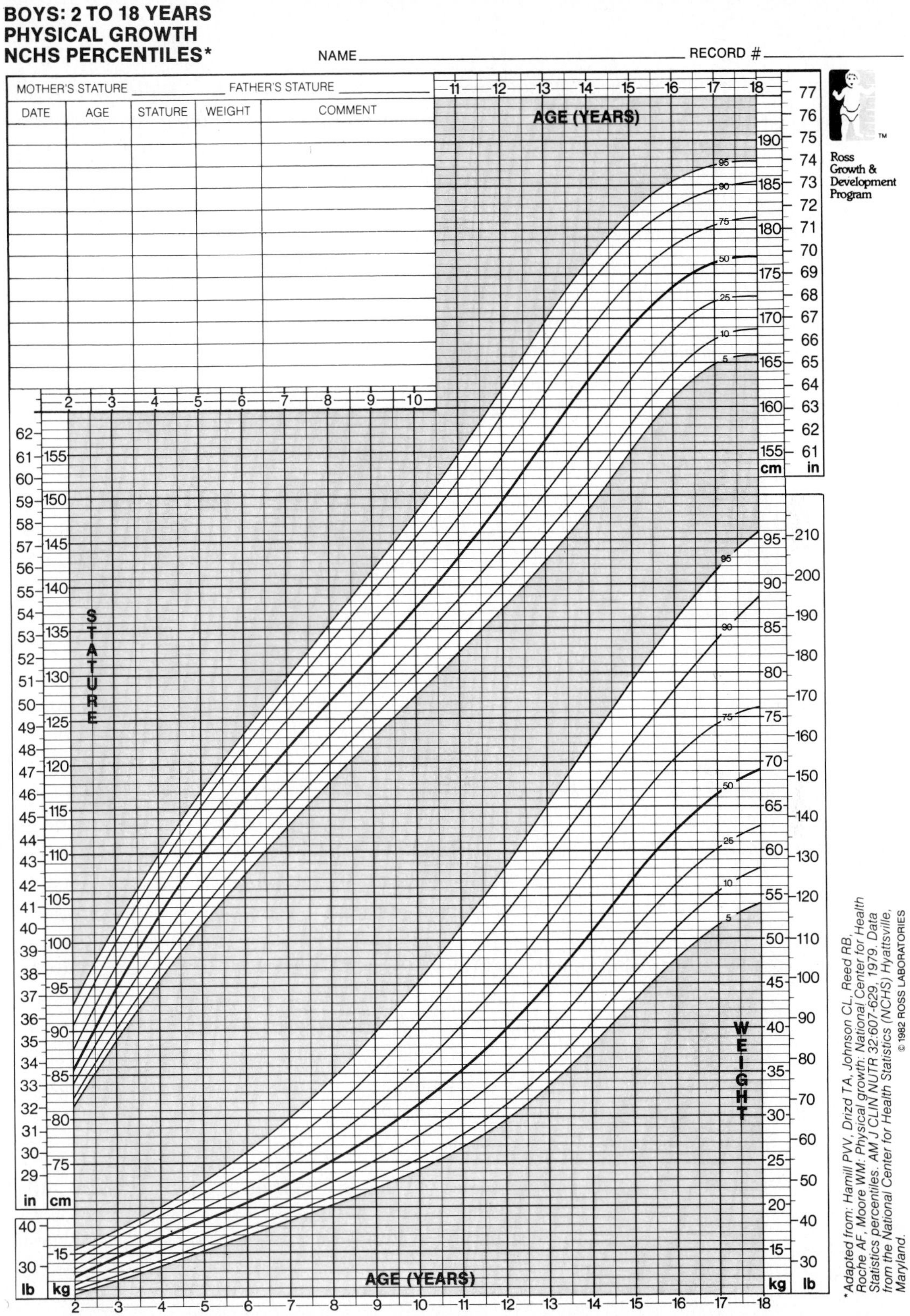

BOYS: 2 TO 18 YEARS
PHYSICAL GROWTH
NCHS PERCENTILES*

NAME _____ RECORD # _____

FIGURE 10-9 *Physical Growth NCHS Percentile Chart for Boys.*

short, light (next 20% and lower 10%). The child's growth is generally considered satisfactory if the plotted points remain within a channel.

Supplies Growth charts can be ordered from the American Medical Association, Order Department OP-311, 535 Dearborn Street, Chicago, IL 60610.

Validity The growth charts were developed after extensive study of the growth record of children at various age levels. They were based on height and weight measurements collected between 1960 and 1975 on boys and girls attending public schools in Iowa and South Carolina. The height and weight channels were obtained by subdividing height and weight distributions at different ages.

Reliability None reported for this specific test.

Comments When the child's growth curve moves from one channel to another, the underlying cause of this change should be determined and appropriate measures taken.

The Ross Laboratory charts (Figures 10-8 and 10-9) provide similar procedures for charting physical growth. Channels representing height and weight were developed for both boys and girls from ages 2 to 18. The channels are based on percentiles including lines drawn at 5%, 10%, 25%, 50%, 75%, 90%, and 95%. Weight may be recorded in kilograms or pounds and height, either centimeters or inches.

SUMMARY

Although informal testing may take place in elementary school physical education programs, few standardized tests of sport and physical activity were developed for this age group in the past. Now, however, the picture is changing. Since youth sports has become a viable area of study, a need has been generated for a wide variety of tests to measure different aspects of the sports environment. To test physical fitness, the AAHPERD Physical Best Test can be used in the lower as well as upper elementary grades. Other national tests are also available. Some of the more recently developed checklists used to assess basic movement patterns are based on sound theory rather than armchair judgement. More tests with substantiated validity and reliability are needed that can be administered in a short period of time. The development of criterion-referenced tests for elementary school physical education would make a valuable contribution to a testing program for young children. Finally, any type of testing program is unlikely to be used with success in the elementary schools unless it is integrated into the instructional program in physical education.

LEARNING EXPERIENCES

1. Form a group with three other students in class. Study the checklist presented in the boxed material on p. 202. Take turns demonstrating each level (step) of arm action and leg action in hopping. Then attempt to use the checklist by evaluating the children in Figures 10-10 and 10-11. Use the detailed description of leg and arm action in the two

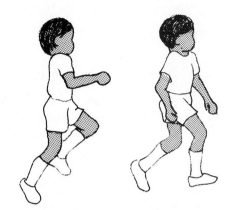

FIGURE 10-10 *Arm and leg action in hopping.*
Redrawn from Roberton, M.A. and Halverson, L.E.

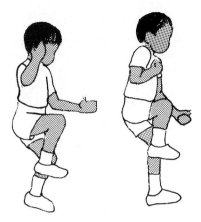

FIGURE 10-11 *Arm and leg action in hopping.*
Redrawn from Roberton, M.A. and Halverson, L.E.

Developmental sequence for leg action in hopping

Step 1. Momentary flight. The support knee and hip quickly flex, pulling (instead of projecting) the foot from the floor. The flight is momentary. Only one or two hops can be achieved. The swing leg is lifted high and held in an inactive position to the side or in front of the body.

Step 2. Fall and catch; swing leg inactive. Body leaning forward allows the minimal knee and ankle extension to help the body "fall" forward of the support foot and, then, quickly catch itself again. The swing leg is inactive. Repeat hops are now possible.

Step 3. Projected takeoff; swing leg assists. Perceptible pretakeoff extension occurs in the hip, knee, and ankle in the support leg. There is little or no delay in changing from knee and ankle flexion on landing to extension prior to takeoff. The swing leg now pumps up and down to assist in projection. The range of the swing is insufficient to carry it behind the support leg when viewed from the side.

Step 4. Projection delay; swing leg leads. The weight of the child on landing is now smoothly transferred along the foot to the ball before the knee and ankle extend to takeoff. The support leg nearly reaches full extension on the takeoff. The swing leg now leads the upward-forward movement of the takeoff phase, while the support leg is still rotating over the ball of the foot. The range of the pumping action in the swing leg increases so that it passes behind the support leg when viewed from the side.

From Roberton, M.A. and Halverson, L.E.

Developmental sequence for arm action in hopping

Step 1. Bilateral inactive. The arms are held bilaterally, usually high and out to the side, although other positions behind or in front of the body may occur. Any arm action is usually slight and not consistent.

Step 2. Bilateral reactive. Arms swing upward briefly, then are medially rotated at the shoulder in a winging movement prior to takeoff. It appears that this movement is in reaction to loss of balance.

Step 3. Bilateral assist. The arms pump up and down together, usually in front of the line of the trunk. Any downward and backward motion of the arms occurs *after* the takeoff. The arms may move parallel to each other or be held at different levels as they move up and down.

Step 4. Semiopposition. The arm on the side opposite the swing leg swings forward with that leg and back as the leg moves down. The position of the other arm is variable, often staying in front of the body or to the side.

Step 5. Opposing-assist. The arm opposite the swing leg moves forward and upward in synchrony with the forward and upward movement of that leg. The other arm moves in the direction opposite to the action of the swing leg. The range of movement in the arm action may be minimal unless the task requires speed or distance.

From Roberton, M.A., and Halverson, L.E.

---

sections of boxed material on pp. 223-224. The correct classifications are included on p. 226. Finally, observe at least two children performing a hop and attempt to classify them, using the checklist. Check with the other members of the group to determine how closely you agreed on your classifications. If there is considerable disagreement, observe the children again and attempt to uncover the sources of disagreement.

2. Observe a group of elementary age children being tested on some aspect of their motor performance. Write a short paper on the problems that can be encountered in administering a test to young children. Suggest ways of avoiding these problems.

REFERENCES

Allison, P.C. 1985. Observing for competence. Journal of Physical Education, Recreation and Dance, **56** (7):50-51, 54.

American Alliance for Health, Physical Education, Recreation and Dance. 1988. Physical Best. Reston, VA: AAHPERD.

Auxter, D., and Pyfer, J. 1985. Adapted physical education and recreation. St. Louis: Times Mirror/Mosby College Publishing.

Barrett, K.R. 1983. A hypothetical model of observing as a teaching skill. Journal of Teaching in Physical Education, 3(1):22-31.

American Medical Association. 1978. Height-weight interpretation folder for boys. Chicago: AMA Medicine/Education Committee.

American Medical Association. 1978. Height-weight interpretation folder for girls. Chicago: AMA Medicine/Education Committee.

Johnson, R.D. 1962. Measurements of achievement in fundamental skills. Research Quarterly, 33:94-103.

Latchaw, M. 1954. Measuring selected motor skills in fourth, fifth and sixth grades. Research Quarterly, 25:439-449.

Roberton. M.A. 1978. Stages in motor development. In Ridenour, M., editor. Motor development: issues and applications. Princeton, NJ: Princeton Book Co., Publishers.

Roberton, M.A., and Halverson, L.E. 1984. Developing children—their changing movement. Philadelphia: Lea & Febiger.

Scott, M.G., and French, E. 1959. Measurement and evaluation in physical education. Dubuque, IA: Wm. C. Brown Group.

Seefeldt, V., Reuschlein, S. and Vogel, P. 1972. Sequencing motor skills within the physical education curriculum, Paper presented at the American Association for Health, Physical Education, and Recreation National Convention, Houston, March 27, 1972.

Thomas, J.R. 1983. Motor development during childhood and adolescence. Minneapolis: Burgess Publishing Co.

Wild, M.R. 1938. The behavior pattern of throwing and some observations concerning its course of development in children. Research Quarterly, 9:20-24.

ANNOTATED READINGS

Hardin, D.H., and Garcia, M.J. 1982. Diagnostic performance tests for elementary school children (Grades 1-4). Journal of Physical Education, Recreation and Dance, 53(2):48-49.

Recommends the use of four performance tests measuring running, jumping, throwing, and ball handling in elementary school physical education; norms are presented for children ages 6 through 9.

Melville, S. 1985. Teaching and evaluating cognitive skills in elementary physical education. Journal of Physical Education, Recreation and Dance, 56(2):26-28.

Describes the development of a written examination on cognitive skill acquisition for third and fourth graders; discusses the benefits of using written examinations in elementary physical education.

Seefeldt, V. 1984. Physical fitness in preschool and elementary school aged children. Journal of Physical Education, Recreation and Dance, 55(9):33-37, 40.

Describes the importance of enhancing children's physical fitness during their early years; discusses the relationship between fundamental motor skills and fitness in preschool years.

Siegel, J. 1988. Children's target heart rate. Journal of Physical Education, Recreation and Dance, 59(4):78-79.

Discusses the importance of using heart rate to control the intensity of children's vigorous physical activity; describes target heart rate range and presents a table of these ranges for children from ages 4 to 18.

Thomas, J.R., and Thomas, K.T. 1983. Strange kids and strange numbers: assessing children's motor development. Journal of Physical Education, Recreation and Dance, **54**(8):19-20.

Identifies important motor behaviors and characteristics to be measured in children; discusses the selection of appropriate tests of the movement performance of preschool and elementary school age children; reviews the circumstances under which the assessments should be made.

ANSWERS TO LEARNING EXPERIENCES

Figure 10-10 represents Leg action, Step 2; Arm action, Step 2. Figure 10-11 represents Leg action, Step 4; Arm action, Step 5.

11
Adapting Tests and Measurements for Special Populations

KEY WORDS *Watch for these words as you read the following chapter:*

anomaly

cerebral palsy

congenital

deaf

disabled

educable

handicapped

hard of hearing

impaired

Individualized Education Program

mentally retarded

motor ability

multihandicapped

needs assessment

orthopedically impaired

paraplegia

reflexes

seriously emotionally disturbed

specific learning disability

speech impairment

visually handicapped

Measurement and evaluation techniques of the **impaired** are frequently used for purposes similar to those used for testing in regular physical education classes. For example, tests may be used to motivate students, to classify them, and for many other reasons (see Chapter 1). However, when students have physical, emotional, or mental impairments that lead to physical **disabilities,** initial testing assumes special significance. Several problems commonly surface when assessing the physical abilities of the individual with impairments (Baumgartner and Horvat, 1988). One, a test battery is needed for each possible combination of handicapping conditions. Each condition can create a different set of limitations in a test setting. Two, it is difficult to develop norms for tests used in handicapped populations, since the size of each subgroup of individuals tends to be small and they may not be readily accessible for testing. Three, individuals with impairments may have problems typically associated with the testing of young children, such as short attention span, limited ability to understand complicated directions, and self-motivation. Indeed, the issue of testing individuals with impairments has become so significant that an entire book has been devoted to this topic (Werder and Kalakian, 1985).

Before initiating a program of physical activity for an individual, a teacher must determine his or her level of physical functioning. Because of the wide variety of handicaps, testing must often take place on an individualized basis. The physical education teacher, working with the appropriate specialists, tests the student to determine the level of psychomotor functioning. This information is used to plan a physical education program based on objectives developed specifically for the individual. The student is then evaluated in light of these objectives. In essence, before a student with impairments is allowed to participate in any form of physical activity in an educational setting, a two-stage approach to testing should take place. A therapist often handles the first stage—determining the extent of the disability. Ideally, a specialist in adapted physical education assists the therapist in this assessment. The results are used to prepare individualized objectives, and the adequacy of these objectives is checked. Are they written at the appropriate level for the child? Are some of the objectives too easy? Too difficult? This analysis represents the second stage of planning, essentially a **needs assessment**—determining the extent to which the student is capable of meeting the individualized objectives. If the child can already meet an objective, it should be modified or rewritten. By this process the objectives are fine tuned. After these assessments are completed, a program of physical activity can be initiated. The long-range goal of the program is to enhance performance in the non-impaired areas and to reduce the level of impairment as much as possible. Many textbooks on adapted physical education stress the importance of using formative evaluation to provide continuous monitoring of performance so that adjustments can be made in the program when necessary (Sherrill, 1981; Seaman and De-Pauw, 1982; Fait and Dunn, 1984). Although norm-referenced approaches to measurement are sometimes advocated, primary emphasis is placed on criterion-referenced testing.

As you might expect, there is no universal agreement on the factors related to motor performance that should be measured in this special population. Kirkendall, Gruber, and Johnson (1987) proposed testing 10 physical factors.

Basic areas
1. Strength
2. Endurance (muscular and cardiovascular)
3. Range of motion
4. Balance

Intermediate areas
5. Body awareness
6. Body sides awareness
7. Space awareness
8. Timing awareness

Advanced areas
9. Coordination
10. Agility

Seaman and DePauw (1982) refer to four broad levels of assessment, ranging from the basic to the complex:

1. Reflex behavior
2. Sensory systems
3. Motor patterns
4. Movement skills

Examples of tests fitting several of these categories are presented later in this chapter. Several of these tests are also appropriate for preschool children without handicaps in a physical education setting. For example, it is not unusual to find the Denver Developmental Screening Test described in textbooks on elementary physical education, motor development, and adapted physical education. However, whether the child is with or without **handicaps,** many of these tests must be administered on an individualized basis, with, of course, certain exceptions. For example, when the handicapping condition is mild, such as mild mental retardation, group testing is possible. When the AAHPERD Motor Fitness Test for the Moderately Mentally Retarded is used, it can be administered to students as a group. As the extent of retardation becomes more severe, individ-

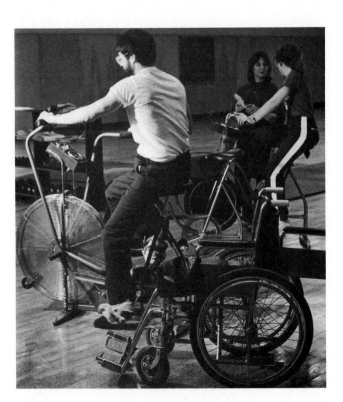

Warm-up for bicycle ergometer test.

ualized testing is more effective. Most of the tests used to screen students for classification purposes require one-on-one testing, regardless of the extent of the handicap.

LEGAL MANDATES AFFECTING EVALUATION

Although it is assumed that good instruction incorporates sound measurement and evaluation practices, the individual with impairments has special needs and thus has been given unique protection by legal action. In effect since 1975, the Education for all Handicapped Children Act (Public Law 94-142) has precise implications for evaluation in physical education. Although many aspects of education are affected by the law, the focus in this chapter is directed to measurement and evaluation in the physical education field.

Public Law 94-142 mandates an **Individualized Education Program** (IEP) for each disabled or handicapped child receiving special education services. The IEP must include documentation about the child's educational program. It must be approved by a committee whose membership, which must include at least one parent, is determined under the law. Assessments must be completed within 30 days of the date of parental permission. Complete assessments are required by law every three years, and the results of assessment must be reported in a formal meeting. Although several adapted physical education textbooks have thorough discussions of this law, the portions of the law affecting evaluation are especially well presented in Fait and Dunn (1984). A summary of part of their review follows.

Due Process

If the child is judged to have impairments requiring a special testing program, the school is required to inform the parents and child of their rights with the provision to challenge educational decisions they feel are unfair. This requirement includes five components:

1. Permission before assessment. The parents must give written permission to have their child evaluated.
2. Results of the assessment. The results must be interpreted in a meeting with the parents.
3. Outside evaluation. The parent may request that an independent evaluation be conducted outside the school. The parent must pay for these expenses unless the results differ from those reported by the school, in which case the school district must cover them.
4. Hearings. If the parents and the school system cannot agree on the evaluation findings, a special hearing must be held.
5. Confidentiality of records. Records of all evaluations must be kept confidential.

Standards for Evaluation

Public Law 94-142 also specifies standards for evaluation, including test selection, test administration, and test examiners.

1. Test selection. The school system must use tests to measure the achievement level rather than the impairment of the child. More than one test procedure must be used. All tests cannot be subjective (such as observational scales), nor can all be objective (like performance tests).

2. Test administration. Tests must be administered to test the student's ability rather than his or her communication skills. This is particularly critical for those with sensory impairments. If the child's native language is not English, the test instructions should be given in the native language, if necessary. If the child is **deaf,** sign language can be used.

3. Test examiners. A multidisciplinary team is required for the testing. Ideally, this team includes a specialist in adapted physical education. All testers must be trained and qualified to administer the measures.

The rest of this chapter contains examples of measures that are frequently recommended by specialists in the field. As you review each test, consider the feasibility of using it in a kindergarten or elementary physical education setting with children who have no handicapping conditions.

OBSERVATIONAL TECHNIQUES

Checklists for assessing the child with impairments are available in adapted physical education textbooks, such as Sherrill (1981), Seaman and DePauw (1982), and Fait and Dunn (1984). Some of these observational techniques were developed by physical educators who have had years of experience working with students having a variety of handicapping conditions, including those with a **special learning disability** and those who are **seriously emotionally disturbed.** However, many of the observational tools are weak measures of the student's physical ability because they lack evidence of validity and reliability. Although logical validity may be self-evident to a certain extent, it does not substitute for the proper establishment of test characteristics. If the techniques are used as quick screening devices before making a thorough assessment, their use is more defensible. If the results of a weak measure are used to make temporary decisions that can be modified in the near future, the consequences of assessment are not as severe as those used to make decisions with long-term implications for the child.

Ulrich (1988) describes several approaches to assessing the quality of movement competence. These include product assessment, qualititative assessment, performance error assessment, developmental task analysis, and a comprehensive analysis. All but the first approach utilize observational techniques and checklists. Several methods (e.g., Roberton and Halverson, 1984; Ulrich, 1985) have sufficient evidence of validity and reliability. The use of criterion-referenced measurement to diagnose and improve student learning in adapted physical education and the virtues of criterion-referenced testing were explored by King and Aufsesser (1988).

PERFORMANCE TESTS
Reflex Testing

Generally, adapted physical education specialists are not expected to test **reflexes** (inborn, involuntary behaviors), although the physical education teacher working in an adaptive setting needs to know the results of reflex testing to analyze the movement deficiencies of the student. This information should be a part of the student's records and is usually obtained by a therapist. Pyfer (1988) has developed a screening test for developmental delays that includes several reflex test items.

Sensorimotor Testing

Sensorimotor or perceptual motor testing samples the function of the underlying sensory system through observable motor performance (Seaman and Depauw, 1982). A description of one test in this category, the Purdue Perceptual Motor Survey, follows. (Sources for obtaining two other tests, the Quick Neurological Screening Test and the Frostig Developmental Test of Visual Perception, are included in Appendix G.)

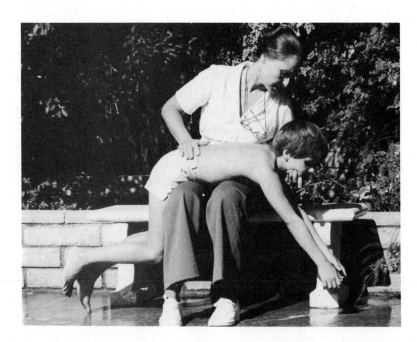

Test of the tonic labyrinthine reflex.
Courtesy Janet A. Seaman.

Purdue Perceptual Motor Survey (Roach and Kephart, 1966)

Test Objective To sample the functions of the sensory systems as they support or contribute to efficient movement.

Description The survey consists of 12 test items:

A. Balance and posture

Test No. 1: Walking Board

Test No. 2: Hopping and Jumping

B. Body image and right-left (R-L) discrimination

Test No. 3: Identification of body parts

Test No. 4: Imitation of movement

Test No. 5: Obstacle course

Test No. 6: Kraus-Weber Test

Test No. 7: Angels in the snow

C. Perceptual-motor match

Test No. 8: Chalkboard activities

Test No. 9: Rhythmic writing

D. Test No. 10: Ocular control

Test No. 11: Ocular pursuits

E. Test No. 12: Form reproduction (drawing simple geometric figures on blank paper)

Test Area A multipurpose room or gymnasium is needed for several items; otherwise, a classroom can be used.

Equipment Chalkboard, chalk, penlight, yardstick or dowel, and visual achievement forms.

Scoring A 4-point rating scale is used.

Validity A validity coefficient of 0.65 was reported between teachers and survey ratings.

Reliability The test-retest reliability was 0.95, with 1 week intervening between test administrations.

Norms Norms have been published for grades 1 through 4, based on the scores of 200 children with 50 randomly selected from each grade.

Comments The Test Manual should be purchased and reviewed before administering the survey. The survey can be administered to an individual in 45 minutes.

Motor Development Profiles

Many qualitative measures of the development of movement patterns have been published. These scales typically assess changes in whole body configurations as the child grows and develops. The Denver Developmental Screening Test (Frankenburg and Dodds, 1967; Frankenburg, Dodds, and Fandel, 1973) follows. (Sources for obtaining the two other tests, the California State University Motor

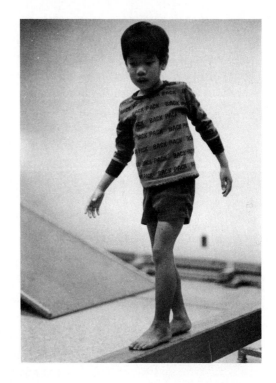

Assessment of asymmetrical tonic neck reflex in an upright position.
Courtesy Janet A. Seaman.

Development Checklist and the Bayley Scales of Motor Development, are presented in Appendix G.)

Denver Developmental Screening Test (Frankenberg and Dodds, 1967)

Test Objective To evaluate children up to age 6 in fine motor, gross motor, social, and language skills.

Description There are 105 tasks selected to identify developmental delays in the above four categories. The tester uses an instruction sheet of 28 items to elicit responses from the examinee. The tester also records behavioral observations (e.g., how the child feels at the time of the test, relation to tester).

Test Area A small room provides sufficient space.

Equipment Small toy, rattle, piece of yarn, paper and pencil, box of raisins, eight small cubes, small bottle, pictures of familiar objects, and small ball.

Scoring Each item is scored in one of four ways—pass, fail, refusal, or no opportunity for child to respond.

Validity A validity coefficient of 0.97 was reported, based on a comparison of the Denver Test with the Yale Developmental Examination, a lengthier, more complex test.

Reliability Reliability coefficient estimates calculated for each of the four categories (fine motor, gross motor, social, and language skills) ranged from 0.66 to 0.93.

Norms Charts have been developed showing the age level at which 10%, 25%, 50%, 75%, and 90% of the children can perform specific tasks. Data from 1043 children through age 6 were used to determine these standards.

Comments Administration time varies, depending on the age and maturity of the child. Test items must be administered individually.

Motor Ability Tests

Motor ability, a rather nebulous term, was originally used to represent one's innate ability to perform motor tasks. However, it was impossible to separate innate ability from learned skills. Motor ability has also been referred to as a predictor of athletic ability. Gradually the term took on a new meaning and is now thought to reflect motor educability, one's ability to learn motor skills. Although it seems intuitively reasonable that individuals possess an innate motor ability, there is no scientific evidence that the tests available at the present time tap this trait. This does not mean that these tests are not at all useful in an educational setting, but rather that labeling these tests as measures of motor ability is questionable. The Bruininks-Oseretsky Motor Development Scale, classified by Sea-

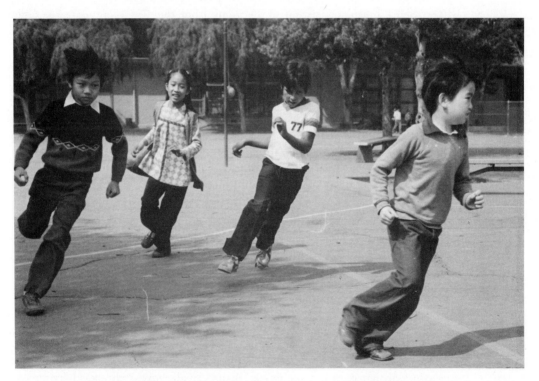

Assessment of quality of running form. Item from Adapted Physical Education Assessment Scale.
Courtesy Janet A. Seaman.

man and DePauw (1982) as a motor ability test often used with disabled students, follows. (Sources for obtaining two other motor ability tests, the Six Category Gross Motor Test and the Basic Motor Ability Test—Revised, are included in Appendix G.)

The Bruininks-Oseretsky Test of Motor Proficiency (Bruininks, 1978)

Test Objective This is an individually administered test that assesses motor functioning from 4½ to 14½ years of age.

Description Both a Complete Battery and a Short Form are available. The Complete Battery includes eight subtests, four to measure gross motor skills, three to measure fine motor skills, and one for both fine and gross motor skills:

Subtest No. 1: Running speed and agility (one item)
Subtest No. 2: Balance (eight items)
Subtest No. 3: Bilateral coordination (eight items)
Subtest No. 4: Strength (three items)
Subtest No. 5: Upper limb coordination (nine items)
Subtest No. 6: Response speed (one item)
Subtest No. 7: Visual-motor control (eight items)
Subtest No. 8: Upper limb speed and dexterity (eight items)

The Short Form, consisting of 14 items from the Complete Battery, follows, along with the respective subtest numbers.

Subtest No. 1: *Item 1:* Running speed and agility
Subtest No. 2: *Item 2:* Standing on preferred leg while making circles with fingers
  Item 7: Walking forward heel to toe on balance beam
Subtest No. 3: *Item 1:* Tapping feet alternatively while making circles with fingers
  Item 6: Jumping up and clapping hands
Subtest No. 4: *Item 1:* Standing Broad Jump
Subtest No. 5: *Item 3:* Catching a tossed ball with both hands
  Item 5: Throwing a ball at a target with preferred hand
Subtest No. 6: *Item 1:* Response speed
Subtest No. 7: *Item 3:* Drawing a line through a straight path with preferred hand
  Item 5: Copying a circle on paper with preferred hand
  Item 8: Copying overlapping pencils with preferred hand
Subtest No. 8: *Item 3:* Sorting shape card with preferred hand
  Item 7: Drawing dots in circles with preferred hand

Test Area Room of any size, as long as space can be cleared for testing.

Equipment All equipment needed for administration of the scale: ball, mazes, scissors, balance rod, matchbook, coins, small boxes, thread, playing cards, matchsticks, ballpoint pen, and paper. The kit can be purchased in a specially designed metal carrying case. In addition to the equipment, the kit includes an

Examiner's Manual, individual record forms for the Complete Battery and the Short Form, and a package of 25 student booklets (for test items that require cutting or paper and pencil responses).

Scoring Scale items are scored on a pass/fail basis. For the Complete Battery, there is a gross motor composite (Subtest Nos. 6 through 8). For the Short Form a single score provides an index of motor proficiency.

Validity Evidence of validity is primarily construct validity.

1. The relationship of test content to research findings in motor development was established.
2. A number of statistical properties of the test were reported: relationship of test scores to chronological age, internal consistency of subtests, and factor analysis of subtest items.
3. Comparisons were made between contrast groups: mildly retarded with normal subjects, moderately to severely retarded with normal subjects, and learning disabled with normal subjects. The interrelationships between subtests were low to moderate, meaning that the subtests tapped different abilities.

Reliability The test-retest reliability was high for composite scores (ranging from 0.68 to 0.86, with only the 0.68 estimate falling on the low side). The coefficients were lower for some of the subtests, where reliability estimates as low as 0.29 were reported; however, the range of estimates was from 0.29 to 0.89. Interrater reliability was generally quite satisfactory, ranging from 0.77 to 0.97. This type of reliability is quite important, since much of the scoring is subjective. The standard error of measurement was also reported for all age groups on each subtest.

Norms Percentile norms were reported for males and females ranging from 6 to 14 years of age.

Comments The Lincoln-Oseretsky version of this test is described in detail in Sloan (1955). The scale has undergone several revisions, with the latest being the Bruininks-Oseretsky Test of Motor Proficiency (1978).* Approximately 45 minutes is required to administer the Complete Battery and 15 to 20 minutes to administer the Short Form. The Bruininks' revision was very well developed. Evidence of an item analysis and standardization of the test is included. Differences between individual standard scores are also reported.

Physical Fitness Tests

Sherrill (1981) notes that, although many children with impairments have low levels of physical fitness, programs to develop their fitness are often neglected.

---

*The Bruininks—Oseretsky Test of Motor Proficiency can be ordered from American Guidance Service, Circle Pines, MN 55014.

TABLE 11-1 *Classifications in selected physical fitness tests*

Test	Classification
Special Physical Fitness (AAHPERD, 1986)	Age, Gender, Type and Severity of condition (mild mental retardation)
Project ACTIVE (Vodola, 1978)	Chronological and Mental Age, Gender, Type of Condition (mental, emotional, learning disability)
Buell Adaptation of the AAHPERD Health and Youth Fitness Test (1982)	Age, Gender, Type and Severity of Condition (blind and partially sighted)
Motor Fitness Test for the Moderately Mentally Retarded (Johnson & Londeree, 1976)	Age, Gender, Type and Severity of Condition (moderate mental retardation)
UNIQUE Physical Fitness Test (Winnick & Short, 1985)	
Visual	Age, Gender, Type of Condition (visual), Severity of Condition (blind, partially sighted), Level of Assistance (unassisted, guidewire or rope assisted, partner assisted)
Auditory	Age, Gender, Type of Condition (Auditory)
Orthopedic	Age, Gender, Type of Condition (cerebral palsy, spinal neuromuscular, congenital anomaly/amputee), Site of amputation or anomaly; Mode of Ambulation (unassisted; cane, crutch or other assistive device; wheelchair), Wheelchair Propulsion (moved with arms, moved with feet forward or backward)

Reproduced by permission of the American Alliance for Health, Physical Education, Recreation and Dance.

One must remember the definition of health-related physical fitness (See Chapter 16) and its emphasis of universal application. Sherrill recommends administering the AAHPERD Health-Related Physical Fitness Test to students with impairments. Adjustments of this test may be necessary, depending on the extent and type of the disability. For example, if a student has severe cognitive disorders, a buddy system might be used effectively in administering distance run tests. If necessary, the distance run can be reduced to 600 or even 300 yards. At these shorter distances the test is no longer a valid measure of cardiorespiratory (CR) function, but nonetheless taps other physiological parameters. Winnick (1988) discusses the classification of individuals with handicapping conditions for physical fitness testing and sport participation. In Table 11-1, examples of various ways of classifying people are provided. Classifications for fitness testing are often based on the type and severity of the medical condition of the individuals.

The AAHPERD Motor Fitness Test for the Moderately Mentally Retarded is presented here in detail. The test for mentally retarded youth parallels two other tests for impaired youth published by AAHPERD, the AAHPERD Youth Fit-

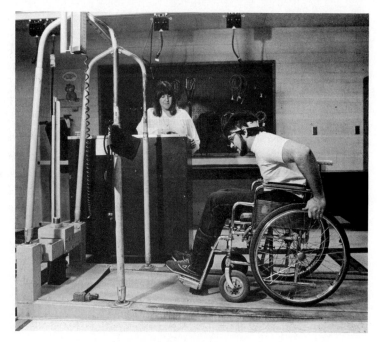

Warm-up for the treadmill test.

ness Test Adaptation for the Blind, and the Special Fitness Test for the Mentally Retarded. The second test—the Project UNIQUE Physical Fitness Test—is presented in less detail but is nevertheless an important contribution to the fitness test area because of its exceptionally sound psychometric underpinnings. Other physical fitness tests and award systems for students with impairments have been described by Stein (1988).

AAHPERD Motor Fitness Test for the Moderately Mentally Retarded (Johnson and Londeree, 1976)

The AAHPERD Motor Fitness Test for the Moderately Mentally Retarded is a modification of the AAHPERD Youth Fitness Test for **educable** (capable of learning) mentally retarded children. Individuals with this level of retardation have IQs ranging from 50 to 70. Included in the Test Manual are 13 items— flexed arm hang, situps, standing long jump, softball throw for distance, 50-yard dash, 300-yard run-walk, height, sitting bob and reach, skipping, tumbling progression, and target throw. The first six items are recommended as sufficient for testing the motor fitness of the moderately mentally retarded, with the other items usable in local situations. In the Test Manual, norms are published for boys and girls, ages 6 through 20, although the norms are based on small sample sizes in many cases. An award system is also available for these age groups.

Flexed Arm Hang

Test Objective Although the objective is not stated in the Test Manual, the Flexed Arm Hang is usually included in a fitness test battery as a measure of arm and shoulder girdle strength and endurance.

Description Adjust the bar to approximately standing height. Instruct the student to grasp the bar with an overhand grip (palms away from the body). The student jumps (and is simultaneously lifted by a tester) to the flexed arm hang position, with the chin above the bar and parallel to the floor. The elbows are held close to the sides, and the chin is just above the bar. Once the student is in motionless, hanging position and is no longer assisted by the tester, the stopwatch is started. Stop the watch when "the chin touches the bar, the head tilts back to keep the chin above the bar, or the chin drops below the bar" (Johnson and Londeree, 1976, p. 16). One trial is administered. Do not allow the student to kick or swing the legs or lift the knees.

Test Area Small indoor area, even a doorway, is adequate.

Equipment In the Test Manual, a metal or wooden bar 1½ inches in diameter is recommended. However, a doorway gym bar or an angled or horizontal ladder would also be suitable. A stopwatch is used to time the test.

Scoring The score is the amount of time, to the nearest tenth of a second, the proper position is held.

Validity Although the manual includes a brief discussion of the validity of the total test battery, there is no reference to the validity of this specific test.

Reliability Test-retest reliability coefficients of 0.90 were reported, with 6 months intervening between test administrations.

Norms Norms are available for moderately mentally retarded boys and girls, ages 6 through 20. However, the norms are based on small sample sizes and should be used only as rough guidelines.

Comments Evidence of validity and reliability for the population of educable mentally retarded youth needs to be obtained for future revisions of the manual. Reliability should be estimated with no more than 2 weeks elapsing between test periods. The most critical issue related to the Flexed Arm Hang Test is whether it can adequately measure differences in strength across all ages and both genders. In the tables of norms for this test, more than 50% of the male samples could not maintain the proper position for any recorded time. At least 50% of the girls were unable to obtain any score at all, regardless of age. The manual stated that children in this group had very low arm strength and endurance. Yet the results suggest that many have no strength in this area, which cannot be true. Stating that the test is not discriminating well is probably more accurate. It lacks a basic characteristic of measurement—that as ability changes, the test score changes correspondingly. Even in a normal population, too many 0 scores were obtained in the flexed arm hang. Other techniques measuring arm and shoulder girdle strength, such as the Baumgartner/Modified Pull-Ups Test, might be considered as substitutes. In cases of more severe impairments, a straight arm hang has been suggested as a reasonable substitute.

Sit-Ups in 30 Seconds

Test Objective Although no objective is stated in the manual, this test is usually used to measure abdominal strength and endurance.

Description The starting position is a back-lying position with knees flexed to less than 90 degrees, feet on the mat, and heels 12 inches from the buttocks. The hands are clasped behind the neck with fingers interlaced, and the elbows are resting on the mat. The feet are held in contact with the mat throughout the test by a partner. To begin the test, use the command "Go!" The student curls to a starting position and touches one elbow to the opposite knee, curls back to the starting position, and curls up again, touching the other elbow and knee. This sequence is continued until a 30-second time period has elapsed.

Test Area For group testing, a gymnasium or multipurpose room can be used; for individual testing a very small area will suffice.

Equipment Tumbling mat and stopwatch.

Scoring The number of sit-ups correctly executed in 30 seconds is the score. The sit-up is not counted if the student does not begin from the starting position, or if the elbow is not touched to the opposite knee. Also, the fingers must remain clasped behind the neck throughout the sit-up. One trial is administered.

Validity There is no reference to the validity of this specific test.

Reliability The Test Manual reports reliability estimates of 0.80 and above for a group of test items, presumably including the sit-ups test.

Norms Norms are available for moderately mentally retarded boys and girls, ages 6 through 20. However, the norms are based on small sample sizes and should only be used as rough guidelines.

Comments The position of the arms and hands should be altered to reflect currently recommended procedures. Therapists have noted that when the hands are clasped behind the neck, a tendency to use the arms in sitting up occurs. Furthermore, this position seems to encourage straight back sit-ups. For these reasons, the Physical Best Test uses a modified position with the arms crossed at chest level and hands placed on opposite shoulders.

Standing Long Jump

Test Objective Although the objective of the Standing Long Jump Test is not stated in the Test Manual, it is usually used as a measure of explosive leg power.

Description In the starting position, the student stands behind the restraining line. The toes must not touch the line, and the feet are several inches apart. Although any preliminary motions may be made as long as the feet are not moved, usually the examinee dips the body several times, swinging the arms backward with one dip and forward with the next. On the actual jump, the arms swing forward at the same time and land at the same time. The object of the test is to jump as far as possible.

Test Area The test can be administered on a floor or a paved, outdoor surface. The manual recommends marking an open area with a restraining line and lines parallel to this line every inch, starting at 12 inches. A testing area of 120 inches is suggested, although this can be modified, if necessary. Each line should be 30 inches long, with the distance clearly marked. Another alternative is to tape a tape measure on the floor perpendicular to the restraining line.

Equipment Tape measure, if the alternate setup is used, and a yardstick to line up the distance on the tape with the student's heels.

Scoring Record the best of three trials to the nearest inch. "Measure the perpendicular distance from the restraining line to the heel or other body part that touches the floor nearest the takeoff line. Be sure to note carefully the point where the heels first contact the floor because there is a tendency for the feet to slide forward" (Johnson and Londeree, 1976, p. 19).

Validity There is no reference in the Test Manual to the validity of this specific test.

Reliability The Test Manual reports reliability estimates of 0.80 or higher for a group of test items, presumably including the Standing Long Jump.

Norms Norms are published for moderately mentally retarded boys and girls, ages 6 through 20. However, the sample sizes are small; thus the norms should be interpreted with caution.

Comments The test developers note that the best jump is often not attained in three trials. They recommend that the youngsters build up to a point where they can perform 20 to 25 jumps with all-out effort. The tester should chart the students' performance over a number of days and determine when the best jump is made. On the actual testing day the student should be given as many practice trials as needed, as determined in previous weeks. The number of trials remains the same for all students, although the number of practice trials may vary. If one student achieved his maximum distance on trial 12, he should be given 10 practice trials before testing.

Softball Throw for Distance

Test Objective Although there is no statement in the Test Manual on the objective of the Softball Throw for Distance Test, it is usually used to measure coordination.

Description The student throws overhand as far as possible, three times in succession. Mark the distance of the first throw. If the next throw is longer, remove the marking of the first throw and mark the better one. If not, leave the marking at the landing point of the first throw. Handle the third throw the same way. Use two or more students to retrieve balls after they hit the ground. Any type of approach may be used as long as the student does not cross the restraining line. The throw must be overhand. Students should warm up before playing catch.

Test Area An open field is recommended for administration of this test, with a width of 50 feet and a length of 250 feet. Use agricultural lime to mark the field. Mark the restraining line first, then start 15 feet from the restraining line and mark lines at 5-foot intervals, up to 225 feet. This distance may be adjusted for different groups.

Equipment A minimum of three softballs (12 inch) in good condition are needed.

Scoring The test score is the best of three trials. The score is the perpendicular distance from the restraining line to the landing point. Record the distance to the nearest foot.

Validity There is no reference in the Test Manual to the validity of this specific test.

Reliability The Test Manual reports reliability estimates of 0.80 or higher for a group of test items, presumably including the Softball Throw for Distance Test.

Norms Norms are published for moderately mentally retarded boys and girls, ages 6 through 20. Because of the small sample sizes of the norm groups, the norms should be used only as rough guidelines.

Comments This test was eliminated from the AAHPER Youth Fitness Test in the 1976 manual because there was no evidence that coordination could be measured by a single item of this type. The softball throw seems to measure a specific skill rather than a general motor fitness trait. Whether it should be retained in this test battery is questionable. Other adapted physical education specialists (Winnick and Short, 1985) have suggested that the Softball Throw for Distance might be used as a substitute for a strength item in special cases. The test item probably measures a specific type of fitness required to perform a softball skill. It is unlikely that this ability generalizes to other sport skills.

The most reliable indicator of the student's ability to throw the softball is the average of three trials rather than the best of three. This is a proven fact in measurement theory. Therefore the scoring procedure for this test should be reexamined.

50-Yard Dash

Test Objective Although there is no statement in the Test Manual on the objective of the 50-Yard Dash, this test is used as a measure of speed.

Description The manual recommends testing two students at the same time. The students take starting positions behind the starting line. The test administrator (at the finish line) raises both arms sideways to indicate the Set position. The Go signal is given by rapidly lowering the arms to the side. The administrator has a stopwatch in each hand, and both watches are started when the arms reach the side of the body. The two students run as fast as possible across the finish line. The watch for a designated runner is stopped when the student's body (not head or arms) crosses the finish line. One trial is taken.

Test Area An outdoor space is usually preferred, although any smooth, solid surface of the appropriate distance may be used.

Equipment The Test Manual recommends using two stopwatches if students are to be tested in pairs. If only one watch is available, the students could be tested individually; however, they could still run in pairs for motivational purposes.

Scoring The score is the time between the Go signal and the moment the student's body crosses the finish line. The time is recorded to the nearest tenth of a second.

Validity There is no reference to the validity of this specific test.

Reliability The Test Manual reports reliability coefficients of 0.80 or higher for a group of tests, presumably including the 50-Yard Dash Test.

Norms Norms are published for moderately mentally retarded boys and girls, ages 6 through 20. These norms should be used with caution because of small sample sizes.

Comments Does the visual signal provide a more accurate start than a verbal signal? Obviously a visual signal requires the examinee to watch the examiner closely. This may lead to a slower start. Further study of these starts would be useful. The advantage of a visual start is that only one tester is needed to administer the test.

300-Yard Run-Walk

Test Objective Although no statement of the objective of the 300-Yard Run-Walk was given in the Test Manual, it is usually used as a measure of CR function.

Description The manual suggests testing five to ten students at a time. Examinees should stand in a single row behind the starting line, using a standard start. On the signal Ready, Go! the students begin running. The 300-yard distance should be run as fast as possible. Walking is permitted but should not be encouraged. As the runner crosses the finish line, the timer calls out the time to the scorer.

Test Area A track is ideal for testing the 300-Yard Run-Walk; however, any paved or smooth, solid surface, either indoors or outdoors, can be used.

Equipment A stopwatch.

Scoring The score should be recorded in seconds.

Validity No evidence of the validity of this specific test is included in the Test Manual.

Reliability No reliability estimates were reported for the 300-Yard Run-Walk.

Norms Norms are published for moderately mentally retarded boys and girls, ages 6 through 20. These norms should be used as rough guidelines because of small sample sizes.

Comments An abundance of scientific evidence now indicates that distances under 1 mile are not effective measures of CR function. Certainly a distance of 300 yards would not tap this parameter. Since CR function is such an important aspect of health-related fitness, strong consideration should be given to increasing the test distance to 1 mile for handicapped students who have been properly trained to run this distance.

Summary of the Test Battery The previous six items were presented in detail as an example of the type of fitness tests available for children with impairments. For additional information on the test battery and the award system, refer to the AAHPERD Motor Fitness Testing Manual for the Moderately Mentally Retarded (Johnson and Londeree, 1976). In general, the test items in this battery measure fitness associated with athletic ability rather than health-related physical fitness. The objectives for using this test should be clearly in mind when it is used in a school setting. The normative data were collected during the spring of 1973. The norms should be updated using substantial sample sizes from a cross section of the United States rather than a single state. Finally the test items should be revised in light of sound measurement principles and scientific evidence on the measurement of physiological parameters. This fine contribution to the testing literature for children with impairments should be continually modified so that it remains useful for teachers in school settings.

Project Unique Physical Fitness Test (Winnick and Short, 1985) In an excellent study of the physical fitness of sensory and orthopedically impaired youth, Winnick and Short (1985) noted that the components of fitness are essentially the same for normal and sensory or orthopedically impaired children, but the performance of the impaired individual generally falls below that of the normal individual. Age, gender, educational setting, and type and severity of handicapping condition must be considered in interpreting the results of physical fitness tests.

Based on a sound psychometric approach, the test battery identifies seven test items. Since all of the items are described elsewhere in this text, only a summary of the battery follows.

Test Objective The battery is designed to measure body composition, flexibility, CR endurance, and muscular strength and endurance.

Description The test battery consists of seven items:

Item 1: Skinfold measures (triceps, subscapular, and sum of triceps and subscapular.)

Item 2: Grip strength (see Figure 11-1)

Item 3: 50 yard/meter dash (see Figure 11-2)

Item 4: Sit-ups (number in 60 seconds)

Item 5: Softball throw (distance)

Item 6: Sit and Reach

Item 7: Long Distance Run (1 mile/9 minute run or 1½ mile/12 minute run)

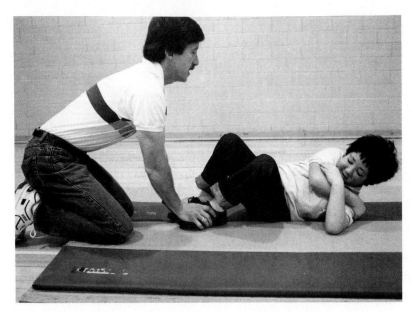

Testing sit-ups.
Courtesy of Dale A. Ulrich.

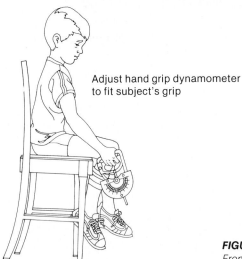

Adjust hand grip dynamometer
to fit subject's grip

FIGURE 11-1 *Measurement of grip strength.*
From Winnick, J.P., and Short, F.X.

Test Area, Equipment and Scoring See Chapters 16 and 17 on fitness testing.
Validity This test is exceptionally well validated. First, the logical validity of each test item is demonstrated. Second, evidence of criterion-related and construct validity is presented. In particular, the factorial validity of the instrument is stressed, forming the basis of this impressive study. Finally, scientific evi-

FIGURE 11-2 *The 50-yard/meter dash.*
From Winnick, J.P., and Short, F.X.

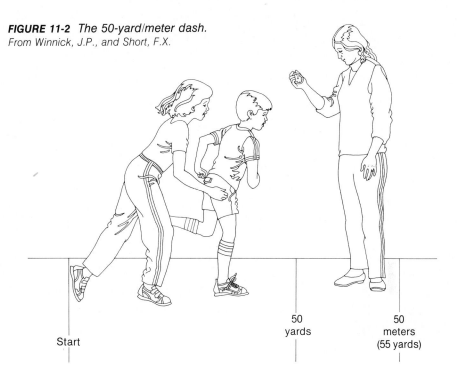

50
yards

50
meters
(55 yards)

Start

dence supporting the validity of the test items is included where appropriate.

Reliability A number of reliability coefficients are presented for each test item. These estimates range from 0.49 to 0.975, although most coefficients are very high—in the 0.90s. Reliability data are presented for **visually handicapped, hard of hearing,** and **orthopedically impaired,** as well as **mentally retarded** individuals. Anyone using these test items should refer to the Project UNIQUE report (Winnick and Short, 1985), which includes one of the best and most thorough tables of reliability estimates for fitness tests.

Norms Means and standard deviations are presented for each age and sex within each subject category. Four major categories of subjects were identified: normal (nonimpaired), visually impaired, auditory impaired, and orthopedically impaired. The sample sizes were too small to convert the data to norms.

Comments Since it is not possible for individuals with certain impairments to take some of the test items, Winnick and Short have recommended substitutions for specific situations. Although a rationale is not presented for the selection of these substitutions, it is apparent that the test developers do not necessarily view the substitute tests as measures of equivalent fitness parameters when compared to original measures. Rather, a testable area of fitness is selected, depend-

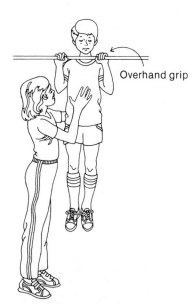

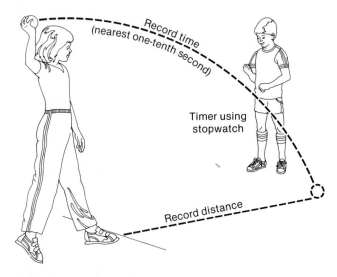

FIGURE 11-4 *Softball throw for distance.*
By permission of Joseph P. Winnick.

FIGURE 11-3 *Measurement of flexed-arm hang.*
From Winnick, J.P., and Short, F.X.

ing on the nature and extent of the handicapping condition. Consider the following examples of substitute tests:

1. For boys with **cerebral palsy,** use an arm hang test instead of grip strength (see Figure 11-3).
2. For boys with **paraplegic** wheelchair spinal neuromuscular disorder, use an arm hang test instead of grip strength.
3. For boys classified as **congenital anomaly**/amputee, use an arm hang test instead of grip strength.
4. For boys and girls classified as paraplegic wheelchair spinal neuromuscular, the softball throw for distance can be used instead of grip strength (see Figure 11-4).
5. For some boys and girls classified as congenital anomaly/amputee, the softball throw for distance may be substituted for sit-ups.
6. For boys and girls who have visual and auditory impairments, the broad jump may be substituted for grip strength.

Summary of Test Battery The soundness of the development of the Project UNIQUE Physical Fitness Test gives it an edge over other physical fitness tests for children with impairments. The test administrator should keep in mind, however, that the items in the battery measure different types of fitness. Several of the items test health-related physical fitness, and a few measure fitness in an ath-

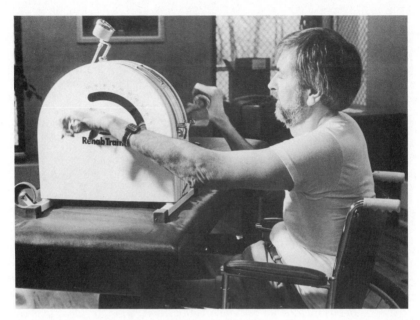

Warm-up for arm ergometer test.

letic performance context. All in all, the physical fitness test batteries for impaired children do not differ markedly from those developed for the nonimpaired child. There is no need for the items to be different, except when a type of impairment prevents performance of an item. Of course, certain modifications of items may be necessary, and norms should be developed for different types of impairments.

MOTOR PERFORMANCE TESTING

Many strategies have been developed to provide initial screening of students in a physical education setting. This screening must be followed by a formal testing program. The Los Angeles Unified School District has developed a scale that can be used to determine appropriate placement of students in physical education. An overview of the Adaptive Physical Education Assessment Scale* follows.

The Adaptive Physical Education Assessment Scale (In Seaman and Depauw, 1982)

Test Objective To place students appropriately in physical education. It measures five areas of motor performance: motor development, motor achievement, perceptual-motor function, posture, and physical fitness.

---

*For more information on the scale, test manual or norms, write to Adapted Physical Education Consultant, Los Angeles Unified School District, 450 North Grand Avenue—Bldg. G, Los Angeles, CA.

Description The scale includes 18 items measuring motor performance:

1. Agility run	10. Vertical jump
2. Throwing accuracy	11. Jumping form
3. Hand preference	12. Ocular control
4. Kick stationary ball	13. Bent knee curl up
5. Foot preference	14. Imitation of postures
6. Catching	15. Standing balance
7. Kicking rolling ball	16. Alternate hopping
8. Running	17. Arhythymical hopping
9. Posture	18. Endurance

A brief description of each of these items can be found in Seaman and DePauw (1982).

Test Area The first eight items should be measured outdoors during a single testing session. The remaining items may be administered either indoors or outdoors during another testing session. The outdoor space requirements are a 4 foot by 18 foot wall target with at least 15 feet by 16 feet of free space in front for throwing, running, and kicking; and a 50-yard rectangular running course.

Equipment In addition to the test manual and scoring materials, equipment needs include an 8½ -inch rubber ball, 18-inch ruler, five bean bags 6 inches by 6 inches, stopwatch, and chalk.

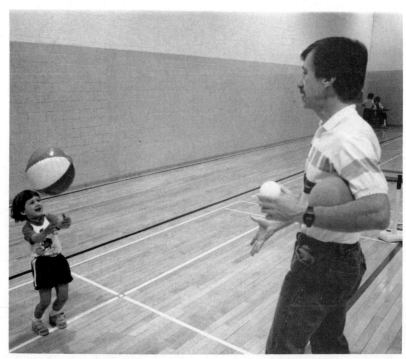

Catching task.
Courtesy of Dale A. Ulrich.

Scoring Eight items are scored using ratios representing distance or repetitions, eight incorporate ratings, and two items yield categorical data. The objectivity of these scoring procedures ranges from 0.39 to 0.96.

Validity The validity as reported in Seaman and DePauw (1982) is "face with literature" (p. 211). Evidence of factorial validity has also been presented by the Los Angeles Unified School District, as well as predictive validity based on a discriminant analysis showing that the scale correctly classifies students 89% of the time.

Reliability Ten of the 18 items have reliability estimates of 0.70 or greater on a test-retest basis (Seaman and DePauw, 1982).

Norms Norms based on scores for 2100 children, ages 5 through 18, from the Los Angeles area, including 1% trainably mentally retarded and 1% severe language delayed children. Percentile ranks are available at 6-month intervals for 5 through 7.11 years and 1-year intervals for 8 through 18 years. These norms were generated during the 1980 revision of the scale.

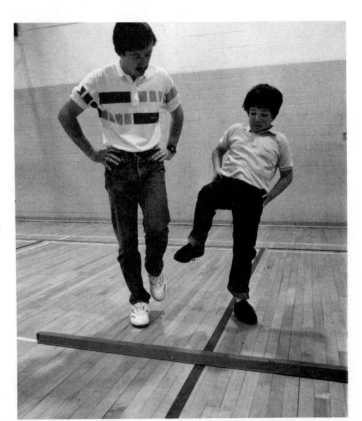

Balance task.
Courtesy of Dale A. Ulrich.

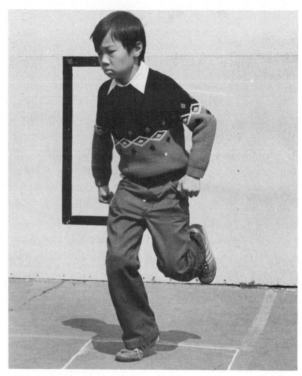

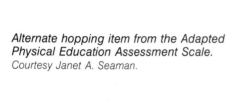

Alternate hopping item from the Adapted Physical Education Assessment Scale.
Courtesy Janet A. Seaman.

Comments Testing time per student is approximately 20 minutes. The primary usefulness of this battery lies in its ability to place students in physical education with what appears to be an impressive degree of accuracy. Of course, the validity is defensible only for the Los Angeles area, but it would be a relatively straightforward matter to validate the procedure in other areas. Reducing the length of the test is highly desirable. If the test is to be used primarily for placement, are 18 items necessary? Despite several low reliability and objectivity estimates, the scale has many positive dimensions. Certainly it provides a useful model for placement in adaptive physical education.

SUMMARY

It is not feasible to present all the motor performance tests developed for children with impairments in a measurement and evaluation textbook. Observational techniques are most frequently used on a daily basis in a field setting. Unless these instruments have acceptable reliability and validity, they should not be used in a more formal situation, as when a child's ability is assessed before developing an individualized education program. Other types of tests, particularly performance measures, have been standardized and can be used with greater confidence in their validity. Some examples of these types are motor proficiency scales, developmental scales, and physical fitness tests. Few tests are available to measure performance in a variety of sport skills. Excellent resources on this topic can be found in Seaman and DePauw (1982). Part II of their book is devoted to assessment, and Chapter 8 provides descriptions of many tests. Furthermore, a quick reference to tests on the market is included in Appendix D. The student interested in adaptive physical education is urged to review other sources of tests in this area.

LEARNING EXPERIENCES

1. Under the direction of your instructor, observe the administration of one or more motor performance tests to children with some type of impairment. What aspects of test administration differ from testing in a physical education setting for the nonimpaired child? Record these considerations and note how the tester handled them.
2. Assume you are working with a paraplegic confined to a wheelchair. How would you test this individual on cardiorespiratory function, body fatness, and low back/abdominal flexibility? First of all, are these important objectives for this person? If so, why? If not, what factors can you test? Why? How would the tests you select differ from those you would administer to a nonimpaired individual?

REFERENCES

Baumgartner, T.A., and Horvat, M.A. 1988. Problems in measuring the physical and motor performance of the handicapped. Journal of Physical Education, Recreation and Dance, **59**(1): 48-52.

Bruininks, R.H. 1978. The Bruininks-Oseretsky Test of Motor Proficiency. Circle Pines, MN: American Guidance Service.

Buell, C.E. 1982. Physical Education and Recreation for the Visually Handicapped. rev. ed. Washington, DC: American Alliance for Health, Physical Education, Recreation and Dance.

Fait, H.F., and Dunn, J.M. 1984. Special physical education. ed. 5. Chicago: W.B. Saunders Publishing Co.

Frankenburg, W.K., and Dodds, J.B. 1967. Denver Developmental Screening Test. Journal of Pediatrics, **71**:181-191.

Frankenburg, W.K., Dodds, J.B., and Fandel, A.W. 1973. Denver Developmental Screening Test manual/workbook for nursing and paramedic personnel. University of Colorado Medical Center, Denver.

Johnson, L., and Londeree, B. 1976. Motor fitness testing manual for the moderately mentally retarded. Reston, VA: The American Alliance for Health, Physical Education, Recreation and Dance.

King, H.A., and Aufsesser, K.S. 1988. Criterion-referenced testing—an ongoing process. Journal of Physical Education, Recreation and Dance, **59**(1):58-63.

Kirkendall, D.R., Gruber, J.J., and Johnson, R.E. 1987. Measurement and evaluation for physical educators. Champaign, IL: Human Kinetics Publishers, Inc.

Pyfer, J.L. 1988. Teachers, don't let your students grow up to be clumsy adults. Journal of Physical Education, Recreation and Dance, **59**(1): 38-42.

Roach, E.G., and Kephart, N.C. 1966. The Purdue Perceptual Motor Survey. Columbus, OH: Charles E. Merrill Publishing Co.

Roberton, M.A., and Halverson, L.E. 1984. Developing children—their changing movement. Philadelphia, PA: Lea & Febiger.

Seaman, J.A., and DePauw, K.P. 1982. The new adapted physical education: a developmental approach. Palo Alto, CA: Mayfield Publishing Co.

Sherrill, C. 1981. Adapted physical education and recreation. ed. 2, Dubuque, IA: Wm. C. Brown Group.

Sloan, W. 1955. The Lincoln-Oseretsky Motor Development Scale. Chicago: C.H. Stoelting Co.

Stein, J.U. 1988. Physical fitness testing and rewards. Journal of Physical Education, Recreation, and Dance, **59**(1): 53-57.

Ulrich, D.A. 1985. The Test of Gross Motor Development. Austin, TX: Pro-Ed Publishing Company.

Ulrich, D.A. 1988. Children with special needs—assessing the quality of movement competence. Journal of Physical Education, Recreation and Dance, **59**(1): 43-47.

Vodola, T.M. 1978. Developmental and Adaptive Physical Education. A.C.T.I.V.E. Motor ability and physical fitness norms: For normal, mentally retarded, learning disabled, and emotionally disturbed individuals. Oakhurst, NJ: Township of Ocean School District.

Werder, J.K., and Kalakian, L.H. 1985. Assessment in Adapted Physical Education. Minneapolis: Burgess.

Winnick, J.P. 1988. Classifying individuals with handicapping conditions for testing. Journal of Physical Education, Recreation and Dance, **59**(1): 34-37.

Winnick, J.P., and Short, F.X. 1985. Physical fitness testing of the disabled: Project UNIQUE. Champaign, IL: Human Kinetics Publishers, Inc.

ANNOTATED READINGS

American Alliance for Health, Physical Education, Recreation and Dance. 1985. Testing for impaired, disabled, and handicapped individuals. Reston, VA: AAHPERD.

Begins with a general introduction to a philosophy and rationale for testing; presents background information to aid in selecting tests; includes brief summaries of physical fitness tests, psychomotor (perceptual motor) scales, and developmental profiles; does not include information about sports skills tests, since the purpose of this publication is to assist others in selecting instruments for diagnostic and descriptive purposes.

Auxter, D., and Pyfer, J. 1985. Principles and methods of adapted physical education and recreation. St. Louis: The C.V. Mosby Co.

Includes chapter on types and purposes of assessment; describes purpose and appropriate usage of each test type; presents examples; also includes chapter on integrating evaluation and programming; provides chart of selected motor tests, including source, population, motor components, and norms.

Brunt, D., and Dearmond, D.A., 1981. Evaluating motor profiles of the hearing impaired. Journal of Physical Education, Recreation, and Dance, **52**(9):50-53.

Describes project in which the motor ability of approximately 150 upper elementary children with hearing impairments was assessed using the Bruininks-Oseretsky Test, including a description of the eight subtests designed for children with severe or profound hearing loss.

Seaman, J.A., and Baumgartner, T.A. 1983. Measurement implications of PL 94-142. In Hensley, L., and East, W. editors. Measurement and evaluation symposium proceedings. Cedar Falls: University of Northern Iowa.

Summarizes the evaluation requirements mandated by Public Law 94-142; discusses efforts to develop a physical fitness test for special populations.

Seaman, J.A. Ed. 1988. Testing the handicapped: A challenge by law. Journal of Physical Education, Recreation, and Dance, **59**(1):32-67.

A series of articles dealing with significant issues in measuring the handicapped; includes articles on classification of individuals, movement quality, measurement problems, physical fitness testing, and criterion-referenced testing.

Ulrich, D.A. 1984. The reliability of classification decisions made with the Objectives-Based Motor Skill Assessment Instrument. Adapted Physical Education Quarterly, **1**(1):52-60.

Examines the reliability of classification decisions made with the Objectives-Based Motor Skill Assessment Instrument based on two different cut-off scores, using a mentally retarded group and a nonhandicapped group; concludes that the instrument consistently assigned examinees to the same mastery state in the fundamental motor skill domain for both mastery levels.

Part Six

Measurement in a Nonschool Setting

A Review of Testing Procedures

KEY WORDS *Watch for these words as you read the following chapter:*

bicycle ergometer

body composition

carotid artery

circumference measure

maximal oxygen uptake
(max $\dot{V}_{O_2}$)

MET

pulse rate

skinfold thickness

step test

Many career options are available to the student who is interested in physical education and exercise science. Teacher preparation for the school setting represents only one of these options; others include fitness center instruction, sports center instruction, athletic training, sports management, sports medicine, and administration. In this chapter the use of measurement and evaluation in several of these roles will be discussed.

Formal instruction in many types of physical activity can take place outside the school setting. Even in the early part of the twentieth century, it was possible to take dance classes in private studios, receive private lessons in sports like tennis and golf, learn a wide variety of skills in summer camps, and participate in activities at a YMCA or YWCA. Today many other opportunities are also available in private sports and fitness centers. In this textbook the instructional aspects of these organizations are considered, as well as the managerial and sports medicine components.

Sound measurement practices are as important in nonschool settings as they are in the school setting. For example, the objectives of a private club may differ from those of a school, but a well-run organization will be accountable for its outcomes. While objectives vary from club to club, the bottom line for each club is to show a profit. This cannot be done unless members are recruited and retained. If a member chooses to enroll in a class, an additional fee is often charged. Once in class the client is presented with the *opportunity* to learn. It is assumed that a level of motivation initially exists, but often it is the instructor's responsibility to maintain this motivation. There is virtually no control over the "students" in these classes. They cannot be required to attend, study rules, practice skills, or take tests, for that matter. However, evaluation cannot be ignored for these reasons. The club, not the client, sets the standards. If the client wishes to ignore the standards, it is his or her prerogative.

MEASURING SKILLS IN SPORTS CLUBS

Joining a sports club for recreational purposes only is not unusual. Advantages include the availability of court space when desired and the offering of instructional programs, which usually include private and group lessons. Undoubtedly each instructor plans objectives for these classes. They may be general or specific, including skills the instructor plans to introduce during the unit of instruction. In some instances these objectives may not be available in written form. Unless the instructional program is rather poor, the instructor has probably thought through the instructional plans and has loosely formed objectives in mind. If the club is part of a franchise, a set of objectives, able to be modified to meet the needs of each club, might be distributed by the home office. Regardless of the source, objectives should be prepared in writing. The small size of the classes and the individualized nature of instruction create an ideal opportunity for tailoring objectives to clients' needs.

Writing objectives for class members in a private club is no different from preparing objectives for students in a school. The major difference is that, because of a smaller class size, the instructor in the private club often has the luxury of formulating objectives for each client. Individualized objectives also support the club as a business. The closer the class comes to meeting the client's needs, the more likely it is that others will enroll in future classes. If a client benefits from a class, the word will be passed on to other prospective clients; some of them will sign up for a future class. Word-of-mouth is a powerful factor in sustaining this type of private enterprise.

Although the process of *writing* objectives is the same in school and non-school settings, the process of *implementing* them can differ. Although objectives have been set and the instructional process delineated, the client may not be concerned about meeting the predetermined objectives. Clients' needs in a class setting may differ. Some sign up for a class simply to learn a little more about the sport; thus developing skills to a specified level may be of little interest to them. They may care little about specific objectives, as long as the basic skills needed for the game are covered. On the other hand, skill development may be important to other individuals, who often respond positively to the use of objectives that include specific evaluation standards. For them, the setups for skills tests provide an excellent opportunity to practice their skills. Furthermore, the client can work toward a set of specific goals. Any published test of a skill can be used in a private club setting, as long as test validity and reliability are adequate for the situation and clientele. In fact, using tests requiring elaborate setup materials in a private club is far more feasible than it is in a school.

Since a private sports club is a business, the needs of the client must be met while ensuring a high-quality program. A multifaceted approach to preparing objectives is recommended. Objectives should be developed for the class as a whole. For example, in a beginning racquetball class objectives could be written for the serve, forehand and backhand drives, playing the game, and so forth. Each of these objectives should include specific evaluation standards. At the first meeting of the class, these objectives should be reviewed. Then the class members could be given choices regarding their own objectives. At the very least, the client should be encouraged to adapt the class objectives to his or her own needs. This allows testing to take place during the unit of instruction, as described in the objectives. Ideally the instructor would work closely with each client to tailor the class objectives to the individual. However, it should be made clear that all clients wishing to progress to a higher-level course must meet the class objectives at the current level. It is possible that individual modifications can be even more stringent than the class objectives. At the other extreme, some class members may not care about being evaluated and may object to taking any type of test and to any formalized rating by the instructor. In small clubs the number of members is often insufficient to allow several classes to take place at the same time, each with different objectives. Flexibility and individualization are the keys to success in the private club.

MEASURING HEALTH-RELATED FITNESS IN FITNESS CENTERS

Many exercise specialists are being trained to assume jobs as instructors and/or directors of private fitness clubs, corporate fitness centers, and other similar organizations. In these settings the objectives tend to be health related rather than skill oriented. Also, objectives are usually individualized, since the fitness level of new clients can vary greatly. A typical objective is the reduction of body fat. The desired amount of weight loss is dependent on the client's distribution of fat and lean body mass at the time he or she joins the program. The client's **body composition,** consisting of bone, muscle mass, and fatty tissue, must be *measured* to determine the individual's current status. Types of measures of body composition vary from one organization to another; however, some methods, such as weighing the person, are not the best measures to use. (Valid measures of body composition are discussed in detail in Chapter 16.) Once the client's body composition has been determined, a reasonable goal can be set for that individual. Note that this is another example of *needs assessment.* The *actual* level of body fatness is compared with the *desired level.*

The testing programs used in fitness centers vary widely, ranging from no tests at all to a relatively sophisticated series of measures. A review of the entrance tests used by several organizations follows. (Refer to Chapter 16 for specific information on the tests mentioned in these sections.)

Private Clubs

Private fitness centers in the United States have proliferated over the past 15 years. Although all clubs have as their goal the improvement of a client's fitness level, various methods are used to achieve this goal. Some clubs merely provide organized workouts for their clients, with no information on the effectiveness of the exercise sessions. Others test basic physiological and physical capacities of all new clients who join their club and, on the basis of these results, prescribe an exercise program for each individual. Obviously the latter approach is preferable. Not only is the program geared to the individual's needs but the client also becomes more knowledgeable about his or her health-related fitness state. The testing programs used in two private clubs are described first.

Vic Tanny International of Wisconsin, Inc. The Vic Tanny clubs in Wisconsin administer two tests of health-related fitness to their new clients. The first is a Body Fat Analysis, in which percent body fat and ideal body weight are estimated from body circumferences. The rationale for using body **circumference measures** to estimate body composition has been discussed by Katch and McArdle (1983). Three body sites are used, although the sites differ with one's gender and age. For women under 30, circumferences are measured at the mid-abdomen, right thigh, and right forearm. The right calf is substituted for the right forearm for women over 30. For men under 30, circumferences are measured at the right upper arm, mid-abdomen, and right forearm. The buttock is substituted for the right upper arm for men over 30. The second test is the Pulse Recovery Step Test, a modification of the **step tests** described in Chapter 16 (see Figure 12-1). The client exercises for 3 minutes on a 12-inch bench, using a cadence of 24 steps per minute. The **pulse rate** is then measured for 10 seconds immediately after the end of the 3-minute period.

Figure 12-2 displays a portion of the form used to record fitness test information. This record is then used to plan an exercise program for the client.

Olympic Health and Racquet Club The Olympic Health and Racquet Club administers the Kasch Pulse Recovery Test. This is another modification of the step test, in which the heart rate is measured during recovery. The bench height is 14 inches for women and 16 inches for men. The duration of the test is 3 minutes, with one step taken every 2 seconds. The heart rate is measured at the **carotid artery.** This rate is recorded in 10-second increments during the first minute of recovery after the completion of exercise. The total score is the sum of the ten 10-second recordings. Body composition measures are made available through other sources.

The score sheet for the Kasch Test is shown in Figure 12-3. Notice that suggested standards for men and women are included on the score sheets used by both clubs.

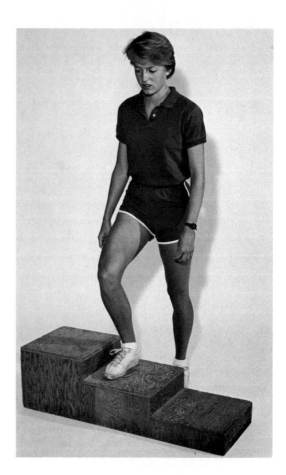

FIGURE 12-1 *Administration of step test.*

Corporate Fitness Centers

Many large corporations provide fitness centers to enable their employees to exercise during working hours as well as before and after work. These centers are often directed by a person with at least a master's degree in exercise physiology. Extensive testing is usually available in these settings.

CUNA Mutual Insurance Group An example of one of these programs is the Exercise Resource Facility of the CUNA Mutual Insurance Group, made available to all employees of CUNA Mutual. The test package includes measurement of body composition, functional capacity, strength, and flexibility. Body composition is assessed by measuring the skinfold thicknesses at three sites. The men's sites are pectoral, abdominal, and thigh; the women's, triceps, suprailiac, and thigh. The **skinfold thickness** values are used to estimate percent of body fat and lean body mass. To measure functional capacity, a **bicycle ergometer** test is used (see Figure 12-4). A bicycle ergometer is a stationary bicycle that can be used to

¤ Facilities   ¤ Workout Floor and Program Explanation

¤ BODY FAT ANALYSIS

¤ I. INTRODUCTION: Body weight as shown on the scale is not a good indi-
         cator of body composition. One does not know what portion of their
         body is fat and or muscle. Therefore, it is necessary to determine
         an individual's % body fat and strive to reduce this percentage by
         proper diet and exercise programs. Percent fat determination using
         selected body circumferential measurements has been scientifically
         proven to give accurate estimates of body fat.

¤ II. MEASUREMENTS: (measurements will be different for each sex and
         age group)

                              WOMEN

           Under 30   Over 30

     (A) Mid-Abdomen: _____   (A) Mid-Abdomen: _____
     (B) Right Thigh: _____   (B) Right Thigh: _____
     (C) Right Forearm: _____   (C) Right Calf: _____
     (D) Age Const: 19.6   (D) Age Const: 18.4

                               MEN

           Under 30   Over 30   BODY BUILDERS

     (A) Rt Upper Arm: _____   (A) Buttocks: _____   (A) WAIST: _____
     (B) Mid-Abdomen: _____   (B) Mid-Abdomen: _____   (B) BUTTOCKS: _____
     (C) Right Forearm: _____   (C) Right Forearm: _____ (C) WRIST: _____
     (D) Age Const: 10.2   (D) Age Const: 14.9   (D) NECK: _____

¤   Locate the constant that corresponds to each of the three
       measurements on reference chart.

¤ III. PERCENT FAT = _____ + _____ - _____ - _____ = [%]
                        A   B   C   D

¤ IV. DETERMINATION OF IDEAL BODY WEIGHT

       1. % fat from formula = _____% Convert to a decimal = [   ]

       2. Fat Weight = Body Weight X % Fat (in decimal form) = [   ]

               = _____ X _____ = [lbs.]

       3. Lean Weight = Body Weight in lbs. - Fat Weight in lbs. = [   ]

               = _____ - _____ = [lbs.]

       4. STANDARDS Endurance Athletes 5-9% Suggested % fat for men = 12-15%

           Suggested % fat for women = 16-20%
           Optimal % fat used = 100 - _____% = [   ]
           (change to a decimal)

Continued.

FIGURE 12-2 *Form used in exercise program planning.*
From Vic Tanny International of Wisconsin.

5. Optimal Body Weight = Lean Weight ÷ Optimal % Fat (in decimal form)
   (assuming lean weight remains the same)

   = _____ ÷ _____ = [_____ lbs.]

6. Pounds of fat to lose = Body Weight - Optimal Body Weight =

   = _____ - _____ = [_____ lbs.]

☐ V. These fat formulas are the exclusive property of Dr. Frank Katch and
      Dr. William McArdle and the Lea & Febiger Publishing Company,
      Philadelphia, Pa. Permission for their use has been exclusively
      given to the Health and Tennis Corporation of America. These formulas
      are protected by U.S. copyright regulations.

      Reproduced by permission
      FRANK I. KATCH and WILLIAM D. McARDLE
      Nutrition, Weight Control, and Exercise
      2nd Ed.
      Lea & Febiger Publishers
      Philadelphia, Pa.
      1983

☐ PULSE RECOVERY STEP TEST

☐   The three minute pulse recovery step test consists of a 12-inch
       bench, 24 per min. stepping rate for exactly three (3) minutes
       duration. Its purpose is to broadly determine the exercise
       tolerance or exercise classification of human subjects. It is not
       intended to be a diagnostic test, but for the screening and classi-
       fication of fitness as a means of prescribing an exercise program;
       (2) evaluating the subject's fitness in comparison to normals; and
       (3) to follow the progress of a person undergoing training or re-
       cuperating from a low fitness level or illness.

☐   Resting pulse rate (beats per minute) _____

☐   Number of heart beats exactly 0 to 10 seconds after the step-up
       exercise _____

☐   "TENTATIVE" CLASSIFICATION OF HEART RATE RECOVERY

Classification	Men	Women
Excellent	17 or less	16 or less
Good	18 to 20	17 to 18
Average	21 to 23	19 to 22
Fair	24 to 26	23 to 25
Poor	27 or more	26 or more

Subsidiary of
HEALTH & TENNIS CORP.
OF AMERICA

FIGURE 12-2, cont'd *Form used in exercise program planning.*

KASCH PULSE RECOVERY TEST

NAME _____

ADDRESS _____

	TEST 1 Date: _____	TEST 2 Date: _____	TEST 3 Date: _____
Resting heart rate	_____	_____	_____
Recovery	0-10 _____	0-10 _____	0-10 _____
Heart rate	11-20 _____	11-20 _____	11-20 _____
0-1 Min	21-30 _____	21-30 _____	21-30 _____
Post exercise	31-40 _____	31-40 _____	31-40 _____
	41-50 _____	41-50 _____	41-50 _____
	51-60 _____	51-60 _____	51-60 _____
	TOTAL _____	TOTAL _____	TOTAL _____

CLASSIFICATION: (Check one)

	TEST 1	TEST 2	TEST 3
Superior	_____	_____	_____
Excellent	_____	_____	_____
Good	_____	_____	_____
Average	_____	_____	_____
Fair	_____	_____	_____
Poor	_____	_____	_____
Very poor	_____	_____	_____

SUGGESTED STANDARDS FOR MEN AND WOMEN

Men (over 30 yrs)	Men (18-30 yrs)	Classification	Women (18 yrs & over)
67	68	Superior	70
68-78	69-80	Excellent	71-82
79-90	81-90	Good	83-94
91-105	91-104	Average	95-109
106-115	105-114	Fair	110-119
116-125	115-124	Poor	120-129
126	125	Very poor	130

FIGURE 12-3 *Kasch Test score sheet.*
From the Olympic Health and Racquet Club.

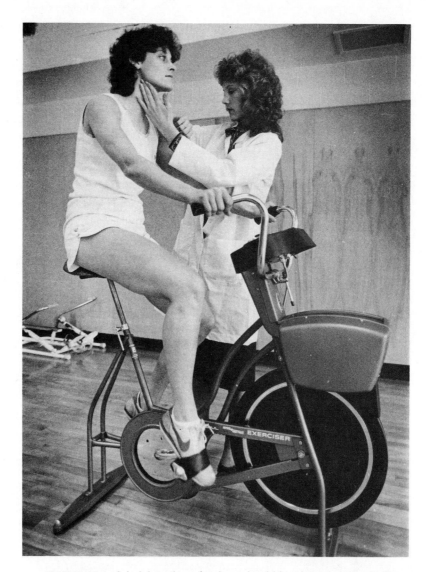

FIGURE 12-4 *Administration of submaximal bicycle ergometer test.*

measure physical work capacity. Since this is a submaximal stress test, the results provide an indirect measure of maximal oxygen uptake (**max $\dot{V}o_2$**). The score is also recorded in **METS,** which is defined as an energy value somewhat like a calorie or, more specifically, the ratio of exercise metabolic rate to resting metabolic rate (1 MET = 3.5 ml/kg). Three measures of strength are administered: a leg press, a bench press, and a sit-up test. To measure flexibility, the Sit and Reach Test is used.

EMPLOYEE TEST DATA

EXERCISE RESOURCE FACILITY

NAME _____   DATE _____/_____/_____

CHECK ONE: Original Test   Retest   Examiner _____

AGE _____ WEIGHT _____ lb _____ kg   OPTIMAL WEIGHT _____ HEIGHT _____
                                                     (Estimate)

BODY COMPOSITION

(Circle one)

MEN	WOMEN	
Pectoral	Triceps	_____
Abdominal	Suprailium	_____
Thigh	Thigh	_____

Sum of three	_____
% Fat	_____
Lean body mass	_____
16% 23%	_____
Abdominal girth	_____
Other: 1.	_____
2.	_____
3.	_____

FUNCTIONAL CAPACITY

Original workload _____

Resting HR   _____

Resting BP   _____

Workload _____ kg@ _____ RPM= _____ KPM

EXERCISE	HR	BP
Min. 1	_____	_____
2	_____	_____
3	_____	_____
4	_____	_____
5	_____	_____
6	_____	_____

Steady State HR

STRENGTH DATA

1.	Leg Press	_____
2.	Bench Press	_____
3.	Sit-Ups Test	_____

FLEXIBILITY DATA

Sit and Reach Test _____

COMMENTS:

TRAINING DATA

METS Max	_____
METS Training	_____
Heart Rate Training	_____/min
	_____/15 sec

FIGURE 12-5 Employee record of training data.
From the Exercise Resource Facility, CUNA Mutual Insurance Group, Madison, WI.

The results of this thorough testing program are used to prescribe an exercise program for the employee. Note the space provided for training data, the level at which the employee should be exercising, on the employee record shown in Figure 12-5.

Sentry World Headquarters The Physical Fitness Center at the Sentry World Headquarters in Stevens Point, Wisconsin, is designed for the benefit of all Sentry Insurance employees. Physical fitness is viewed as a key element in maintaining personal health. The Sentry Wellness Program was developed to improve the quality of life of employees. It provides for an appraisal of the employee's current state of health as well as education regarding exercise, rest, nutrition, and other elements affecting one's health. Screening for potential problems such as high blood pressure is available on an ongoing basis. Assistance is provided for well and relatively well people, those with acute illness or injury, and those suffering from a chronic disability. A "flexible time" principle permits the employee to arrange working hours to allow scheduling of health promotion activities during a regular work day.

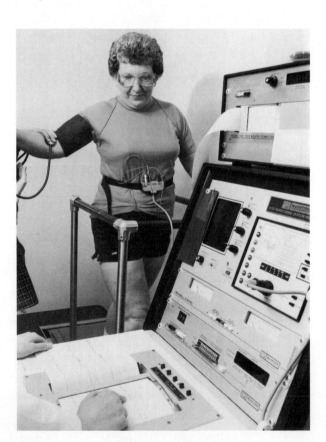

Employee taking treadmill test at Sentry World Headquarters, Stevens Point, WI.

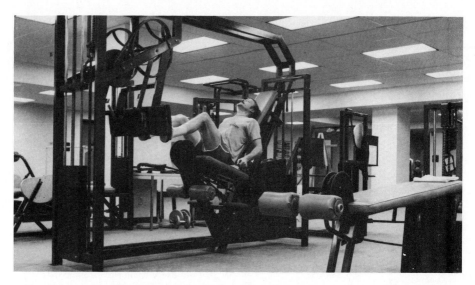

Employee using Nautilus equipment for self-testing at Sentry World Headquarters.

Three steps must be completed by any employee wishing to use the Physical Fitness Center. First, an orientation program is undertaken to instruct the employee in identifying good health habits and taking control of his or her personal fitness program. Next, the employee receives a medical screening, completes the form shown in Figure 12-6, and takes the form to the medical department before participating in an organized program. This form is typical of the inventories designed to assess lifestyle, including both physical and mental health. Finally, a trained physical fitness specialist provides the employee with specific instructions for an individualized program consisting of two parts—Cardiovascular and Nautilus Strength and Flexibility training (Sentry World Headquarters, 1979). Each participant keeps a daily record of personal activities using the form shown in Figure 12-7.

Other Organizations

Many hospitals have their own fitness center that includes an exercise physiology laboratory. These facilities are frequently available only to patients with cardiac disease or hypertension and employees of the hospital. However, services are sometimes extended to special groups of patients such as pregnant women and elderly individuals. It is not unusual for hospitals to promote a wellness program, although exercise facilities may not be provided for those in reasonably good health. A physical education department in a university may provide fitness programs for faculty and staff. Basic assessments such as stress testing and skinfold

FITNESS AND STRESS TEST PROTOCOL

Date_____

This form is to be completed and brought to the Medical Department prior to participating in an organized program in the Physical Fitness Center or a stress test.

1. Name _____ Address _____

2. Sentry employee _____ Spouse/Dependent (State employee's name) _____
   Other _____

3. Age _____ 4. Sex _____ 5. Phone: (Home) _____ (Bus.) _____
   Location _____

6. Exercise program interested in _____

7. Previous stress test? _____ If so, date: _____ A copy should be on file in the Medical Department.

8. **HABITS THAT AFFECT QUALITY AND QUANTITY OF LIFE:**   **PLEASE LIST TYPE OF EXERCISE**

   A. **Exercise** _____ At least 3-5 times weekly for at least 15 minutes of vigorous exercise each time.   _____

   _____ Less than above.   _____

   _____ None   _____

   B. **Rest:** Average number of hours of sleep per night_____

   C. **Smoker:** _____ If so, what? _____ For how long? _____

   How much have you been averaging per day? _____

   If you quit smoking, CONGRATULATIONS! How long ago? _____

   D. **Nutrition:** Do you eat breakfast? _____
   Do you eat at least three meals per day? _____
   Do you snack between meals? _____
   Average number of alcohol drinks per week? _____
   (1 drink = 1 can of beer, 1 glass of wine, 1 shot of hard liquor)

   Average number of cups of caffeinated coffee per week _____
   Average number of 8 oz. cola drinks per week _____

   E. **Stress:** Do you feel you take adequate relaxation time? _____
   Do you usually feel you are "in control" of how life is going? _____

9. Allergies to materials or drugs? _____ If so, what? _____

   _____

10. Use of medications, pills or shots? This would include either prescription drugs or "over the counter" prescriptions such as sleeping aids, tension-reducers, diet pills or vitamins. No _____ Yes _____ Please list: _____

   _____

11. Presently receiving care for any conditions? No _____ Yes _____

   Explain: _____

FIGURE 12-6 *Fitness and stress protocol form.*

12. If you have ever had problems with any of the following, please describe below:
Heart or blood vessels (blood clot, murmur, rheumatic fever, chest pain, irreg. heart beat) _____

_____

High blood pressure _____

Lungs, asthma, chronic bronchitis _____

Seizure disorder/epilepsy _____

Muscles, joints, or back _____

Thyroid gland or metabolism _____

Diabetes _____

Balance or dizziness _____

Any previous surgery/pregnancy _____

13. Have any blood relatives (parents, brothers, sisters) died before age 60 of any of the above problems? Yes _____ No _____ Explain: _____

_____

14. Do any living blood relatives have any of the above health conditions? _____
Explain: _____

15. Have you ever had a cholesterol or triglyceride test? _____ If so, when and what were the results? _____

_____

I understand that the information on this form will be released to the Physical Fitness Center.
Signed_____

— —

THIS PORTION TO BE FILLED OUT BY MEDICAL DEPARTMENT STAFF

Height _____   Weight _____   Ideal Weight _____

Blood Pressure _____   Resting Heart Rate _____

Stress Test Date _____   Physical Condition _____

Age-Adjusted Maximum Heart Rate (220-Age) _____

65% _____   75% _____   85% _____

RECOMMENDED INITIAL TARGET HEART RATE _____

Conditions to be Aware of: _____

_____

_____

Restrictions: _____

_____

Reviewed by _____
Date sent to PFC _____

FIGURE 12-6, *cont'd*

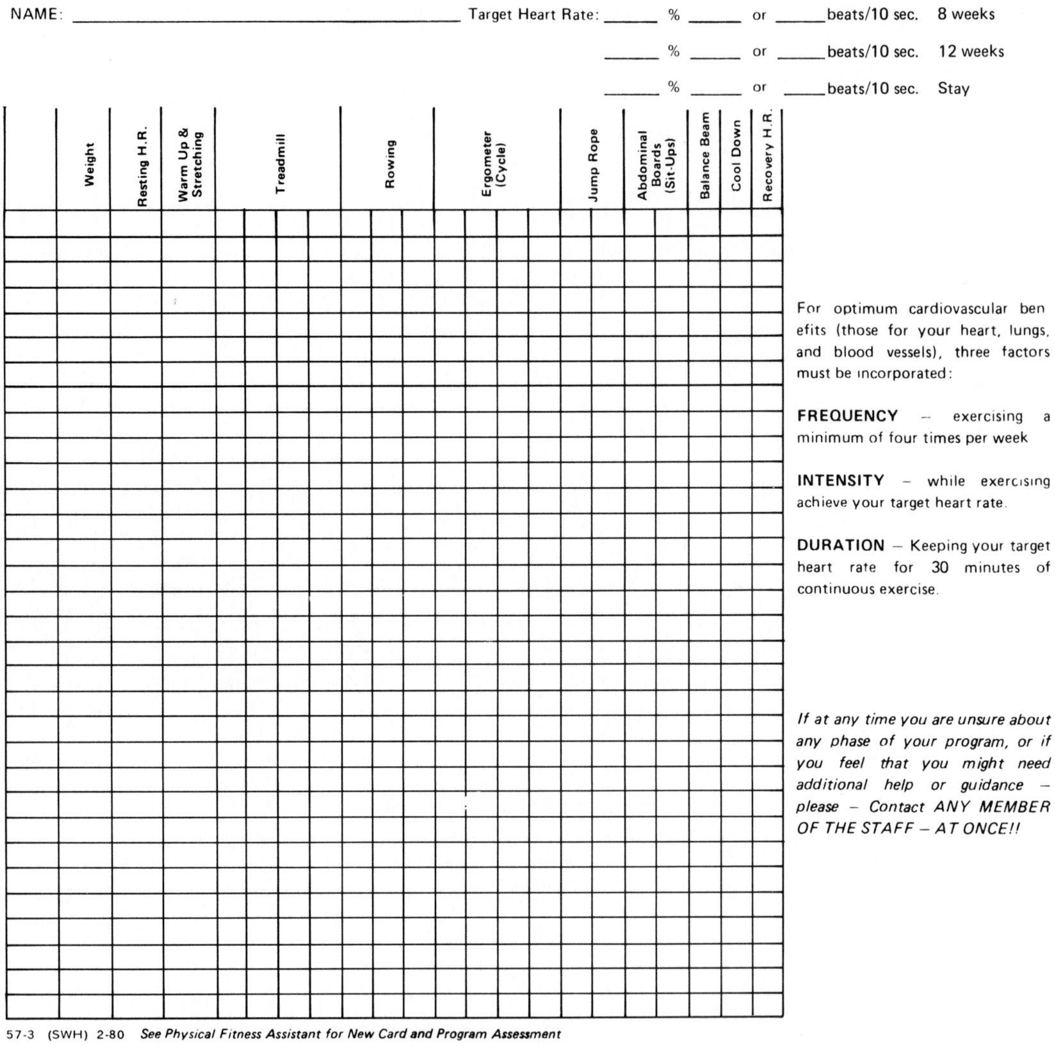

NAME: _____ Target Heart Rate: _____ % _____ or _____beats/10 sec. 8 weeks

_____ % _____ or _____beats/10 sec. 12 weeks

_____ % _____ or _____beats/10 sec. Stay

	Weight	Resting H.R.	Warm Up & Stretching	Treadmill		Rowing		Ergometer (Cycle)		Jump Rope	Abdominal Boards (Sit-Ups)	Balance Beam	Cool Down	Recovery H.R.

For optimum cardiovascular ben
efits (those for your heart, lungs,
and blood vessels), three factors
must be incorporated:

FREQUENCY – exercising a
minimum of four times per week

INTENSITY – while exercising
achieve your target heart rate.

DURATION – Keeping your target
heart rate for 30 minutes of
continuous exercise.

*If at any time you are unsure about
any phase of your program, or if
you feel that you might need
additional help or guidance –
please – Contact ANY MEMBER
OF THE STAFF – AT ONCE!!*

57-3 (SWH) 2-80 *See Physical Fitness Assistant for New Card and Program Assessment*

FIGURE 12-7 *Each participant keeps a daily record of personal activities.*

measurement are often provided. If collaboration with a nearby hospital is solid-
ified, a cardiac rehabilitation program may be established.

YMCA The YMCA uses an extensive battery of tests in the Y's Way to Physical Fitness. Body composition is determined by measuring skinfold thicknesses
at either four or six sites for men and three or five sites for women. The number
of sites measured depends on the formula to be used in estimating percent fat.
The measures of skinfold thickness are summed across the sites, and an estimate
of percent body fat is calculated. Furthermore, percentile norms for each skin-

LEGS: Progress to 20 repetitions then increase weight unit by one the next session while decreasing the repetitions.

ARMS: Progress to 15 repetitions then increase weight unit by one the next session and decrease repetitions.

Hip & Back		Compound Leg						Pullover		Double Chest				Double Shoulder				Bicep-Tricep				4-Way Neck		Multi-Exercise						Balance Beam	Cool Down	Recovery H.R.
		Leg Ext.		Leg Press		Leg Curl				Arm Cross		Decline Press		Lateral Raise		Overhead Press		Bicep Curl		Tricep Extension				Chin Ups	Calf Raises	Dips	Wrist Curl	Side Bends	Knee Tucks			
Wt	Rep	Wt	Rep	Wt	Rep	Wt	Rep	Wt	Rep	Wt	Rep	Wt	Rep	Wt	Rep	Wt	Rep	Wt	Rep	Wt	Rep	Wt	Rep									

(Seat No. columns indicated above Pullover, Arm Cross, and Lateral Raise)

FIGURE 12-7, cont'd

fold site are available. The Body Composition Rating Scale for males 35 years and younger is shown in Figure 12-8.

A physical work capacity (PWC) test is included as a measure of cardiorespiratory function. The male client begins exercising on a bicycle ergometer at 300 kilometers per minute (kpm) (150 kpm for the female client), and the workload is increased as dictated by the client's level of fitness (See Figure 12-9). Two scores are calculated: max $\dot{V}O_2$ and METS. To measure flexibility, a trunk flexion test is administered. Two measures of muscular strength and endurance are included:

Y's WAY TO PHYSICAL FITNESS

Rating Scale

Norms Males 35 Years and Under

Name _____

Dates: T_1 _____ T_2 _____ T_3 _____

Percentage ranking	Rating	Percent fat	Skinfolds						
			Chest mm	Abdomen mm	Ilium mm	Axilla mm	Tricep mm	Back mm	Thigh mm
95	Very lean	6	3	4	4	4	3	4	4
85	Lean	9	7	8	6	8	6	8	6
75	Leaner than ave.	14	12	16	11	13	10	12	10
50	Average	18	15	21	16	17	11	15	14
30	Fatter than ave.	22	18	27	20	21	13	19	16
15	Fat	25	22	34	26	25	16	24	21
5	Very fat	30	28	44	33	33	21	33	33
YOUR SCORE	T_1	___	___	___	___	___	___	___	___
	T_2	___	___	___	___	___	___	___	___
	T_3	___	___	___	___	___	___	___	___

FIGURE 12-8 *Body Composition Rating Scale.*

From Y's Way to Physical Fitness. Lawrence A. Golding, Ph.D., Clayton R. Myers, Ph.D., and Wayne E. Sinning, Ph.D., editors. Published by National Board of YMCA of USA, 1982, Chicago. Copies available YMCA of the USA, Program Resources, 6400 Shafer Court, Rosemont, IL 60018. By permission of the YMCA.

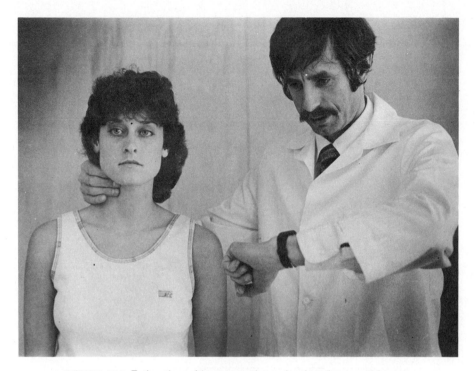

FIGURE 12-9 *Estimation of heart rate by palpating the carotid artery.*

an 80-pound bench press and a 1-minute timed sit-up test. These scores are recorded on the Physical Fitness Evaluation Form reproduced in Figure 12-10. This version of the form includes the norms for females 35 years and under. The YMCA has developed separate norms for males 35 years and under, females 35 years and under, males 36 to 45 years, and females 36 to 45 years.

Once all tests have been administered, scores are recorded on a master score sheet, shown in the version for women in Figure 12-11, and then transferred to the Physical Fitness Profile.

At this point the steps used in determining fitness objectives for a client should be understood. The client's *desired* level of physical fitness is compared with his or her *actual* level. Then a program of physical activity is prescribed. The appropriate physiological parameters are monitored on a regular basis to determine progress toward the desired level of fitness. *Remember that the general procedure is no different in a private sports club or a school setting.* The *implementation* of the objectives may differ because the client chooses to join a private club, while the student is required to be in school. Evaluation assumes an important role in instruction in school and nonschool settings.

Accountability is as important in a nonschool setting as it is in the schools.

Y's WAY TO PHYSICAL FITNESS

Rating Scale

Norms   Females 35 Years and Under

Name _____

Dates: T_1 _____ T_2 _____ T_3 _____

Percentage ranking	Rating	PWC max kgm	Liters/ min	ml/kg	Mets	Trunk flexion ins	Bench press repetitions	Sit-ups 1 min reps	3-Min step test post Ex. HR 1 min BPM	Resting HR BPM
95	Excellent	1700	3.32	55	15.	23	30	39	79	59
85	Good	1500	2.74	45	13.	21	24	34	94	63
75	Above Av.	1300	2.42	39	11.	20	20	30	109	68
50	Average	1100	2.09	34	10.	18	16	25	118	72
30	Below Av.	900	1.76	30	9.	15	13	20	122	80
15	Fair	700	1.44	26	7.	14	10	15	129	84
5	Poor	500	.86	20	6.	11	5	10	137	92

YOUR SCORE
T_1 ___ ___ ___ ___ ___ ___ ___
T_2 ___ ___ ___ ___ ___ ___ ___
T_3 ___ ___ ___ ___ ___ ___ ___

	Test 1	Test 2	Test 3
Target Weight	_____	_____	_____
Actual Weight	_____	_____	_____
Difference	_____	_____	_____
% Body Fat (23% Target)	_____	_____	_____
Blood Pressure	___/___	___/___	___/___

Your actual weight should be within 10% of your target weight.

Any values over 140/90 are considered high, and below 110/65 are considered low. Values exceeding 160/95 are labeled as hypertensive.

FIGURE 12-10 *Physical Fitness Evaluation Form.*

From Y's Way to Physical Fitness. Lawrence A. Golding, Ph.D., Clayton R. Myers, Ph.D., and Wayne E. Sinning, Ph.D., editors. Published by National Board of YMCA of USA, 1982, Chicago. Copies available YMCA of the USA, Program Resources, 6400 Shafer Court, Rosemont, IL 60018. By permission of the YMCA.

Y's WAY TO PHYSICAL FITNESS

SCORE SHEET FEMALES

NAME _____   DATE _____

TIME _____

Temp. F°

    Age _____ years   Weight _____ lbs _____ kg   Height _____ ins

    Resting Blood Pressure _____/_____ mm Hg   Resting Heart Rate _____ bpm

---

1. SKINFOLDS

    Chest   _____ mm

    Abdomen _____ mm

    Ilium   _____ mm

    Axilla _____ mm

    Scapula _____ mm

    Tricep _____ mm

    Thigh   _____ mm

2. PERCENT FAT

	Sum of 5	(or)	Sum of 3
Thigh	_____	Ilium	_____
Ilium	_____	Abdomen	_____
Abdomen	_____	Axilla	_____
Tricep	_____	Sum	_____
Scapula	_____		
Sum	_____		

    Percent fat ____ %   Percent fat ____ %

3. TARGET WEIGHT (23%) _____ lbs

4. PHYSICAL WORK CAPACITY TEST

    Seat Height _____ Predicted Max Heart Rate _____ B/M

    85% of Predicted Max Heart Rate _____ B/M _____ Seconds for 30 Beats

        WORKLOADS   HEART RATE

        1st Workload 150 kgm   _____ 2nd min

                                  _____ 3rd min

                                  _____ 4th min (if needed)

        2nd Workload _____ kgm   _____ 2nd min

                                  _____ 3rd min

                                  _____ 4th min (if needed)

        3rd Workload _____ kgm   _____ 2nd min

                                  _____ 3rd min

                                  _____ 4th min (if needed)

        NOTE: Transfer above results to the PWC Graph and Compute

5. FLEXIBILITY

    Trunk flexion _____ ins

6. MUSCULAR STRENGTH & ENDURANCE

    Bench Press (35 lbs) _____ reps

    1 min Timed Sit-ups _____ reps

        Transfer all results to Physical Fitness Profile

FIGURE 12-11 *Master score sheet.*

From Y's Way to Physical Fitness. Lawrence A. Golding, Ph.D., Clayton R. Myers, Ph.D., and Wayne E. Sinning, Ph.D., editors. Published by National Board of YMCA of USA, 1982, Chicago. Copies available YMCA of the USA, Program Resources, 6400 Shafer Court, Rosemont, IL 60018. By permission of the YMCA.

Because private clubs are profit-making organizations, they must gear their operation to attracting a large membership contingency. To retain this appeal the club is often evaluated at several levels. For instance, the cleanliness and decor of the club are factors in retaining new members, as is the efficiency of the day-to-day operation. The nature of the publicity and the attractiveness of club membership packages affect the club's ability to secure new members. All these elements must be evaluated periodically by the club manager. One of the best ways to retain members is to improve their skills. Theoretically, if individuals can play better, they will enjoy it more. This is why it is so important to attempt to individualize objectives in instructional settings in a private club. By creating a more personal atmosphere, the instructor is providing a rare opportunity for the member to receive individual attention from the club staff. Furthermore, the private club that is part of a franchise will be expected to demonstrate its accountability to the home office. Every effort should be made to satisfy the needs of the member while retaining high standards set by the club.

MEASURING HEALTH-RELATED FITNESS IN PROGRAMS FOR OLDER ADULTS

Measurement techniques developed for younger populations are not always suitable for older adults. In assessing the physical fitness of the older adult, the functional age of the examinee rather than the chronological age is of interest (Osness, 1986). Functional age is physiological, although it is affected by genetics, the absence or presence of disease, lifestyle, and a person's day-to-day decisions.

A functional fitness test for older adults is being developed by an AAHPERD committee. The test has not yet been published, pending the collection of data to establish norms. All items have been administered to a small number of examinees. Evidence of reliability and validity has been obtained for some of the test items, but specific information is not available at the present time.

The following guidelines were used during the development of this test (AAHPERD Ad Hoc Committee, 1988; p. 1):

1. The test must relate to the full range of age among older people. Options may be used for subgroups.
2. The test would not relate to follow-up prescriptions at this point in time.
3. The test would be nondiagnostic from a pathological point of view.
4. The test is a physical function evaluation only.
5. The test would be drug independent.
6. The test will not need physician approval—no more risk than life itself.
7. The test will be prepared for paraprofessional use.
8. The test will require only normally available equipment.

Before administering the test items, measurement of the examinee's weight and standing height is recommended. The test consists of five items, briefly described below:

Item 1: Trunk/Leg Flexibility This item is often referred to as the V-sit and reach. The examinee sits on the floor with legs extended in a V position and reaches as far as possible along the top of a yardstick taped to the floor.

Item 2: Agility/Dynamic Balance A chair is taped to the floor, and two cones (one to each side) are placed 6 feet to the side and 5 feet behind the chair. The examinee begins fully seated in the chair. He/she rises and moves to and around a cone and returns to a seated position in the chair. The same movement is repeated around the other cone. Another complete circuit is executed to complete a trial of the test.

Item 3: "Soda Pop" Coordination Test A strip of tape is placed on a table top and marked at six 5-inch intervals. The examinee sits comfortably in front of the table. Three unopened (full) cans of soda pop are placed in squares 1, 3, and 5 on the table. When the test begins, the examinee turns each can upside down and places it in the adjacent square as rapidly as possible. Then the cans should be returned to their original placement.

Item 4: Strength/Endurance Test The examinee sits in a chair with the non-dominant hand resting in the lap and the dominant hand hanging to the side. A weighted milk bottle (plastic) is placed in the dominant hand. A 4-pound weight (quart container) should be used for women and an 8-pound weight (gallon container) for men. The tester stands to the side of the examinee and places one hand on the dominant bicep and the other under the bottle to assist in supporting it. When the test begins, the examinee attempts to contract the bicep through the full range of motion. If this movement can be completed, the examinee is given a 1-minute rest and then asked to make as many repetitions as possible in thirty seconds.

Item 5: Half-Mile Walk (or 880-Yard Walk) This is the usual timed walking test. Running is not permitted.

Rockport Fitness Walking Test The Rockport Fitness Walking Test has been developed for both younger and older adults. This test can be self-administered. Before taking the test, the examinee goes through a pretest warm-up. After walking in place for 30 seconds, the resting pulse is determined.

The test requires walking a mile as fast as possible. Record time to the nearest second. Record heart rate immediately at the end of the mile. The examinee should stretch for 5-10 minutes before beginning the test.

Refer to the Rockport Fitness Walking Test chart (The Rockport Company, 1986) for the examinee's age and sex-relative fitness level. Use the chart to evaluate test performance. One strong point of this test is that, after the self-test has taken place, an exercise program is recommended for the examinee's age and sex. A 20-week walking program is recommended, followed by a repetition of the Rockport Fitness Walking Test.

Measurement in Other Career Options

Earlier in this chapter, the uses of evaluation by instructors and managers in sports or fitness centers were discussed. The managerial role is only one of the career options a *sports management* major would be prepared to undertake. Other alternatives include a front-office position with a sports team, event organizer, athletic director, and similar administrative positions. Evaluation is an important part of these jobs. Programs must be evaluated as well as personnel. The needs and interests of those likely to attend the sports events might be surveyed. Instruments such as questionnaires or inventories are often employed in these settings. If rating scales are developed, they should possess valid content and should be based on knowledge of the appropriate underlying measurement methodology.

In the National Athletic Trainer's Association Handbook, many evaluation competencies are listed. Even the fledgling *athletic trainer* must know how to assess the extent of an injury and decide on a course of treatment. Most of the decisions made by an athletic trainer require the use of evaluation techniques. To be certified, the basic skills the trainer should possess are carefully evaluated. He/she must be evaluated on the ability to tape body parts properly. The ability to choose the best exercises to prescribe for rehabilitation must also be assessed. Extensive knowledge of measurement and evaluation are required of the athletic trainer.

There are many medical aspects of measurement, as for example in *physical therapy* and *sports medicine.* One of the most common types of measurement in these areas is the use of the goniometer to measure joint angles. Also frequently used is the Cybex machine to measure strength of specific parts of the body. These professionals are often called upon to assess the effectiveness of a rehabilitation program for a specific client, for instance, whether the program has been effective enough to allow the client to return to work. These types of decisions are critical both for the client and the hiring agency.

SUMMARY

Many instructional opportunities exist in nonschool settings. The process of writing objectives for these classes is similar to preparing objectives in a school setting. Individualizing objectives in a private club is often easier, however, and these objectives may be implemented differently in this setting. In a private sports club the objectives might be tailored to the skill level of class members having similar skill levels. In a fitness center objectives are expected to be individualized, since the level of fitness of the clients typically varies markedly. Any test of sports skills or physical fitness can be adapted for the nonschool setting. In practice some organizations evaluate their clients' progress only in the most subjective manner, while others have instituted formal testing programs.

LEARNING EXPERIENCES

1. Visit a private fitness or sports club in your community and ask for information on the entry-level testing for new clients. Secure the printed evaluation form from the club manager, if possible. Ask for clarification of any aspect of the testing you do not understand. Bring this information back to class, and report it to your classmates.
2. Write one behavioral objective for a hypothetical new member of a private fitness club. Be sure to include all the important components of a behavioral objective as described in the previous chapter.
3. Write one behavioral objective for a beginning tennis class in a private club. Then modify the objective for a new member of the class who seems to have natural ability in tennis and is highly motivated.
4. Assume you are the manager of a fitness center. How many aspects of the club would you evaluate? List these aspects, and suggest one way of evaluating each one.

REFERENCES

AAHPERD Ad Hoc Committee. 1988. AAHPERD Functional Fitness Test for Older Adults. Unpublished material.

Golding, L.A., Myers, C.R., and Sinning, W.E. 1982. The Y's way to physical fitness. Chicago: National Board of YMCA.

Katch, F.I., and McArdle, W.D. 1983. Nutrition, weight control, and exercise, ed. 2, Philadelphia: Lea & Febiger.

Osness, W.H. 1986. Physical assessment procedures—the use of functional profiles. Journal of Physical Education, Recreation, and Dance, **57:** 35-38.

Pollock, M.L., Schmidt, D.H., and Jackson, A.S. 1980. Measurement of cardiorespiratory fitness and body composition in a clinical setting. Comprehensive Therapy, **6:**12-27.

Sentry World Headquarters. 1979. Sentry physical fitness handbook. Stevens Point, WI: Sentry World Headquarters.

The Rockport Company. 1986. The Rockport Fitness Walking Test. Walboro, MA: The Rockport Company.

SUPPLEMENTARY READINGS

Heyward, V.H. 1984. Designs for fitness. Minneapolis: Burgess Publishing Co.

Pollock, M.L., Wilmore, J., and Fox, S.M. 1984. Exercise in health and disease: evaluation and prescription for prevention and rehabilitation. Philadelphia: W.B. Saunders Co.

ANNOTATED READINGS

Baun, W., and Baun, M. 1984. A corporate health and fitness program. Journal of Physical Education, Recreation and Dance, **55**(4):42-45.
Describes the use of a computer system to achieve objectives in a corporate fitness setting; discusses the use of initial screening of employees followed by daily assessments; provides immediate feedback to the participant as well as a monthly activity program; uses monthly statistics to evaluate the program continuously and to develop a data base for longitudinal analysis.

Baun, W.B., and Landgren, M.A. 1983. Tenneco health and fitness: a corporate program committed to evaluation. Journal of Physical Education, Recreation and Dance, **54**(8):40-41.

Lists the objectives of the model fitness program at Tenneco Inc. in Houston; describes the program and program statistics; emphasizes the evaluation process, which includes four principal areas: (1) health and fitness monthly statistics, (2) fitness and wellness program evaluation, (3) special projects, and (4) longitudinal projects; uses information from the evaluation process to increase awareness of and commitment to positive health habits and improve the overall quality of life.

Cooper, K.H., and Collingwood, T.R. 1984. Physical fitness: programming issues for total well-being. Journal of Physical Education, Recreation and Dance, **55**(3):35-36, 44.

Describes the involvement of the Institute for Aerobics Research in developing and evaluating employee health and fitness programs within the private and government sectors; notes that accountability is the major issue in program implementation; based on their evaluations of many programs, identifies several factors contributing to the success of a program, thereby facilitating participant adherence to the program; describes several program models.

Crossley, J.C., and Hudson, S.D. 1983. Assessing the effectiveness of employee recreation/fitness programs. Journal of Physical Education, Recreation and Dance, **54**(8):50-52.

Discusses a practical approach to assisting the effectiveness of employee recreation/fitness programs; labels this type of approach as *controlled comparison:* describes data collection (1) to construct an employee profile and (2) to measure employee perceptions of program benefits; substitutes survey questions for objective data; data collection also includes employee perceptions of the effectiveness of a recreation/fitness program; discusses how the data can be used to improve the program.

Farley, M. 1984. Program evaluation as a political tool. Journal of Physical Education, Recreation and Dance, **55**(4):65-67.

Examines program evaluation as it applies to public service agencies; suggests program evaluation can become a persuasive political tool if viewed as a communication device; proposes ways of using program evaluation as a political tool; discusses evaluation as a means of linking the agency and elected officials in the tasks of planning and delivering services and accounting for the use of public funds.

Howell, J. 1983. Wellness for the practitioners. Journal of Physical Education, Recreation and Dance, **54**(8):37, 55.

Describes hospital wellness program for hospital employees; uses an aerobic circuit modeled after Kenneth Cooper's concept; discusses fitness advisor assisting participants in establishing personal goals and monitoring progress; uses two fitness assessments as a part of membership: initial testing and the Lifestyle-Health Audit; evaluates program using class evaluations and existing questionnaires.

13

Special Issues in Testing Motor Behavior

KEY WORDS   *Watch for these words as you read the following chapter:*

course evaluation   instructor evaluation   program evaluation

Measurement and evaluation do not occur in isolation. Scores must be interpreted in some meaningful way, and three major interpretive issues are examined in this chapter. The first issue focuses on testing minority students. The second issue encompasses several evaluation topics, including objective assessments of instructional effectiveness, programs, and curricula. In the third section, sex differences in motor performance and their impact on standard setting are discussed.

TESTING MINORITY STUDENTS

Testing minority students on motor skills is a little-discussed topic. Numerous discussions have been held on the appropriateness of certain cognitive and affective tests for those coming from a minority culture. Studies of test bias provide information to be used in evaluating tests. A widely held view is that most tests are based on white middle-class values; therefore, whites score higher than blacks (for example). On the surface, it would appear that tests of motor performance may be devoid of these concerns. However, this is largely an unexplored area. It is possible that, even if the tests themselves are not biased, the instructions for test administration should be examined closely for possible bias.

Certainly when cognitive and affective tests are used in physical education and the exercise sciences, their usefulness with minority children should be analyzed. Many authors have proposed ways of dealing with potential bias in testing (e.g., Isen, 1986; Sharma, 1986). In addition to studying test bias, strategies include the use of multiple assessment procedures, an increase in motivation, a perception of learning difficulties as culturally derived, use of test administrator from same ethnic group, and administration of the test in both languages (if the child is bilingual).

The potential for test bias in physical education and exercise science has rarely been discussed, much less studied systematically. This is an especially important consideration for tests recommended on a national basis, such as the recently proposed national physical fitness tests.

EVALUATION TOPICS

As you recall from Chapter 1, *measurement* involves the administration of a test and *evaluation* pertains to the interpretation of test scores. A test has many purposes, including assessment of the effectiveness of a course, teacher, curriculum, or program.

The *formative evaluation* approach is emphasized in this chapter. When courses or programs dealing with sport or physical activity are evaluated, the traditional approach is to evaluate at the end of the designated period. If weaknesses are detected, plans are usually made to correct these weaknesses during the coming year. However, the next time the evaluation takes place, the same weaknesses may exist; thus an entire year has been consumed in applying ineffective solutions. If the evaluation had been of the formative type, determining that the proposed solutions were ineffective and in need of modification or replacement, this would have been possible early in the school year. Keep in mind that the purpose of evaluation is to improve the course or program, not to judge it. Of course, evaluation techniques must be used to make judgments sometimes, but in most cases passing judgment should not be the primary reason for evaluation.

Accepting the premise that the use of formative evaluation is an appropriate method for improving effectiveness, what techniques can be used to obtain data over time? Essentially the evaluator must ask three basic questions:

1. Is the program, teacher, student, or administrator functioning successfully?
2. If not, how should one intervene?
3. Is the intervention successful?

Course and Instructor Evaluation

In the 1970s the emphasis on evaluating the effectiveness of courses and instructors increased a great deal, particularly in colleges and universities. Many institutions of higher learning required or strongly encouraged faculty members to obtain periodic evaluation of their courses and teaching. Much effort has been expended in the development of instruments that can be used for this purpose; the most popular type is an evaluation form using a Likert-type scale. Usually administered at the end of a unit or a year of instruction, this instrument represents the summative approach to evaluation. Although certain items on the scale would apply to any course, the evaluation forms are generally not applicable to activity courses in sport and physical activity. Efforts to develop a form for activity courses usable nationwide have not been successful, probably because institutions have different missions and course objectives.

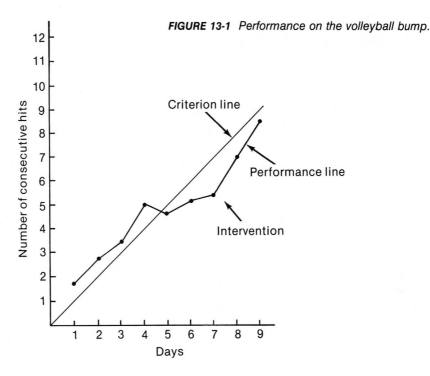

FIGURE 13-1 *Performance on the volleyball bump.*

In the following sections a formative approach to course and instructor evaluation able to be used in elementary and secondary schools, private clubs, colleges, and universities is demonstrated. The underlying goal is to provide evidence of the effectiveness of a course or an instructor by monitoring behavior on a regular basis. When satisfactory progress is not being made, an intervention should take place. Three examples are used to illustrate this approach.

Example 1—Volleyball Unit A physical education teacher establishes a goal for her students in learning the bump. The goal is to execute 10 consecutive, legal bumps within a given height range and area by the middle of the volleyball unit. Achievement of the goal would indicate that the students have developed adequate control and are ready for more refined work on the skill. Figure 13-1 shows the results obtained in a beginning class. The solid line is the criterion line, indicating a hypothetical line of improvement from 0 to 10 consecutive hits. The criterion line is used only as a guide, since the performance curve would not necessarily be expected to be linear. The solid line connecting the dots is the actual performance curve for the class. Note that the performance line drops below the criterion line on day 5 and falls further away on days 6 and 7. Since we do not know the learning curve for students on this skill (perhaps research will show this drop to be expected), we must assume that the students are not going to reach the criterion unless the teacher intervenes in some way. The mark at day 7 represents a planned intervention, which might consist of additional instruction by the teacher, close supervision by a partner, use of instructional materials, or varying teaching methodology. In this case the performance line begins to move toward the criterion line again, revealing the intervention as successful. By monitoring progress daily the course itself or one aspect of it is evaluated on a ongoing basis.

Example 2—Class Management A physical education teacher senses that he spends too much time in class talking to his students (e.g., giving directions and discussing mechanical principles). Although he feels the information he provides is important, he would like to impart it more efficiently, that is, in less time. He would like to increase the amount of active learning time his students have in class. First, he needs to know how much time he actually spends in class on verbal presentations. This information may be obtained in several ways—by audiotaping his classes or by having someone, perhaps a student from study hall, monitor the amount of time he spends talking in his class for a week. These results would provide him with a baseline from which to work. In this case the teacher spent an average of 40% of the total class time talking. This is shown in Figure 13-2 as the baseline. The teacher decides that 25% of class time should be adequate for class discussion. This is represented in Figure 13-2 by the dashed line, the criterion line set by the teacher. How can this designated criterion be met? Perhaps some of the material could be presented by preparing handouts and by

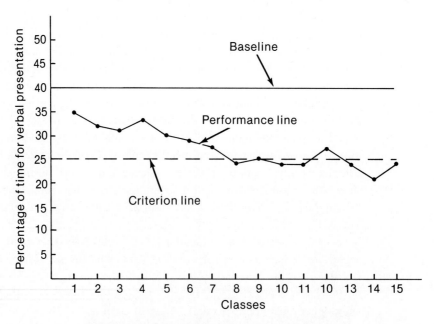

FIGURE 13-2 *Time devoted to verbal presentations.*

using loopfilms on an individualized basis. If his talk time decreases to 25% and remains there, he has achieved his goal. If the percentage of time increases again, another method of intervening should be used. In Figure 13-2, the solid line connecting dots represents the teacher's performance. Since talk time is being decreased in the desired direction and reaches the criterion line during class 8, no intervention is necessary. The performance curve remains around the 25% level for the next seven sessions; therefore, the teacher has some assurance that he will be able to maintain this amount of talk time. Using this approach, a teacher may monitor any aspect of instructional effectiveness on a continual basis. Problems can be identified and corrected before the end of the unit, course, or year when modifying the teacher's behavior would essentially be ineffectual.

Example 3—*Instructor Evaluation* A college instructor in a theory class administers a course evaluation form at the end of each semester and finds that the students consistently rate the clarity of her instruction from average to below average. If the material is not being presented clearly, the students cannot be expected to understand and apply it. The instructor does not wish to wait until the end of the next semester to find out whether her presentations are improving in clarity. An evaluation procedure consisting of a rating scale (see Figure 13-3) is devised. The student picks up the rating form at the end of each class, circles the number best reflecting the perceived degree of clarity of instruction, and turns in the form to another student who collects and returns it to the instructor. This process assures the student of an anonymous response.

The ratings are averaged each day and plotted, as in Figure 13-4. The solid line represents the baseline, the average end-of-semester rating the instructor has been receiving. She decides to strive for an average daily rating of 6 or higher, represented by the criterion (dashed) line. The solid line connecting the dots is the teacher's performance curve, measured by the daily rating of students. By organizing the structure of the classes more carefully, the instructor is able to maintain clarity ratings at a satisfactory level. If the performance curve had fallen below 6 for two or more consecutive classes, possibilities for intervention would have to be explored. One approach might be to ask the students why

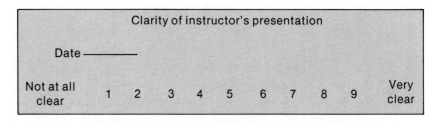

FIGURE 13-3 *Rating scale to monitor clarity of instruction.*

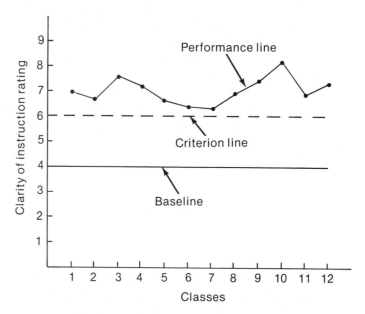

FIGURE 13-4 *Ratings of clarity of instruction.*

the presentation did not seem clear. Another approach would be to prepare at least two examples of each concept presented in class and discuss these examples. A low clarity rating might simply indicate that the instructor needs to present the same material again during the next class session. Unless experimental evidence on the best method of intervening is available, the instructor must intervene on the basis of a logical analysis.

Although the evaluation procedures described in the previous examples are useful, the measures used in all three examples are weak measures. For instance, a student rating of clarity of instruction may reflect something other than clarity, such as the instructor's personality. This effect can be controlled to some extent by obtaining two different measures of the same attribute. Student ratings of the clarity of instruction might be accompanied by an observer's rating of the clarity of instruction or a rating of tape recordings of class sessions. Unobtrusive measures such as content analysis of lesson plans or instructional materials might also be used. This approach lacks the controls necessary in an experimental study. No control groups are used, only one teacher is involved, and factors other than the planned intervention might account for the desired performance.

Even with the foregoing limitations, if this informal approach assists a teacher or exercise scientist in achieving personal goals, it seems to be a worthwhile evaluation tool. It forces one to identify problems, work actively to alter behavior in the desired direction, and increase awareness of strengths and opportunities for improvement. It enables the professional to perform and somewhat control his or her self-evaluation in a nonthreatening environment.

In the sport arena, the evaluation of coaching is a vital component of the assessment of an athletic department. Often this evaluation is based on the sole criterion of wins and losses. However, in an educational setting, placing such a heavy emphasis on a product-oriented goal has been widely criticized. A performance analysis system has been proposed as a means of evaluating a coach's role in enhancing the entire athletic program. The five-step process includes: (1) statement of departmental goals; (2) review of position guide, (3) review of performance criteria and development of performance standards, (4) performance analysis, and (5) recognition of achievement.

Program Evaluation

The **evaluation of programs** dealing with sport and physical activity incorporates the same techniques used to evaluate any program. Two examples of evaluating program goals in the school setting are provided to emphasize important aspects of program evaluation and to describe approaches to the use of formative evaluation techniques. The first example was developed for a high school physical education program and the second for a middle-school physical education program.

A basic assumption is that all physical education teachers have a list of program goals stated in some fashion. If program goals are stated in general rather than behavorial terms, the evaluation of their effectiveness may be imprecise. For example, a high school program goal might be stated as follows.

Goal 1 (general): To develop and maintain an optimal level of physical fitness needed to function in everyday life.

To evaluate this goal, more specific information is needed. What is an optimal level of physical fitness? Also, what type of physical fitness is of concern? Let's assume that cardiorespiratory (CR) endurance was identified as the most important type of fitness. A more explicit statement of this goal follows:

Goal 1 (specific): All high school students will develop an above-average level of CR endurance by the end of the school year. An "above-average" level is defined as Cooper's category labelled "Good" for 12-minute run performance; 80% of the students are expected to achieve this goal.

When the program goal is stated in behavorial terms, the procedure for evaluating the goal is precisely described.

Of course it seems logical to assume that the students cannot meet this goal already, or it would not be identified this way initially. Sometimes test users are not sure, however. A needs assessment can then be conducted, in which the actual status of the students is compared to the desired status. If no discrepancy

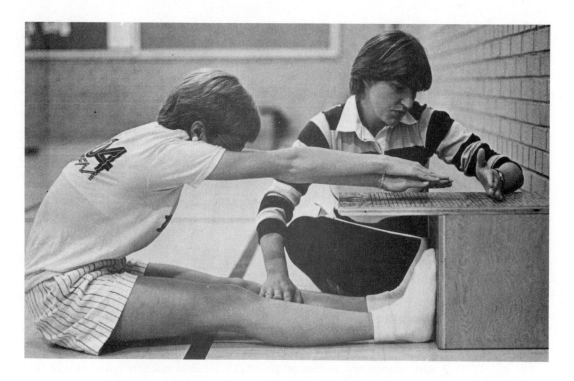

exists, the goal should be rewritten. In this example, the 12-minute run test would be administered to all students. Their performance represents their actual status on CR endurance, and the teacher's standard represents the desired status. Since Cooper identified separate standards for males and females, the actual status of boys and girls is recorded in Table 13-1 and compared to the desired status.

According to this comparison, the students' performance level is far from the desired status. Only 16% of the boys and 22% of the girls perform well enough to be classified in the Good or Excellent categories. Using a formative evaluation approach, one can assess the students' average monthly performance on the 12-minute run and plot the results, as shown in Figure 13-5.

Now we can determine the monthly progress being made toward the desired status. If the average performance levels off in 2 or more months and it becomes clear that the desired status will not be reached at the present rate of improvement, the physical education teacher must intervene. Intervention may take the following forms: increasing the class time devoted to improving CR endurance, determining how the presently allocated time for improving CR endurance is being used, or using different ways to motivate students.

Once a program goal has been stated in behavorial terms, actual status can be determined and ways to monitor progress toward the desired status can be developed. However, the physical education teacher may also wish to identify concomitant concerns that should not be sacrificed for the sake of achieving the goal. For example, it is reasonable to ask what kind of conditioning program is necessary to effectively improve CR endurance. Certainly the students must exercise regularly, at least three or four times a week. If the activity is jogging, the amount of distance run should be gradually increased within a given time limit. Thus the physical education teacher must commit a part of every class period to this goal, since the typical activity in class (even basketball and football) will not

TABLE 13-1 *Discrepancy between actual and desired status on 12-minute run (percent)*

12-minute run categories	Actual status		Desired status	
	Boys	Girls	Boys	Girls
Excellent (V)	6	7	80	80
Good (IV)	10	15		
Average (III)	27	33		
Fair (II)	33	25	20	20
Poor (I)	24	20		

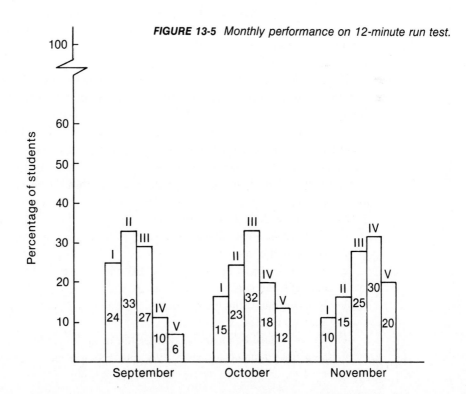

FIGURE 13-5 *Monthly performance on 12-minute run test.*

contribute to a CR endurance goal to any great extent. Is the teacher willing to spend the time necessary to develop CR endurance? How much class time is presently devoted to improving CR endurance? Plotting the way class time is allocated in physical education is possible. A student aide could easily record this information. After reviewing this chart, the teacher may decide that a goal involving improvement of CR endurance in class is not realistic because the achievement of this goal would require too much class time. The goal might be rewritten so that students are expected to understand the need for developing and maintaining CR endurance and be aware of ways of achieving an optimal level of endurance. On the other hand, the teacher may decide that this goal is so important that it warrants using whatever class time is necessary.

A second example of setting goals in a school setting deals with lifetime sports. This goal for middle school physical education students might be stated as follows:

Goal 2 (general): To develop skills in lifetime sports.

Again, more information is needed. How many lifetime sports? What level of skill is expected? How many students are expected to meet the standard? A better statement of the goal follows:

Goal 2 (specific): All middle school students will demonstrate skill attainment in at least one lifetime sport each year by achieving either a beginning or an intermediate competency level for four of the five subunits for that sport; 75% of the students are expected to achieve this goal.

To write the specific goal in this way, the teacher would have to establish beginning and intermediate standards for each sport; however, this is not unrealistic. For example, Memorial High School in Madison, Wisconsin, has established competency levels for all activities—not just for lifetime sports. To monitor student progress toward this goal, daily performance could be plotted. The teacher might wish to review individual charts weekly or perhaps monthly.

Here again there may be concomitant factors that the teacher wishes not to forgo in achieving a goal. These factors should be noted in writing by the teacher. Some of these goals follow:

1. The student must have a positive attitude toward, and feel satisfied about, achieving the goal.
2. The teacher must have a positive attitude toward, and feel satisfied about, achieving the goal.
3. Opportunities should be provided for using varied instructional approaches in classes.
4. Classes should be balanced, with some time devoted to learning skills and some time devoted to using skills and strategies in a game setting.

5. The teacher should provide each student with some individual attention at least every other class period.

Formative evaluation procedures could be developed for each of these factors to monitor them throughout the year.

If there is more than one physical education teacher in a school, all must agree on the most important program goals. Usually this can be resolved informally. However, if citywide consensus is expected, more formal techniques can be adopted to aid the group in reaching an agreement. In the Delphi technique, each staff member ranks goals individually. These rankings are then summed for each goal and averaged. Each member is given the average rankings, and all members rank the goals again. If one member of the group ranks a goal very differently from the group ranking, a written rationale is submitted for retaining it. This process is continued until consensus is achieved. A second and perhaps more efficient technique in a school setting is the nominal group method. Using this method, the staff members form a group but work independently within that group. In other words, the individuals do not interact with one another in the early stages, even though they are physically together in a group. Again, feedback is given to the group, and gradually group interaction increases. Once a list of program goals has been generated, the group works toward agreeing on priorities. Although these techniques may be more effective if conducted by someone not on the physical education staff, good results can be obtained using a staff member who has had some experience in working with small groups.

By planning in advance how progress toward the achievement of program goals can be monitored, the chances of actually achieving the goals are greatly enhanced. Teachers evaluate to detect weaknesses and determine ways of correcting those weaknesses. Evaluation, then, becomes an integral part of the educational process.

Curriculum Evaluation

Although evaluating many aspects of the physical education curriculum is possible, this section discusses the evaluation of the overall merit of the curriculum. (The more familiar process of evaluating specific objectives within the curriculum receives extensive examination on pp. 162-164.) Let's assume that a staff of physical education teachers has decided to use the Purpose Process Curriculum Framework (PPCF) as a guide for making curricular decisions (Jewett and others, 1971). One approach to implementing this framework might be to use the grid shown in Table 13-2. Only one of the major categories of purposes for moving is included in Table 13-2 to exemplify this evaluative procedure. The first task of the physical education staff would be to select combinations of purposes and processes that are to receive emphasis in their physical education program. (The purposes for moving are represented across the top of the grid; the movement

TABLE 13-2 *Portion of grid for evaluating Purpose/Process Curriculum Framework*

| | Man master of himself | | | | | | |
| | Physiological efficiency | | | Psychic equilibrium | | | |
Process	C-R efficiency	Mechanical efficiency	N-M efficiency	Joy	Self-knowledge	Catharsis	Challenge
Perceiving							
Patterning	X						
Adapting							
Refining							
Varying							
Improvising							
Composing							

processes, along the side.) These purpose/process combinations can be viewed jointly by marking the appropriate cells in the grid. For example, in Table 13-2, an X has been placed in the cell representing a combination of circulorespiratory endurance (purpose) and patterning (process). When all purpose/process combinations of interest have been recorded on the grid, the overall framework of the physical education curriculum has been identified.

However, the selections within the PPCF should be justifiable in the eyes of physical educators who are qualified to make such judgments. Otherwise, curricular choices may be merely a reflection of the personal biases of the physical education staff. If, for example, a curriculum is considered too broad or too narrow by the physical education curriculum experts, the staff has not established sufficiently the merit of the curriculum.

How can physical education teachers evaluate the merit of a curriculum? First, a written rationale should be set forth for the choices made within the PPCF. This step provides the outside observer with the staff's philosophical orientation toward physical education. It also helps to ensure that curricular choices are made on a logical basis. This rationale would provide input to the curriculum evaluator. One might disagree with the philosophical approach but at the same time judge the curricular choices appropriate.

Bringing in outside evaluators to assess the physical education curriculum is not always possible. A team of teachers and administrators within a school system might be asked to review the rationale and subsequent curricular choices. A needs assessment might be conducted to determine whether these choices meet the needs of students, parents, other community members, teachers, and administrators. It cannot be overemphasized that these curricular choices are not arbitrary; they must be fully justifiable. Once the purpose/process combinations have been selected, the activities that will contribute to these combinations must be identified. Presumably different approaches could be taken at this stage. A variety of activities might be used to meet a given purpose at an identified process level. For example, if the purpose for moving is object projection, the student might experience throwing, striking, and kicking a variety of objects in a structured environment. As an alternative approach, a single sport might be selected as a means of emphasizing a purpose. Softball might be an appropriate sport for providing many opportunities for a variety of object projection tasks. Regardless of the approach to selecting activities, these activities must be justified as bona fide contributors to the designated purpose/process combinations.

The first step in justifying the selection of activities is to review the literature to obtain supporting evidence from research studies. Consider CR endurance as a purpose of interest. Evidence supports the selection of running as an activity that contributes to circulorespiratory endurance, assuming the run takes place over a reasonably long distance. If the distance is too short (½ mile, for instance), running would no longer be an appropriate activity for this purpose. The literature review may not be fruitful in many cases, since experimental studies have been conducted only on a small number of purposes. If this is the case, the next best source to use in justifying the selection of activities is the content specialist in physical education. If the purpose is psychological (e.g., catharsis), the sport psychologist would be the appropriate content specialist to contact. The biomechanics specialist would be called on to deal with purposes such as object projection. If research evidence does not exist, at least the best possible logical judgment can be made.

In a curriculum evaluation the merit of the total curriculum as well as the worthiness of specific goals must be examined. Only then is it appropriate to assess the extent to which curricular goals are being attained. However, even this assessment cannot be conducted in isolation but must be conducted in conjunction with other factors that the physical education staff views as important.

SEX DIFFERENCES IN MOTOR PERFORMANCE

That sex differences exist in motor performance cannot be denied. However, to what extent are these differences culturally induced or genuinely physiological? This question has been widely discussed for many years and remains controversial in the exercise science field.

Research has shown that, in general, boys have more strength, height, weight, and CR endurance than girls. In addition, they tend to have a smaller

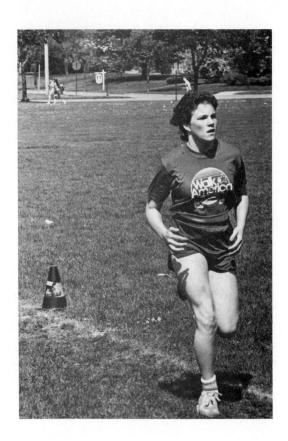

percentage of body fat. The gender gap may be narrowing for some aspects of strength. While there is a clear difference in arm and shoulder girdle strength, performance on leg strength measures demonstrates considerable overlap. Even so, the strongest individuals are usually male and the weakest, female. Girls generally possess greater flexibility, rhythmic ability, and buoyancy. However, there are certainly exceptions to this delineation of sex differences, in particular among upper elementary school age boys and girls and highly skilled versus poorly skilled performers.

Sex differences have also been reported in sports skills. For example, Stamm (1979) noted differences in the test scores of college men and women in tennis and bowling classes. This suggests the need to consider separate performance standards for men and women. However, separate standards are not always appropriate for all activities. At the U.S. Air Force Academy (1978), the same performance standards were used for both male and female cadets in swimming classes. In this situation, men and women were equally capable. Drawing conclusions about sex differences in motor performance is difficult without a substantial, recent data base for all ages, girls and boys.

Implications for Ability Grouping

Ability grouping is neither required nor prohibited by the Title IX regulation. However, if it is used, group membership cannot be determined on the basis of sex. On the other hand, the assignment of an equal number of boys and girls to a group does not necessarily yield a sex-fair grouping. Group membership must be determined objectively. During the practice or competition of contact sports, students must be separated by sex. However, this grouping may not be permissible during the instructional portion of the class.

What are the implications for ability grouping? In a report prepared by the state of Illinois, the use of sports skills tests was recommended for ability grouping when these skills were incorporated into the unit objectives. If the objective involves physical fitness, a number of fitness tests are available to be used in grouping. Motor ability tests are not recommended to ability group students. "There is no evidence that a phenomenon such as motor ability is measurable or even that the phenomenon exists" (Illinois State Board of Education, 1982, p. 5). Random assignment to groups is recommended when the objective is to help students learn to appreciate the skill level of others.

When students of similar ability compete, the same standard should be used for ability grouping. When excellence in performance is the primary goal, separate standards should be used, in particular for fitness and sports skill objectives. With traditional mass instruction, a single standard is recommended. With an individualized approach, separate standards are recommended.

Implications for Performance Evaluations

The Illinois report also makes recommendations on sex-fair performance evaluation. Separate (higher) standards are proposed for boys when performance is based on strength, endurance, height, weight, or lean body mass. Separate (higher) standards for girls are recommended when performance is based on flexibility, buoyancy, or rhythm.

When an accuracy test is administered, where strength and power are not factors, a single standard should be used. A single standard is also proposed for wall volley tests not dependent on strength or power and for the assessment of form and game strategy.

SUMMARY

To interpret scores on motor behavior tests, several factors should be taken into account, including course and program objectives and gender differences. Actual status of student ability as well as desired status must be considered in determining objectives. Typically, desired status is reflected in course and program objectives. Gender differences, in particular physiological ones, may lead to a different interpretation of scores for males and females. In general the process of interpreting test scores should be handled as conscientiously as the process of selecting and administering the test.

LEARNING EXPERIENCES

1. Assume one of the goals for female members of your fitness club is to increase arm and shoulder girdle strength. Your club owns a Universal gym machine (or something similar). Write a specific objective for this goal, including a performance standard. Note how you could monitor the progress in achieving the objective on an ongoing basis. If a client does not progress as expected, what type of intervention would you propose? Draw a hypothetical graph of your formative evaluation.

2. Assume you are a physical education teacher working with high school boys. Lately you have observed some problems with sportsmanship in your classes. You would like to monitor this behavior on an ongoing basis to determine its severity. Describe a simple procedure you might use to monitor sportsmanship on a daily basis. Propose several methods of intervening if the behavior problems become severe. Draw a hypothetical graph of this evaluation. Be specific in stating your evaluation objective, including a standard of performance for the class as a whole.

REFERENCES

Jewett, A.E., and others. 1971. Educational change through a taxonomy for writing physical education objectives. Quest, **15**:32-38.

Illinois State Board of Education. 1982. Tips and techniques: ability grouping and performance evaluation in physical education. Springfield, IL: Illinois State Board of Education.

Isen, H.G. 1986. Assessing the black child: a strategy. Journal of Non-White Concerns, **11**:47-58.

Sharma, S. 1986. Assessment strategies for minority groups. Journal of Black Studies, **17**:111-124.

Stamm, C.L. 1979. The evaluation of coeducational physical education activity classes. Journal of Health, Physical Education, and Recreation, **50**:68-69.

United States Air Force Academy. 1978. Women's integration research project-phase III. Department of Athletics, April 10.

United States Department of Health, Education, and Welfare. 1975. Federal Register, **40**(108), June 4.

ANNOTATED READINGS

Finke, C.W. 1972. Use evaluation positively. Journal of Health, Physical Education, and Recreation, **43**:16.
Suggests that too many testing procedures in physical education produce anxiety; believes that evaluation should build the learner's self-reliance and increase the desire and ability to move; supports the concept of continuous evaluation, using both teacher evaluations and self-evaluation.

Kneer, M.E. 1982. Ability grouping in physical education, Journal of Physical Education, Recreation, and Dance, **53**(9):10-13, 68.

Discusses the identification of performance standards to be used in grouping students in physical education on the basis of their ability; prescribes curricular and instructional approaches to accommodating these abilities.

Kosekoff, J., and Fink, A. 1982. Evaluation basics: a practitioner's manual. Beverly Hills, CA: Sage Publications, Inc.

Provides a thorough introduction and overview of the techniques needed for a do-it-yourself evaluation; offers guidelines, checklists, and key points to watch at every step of the evaluation process; uses almost 100 examples to illustrate its practical advice; invaluable to anyone who needs to know the basics of evaluating programs.

Loughrey, T.J. 1988. Evaluating program effectiveness. Journal of Physical Education, Recreation and Dance, **59**(1): 63-64.

Describes the goals of program evaluation identified by the Evaluation Research Council; lists program factors and products to evaluate in physical education.

McDonald, D., and Yeates, M.E. 1979. Measuring improvement in physical education. Journal of Physical Education and Recreation, **50**:79-80.

Discusses problems encountered in measuring improvement; reviews the Hale and Hale method for adjusting raw improvement scores so that the inequality of scale units is taken into account; presents a simplified procedure, in tabular form, for calculating the improvement score.

McGee, R. 1989. Program evaluation. Chapter in M.J. Safrit and T.M. Wood (eds.), Measurement Concepts in Physical Education and Exercise Science. Champaign, IL: Human Kinetics Publishers.

Identifies and describes a variety of program evaluation models; provides numerous examples in physical education and exercise science settings.

Potter, G., and Wandzilak, T. 1981. Youth sports: a program evaluation. Journal of Physical Education and Recreation, **53**(3):67-68.

Describes the evaluation of a basketball program for seventh- and eighth-grade boys; use of preseason and postseason questionnaires to determine whether program objectives were met; includes discussion of results.

Stringfellow, M.E. 1976. Competency-based instruction in measurement and evaluation. Journal of Physical Education and Recreation, **47**:50-51.

Describes the use of a competency-based approach to teaching a traditional undergraduate course in measurement and evaluation at the university level; prepares students to become critical test analyzers; includes samples of course outlines; general objectives, behavioral objectives, and grade criteria.

Zakrajsek, D.B. 1979. Student evaluations of teaching performance. Journal of Physical Education and Recreation, **49**:64-65.

Presents a method of collecting objective evidence to evaluate instruction; discusses the validity of student ratings; measures students' perceptions of effective instruction using an opinionnaire; presents a 20-item example of a student opinionnaire.

Part Seven

Principles of Test Construction

14

Constructing Sports Skills Tests

KEY WORDS   *Watch for these words as you read the following chapter:*

components of skill   rating scale   test battery

game statistics

Whenever you need a test in physical education or exercise science, try to find an appropriate one from the many already available. Test development is a time-consuming process that must be handled with care and thoroughness. There is nothing magical about the process, but full-time teachers and exercise specialists often do not have sufficient time for this purpose. If you work in a fitness club, you will already have at your fingertips a number of tests you can administer to your clients. In a school setting you may not always be able to find the type of test you need, partially because of the variety of physical activities taught. Consider the number of sports alone that are included in many physical education curricula. In each of these sports, many skills must be learned and, theoretically, tested; however, administering a great number of tests would not be very practical. Therefore a decision on what to test must be made, taking into consideration the most important skills and which will receive the greatest emphasis.

The first step is to review the available tests of the skills that will be given the most emphasis. Looking through a variety of textbooks in measurement and evaluation is a cumbersome and time-consuming process. However, two available sources should provide a comprehensive overview of sports skills tests: a book by Collins and Hodges (1978), which is devoted to descriptions of sports skills tests, and a series of manuals, published by AAHPERD, each dealing with skills tests for a specific sport. These manuals are currently being revised, with greatly improved tests (see Chapter 18).

Developing a clear idea of the most appropriate type of test saves a lot of time when reviewing test literature. A test can be designed to measure a specific skill, a combination of skills, or playing ability. It may be developed as part of a **battery** of tests. For example, assume that a dribbling skill has been emphasized in a basketball class and that Mr. Masters, the teacher, is going to test the students on this skill. He finds a test that measures a combination of dribbling and shooting. This seems to be a legitimate basketball test, since the dribbling-shooting combination of skills occurs all the time in basketball. However, Mr. Masters reasons that a test measuring only dribbling would be more desirable. Using a test of dribbling alleviates any questions about interpreting the test score. It will reflect only dribbling ability. A test measuring both dribbling and shooting might yield a score that could have several interpretations. In another situation the dribbling-shooting combination test might be most appropriate. The test's appropriateness depends on the reason for using the test.

Perhaps after you have looked through the literature and have been unable to find a good, suitable test, you decide to develop your own test. The remainder of this chapter provides guidance in developing a test.

STEPS IN DEVELOPING A SPORTS SKILLS TEST

Be forewarned that test development is a lengthy process. Developing a good test takes, at best, several months. The following test-construction procedures are for a test of a sport skill such as the volleyball serve, baseball throw, or badminton short serve. Seven steps should be followed in developing this type of test:

1. Write the test objective.
2. Review the test literature.
3. Design the test.
4. Standardize test directions.
5. Administer the test on a pilot basis.
6. Determine validity and reliability.
7. Develop norms.

Obviously, following this process is not recommended, unless important decisions will be made on the basis of the test score and the test will be used on a regular basis. For simple testing during a class session (similar to a drill) where the test is used only in a practice setting and no major decision is made using the test score, strictly following these steps is not necessary. A quick-and-easy test can be developed for this purpose.

Test Objective

The first step in constructing a skill test is to write the objective of the test. This process is not difficult, but it does require careful thought. Which **components of the skill** have been emphasized? The test should be designed to measure these components. Note, for example, the Brumbach Volleyball Serve Test (1967) described in Chapter 18. The test objective is to measure the ability to serve the volleyball low and deep into the opponent's backcourt. Obviously, Brumbach felt that two components of skill in serving the volleyball were important—hitting the ball low (close to the net) and deep (close to the baseline). Do not try to incorporate too many components of the skill in your objective. Remember that the test is supposed to measure each of these components. As the number of components increases, so does the complexity of the test. You may produce a test that is not practical for a school setting. A compromise is in order. Select only the most important components to be measured.

Review of Literature

After writing the test objective, review the test literature for the sport. Presumably you have already done this for the specific skill, since you would not develop a new test if a suitable one were already available. Familiarize yourself with *tests of other skills* used in the same sport, which may provide useful ideas in developing your own test. Review books and pamphlets on the sport written by experts, including successful teachers, coaches, and outstanding players. Their assessment of the important components of the skill you wish to test might be useful in designing the test. Journals might also be useful sources of tests. Three journals which occasionally publish tests are *Research Quarterly for Exercise and Sport*, *Journal of Physical Education, Recreation and Dance*, and *Journal of Teaching in Physical Education*. Textbooks dealing with measurement and evaluation in our field can provide additional information about available tests. See, for example, the list of sources for tests presented in Appendix D. One other source of skills test is the series of test manuals published by the American Alliance for Health, Physical Education, Recreation and Dance. Although some

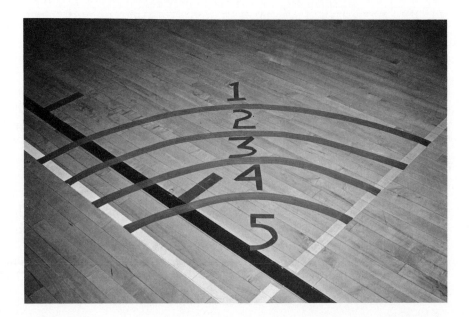

of these manuals have not been updated recently, they nonetheless provide some good ideas about tests that can be used by the test developer.

Design of Test

Now you are ready to design the test. Each component of skill mentioned in the test objective should be measured in the test. For example, in the Brumbach Volleyball Serve Test a rope is strung above the volleyball net to determine whether the ball is hit low over the net. Then a target is placed on the floor of the court opposite the server, with higher point values closer to the baseline, to assess the depth of the serve. The test was designed so that both components of volleyball serve skill—ball hit low over the net and deep into the backcourt—were measured. Specific dimensions of the test layout should be determined at this time. How high should the rope be placed above the net? What are the dimensions of the target? Determine ways of marking the gymnasium floor that will not damage the floor or the permanent markings, such as special tape or water colors. Set up the test and ask one or two students to try it. Their performance will help you decide if the test is too difficult or too easy. Make the necessary modifications before proceeding to the next step.

Standardization of Directions

Before administering the test, even on a trial basis, think through the instructions for administration of the test. These should be written as precisely as possible. Consistency in test administration is essential. Where should the examinee stand? How many practice trials are allowed? How many test trials does the test include? What faults can occur during testing? How are the faults scored? The entire scoring process should be clearly delineated.

Administration of Test

Try the test out first in a pilot study. Use your own students, if you wish, or a group that is similar to ones you will be testing in the future. This will allow you to work out any problems in advance of the actual testing. Although a test may appear to be straightforward and easy to administer, it may have deficiencies that do not show up until the test is administered to a group of examinees. The larger the number of students you can test, the better. If possible, administer the test to the same group of students on two different days (especially if your test consists of only one trial). This will allow you to estimate the test-retest reliability of the test. Be sure to follow the test instructions closely.

Validity and Reliability

The next step in test development is to establish the validity and reliability of the test. (All the procedures recommended in this section are described in detail in

Chapters 6 and 7. Refer to these chapters for additional information and examples.)

If the test is designed so that it measures each component of skill in the test objective, *logical validity* can be claimed for the test. However, this does not mean your test objective cannot be questioned by others. Maybe an important component of the skill in the test objective was omitted. What if Brumbach had mentioned only one component of the volleyball serve—that the ball be hit deep into the opponent's backcourt. All his test would require is a target measuring the landing point of the ball. However, many volleyball teachers might question this objective, noting that a great difference exists between a serve that passes close to the net and one that loops high over the net. Yet both could receive the same score. Your test objective, then, must not only lead to a practical test but also should include the components that others would agree are essential. Since you are developing this test for the objectives of your school system or sports club only, you may think this does not matter. However, the basic essentials of a skill ought to be taught, and the objective should be rewritten to ensure that this actually happens. Establishing evidence of logical validity is essential in developing a test, either norm-referenced or criterion-referenced.

Establishing *concurrent validity* as well as logical validity is useful if you are developing a norm-referenced test. (See Chapter 6. Types of statistical validity for a criterion-referenced test are described in Chapter 7.) Remember that to establish concurrent validity, a *criterion test* must be administered to the group in your pilot study. The criterion test might be *subjective* ratings of the ability to use the skill in a game setting. This may sound simple and straightforward, but it requires the development of a rating scale, which is discussed later in this chapter. Once a rating scale has been developed, raters must be trained to use it. You can see why good test development cannot be accomplished in a short time! To determine concurrent validity, the test scores are correlated with the ratings of skill. Sometimes a measure of playing ability (e.g., ratings in game setting or tournament rankings) is used as the criterion test for a test of skill. This is not a desirable criterion measure. Not surprisingly, the validity coefficients that result from this method of test development are often low.

Evidence of statistical validity is determined by correlating scores on the test being developed with criterion test scores. The higher the validity coefficient, the greater the validity of the test. The familiar *Pearson product-moment correlation* procedure is used to calculate the validity coefficient. The establishment of concurrent validity, while not always essential, is highly desirable, since it provides strong supportive evidence of test validity.

Next, the reliability of the test should be established. If you were able to administer the test twice, a test-retest reliability coefficient can be calculated (see Chapter 6). In brief, two approaches to estimating test-retest reliability were described. One was the interclass reliability coefficient ($r_{xx'}$), which is also calculated using the Pearson product-moment correlation method. The other was the intraclass correlation coefficient ($R_{xx'}$), which is estimated using a statistical technique known as analysis of variance. (An example of the interclass method is presented in Chapter 6.) If you only administered the test once and your test consists of more than one trial, the reliability of the single test administration can be calculated. One such approach is described in Chapter 6 as the split-half method for estimating reliability. Essentially, the test is split into two equal sets of trials, and the averages of each set of trials are correlated. Then, the reliability coefficient must be "stepped up" using the *Spearman-Brown Prophecy formula*. (An example is provided in Chapter 6; one of the learning experiences at the end of this chapter also focuses on this process.)

Revise the Test

If the reliability, validity, or objectivity of the test is not satisfactory, it should be revised. Validity can be enhanced by developing a closer match between the components measured by the test and the ones identified in the test objective. Or, the criterion test might include extraneous elements. If so, a criterion test including the important components of skill should be sought. Reliability can be increased by increasing the number of trials or simplifying the test so that it is less affected by outside elements. Objectivity can be improved by simplifying the scoring system. If a subjective measurement is used, the rating scale might be scaled down so that it is more manageable. Or, the rater(s) might be trained more carefully.

Development of Norms

If the test is to be used as a norm-referenced measure, developing a table of norms is desirable. (The calculation of both percentiles and T-scores is described in Chapters 2 and 3.) A simple method for developing a table of T-scores is the constant-value method, which is exemplified in Chapter 3. Test scores for several hundred students are needed for each table. That amount of test data may not be available from your pilot testing, but test scores for a year or two can be accumulated, if necessary. Developing separate norms for boys and girls may be necessary, depending on the nature of the particular skill. A federal law mandates that, when appropriate, separate performance standards must be set for boys and for girls. This was discussed in greater detail earlier.

DEVELOPMENT OF A BATTERY OF SKILLS TESTS

Often a battery of skills tests is developed to measure the most important skills in a sport. A good example of this type of test battery is the basketball skills test series (Hopkins, Shick, and Plack, 1984) published by AAHPERD. (See Chapter

18. See also the hypothetical softball test battery described by Mood, 1980, and the battery of defensive softball skills tests by Shick, 1970). Developing the individual tests in a battery is no different from the method described in the previous section. However, the validity is determined, in part, on logical grounds. A good, strong rationale should be presented for the inclusion of a specific set of skills in the battery. This logical appraisal can be substantiated using a statistical procedure known as factor analysis. Statistical validity can also be determined by comparing the combined tests with a criterion test of playing ability. This is beyond the scope of this book, since a multiple correlation coefficient must be calculated to estimate validity. The reliability of the test battery should also be estimated, but the appropriate procedures are also beyond the scope of this book, since they require knowledge of multivariate statistics.

DEVELOPMENT OF RATING SCALES

Rating scales are frequently used in the physical education field to measure skills that are difficult to measure in the more traditional manner. Since these scales are usually associated with subjective measurement, they must be carefully developed so that the examinee clearly understands the basis of the ratings. For instance, suppose Ms. Miller, a physical education teacher, decides to measure her students' playing ability in badminton. She observes each of them as they play games and uses the following scale to rate them:

5 Excellent
4 Good
3 Average
2 Fair
1 Poor

The problem with this scale is that no one except Ms. Miller knows what she means by *excellent, good,* and so forth, and perhaps Ms. Miller does not have a clear distinction between ratings. If John received a 4 and Mary a 5, in what ways was John's performance inferior to Mary's? In an educational setting test scores should have meaning to students as well as teachers. Granted, expecting a rating scale to incorporate every aspect of the ability being rated is unreasonable, but general descriptors should certainly be written for each category.

Review a rating scale for the badminton short serve, as shown in the boxed material. A rating of 5, which could still be viewed as excellent, now has specific meaning to the player. A student receiving a rating of 4 knows that his or her ability to place the serve needs more work. Sometimes it is not possible to be this specific in rating more general abilities, since a combination of factors must be considered. However, if a rater is able to judge the examinee's ability by taking these factors into account, it should be possible to write descriptors for each rating used in the scale.

Rating scale for badminton short serve

---

5 No faults*; serve close to net; serve close to short service line; placement appropriate for opponent's weaknesses or position.
4 No faults*; serve close to short service line; no evidence of placement.
3 No faults*; serve either close to net or close to short service line; no
   apparent placement.**
2 No faults*; serve neither close to net or close to short service line; no
   apparent placement.**
1 One or more faults; serve neither close to net nor close to short service
   line; no apparent placement.**

---

*If one or more faults occur, lower the score by 1 point.
**If placement is considered satisfactory, raise the score by 1 point.

Rating scales do not necessarily have to be complex and elaborate. In beginning badminton a teacher may have few expectations of the student in a game
setting, especially if the unit of instruction is short. However, the teacher has
every right to expect the students to meet these expectations; thus, a rating scale
could be devised to measure the aspects of playing ability deemed important.
These aspects might include the following abilities: to hit the shuttle away from
one's opponent, to use a variety of basic skills in the game, and to maintain good
court position during the game. This type of rating scale would be fairly simple
to develop and use, and the players would know what is expected of them.

Of course, a rating scale, no matter how well developed, must be used by
one or more raters. This introduces an element of subjectivity into the measurement process. However, subjectivity can be reduced by practicing the use of a
rating scale before using it in an actual testing setting. If more than one rater is
used, the ratings should be compared in a practice setting before actual testing.
In Chapter 6 some of the problems associated with the use of rating skills and
abilities in diving and gymnastics are discussed, along with procedures for determining the objectivity of raters.

Rating scales constitute an important approach to measurement in the physical education field, especially when the form used by the participant in executing
a skill is of primary concern. This is probably the most abused testing procedure
in physical education because it can be misused so easily. If the scale is too subjective, the rating might be influenced by factors totally unrelated to the examinee's skill. For example, teachers have been known to be influenced in their
ratings by students' personalities. Judges at Olympic events may modify their
ratings depending on the nationality of the performer. However, rating scales

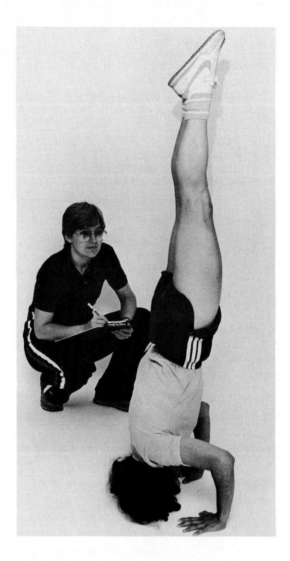

should not be avoided; a properly developed and carefully used scale can be a valuable measurement tool.

To summarize, the following steps should be followed in developing a rating scale:

1. *Determine the purpose of the scale.* Why is the rating scale needed? A variety of reasons for measuring motor performance were delineated in Chapter 1, such as motivation, diagnosis of weaknesses, and grading. How important is the decision that will be made on the basis of the rating scale? If the decision is important, the rating scale should consist of at least five categories. Perhaps the scale is to be used to assess progress at one stage

of learning, and the decision is not as major. Then a rating scale with two or three categories might suffice. Some attributes are well suited to a two-category scale. If a child is asked to demonstrate the ability to balance on two body parts in eight or more different combinations, a two-category (can achieve/cannot achieve) scale might be adequate. However, if the quality of the balance is important, additional categories would probably be more suitable.

2. *Identify the most important components of the motor task.* It is rarely possible to rate every aspect of a sport skill, movement pattern, or some other motor task. This difficulty is magnified when attempting to rate overall performance, such as playing ability in a game. First, the most important skills in the sport should be identified. This is not an easy task, as the measurement of all skills in the game would be prohibitive. In basketball, for example, a long list of skills and combinations of skills could be generated, including passing, dribbling, shooting, defensive skills, and so forth. Subcategories of the rating scale might be developed for the skills identified as most important. Other aspects of the game, such as use of strategy, might form a separate subcategory.

   Even with the breakdown into subcategories, the rating scale will be rather general. Consider that each subcategory can be broken down even further by identifying the types of passes or shots emphasized most during the unit. The level of specificity of the scale depends on the purpose of the scale. In a school setting, it is difficult to use a rating scale with many subcategories due to time constraints. A researcher, on the other hand, might videotape a performance and use a complicated rating scale to evaluate it.

3. *Weight the components to be rated.* All components of skill or playing ability may not be of equal importance. In badminton, the serves and the overhead clear might be emphasized more than the drop shot. If so, the rating for the first two skills should be weighted more heavily than the latter one. One way of accomplishing this is to multiply the ratings of the serves and clear by 2 and the rating of the drop shot by 1. Another possibility is to assign higher values to the rating scale for the serves and the clear. In gymnastics and diving competition, the ratings of events are routinely weighted, although with much greater precision than in the examples given above.

4. *Identify the number of categories.* Several factors affect the selection of the number of categories in the rating scale. One is the importance of the decision to be made based on the scale. Another is the complexity of the skill or ability to be rated. A simple skill might be rated with fewer categories than a complex ability. However, it is difficult for a rater to effec-

tively use more than seven or eight categories, especially in a practical setting. If a teacher wishes to rate all her students on their playing ability in basketball, the use of a large number of categories would not be feasible. This difficulty has sometimes led to the use of simplified (earlier identified as weak) versions of the rating scale that provide little or no information to the user or the examinee. Simply using good, average, fair, and poor (for example) with no descriptors provided for each category is poor practice. Rating scales are valuable methods of describing performance, but only if the ratings can be interpreted clearly. Why did one examinee receive a lower rating on shooting than another? This should be evident from the rating scale and its descriptors.

5. *Identify numerical values for scale.* Although qualitative data are useful in some situations, it is often more convenient to assign a numerical value to each scale point. Then the scores can be analyzed descriptively. In Chapter 22, a variety of rating scales are described. Refer to this chapter for examples of scales with numerical values.

6. *Develop rating sheet.* Development of the rating sheet is an extremely important step in preparing to use the rating scale. The rating sheet should be designed so that the rater can record ratings in the simplest possible way. A checklist in which the checks can later be converted to numerical scores is often the most practical version. A good rating sheet is clearly laid out and simple to use. The descriptors of each category should be printed on the rating sheet as an aid to the rater.

7. *Prepare raters.* Often, at least in practical settings, only one rater is available. The rater should practice using the scale on several occasions before using it in an actual rating situation. This will allow him/her to develop a consistent pattern of rating prior to the actual setting. Otherwise, the rater may be easier or harder on the first few examinees compared to later examinees, resulting in a lack of objectivity in using the scale. When more than one rater will be used, the raters should use the scale in a practice setting and compare their ratings periodically. If there are discrepancies in the ratings, the raters should discuss the problems and continue practicing until reasonable agreement is attained. High levels of agreement between raters are expected for high levels of competition as well as in a research setting.

After the rating scale has been developed and used in an actual setting, information about the ratings should be conveyed to the examinees or other relevant individuals. The results should be linked to the purpose of the scale, and the information should be analyzed and reported in a meaningful way. Several examples of rating scales are presented in the Instructor's Manual accompanying this book.

OTHER APPROACHES TO MEASURING SKILL

Sometimes tournament rankings are used as an indicator of specific skills or playing ability in a sport. This is a much weaker measure than a well-developed rating scale. Tournament play incorporates not only skills and abilities but also elements of competition and chance factors that may not be of greatest concerns in an educational setting. Notice that the suggestions for a rating scale of playing ability in badminton described in the previous section did not take into account who won the game. Of primary interest was the student's ability to employ basic game strategy, even if this resulted in losing the game. At more advanced levels of skill, a rating scale may incorporate a won-loss component, but this would not be recommended as the sole indicator of playing ability. Tournaments in an educational setting should be educational, not simulations of the competitive circuit. **Game statistics** can also be used to supplement the rating of playing ability. If desired, this can be done at a very simplistic level. With the increasing popularity of microcomputers a student or teacher who is a computer buff could easily computerize a system for recording and summarizing data during a game that would make this type of data gathering much more feasible for the average physical educator. Simple microcomputer programs to record and summarize game statistics can be purchased from several commercial firms. Much more sophisticated systems are being developed for the coach. In addition to gathering game statistics, microcomputer programs are being written to assist coaches in making decisions by calculating the probability of success of a play after a specified sequence of events has occurred.

SUMMARY

Test development is a time-consuming process. Whenever possible, a test should be selected from the existing test literature. If an appropriate test cannot be found, use the seven-step approach to develop the desired test. These steps include identifying the test objective, reviewing the test literature, designing the test, standardizing directions, administering the test on a pilot basis, determining test validity and reliability, and developing norms. A process is also described for developing rating scales and test batteries. Several excellent sources of tests are available.

LEARNING EXPERIENCES

1. Select your favorite sport. Choose one skill in this sport and review the literature to examine tests of this skill. Write an analysis of *one* of these tests. Is the test objective acceptable? Is the test valid? Reliable? Discuss ways in which the test could be improved.
2. Identify a sport skill for which *no* test is available. Carry out steps 1 through 4 of the process recommended for the development of a skill test. Also, discuss how validity and reliability could be determined. This can be done either as an individual or a

group project. If a group project is chosen, *all* members of the group should review the test literature.

3. Draw three targets that could be used to measure the accuracy of a volleyball serve. The first target should be drawn so that a beginner, at the end of a course, could hit it and obtain a high score. Do not oversimplify, however. The second target should be of medium difficulty and the third, very difficult (but not so difficult that even highly skilled volleyball players could not obtain a high score). Include the dimensions of each target in feet and inches. Describe the elements of targets 2 and 3, and discuss how these elements increase the difficulty level of the targets. Explain when you would use each of these three targets. Describe each situation specifically.

REFERENCES

Collins, D.R., and Hodges, P.B. 1978. A comprehensive guide to sports skills tests and measurement. Springfield, IL: Charles C Thomas, Publisher.

Hopkins, D.R., Shick, J., and Plack, J.J. 1984. Basketball for boys and girls: skills test manual. Reston, VA: American Alliance for Health, Physical Education, Recreation, and Dance. (Note: This is a recent revision of one of the AAHPERD skills test series. Test manuals are also available for other sports.)

Mood, D.P. 1980. Numbers in motion. Palo Alto, CA: Mayfield Publishing Co.

Shick, J. 1970. Battery of defensive softball skills tests for college women. Research Quarterly, 41(1):82-87.

ANNOTATED READINGS

Bobo, M. 1978. Skill testing—a positive step toward interpreting secondary school physical education. Journal of Physical Education and Recreation, 49:45.
Discusses students' need for meaningful feedback from skills testing; stresses the importance of using valid and reliable skills tests to develop a positive attitude among students toward physical education; lists steps that can be taken by a teacher to provide functional, reliable, and enjoyable skills tests; recommends use of individual school norms for these tests.

Brown, E.W. 1982. Visual evaluation techniques for skill analysis. Journal of Physical Education, Recreation, and Dance, 53(1):21-26,29. Describes visual evaluation techniques for observing physical skills; techniques grouped into five categories—vantage point, movement simplification, balance and stability, movement relationships, and range of movement; provides examples of the technique applied to the tennis serve, a wrestling takedown, batting, soccer instep kick, and other skills.

Davis, M.W., and Hopkins, V.L. 1979. Improving evaluation of physical fitness and sport skill performance. Journal of Physical Education and Recreation, 50:76-78.
Describes problems of evaluating student performance in physical education; stresses importance of improving performance in a variety of sports skills and physical fitness; recommends using profiles for feedback to students and parents; includes graphic example of a tennis student's profile representing performance on tests of skill in tennis.

Hensley, L.D. 1983. Biomechanical analysis. Journal of Physical Education, Recreation, and Dance, 54(8):21-23.
Demonstrates how a rating scale can be developed through a biomechanical analysis; uses basic process evaluation techniques to identify the underlying components of a movement; presents an example of a kinesiogram, a biomechanical profile analysis.

15

Constructing Knowledge Tests

KEY WORDS *Watch for these words as you read the following chapter:*

correction for guessing	item analysis	multiple-choice item
essay item	item difficulty	short-answer item
halo effect	item function	table of specifications
index of discrimination	matching item	true-false item

The motor performance of an individual is of primary concern to physical educators and exercise scientists; therefore, the major portion of this textbook is devoted to the measurement of various forms of sport and physical activity. However, educators also teach people the principles underlying the efficient use of their bodies as well as a knowledge of the relationship of physical activity to health and well-being. Educators teach rules that must be learned to participate in a sport, steps to be followed in carrying out life-saving skills, and game strategies. Students are expected to learn these knowledges. It is hoped that clients in fitness clubs do more than participate in physical activity—that they learn more about the short-term and long-term effects of exercise and the scientific principles upon which an exercise prescription is based. In private sport clubs members should be taught principles of conditioning for a specific sport as well as skills and rules. Thus, there is a need to develop and use knowledge tests. If knowledge tests are administered in a private club, they are often used in a self-testing capacity. However, in either setting, a knowledge test is a good way to reinforce learning.

In this chapter the development of various types of written test items is described. Items may be generated for norm-referenced or criterion-referenced tests (Roid, 1984). Most likely, you will have taken tests exemplifying all these types of items, so you will be familiar with them. As you might recall from the discussion of content validity in Chapter 6, developing a knowledge test must be undertaken in as careful a manner as any other type of test. A list of sources of physical education written tests can be found in Mood (1980) and Johnson and Nelson (1986). The best source of test items for various sports and other forms of physical activity is a book prepared by McGee and Farrow (1987).

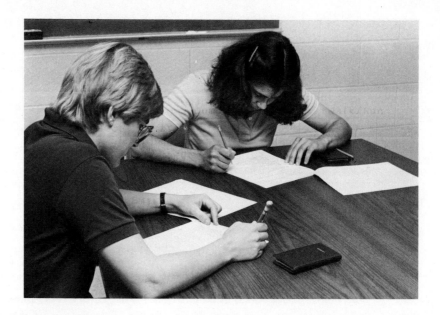

TABLE OF SPECIFICATIONS

The first step in devising any type of knowledge test is to develop a **table of specifications,** in which the basic categories of knowledge are identified and a decision is made on the relative importance of each. Without this plan the efforts of the test writer tend to be haphazard. Deciding how many items should be included to test memorization of facts and application of facts is also a good idea. The table of specifications is then set up as described in Chapter 6. The relative importance of each category is reflected in its weighting, which dictates the number of items to be written for the category. For example, in an exercise class the scientific principles of exercise might be viewed as twice as important as the knowledge of basic exercise prescriptions. If so, twice as many items should be written on principles. In a basketball class rules may be more important or less important than knowledge of game strategies; the number of items should be adjusted accordingly.

Of course, other factors affect the length of the test. For example, an examinee should be able to answer the total number of items in the time available for testing. As a general rule of thumb, allow 45 seconds for each multiple-choice item and 30 seconds for each true-false item. However, practical experience with the test provides more definitive feedback on test length.

TEST ADMINISTRATION

The directions for test administration should be clearly stated. The most desirable method of presenting test directions is to print them on the test itself, which enables the test taker to read and reread them. At the beginning of the testing period, these directions should be read aloud by the administrator, since it is well known that some examinees do not read directions carefully. The following example of directions might be used for a written test:

Directions: Read the following directions carefully before beginning the test. This is a six-page test consisting of 35 multiple-choice items. Be sure your test contains six pages and that all pages are in correct sequence. Circle the response that represents the *best* answer to the question or lead statement. Only one answer is correct for each item. Each item counts two points. Write your name at the top of this page and begin the test.

The administrator should also inform the examinee if a correction for guessing will be used. (The concept of correcting for guessing is explained later in this chapter.) The student should be notified if guessing will be penalized.

The test taker's attention should be called to anything else that will help the individual to interpret the test. For example, how much time will be allowed for the test? At periodic intervals the examinee should be informed of the amount of time remaining. Are there multiple pages of the test? If so, the group should be asked to count the number of pages to be sure no page is missing or blank. Are certain sections of the test weighted more heavily than others? If so, note this at the beginning of the test period so the examinee can allocate time wisely. The number of points allocated to each section should also be printed on the test.

With the widespread availability of microcomputers, developing tests is easier using a test writer program. A number of these types of programs can now be purchased. Items are entered into the computer and then printed. Modification of test items is then a simple matter. Sometimes a test user might not realize an item is poor until it has been used once; thus the item must be either revised or discarded. This can be done by changing that item on the computer without retyping the whole test. Sometimes an educator does not teach every concept covered in the previous year's unit, so last year's tests may be inadequate this year. The items not covered can be eliminated on the computer, and a new version of the test can be printed. Better yet, a bank of items can be entered, and specific items can be requested. A random sample of items can also be drawn from each category of items (with the number of items designated by the teacher) that is different for each student's test. In other words, if the test is being administered to 20 people, 20 different versions of the test could be randomly generated. This facilitates monitoring an examination in a school setting, since copying someone else's answer to a different examination makes no sense.

The administration of a test, then, requires careful consideration before the actual testing period. Educators are primarily interested in how well the test taker can deal with the *content* of the test and not in the trappings of the test.

TYPES OF TEST ITEMS

Five types of knowledge test items are commonly used: true-false, multiple choice, matching, short answer, and essay. Generally the multiple-choice items are the hardest to write, since a number of choices must be prepared for each item. However, they are easy to score. The essay item, on the other hand, is often considered easy to write, yet it is difficult to grade because of the subjective nature of the test response. A review of each type follows.

True-False

Since the **true-false item** consists of a single statement, it seems relatively easy to write. It is a familiar type of test item and is widely used. Although there are several variations of the true-false item, none is appreciably different from the standard true-false version. Examples of several of these versions are presented in the boxed material. The *correction* variety, last in the box, requires the test taker to correct the statement, with the correction limited to the underlined word(s).

The true-false item has been criticized in the past for several reasons. First, some teachers have developed true-false tests by merely taking complete sentences out of a textbook, either leaving them as they are or changing one or two words. This, of course, encourages students to study for these types of test by memorizing portions of the textbook, causing some to think that the true-false test has become associated with the lowest level of cognitive behavior (memorization). However, well-written test items can tap higher levels of cognitive be-

---

Samples of true-false items

The true-false variety.
The mean is a measure of central tendency. <u>T</u>　F

The right-wrong variety.
When aiming in field archery, the correct anchor point for the hand is directly under the chin. R　<u>W</u>

The yes-no variety.
Is "dunking" the ball legal in college basketball? <u>Y</u>　N

The cluster variety.
A badminton serve that lands in the proper court is legal when the shuttlecock is hit:

<u>T</u>　F　1. By the frame of the racket
T　<u>F</u>　2. Above the racket hand
T　<u>F</u>　3. Below the waist
<u>T</u>　F　4. While on one foot

The correction variety.
The skill with which a tennis serve is executed can be measured by determining the *accuracy* of the serve. *(accuracy and force)*

havior. (Refer to Chapter 8 for more information on levels of cognitive behavior.) Second, the true-false item is often ambiguous, since, with no standard of comparison, it must be judged in isolation. It must be *clearly* true or *clearly* false, rather than subject to multiple interpretations. A carefully written item leaves little or no room for ambiguity. A third objection to the true-false item is that it is less reliable than the multiple-choice item. However, more true-false items than multiple-choice items can be answered during a given time period. By increasing the number of true-false items, the reliability of the total test is improved.

Critics of the true-false test item often note that an examinee could receive a good score merely by guessing the answer. By guessing on every item, there is a 50-50 chance of answering each item correctly. However, it is not likely that many test takers actually guess blindly on all questions. Think of your own test-taking behavior. You may not be certain you know the correct answer, but you can frequently take an educated guess. Based on your overall knowledge of the test content, you may make a plausible response, although you are not sure it is correct. Thus the probability of answering correctly is no longer 50-50. Although a correction for guessing can be applied, as you will see later, it may not be desirable.

Suggestions for Writing True-False Items As noted earlier, the process of writing a true-false item can seem deceptively simple. In reality, it is one of the more difficult items to write *well*. The following list summarizes a number of suggestions for writing good true-false items:

1. Avoid trivial items. Write items that measure meaningful content and that require application of concepts. Consider, for example, the following item from a volleyball test written for beginning players at the high school level:

   T F   The dimensions of a volleyball court are 20 feet by 50 feet. (F)

   How important is this content for a beginning volleyball player in a high school physical education class? It is questionable whether a student at this level of skill needs to know this information at all. Of far greater value would be items dealing with skill execution and rules of the game, along with simple game strategies.
2. Avoid using sentences from textbooks or stereotyped phrases as items.
3. Avoid ambiguity.
4. Include an equal number of true and false items, or more false than true. (The tendency in constructing true-false tests is to include more true items than false, yet evidence shows that examinees tend to mark an item true when uncertain of the correct answer. False items discriminate better than true ones.)

5. Reorder the test items randomly after completing all of them. Otherwise, you might generate a pattern of responses that can be detected by the test-wise student.

6. Express only a single idea in each item statement. Examine, as an example, the following item from a badminton test:

> T   F   A serve is illegal if the shuttlecock touches the net before landing in the proper court or if the server steps over the service line.

This item refers to two rules affecting service. The first hypothesis is false and the second is true. How should the test taker respond? This item should be divided into two separate items, so that a clear-cut, correct response is possible for each one.

7. Avoid negative statements. If an occasional item lends itself to the negative form, underline the negative term(s) in the statement. Consider the following example:

> T   F   The Kraus-Weber Test is *no longer* viewed as a valid test of the physical fitness of school children. (T)

In this case the negative form is justifiable because it accurately reflects a change in the way the test has been interpreted over the past 30 years. It was accepted (although erroneously) as a valid test of fitness for children, but now the test is correctly interpreted as a test of minimum strength.

8. Avoid the use of words such as *sometimes, usually,* or *often* in true statements, or *always, never,* or *impossible* in false statements.

9. Make false statements plausible.

10. Make true statements clearly true.

Multiple Choice

The **multiple-choice item** contains a **stem**—an introductory question or incomplete statement—and a set of *alternatives*—or suggested options, sometimes referred to as *foils*. The correct alternative is referred to as the *answer;* the incorrect alternatives are called *distractors*. Several varieties of the multiple-choice item are shown in the boxed material. In the *correct-answer* variety only one alternative is correct. More than one answer is correct, but one answer is better than the other in the *best-answer* variety. In the *multiple-answer* variety more than one answer may be correct.

The Stem The stem is written either as a direct question or as an incomplete sentence. Usually the incomplete sentence consists of fewer words than the direct question and thus is more economical. However, the direct question is often easier to use effectively. When the stem is an incomplete sentence, each alternative must be written to conform satisfactorily to the stem. When the stem is a

---

Samples of multiple choice items

The correct-answer variety

When a fencer attacks to the high left side of an opponent's target area,
the appropriate defensive action is
a. Parry 2
b. Parry 4
c. Parry 6
d. Parry 8   (b)

The best-answer variety

To develop skill in shooting a basketball from a given distance, a player
must learn to reproduce the correct
a. Vertical angle of projection
b. Horizontal angle of projection
c. Trajectory
d. Velocity   (c)

The multiple-answer variety

The reliability of a written test can be raised by increasing the
a. Range of ability
b. Length of the test
c. Number being tested
d. Level of ability   (a,b)

---

direct question, the task is simplified somewhat because the alternatives are written only to conform with each other.

The stem should present the problem clearly and briefly. Be aware that if the stem is too long, the test taker may forget what he or she has read by the time the alternatives are reached. On the other hand, do not be so brief that no message is conveyed, as in the following:

Conscious relaxation is . . .

An exact, more meaningful statement follows:

The major characteristic of conscious relaxation is . . .

As is true with true-false statements, stereotyped phrases should be avoided. Generally, the stem should be written in the positive, not the negative, form.

The Alternatives Usually between three and five alternatives are written for a multiple-choice item. Using the same number of alternatives with all items is not absolutely necessary. Writing five alternatives might be easy for one test item but difficult for another. Developing fewer, well-written alternatives is better than adding one or two poorly written ones for the sake of generating a predetermined number of alternatives. There is an advantage, however, to preparing five alternatives for each item. As the number of alternatives increases, the reliability of the item increases and the chance level for getting an answer correct is reduced. Regardless of the number of alternatives used, plan to spend considerable time writing good ones.

Some test users find the distractors harder to write than the correct answer. It is only logical that the distractors should seem plausible to the test taker. One way of generating ideas about possible distractors is to administer a set of open-ended questions to a group similar to those who will be tested. There will, of course, be a number of correct answers, but there will also be a variety of incorrect responses. These can be used as a basis for developing good distractors.

The distractors should be parallel in grammatical form and of the same approximate length. Note the length of the alternatives in the following item from an archery knowledge test:

How many arrows are shot in a Columbia Round? (b)
a. 12   c. 36
b. 24 at 50, 40, and 30 yards   d. 48

The difference in the length of *b* compared with the other three alternatives suggests that it might be the correct answer, which it is. The general format of all four alternatives should conform. Furthermore, the smallest and largest number of arrows in *a* and *d* do not appear to be as plausible as *b* and *c* are. A better version of this item follows:

How many arrows are shot in a Columbia Round? (b)
a. 24 at 40, 30, and 20 yards   c. 36 at 40, 30, and 20 yards
b. 24 at 50, 40, and 30 yards   d. 36 at 50, 40, and 30 yards

As is true with true-false items, words such as *always* and *never* should be avoided. *None of the above* and *All of the above* should be used sparingly as distractors and not used as substitutes for the alternative that is difficult to write.

Be sure that no pattern to the correct responses exists. Sometimes a patterning occurs even though the test writer is unaware of it. An easy way to prevent this occurrence is to order the alternatives randomly. If an item has four alternatives, drop slips of paper numbered 1 through 4 into a container, and draw them out one by one. This represents the random ordering of the alternatives.

Multiple-choice items, like any other type of item, can easily be written in an ambiguous way. The only way ambiguity can be reduced is by writing and rewriting the item until there is a general agreement on the interpretation of the item and the feasibility of the alternatives.

Matching

A **matching item** consists of two columns of words or phrases, with the column on the right containing the alternatives. The examinee is instructed to select one alternative from the right column to correspond with each item in the left column. Two examples of matching questions are given in the boxed material.

Sample matching items

Directions: Place the *letter* of the appropriate organization in the space.

____ 1. Organization governing amateur sports in America	(a) AAHPERD
	(b) AAU
____ 2. Organization governing college athletics in America	(c) AIAW
	(d) NCAA
	(e) USGA
____ 3. National professional physical education association	(f) USLTA
____ 4. Governed women's collegiate athletics	
____ 5. Rules governing body for golf	

Directions: Place the *letter* of the appropriate person in the space provided to the left of each statement.

____ 1. Grandfather of physical education

____ 2. First president of physical education professional organization

____ 3. Thought aim of education was happiness

____ 4. Instrumental in growth of measurement in physical education

____ 5. Developed athletic achievement tests with YMCA

____ 6. Founded interpretive dancing

____ 7. Gave first "modern dance" concert

____ 8. Day's order of exercises in public schools

(a) Aristotle
(b) Catherine Beecher
(c) Isadora Duncan
(d) Martha Graham
(e) Luther Gulick
(f) Guts Muth
(g) Margaret H'Doubler
(h) Edward Hitchcock
(i) Dio Lewis
(j) Dudley Sargent
(k) Jesse F. Williams

From Haskins, M.J.

It is desirable to include a larger number of alternatives in the second column than the number of items in the first column, as depicted in the example in the boxed material on p. 323. If the number of alternatives is equal to the number of items, answering the last one or two items merely through the process of elimination may be possible. Between 5 and 15 items per test section is recommended.

Many variations of the matching item exist. A popular version in physical ed-

---

Sample of variation of matching question

Volleyball

Directions: Indicate the official's decision in the following situations, using the key letters for your answers. There is only one best answer. Assume that no conditions exist other than those stated.

P – point   L – legal, or play continues
SO – side out   R – re-serve, or serve over

____ 1. Server steps on the end line as the ball leaves hand.

____ 2. On the service, the ball touches the top of the net and lands on the boundary line of the receiving team's court.

____ 3. A player on the receiving team spikes the ball before it crosses to his/her side of the net. Player does not touch the net.

____ 4. A front line player on the serving team, in spiking the ball, returns to the floor across the center line. On the same play, a front line player of the receiving team who attempts to block the ball steps on the center line.

____ 5. As a player on the serving team attempts to contact the ball, it touches the upper arm.

Soccer

Directions: Place the appropriate letter in the space provided.

A—Free kick for opposing team   E—Free kick on penalty cir-
B—Kick-in for opposing team   cle
C—Roll in   F—Penalty kick
D—Corner kick   G—No penalty
                                                                  H—Score

____ 1. On a kick-in player A dribbles the ball rather than kicking it.

____ 2. A team "B" player, taking a kick-in, sends the ball between the goal posts.

____ 3. "A" is tackling "B" who has the ball; it goes out of bounds off both players.

____ 4. During play the ball is lofted into the air, and the left inner bounces it off his knee through the goal posts.

From Haskins, M.J.

ucation is the use of a small number of alternatives, each of which can be used more than once. See the boxed material on p. 324 for two examples of this variation.

Short-Answer

The **short-answer item** is undoubtedly the easiest of all items to construct; however, there are drawbacks. More than one response may be correct. The test taker often has the difficult task of trying to think of the answer the *test developer* has in mind. Several words or phrases may be appropriate. Furthermore, this type of item often measures simple recall. Examples of three versions of short-answer items are shown in the boxed material below: the *question* variety, consisting of a direct question; the *completion* variety, written as an incomplete statement; and the *identification* or *association* variety, containing a list of words or phrases that the examinee must identify in the designated way.

Short-answer items should only be used when the desired answer is clear to experts and when the answer can be given in one or two words. These items are often used in tests of first aid and cardiopulmonary resuscitation (CPR), where the series of steps that should be followed in an emergency setting has been established by experts.

Samples of short-answer items

The question variety

If a bowler gets a strike in the first frame and six pins in the second frame, what is his second frame score?

(22)

The completion variety

The extension of the foil arm in fencing is called the

(thrust)

The identification or association variety

After each name write the sport in which her (or she) achieved fame.

Larry Bird	(Basketball)
Bobby Jones	(Golf)
Knute Rockne	(Football)
Steffi Graf	(Tennis)
Jane Blalock	(Golf)
Vida Blue	(Baseball)

Essay Items

An essay test usually contains a small number of **essay items,** each one requiring the examinee to construct a response at least several sentences long. Often an interpretation of facts is expected; therefore, no one response is correct, and a variety of responses might be acceptable.

One of the major limitations of an essay item is the lack of consistency that may occur in evaluating the answer. Various raters might assess the same response differently, and one rater might judge a response differently on two separate occasions. The lack of objectivity on the part of raters exists for several reasons. First, some raters are more severe than others and will always assign lower ratings. Second, some raters tend to give "middle-of-the-road" ratings, and others use the full range of ratings. If a rater predominantly uses the "middle-of-the-road" range, the best responses are penalized and the poorest ones are unduly rewarded. Third, raters may differ in the relative values they assign to different responses because each rater uses a separate criterion. One rater may emphasize writing form and style; another looks primarily for content.

Other factors also affect the consistency of ratings of essay items. The **halo effect,** where the rater is affected by the examinee's previous performance, can lower objectivity. For example, a good essay written by a usually poor student may receive a lower rating than a paper of the same quality written by a generally good student. One way of controlling this source of error is to ask that the examinee's name be placed only on the first page of the test. Then this page can be folded back out of sight until all examinations have been graded. Extraneous factors such as handwriting, spelling, and organization can contribute to less objective ratings. Carefully describe the degree to which these factors will be taken into account when the test is scored. Otherwise, the examinee may assume only content is being evaluated.

Since including a large number of items on an essay examination is not possible, the reliability of the test may be low. Because of time limitations, sampling a wide range of content on an essay examination is usually not feasible. For this reason, students sometimes feel penalized by the particular set of questions included on an essay test.

Construction of Essay Items At first glance, the essay test seems much easier to develop than an objective test. It is tempting to put together a few items in the shortest possible amount of time, but this often leads to a vague test that does not tap the desired knowledges. To avoid this, the objectives of the test should be carefully defined, and the items should be formulated based on these objectives. General questions, such as the following, should be avoided.

Discuss the mechanical principles of swimming.

There is no reasonable focus to this question; thus, it might be answered in a broad, surface manner. The question should be delimited, perhaps in the following way:

Discuss the principles of buoyancy as it applies to the breast stroke. Include the following points:

1. Definition of principle of buoyancy
2. Application with regard to coordination of body parts
3. Application with regard to position of body parts

Including from 10 to 15 questions that require relatively short answers is preferable to asking two or three questions needing longer responses. The greater the number of questions, the better the sampling of content will be.

After the items have been written but before the test is administered, a model answer should be constructed for each item. The model answer can be prepared in outline form, including all major points the student would be expected to make. These responses should be prepared in less than the amount of time the examinees will have to complete the test, since the student will have to compose an answer rather than merely formulate an outline. If problems arise in writing the model answer, perhaps the items need revision.

Sometimes the test taker is allowed to choose a number of items out of the total number available. If the test is tailormade for a specific individual, this is not unreasonable. However, if the test is being administered to a group, allowing a choice might not be as fair as it seems. When examinees select different sets of items, each with different difficulty levels, comparing performances on the test is difficult. This is a problem especially when the tests are to be graded in a school setting.

Scoring Essay Items Ebel (1972) has described six deficiencies that commonly occur in the response to an essay item:

1. Incorrect statements were included in the answer.
2. Important ideas necessary to an adequate answer were omitted.
3. Correct statements having little or no relation to the question were included.
4. Unsound conclusions were reached, either because of mistakes in reasoning or because of misapplication of principles.
5. Bad writing obscured the development and exposition of the student's ideas.
6. A number of errors occurred in spelling and the mechanics of correct writing.

For maximum objectivity in scoring, evaluate one question for all examinees before moving to the next question. As discussed earlier, do not look at the examinee's name until the scoring of all tests is completed. Sometimes the rater's standards will change after scoring the first few items. Occasionally turning back and rechecking the first item on the tests initially scored is wise to be sure consistent standards have been applied. An even better approach is to skim through all answers to an item before scoring it to arrive at a feeling for the range of responses; this can lead to greater consistency in grading from the outset.

WEIGHTING TEST COMPONENTS

Earlier in this chapter the relationship of the number of items to the importance of the content area was discussed. In general, if more items are included on a given topic than any other one, this topic is automatically weighted more heavily. Although this may seem obvious, sometimes test developers neglect to examine the proportion of items per topic on a test.

Other factors also affect the weighting of test components. If a test is answered correctly by all examinees, then it is essentially weighted 0. The item does not discriminate among examinees. The same effect occurs if *no* examinee can answer an item correctly. The weighting of test components, then, is affected not only by the number of items per component but also by the ability of the items to discriminate.

CORRECTION FOR GUESSING

When an objective knowledge test is used, it is possible to apply a **correction for guessing.** In some test settings, examinees are encouraged not to answer an item by guessing. If the answer is not known, the examinee is asked to leave the item unanswered. Then the total test score is corrected for guessing. For the true-false test Formula 15-1 is used.

$$S = R - W$$

where S = corrected *score*
R = number of *right* answers
W = number of *wrong* answers

Formula 15-1

Clearly, when using this formula, one assumes that wrong answers are a function of guessing. This, of course, may not be true.

For multiple-choice tests, Formula 15-2 is used to correct for guessing.

$$S = R - \frac{W}{n - 1}$$

where n = *number* of alternatives per items

Formula 15-2

Note that Formula 15-1 is a special case of Formula 15-2 when n = 2.

When an objective knowledge test is developed so that all examinees should be able to finish in a given time period, a correction for guessing formula is often not necessary. This covers the majority of tests used in physical education and exercise science. However, when speed is an important part of the test, a correction formula should be used. Certain types of tests include so many items that the typical examinee is not expected to complete the test in the designated time period. In the physical education field these tests might be included in perceptual-motor learning test batteries and sport psychology test batteries. Here the use of a correction formula is recommended.

RELIABILITY AND VALIDITY

The reliability of a written test is sometimes determined by correlating scores on equivalent forms of the test. Although the items on the two tests differ, they cover the same content. The test-retest method is not appropriate because the examinee is likely to remember items from the first administration of the test.

Perhaps the most frequently used method of determining the reliability of a written test is a measure of internal consistency. This can be calculated by administering the test on only one occasion. A split-half coefficient is one example of this method. However, there are many ways to split a test into two halves. A procedure known as the Kuder-Richardson method was developed to provide a reliability estimate of the average of all possible split-halves. The simplest of the Kuder-Richardson formulas is shown in Formula 15-3.

$$r_{kr21} = \frac{k\,(s^2) - \overline{X}\,(k - \overline{X})}{(k - 1)\,(s^2)} \qquad \text{Formula 15-3}$$

where r_{kr21} = Kuder-Richardson 21 reliability coefficient
k = number of items on the test
$\overline{X}$ = mean score on the test
s^2 = variance of the test scores (standard deviation squared)

Assume $k = 20$, $s^2 = 8$, and $\overline{X} = 12$. Using Formula 15-3, the Kuder-Richardson formula 21 reliability coefficient is calculated as shown below:

$$r_{kr21} = \frac{20(8) - 12(20 - 12)}{(20 - 1)\,(8)}$$

$$= \frac{160 - 12\,(8)}{(19)\,(8)}$$

$$= \frac{160 - 96}{152} = 0.42$$

The interpretable range of the KR 21 coefficient is $.00 - 1.00$. It is possible to have some reliability or no reliability (.00), but a negative coefficient lacks meaning. A negative reliability coefficient suggests that the test has less than no reliability. If all else is equal, the larger the standard deviation, the higher the reliability coefficient.

One procedure for determining the validity of a written test has already been discussed. This is the development of a table of specifications, which can be used as the basis for establishing content validity. Item analysis procedures can be used to provide information on the validity of the individual test items.

ITEM ANALYSIS

An **item analysis** is a procedure for determining the usefulness of each individual item as a part of the total test. It is applied after the test has been administered to a group of examinees. Overall, the results of an item analysis provide information on the effectiveness of the total test. It is a good idea to accumulate test scores for approximately 100 students before undertaking an item analysis. However, an informal analysis can be used with smaller numbers, especially if a rough indicator of how the items are working is needed. Two aspects of an item analysis are described—item difficulty and item discrimination.

Item Difficulty

How difficult was a particular item? **Item difficulty** can be determined quite easily by calculating the proportion of examinees answering the item correctly.

$$P = \frac{\#R}{N} \qquad \text{Formula 15-4}$$

where P = item *difficulty*
$\#R$ = *number* answering correctly
N = total *number* in group

Overall the item should not be too easy or too difficult because both extremes do not provide very much information on the achievement of the examinees. A general range of .30 − .70 is recommended (Ebel, 1972). However, difficulty levels slightly above or below this range may be acceptable if the item discriminates well. It is not uncommon to observe one or two easy items at the beginning of a test, deliberately chosen to set the examinee at ease.

Knowing something about the level of difficulty of the item does not relate anything about the people who answered correctly. Did people who answered the item correctly also receive higher scores on the test, and vice versa? This is unknown, based on *P* alone. The next step is to calculate *D*, the index of discrimination.

Item Discrimination

If an item discriminates well, more high scorers answer the item correctly than low scorers. If the reverse occurs (i.e., more low scorers answer the item correctly), the item is poorly constructed. The statistic used to determine item discrimination is known as the **index of discrimination**. The index of discrimination, D, compares the proportion of high scorers and low scorers who answer an item correctly.

The following steps are used to calculate the index of discrimination:

1. Separate two subgroups of test papers, an upper group (approximately 27% of the total group) who received highest scores on the test and a lower group (same percentage of total group) who received the lowest scores.
2. Count the number of times the correct response to each item was chosen on the papers of the upper group, then do the same for the lower group.
3. Tally these response counts on a copy of the test.
4. Subtract the lower group count of correct responses from the upper group count of correct responses. Divide this difference by the maximum possible difference, that is, the total number of people in the upper (or lower) group. This is essentially Formula 15-5.

$$D = \frac{R_u - R_l}{N_u}$$

Formula 15-5

where D = index of *discrimination*

R_u = number of correct *responses* in *upper* group

R_l = number of correct *responses* in *lower* group

N_u = total *number* in *upper* group

Although taking 27% of the upper and lower extremes is often recommended to maximize the differences between the extremes, any percentage between 25% and 33% is acceptable (Ebel, 1972). If the total group size is small, the top 9% and bottom 9% may be counted twice.

Theoretically, the index of discrimination can be as high as 1.00. In reality, an index this high is rarely obtained. If $D > 0.40$, the item discriminates well. Refer to Table 15-1 for an evaluation of the size of the index of discrimination.

Other Item Discrimination Methods In a classroom setting there is a simpler way of obtaining the numbers of high and low scorers answering an item correctly. The teacher can identify the test score that represents the cutoff score for the high group and the cutoff score identifying the low group. Then, for each item, the teacher asks those in the high group who answered the item correctly to raise their hands. The number is counted and recorded, and the same request

TABLE 15-1 *Evaluation of the size of the index of discrimination*

Index of discrimination	Item evaluation
0.40 and up	Very good items
0.30-0.39	Reasonably good but possibly subject to improvement
0.20-0.29	Marginal items, usually needing and being subject to improvement
Below 0.19	Poor items, to be rejected or improved by revision

From Ebel, R.L.

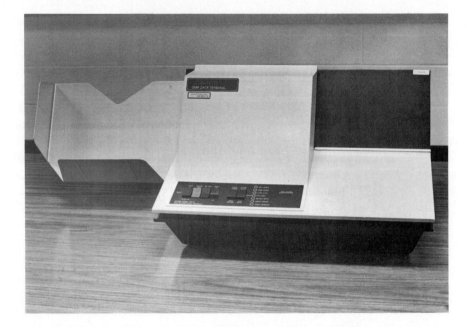

is made of the low group. The groups can be labeled A and B instead of high and low to avoid possible embarrassment of the low scorers. The middle group could even be asked for a show of hands on each item to allow total class participation, although this information would not actually be used. The number of students in the low group who answered the item correctly should be subtracted from the number in the high group answering correctly and divided by the total number in either group, as shown in Formula 15-5.

A computer can provide much more technical information, however. Many computer programs have been written to conduct an item analysis on a set of test scores. Although the results may be in more technical form, they nonetheless consist of item difficulty, item discrimination, and total test reliability.

Also of interest is the degree to which each alternative functions, referred to as **item function.** This is determined by the percentage of examinees choosing a given alternative. Tally the number of students who responded to each alternative. Each alternative should be plausible enough to be selected by 2% to 3% of the examinees. If not, it should be revised.

SUMMARY

Knowledge tests should be carefully constructed to ensure content validity. Before the test items are written, a table of specifications is prepared to provide the guidelines for test development. Test items are written according to this plan. The usefulness of individual items can be checked by conducting an item analysis. Additional validation techniques, as well as reliability estimation procedures, are described in Chapter 6.

LEARNING EXPERIENCES

1. Develop a table of specifications for a test of a sport or principles of exercise. Indicate content areas and levels of cognitive behavior on the table. Specify the number of items that should be written for each cell of the table.
2. Write 10 multiple-choice items, using the table of specifications you developed in 1 above. Exchange items with one of your classmates, and carefully analyze his or her items. Note ambiguous items that need rewriting. Revise your items according to his or her suggestions and give them to your instructor to be evaluated.
3. Use the 10-item test you developed in 2. Another revision may be necessary once the instructor has evaluated your items. Administer the test to 30 students on your campus. Group administration is not necessary; the test may be taken by one, two, or more students at a time. However, each student should have *some* knowledge of the sport or exercise principle measured by the test. When 30 students have completed the test, determine the score for each test and conduct an item analysis. Use the 10 top scores for the upper group and the 10 lowest scores for the lower group. Prepare a list of results as shown below.

Item number	Item difficulty	Item discrimination	Item function
1			
2			
3			
4			
5			
6			
7			
8			
9			
10			

Discuss any items that do not discriminate well. How might they be improved? Keep in mind, however, that a group of 30 people is too small for a definitive item analysis. Therefore, results should be interpreted somewhat tentatively.

REFERENCES

Ebel, R.L. 1972. Essentials of educational measurement. Englewood Cliffs, NJ: Prentice-Hall, Inc.

Haskins, M.J. 1971. Evaluation in physical education. Dubuque, IA: Wm C Brown Group.

Johnson, B.L., and Nelson, J.K. 1986. Practical measurements for evaluation in physical education. Minneapolis: Burgess.

Mood, D.P. 1980. Numbers in motion. Palo Alto, CA: Mayfield Publishing Co.

Roid, G.H. 1984. Generating the test items. In R.A. Berk, editor. A guide to criterion-referenced test construction. Baltimore: The Johns Hopkins University Press.

ANNOTATED READINGS

Hambleton, R.K. 1984. Using microcomputers to develop tests. Educational Measurement, 3(2):10-14.

Discusses the advantages of item banking, a collection of test items uniquely coded for easy retrieval; describes an item banking and test assembly system for microcomputers; points to the need to identify situations where computer testing enhances the quality of testing in appropriate and cost-effective ways.

Hopkins, K.D., and Stanley, J.C. 1981. Educational and psychological measurement and evaluation, ed. 6, Englewood Cliffs, NJ: Prentice-Hall, Inc.

Describes Bloom's taxonomy of educational objectives for the cognitive domain in simple, straightforward language; provides many practical suggestions for preparing a test, including the readability (reading difficulty) of the test; excellent illustrations of test items.

Melville, S. 1985. Teaching and evaluating cognitive skills in elementary physical education. Journal of Physical Education, Recreation and Dance, 56(2):26-28.

Describes efforts to measure cognitive skill acquisition of third and fourth graders using a written examination; discusses strategies for testing young children, such as reading questions and using pictures; delineates several benefits of written exams in elementary school physical education; points to the need for an incremental, hierarchical list of cognitive skills for K-6 students.

Millman, J. 1984. Individualizing test construction and administration by computer. In R.A. Berk, editor. A guide to criterion-referenced test construction. Baltimore: The Johns Hopkins University Press.

Addresses computer-assisted testing (CAT); compares various approaches to individualized testing; includes guidelines for practitioners.

Popham, W.J. 1981. Modern educational measurement. Englewood Cliffs, NJ: Prentice-Hall, Inc.

Includes an excellent section on developing educational tests, chapters on test specifications, construction of test items, improvement of test items, observations and ratings, and creation of affective measures; differentiates between norm-referenced and criterion-referenced test items.

Shick, J. 1981. Written tests in activity classes. Journal of Physical Education, Recreation, and Dance, 52(4):21-22, 83.

Presents examples of various types of test items, including true-false, multiple choice, multiple response, rearrangement, and multiple choice with constant alternatives; sample items are provided for bowling, golf, archery, badminton, and fencing.

Part Eight

Measures of Physical Fitness

16

Tests of Health-Related Physical Fitness

KEY WORDS *Watch for these words as you read the following chapter:*

AAHPERD Physical Best Program

body composition

field test

FITNESSGRAM

health-related physical fitness

hydrostatic weighing

Kraus-Weber Test

max $\dot{V}o_2$

Presidential Physical Fitness Award Program

skinfold caliper

step test

Never in the history of the United States of America has so much attention been devoted to the status of physical fitness in children and youth as in the 1980s. Several national surveys have been conducted, a number of nationally known fitness tests have been revised, the merits of health-related versus motor performance–related fitness have been debated extensively, fitness tests have been incorporated into fitness programs, concepts and knowledge about fitness have been stressed, and criterion-referenced standards have been introduced into the realm of fitness testing.

Although many physical fitness tests have been published in the United States, only a handful have been developed with an adequate concern for type of fitness, test validity, and test reliability. In addition to having these characteristics, a sound test should be accompanied by a table of norms that is useful on a national scale. Throughout most of the twentieth century, physical fitness has received its greatest emphasis during times of war. The focus on fitness was a result of the drafting of young men into the armed forces; inevitably a substantial number of men were not able to meet the physical requirements of the draft. Each time this occurred, government officials expressed dismay about the level of physical fitness of American citizens. After World War II, President Eisenhower became a strong advocate of the development of physical fitness throughout the United States. His support was largely due to the results of the **Kraus-Weber Test,** which was administered to elementary school children in the United States and Europe. President Eisenhower was distressed that American children fared poorly on the test in comparison with European children.

Although the presidential support of physical fitness generated by the poor

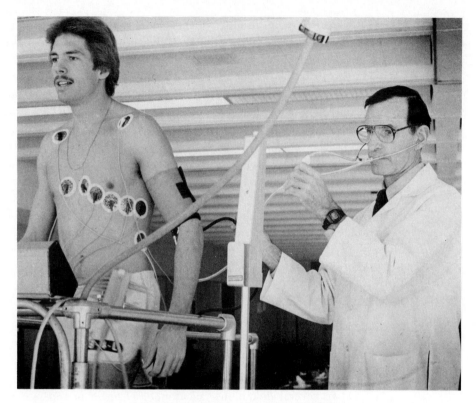

Administration of the Balke Treadmill Test.

results on the Kraus-Weber Test was beneficial, it is rather curious in one sense in that the Kraus-Weber Test was not designed as a measure of overall physical fitness. It was developed as a measure of minimal functioning of the low back area. Individuals who could pass the test were considered unlikely candidates for developing low back problems but were not judged physically fit in a broader context. A brief examination of two of the six test items will verify the actual purpose of this test, which is still used today in clinical settings.

One item consists of a sit-up test with the examinee in a supine position, hands behind the neck. The feet are held down by an examiner. The objective of the test is to perform one sit-up. Another item requires the examinee to lie prone with a pillow under the hips and lower abdomen. The hands are clasped behind the neck, and the feet are held down by the examiner. The examinee raises the chest, head, and shoulders and holds this position for 10 seconds. It is evident that these two tests are not high-powered indicators of strength and endurance, but this was not the intent of the test developers. Thus even though the test was inappropriately used as a measure of physical fitness, it generated nationwide interest in fitness. Furthermore, it led to another positive outcome under the leadership of President Eisenhower—the initiation of a conference to consider ways of promoting physical fitness throughout the United States.

In the 1970s a surge of interest in physical fitness was observed throughout the United States, only this time the emphasis was more closely tied to personal health and well-being than to fitness for fighting wars. To what extent does physical fitness contribute to a healthy life-style? This question has been studied extensively in recent years by exercise scientists, including doctors, physical educators, exercise physiologists, health specialists, and others. The answer to this question is quite complex and not yet fully known. However, there is considerable evidence to support the value of maintaining an adequate state of physical fitness. How, then, can this state of fitness be assessed? The focus of this chapter is on tests developed to measure one or more components of health-related fitness. This type of fitness is related to one's positive health state rather than one's athletic ability, acknowledging that there is some overlap between the two.

DEFINITION OF HEALTH-RELATED PHYSICAL FITNESS

Many versions of a definition of physical fitness have been published. A common denominator across most of these definitions is that physical fitness is viewed as a multifaceted ability. Sometimes the multifaceted nature of fitness is explicit in the definition; in others it is implied by the types of tests included in the test battery. In several definitions, an attempt is made to separate health-related physical fitness from performance-related fitness. However, the tests used to measure physical fitness usually tap both health-related and performance-related abilities. In some cases the health-related element is predominant, while in others, the performance-related ability prevails.

The American Alliance for Health, Physical Education, Recreation and Dance (AAHPERD) has gone on record in support of physical fitness tests and programs that emphasize the relationship between health and physical activity. According to AAHPERD, **health-related physical fitness** can be viewed thus:

> Physical fitness is a multifaceted continuum extending from birth to death. Affected by physical activity, it ranges from optimal abilities in all aspects of life through high and low levels of different physical fitness, to severely limiting disease and dysfunction (AAHPERD, 1980, p. 3).

Most physical educators and exercise scientists are not medical doctors and thus are not qualified to work independently with the physical activity needs of the person in a disease state. Although exercise physiologists may be associated with cardiac rehabilitation programs, their work is under the supervision of a cardiologist. Generally, it is the job of the physical educator to work with the healthy person using physical activity as a medium for maintaining and improving that person's health state and preventing disease. This global statement must be qualified by noting that lack of physical activity is only one of the risk factors associated with certain diseases. Certainly other factors such as nutrition must be taken into account. At the same time, our unique function in physical education and exercise science is our training and background in sport and physical activity. Specialists in these areas should be qualified to provide exercise prescriptions for the healthy person.

To determine the level of physical fitness of an individual, a test that reflects an accurate definition of physical fitness should be used. In the context of health-related physical fitness, a test measuring short-distance runs (e.g., 100 yards) would not be valid, since it is the longer distances that affect one's capacity to use oxygen. The remainder of this chapter is devoted to an overview of tests of physical fitness that are typically used in school and laboratory settings. (For fitness testing in a nonschool setting, see Chapter 12.)

MEASURING HEALTH-RELATED FITNESS

In a laboratory setting fairly precise measures of health-related fitness can be made. Usually students are exposed to some of these measures in an exercise physiology course. Since using laboratory tests in a practical setting is not feasible, **field tests** are used. A good field test does not require expensive equipment that can only be used by highly trained personnel in controlled settings. There must be evidence that the test is a valid measure of some aspect of physical fitness, perhaps not as valid as the laboratory test but with acceptable validity nonetheless. The majority of the field tests of health-related physical fitness can be used in a variety of settings, including schools, private clubs, YMCAs, YWCAs, and so forth. Although this section focuses on measures that are appropriate in a school setting, their applicability extends beyond the schools.

Historical Perspective

During the early 1950s the American Association (now Alliance) for Health, Physical Education, and Recreation began exploring tests that could be used to measure fitness on a broad scale in the public schools and that could be standardized, including tables of norms. The outcome of this exploration was the development of the AAHPER Youth Fitness Test, which is no longer sponsored by the AAHPERD. Although the developers of this test did not define physical fitness before developing the test, the last version of the test manual (AAHPER, 1976) stated that one criterion was that the test measure different components of fitness. The manual further noted that it measures elements of strength, agility, and endurance as well as proficiency in running and jumping. This test has become very popular in the United States. It has been sponsored by the FITNESS-GRAM program and the President's Council on Physical Fitness and Sports as well as the Alliance. The test items are reasonably familiar, require little or no equipment, can be administered to both boys and girls, can be administered to the entire range of grades 5 through 12, and allow self-testing by students (AAHPER, 1976, p. 10). On the other hand, the test has been criticized as a test of health-related physical fitness because of the types of items included. These criticisms became pronounced in the early 1970s when physical educators and exercise scientists became more concerned about the health-related fitness of Americans. The AAHPER Youth Fitness Test was generally viewed as a measure of physical performance related primarily to athletic ability. Furthermore, the test did not convey a definition of fitness that would be appropriate across the life span. In other words, a test measuring health-related fitness should be appropriate for persons of any age whether young, middle-aged, or elderly. The Youth Fitness Test includes items such as the standing long jump and the 50-yard dash. Although these items are useful as measures of athletic performance-related fitness, they are not valid indicators of health-related fitness.

As a result of these concerns, the AAHPERD Health-Related Physical Fitness Test (HRPFT) was developed in 1980. This test has been sponsored by the Alliance and the FITNESSGRAM program. Specific criteria were identified for choosing test items:

1. A physical fitness test should measure a range that extends from severely limiting dysfunction to high levels of functional capacity;
2. It should measure capacities that can be improved with appropriate physical activity; and
3. It should accurately reflect an individual's physical fitness status as well as changes in functional capacity by corresponding test scores and changes in these scores (AAHPERD, 1980, pp. 4-5).

Three areas of physiological function appeared to be related to the above criteria: cardiorespiratory (CR) function, body composition (leaness/fatness), and abdominal and low back–hamstring musculoskeletal function. Recently, national tests of physical fitness have added a measure of arm and shoulder strength and endurance, using the rationale that fitness in this area may aid in the prevention of bone deterioration in later life. From a more practical standpoint, sufficient fitness in the arm and shoulder area is essential to participate effectively in many forms of physical activity.

In the mid-1980s, physical educators and exercise scientists around the country attempted to gain support for one national physical fitness test for children and youth. These efforts failed, and several organizations have developed and promoted their own tests. Six tests have been selected for review in this chapter. These are the AAHPERD Physical Best Program, the Chrysler/AAU Test, the Fit Youth Today Test, the FITNESSGRAM System, the NCYFS Test, and the Presidential Physical Fitness Award Program.

AAHPERD Physical Best Program

The **AAHPERD Physical Best Program** (American Alliance for Health, Physical Education, Recreation and Dance, 1988) defines physical fitness as "a physical state of well being that allows people to perform daily activities with vigor, reduce their risk of health problems related to lack of exercise, and provide a fitness base for participation in a variety of physical activities" (p. 12). The major emphasis is on components of fitness that promote health: aerobic capacity, body composition, flexibility, and muscular strength/endurance. Each component is defined as follows:

1. Aerobic capacity is the ability to perform large muscle, whole body physical activity of moderate to high intensity over extended periods of time.
2. Body composition is the division of the total body weight into two components: fat weight and lean weight.
3. Flexibility is the ability to move muscles and joints through their full range of motion.
4. Muscular strength and endurance is the ability of muscles to produce force at high intensities over short intervals of time (strength) and to sustain repeated productions of force at low to moderate intensities over extended intervals of time (endurance) (AAHPERD, 1988, p.12).

The Physical Best Program consists of three dimensions: an educational component, a health-related fitness assessment, and a set of awards. The test items shown in Table 16-1 are used to measure physical fitness.

The award system, called the American Alliance Physical Best Recognition System, consists of three types of awards. One is the Fitness Activity Award, which is a recognition for participation in appropriate physical activity beyond the requirement of physical education. The participant is required to maintain a log of activity related to physical fitness. Two is the Fitness Goals Award, which involves recognition for the attainment of individual goals developed by the stu-

---

TABLE 16-1 *The AAHPERD Physical Best Test Battery*

Item	Component of fitness
One Mile Walk/Run (or any test 6 minutes or longer)	Aerobic capacity
Sum of Tricep and Calf Skinfolds (or sum of tricep and subscapular or Body Mass Index) BMI = Body Weight (Kg) / Height (mm)^2	Body composition
Sit-and-Reach Test	Flexibility
Modified sit-ups	Muscular strength/endurance
Pull-ups	Muscular strength/endurance

TABLE 16-2 Health fitness standards

Age	One-mile walk/run (min)		Sum of skinfolds (mm)		Body mass index		Sit and reach (cm)		Sit-up		Pull-up	
	Girls	Boys	Girls	Boys	Girls	Boys	Girls	Boys	Girls	Boys	Girls	Boys
5	14:00	13:00	16-36	12-25	14-20	13-20	25	25	20	20	1	1
6	13:00	12:00	16-36	12-25	14-20	13-20	25	25	20	20	1	1
7	12:00	11:00	16-36	12-25	14-20	13-20	25	25	24	24	1	1
8	11:30	10:00	16-36	12-25	14-20	14-20	25	25	26	26	1	1
9	11:00	10:00	16-36	12-25	14-20	14-20	25	25	28	30	1	1
10	11:00	9:30	16-36	12-25	14-21	14-20	25	25	30	34	1	2
11	11:00	9:00	16-36	12-25	14-21	15-21	25	25	33	36	1	2
12	11:00	9:00	16-36	12-25	15-22	15-22	25	25	33	38	1	2
13	10:30	8:00	16-36	12-25	15-23	15-23	25	25	33	40	1	3
14	10:30	7:45	16-36	12-25	17-24	16-24	25	25	35	40	1	4
15	10:30	7:30	16-36	12-25	17-24	17-24	25	25	35	42	1	5
16	10:30	7:30	16-36	12-25	17-24	18-24	25	25	35	44	1	5
17	10:30	7:30	16-36	12-25	17-25	18-25	25	25	35	44	1	5
18	10:30	7:30	16-36	12-25	18-26	18-26	25	25	35	44	1	5

Test Item

Reproduced from *Physical Best* (pp. 28-29). Reston, VA: The American Alliance for Health, Physical Education, Recreation and Dance, 1988. By permission of the publisher.

dent with the help of the physical education teacher. Three is the Health Fitness Award which is recognition of mastery of health fitness standards. Mastery reflects achievement of a standard associated with minimal risk of health problems. To receive this award, the participant must attain a minimal level of fitness on all items in the battery. Criterion-referenced standards are presented for each test. These standards are reproduced in Table 16-2.

No tables of norms are included in the test manual. However, normative data are available from the National Children and Youth Fitness I and II studies. Percentile norms from these studies are presented later in this chapter.

The Chrysler Fund-AAU Physical Fitness Program

The AAU Physical Fitness Program is currently being cosponsored by the Chrysler Corporation. A test manual is available for test users. The test battery, shown in Table 16-3, consists of four required items plus one optional item. Several variations should be noted in the test items. The distances used in the Endurance Run vary by age, with ¼ mile for ages 6-7, ½ mile for ages 8-9, ¾ mile for ages 10-11, and 1 mile for age 12 and over. The Flexibility Test is a V-sit reach.

In the test manual, a distinction is made between physical fitness and motor skill. "Unlike physical fitness, skill may be retained at reasonably high levels even without regular practice. Both physical fitness and motor skill are important in physical performance, but they are developed in different ways. In general, physical fitness is *earned*—skill is *learned*" (The Chrysler Fund-AAU, 1987, p. 2).

TABLE 16-3 *The Chrysler Fund-AAU Fitness Test*

Item	Component of fitness
Endurance Run	Cardiorespiratory endurance
Bent-Knee Sit-ups	Trunk strength and endurance
Sit and Reach Test	Flexibility in hamstrings/lower back region
Pull-ups (Boys)	Upper body strength and endurance
Flexed Arm Hang (Girls)	Leg strength; efficiency of control of body mass
Isometric Pushup	Upper body static endurance
Push-ups, Modified (Girls)	Upper body strength and endurance
Isometric Leg Squat	Static leg endurance
Shuttle Run	Agility and quickness
Sprints	Speed, quickness, and anaerobic ability

Three awards are given in this program, each based on a normative standard. The Outstanding Award is given to students who score at the 80th percentile or higher. Students who score in the percentile range 45%-79% are eligible for the Attainment Award. Those who score below the 45th percentile are given the Participation Award. In 1986-87, 6% of the students taking the test received the Outstanding Award; 23%, the Attainment Award; and 71%, the Participation Award. An attractive feature of the AAU program is that all materials, including awards, are free with the exception of shipping and handling charges.

The Fit Youth Today Program

The Fit Youth Today Program is sponsored by the American Health and Fitness Foundation. In the test manual (American Health and Fitness Foundation, 1986), physical fitness is not specifically defined, although four components of fitness are emphasized: cardiorespiratory endurance, muscular strength and endurance, flexibility, and body composition. These components are defined as follows:

1. Cardiorespiratory endurance is the ability of the heart, blood vessels, and lungs to respond effectively to the oxygen and energy demands of increasing muscular activity. (p. 8)
2. Adequate strength refers to the level of muscular strength necessary to enable you to perform all normal daily activities in an efficient manner and maintain a sufficient reserve to confront emergencies. (p. 11)
3. Muscular endurance refers to the ability of specific muscle groups to continue contracting for extended periods. (p. 11)
4. Flexibility is the measure of the range of movement possible at each joint in the body. (p. 14)
5. Body composition was not defined.

Four tests, listed in Table 16-4, are included in the Fit Youth Today (FYT) test. The test of cardiorespiratory endurance is called the Steady State Jog, which is a measure of the distance an examinee can run in 20 minutes. Otherwise, the tests are comparable to those used in other testing programs.

TABLE 16-4 *Fit Youth Today test*

Item	Component of fitness
Steady State Jog	Cardiorespiratory endurance
Bent-Knee Curl-up	Muscular strength/endurance
Sit-and-Reach	Flexibility
Body Composition (Triceps and Calf)	Body composition

TABLE 16-5 *Fit Youth Today: Criterion-referenced standards*

20-MINUTE STEADY STATE JOG TEST

	Distance covered in 20 minutes					
	Males			Females		
Grade level	Miles	Yards	Meters	Miles	Yards	Meters
4	1.8	3,170	2,900	1.6	2,820	2,570
5	2.0	3,520	3,220	1.8	3,170	2,900
6	2.2	3,870	3,540	2.0	3,520	3,220
7-12	2.4	4,220	3,860	2.2	3,870	3,540

BENT-KNEE CURL-UP TEST— NUMBER OF CURL-UPS COMPLETED IN 2 MINUTES

	Grade level			
Sex	4	5	6	7-12
Males and females	34	36	38	40

SIT-AND-REACH TEST

All grade levels and both
sexes = 9.0 inches

BODY COMPOSITION—SUM OF CALF AND TRICEPS SKINFOLD

	Males		Females	
Grade	Sum of calf and triceps	Approximate % body fat	Sum of calf and triceps	Approximate % body fat
4	23	19	32	26
5	26	21	32	26
6	29	23	33	27
7	29	23	34	28
8	29	23	34	28
9	27	22	34	28
10	25	20	34	28
11	23	19	34	28
12	23	19	34	28

Reproduced from *Fit Youth Today Program Manual* (1988). Austin, TX: American Health and Fitness Foundation, pp. 61, 65, 59, 75. By permission of the publisher.

The FYT awards program consists of three levels of awards. Level 1 is the All Star Award, which requires participants to meet all four criterion standards. Level 2 is the FYT Star Award, given to the participant who achieves the criterion standard on the Steady State Jog and one other test. Level 3 is the FYT Award, given for significant improvement toward the accomplishment of a participant's personal fitness goal.

The manual presents criterion-referenced standards but no tables of norms. The criterion-referenced standards are presented in Table 16-5. Suggestions are included for an FYT curriculum, and questions and answers are provided for teachers and students in various grade levels. Methods of conditioning are described.

The FITNESSGRAM System

The **FITNESSGRAM** test manual identifies four components of physical fitness that are related to overall health status and optimal function: aerobic capacity, body composition, flexibility, abdominal strength and endurance, and upper body strength and endurance. Of these components, only one is defined precisely. Aerobic capacity is defined as the highest rate at which aerobic metabolism can proceed in muscle cells during dynamic exercise involving large muscle groups (Institute for Aerobics Research, 1987, p. 7-3).

The fitness tests used in the FITNESSGRAM program are shown in Table 16-6. Note that the shuttle run is included in the battery. This is described as a fun, motivational test item for children in grades K-3 and not a health-related fitness item.

Criterion-referenced standards are presented in the manual, but no norms tables are given. The standards are reproduced in Table 16-7. Modifications of the test battery are recommended for special populations. An extremely well-developed component of this program is its system of computerizing test results and

---

TABLE 16-6 *FITNESSGRAM test*

Item	Component of fitness
One-Mile Walk-Run	Aerobic capacity
Sit-Ups	Abdominal strength/endurance
Pull-up/Flexed Arm Hang	Upper body strength/endurance
Sit-and-Reach	Low back flexibility
Skinfold Test or Body Mass Index	Body composition
Shuttle Run Test (Grades K-3)	Agility

TABLE 16-7 *FITNESSGRAM health-referenced standards*

| Age | One mile run/walk* | Body composition | | Sit and reach | Sit-up | Pull-up | Flexed arm hang |
		% Fat*	Body mass index*				
				Girls			
5 yrs	17:00	32%	20	10.0	20	1	5
6 yrs	16:00	32%	20	10.0	20	1	5
7 yrs	15:00	32%	20	10.0	20	1	5
8 yrs	14:00	32%	20	10.0	25	1	8
9 yrs	13:00	32%	20	10.0	25	1	8
10 yrs	12:00	32%	21	10.0	30	1	8
11 yrs	12:00	32%	21	10.0	30	1	8
12 yrs	12:00	32%	22	10.0	30	1	8
13 yrs	11:30	32%	23	10.0	30	1	12
14 yrs	10:30	32%	24	10.0	35	1	12
15 yrs	10:30	32%	24	10.0	35	1	12
16 yrs	10:30	32%	24	10.0	35	1	12
16+ yrs	10:30	32%	25	10.0	35	1	12
				Boys			
5 yrs	16:00	25%	20	10.0	20	1	5
6 yrs	15:00	25%	20	10.0	20	1	5
7 yrs	14:00	25%	20	10.0	20	1	5
8 yrs	13:00	25%	20	10.0	25	1	10
9 yrs	12:00	25%	20	10.0	25	1	10
10 yrs	11:00	25%	21	10.0	30	1	10
11 yrs	11:00	25%	21	10.0	30	1	10
12 yrs	10:00	25%	22	10.0	35	1	10
13 yrs	9:30	25%	23	10.0	35	2	10
14 yrs	8:30	25%	24	10.0	40	3	15
15 yrs	8:30	25%	24	10.0	40	5	25
16 yrs	8:30	25%	25	10.0	40	5	25
16+ yrs	8:30	25%	26	10.0	40	5	25

*Lower scores indicate better performance.
Reproduced from *FITNESSGRAM User's Manual* (p. 2-14). Dallas, TX: Institute for Aerobics Research, 1987. By permission of the publisher.

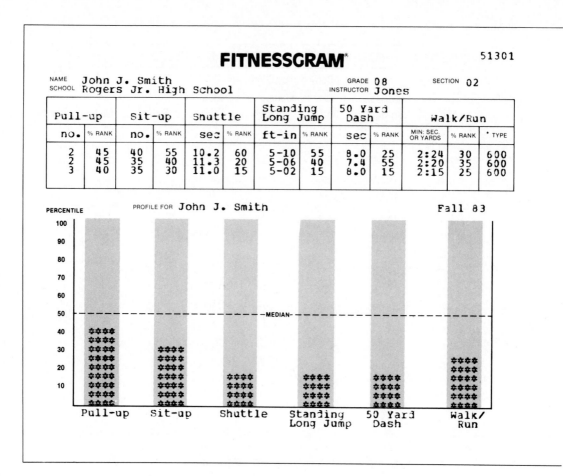

FIGURE 16-1 *Sample of FITNESSGRAM.*
By permission of the Institute for Aerobics Research.

sending a "fitnessgram" to parents. A sample FITNESSGRAM is shown in Figure 16-1.

The national program model includes program delivery at three levels: direct service, in which the Institute for Aerobics Research produces the fitness report cards for the school district; development of microcomputer software for use by a school district to produce FITNESSGRAMs locally; and availability of consultants to help selected districts program large computer systems to produce the cards and do statistical analyses locally (Institute for Aerobics Research, 1987).

The award system consists of four types of awards. The "Get Fit" Award is given to participants who complete a 6-week development program. An exercise log is maintained for this award. The Honor Award is given to students who

TOTAL PHYSICAL FITNESS SCORE	
EXCELLENT	352 +
ABOVE AVERAGE	316-351
AVERAGE	287-315
BELOW AVERAGE	251-286
WELL BELOW AVERAGE	0-250

DATE	HEIGHT	WEIGHT	TOTAL FITNESS SCORE
SEM - YR	FT - IN	LBS	
Fa 82	5-02	157	295
Sp 83	5-03	160	283
Fa 83	5-04	163	259

These activities are recommended:

To improve your cardiorespiratory endurance: jogging, swimming, rope jumping, walking, and cycling.

To improve your abdominal strength: bent knee sit-ups and leg lifts.

* WALK/RUN TYPE
600 = 600 YARD (MIN:SEC)
1 mi = 1 MILE (MIN:SEC)
1.5 = 1.5 MILE (MIN:SEC)
9 = 9 MINUTE (YARDS)
12 = 12 MINUTE (YARDS)

Dear Parent:

We are pleased to send you this FITNESSGRAM to provide information on your child's level of physical fitness as indicated by his/her performance in the AAHPERD Youth Fitness Test recently administered in our school. This test was developed by the American Alliance for Health, Physical Education, Recreation and Dance.

Your child participates in the test in the fall and spring. The FITNESSGRAM will show you any progress in his/her growth and development over the school years.

The FITNESSGRAM provides the following information:

1. A total physical fitness score for your child based on assessments of
   - upper body strength and endurance--measured by flexed-arm hang or pull-up test;
   - abdominal strength and endurance--1 minute sit-up test;
   - speed with change of direction--shuttle run;
   - explosive power--standing long jump test;
   - speed--50 yard dash;
   - cardiovascular fitness--600 yard, 1-mile, 1.5-mile, 9-minute, or 12-minute walk/run.

2. A percentile rank (% RANK) for each test item is computed based on a national norm developed over the last 20 years. You can see both your child's score and the national average (50%) of students of his/her age who have taken the test.

3. An exciting feature of the FITNESSGRAM is the recommendation for activities which can help improve your child's individual scores.

4. The FITNESSGRAM reflects past performances which will allow the monitoring of improvement from test date to test date!

We hope you will find the FITNESSGRAM a useful tool to assess your child's fitness level, height and weight development--and to encourage your entire family to enjoy the benefits of an active lifestyle.

Mr. Jerry G. Jones
Physical Education Instructor
Rogers Elementary

FIGURE 16-1, cont'd

meet fitness contracts that have been established with teachers. The "I'm Fit" Award can be obtained by meeting 5 of the 6 criterion-referenced standards. The "Fit for Life" Award is available for individuals outside the school program who have displayed commendable exercise behavior. This award may be given to a child or an adult.

The National Children and Youth Fitness Studies I and II

The most recent studies of youth fitness, the National Children and Youth Fitness Studies (NCYFS) I and II, were published in 1985 and 1987 by the Department of Health and Human Services (Ross and Gilbert, 1985; Ross and Pate, 1987). The purposes of the studies were to describe the current fitness status of children and youth of the United States and the patterns of participation in physical activity and to evaluate the relationship among physical activity patterns and measured fitness. The HRPFT and a chin-ups test were used to measure health-related fitness.

Fitness test items were administered to 8800 boys and girls ages 10 through 17 and 4853 boys and girls ages 6 through 9 across the country. Excellent sampling techniques were used in that these children and youths were selected on a probability basis guaranteeing that they were representative of all American boys and girls in the 6 to 17 age group. The fitness norms developed from the data of this national sample represent the most recent norms available for health-related physical fitness, although sound normative data for a variety of fitness tests are also available from Reiff and others (1985). The sex/age norms for the NCYFS test items are reproduced later in this chapter.

In general the NCYFS I data revealed that boys and girls showed continual improvement in most of the fitness test items as they advanced in age from 10 to 17. However, the sum of skinfold data demonstrated a tendency for all age groups to be fatter than comparable groups in the 1960s. Other results of the study pertained to the activity patterns of boys and girls. Over 80% of the students in this study were enrolled in physical education classes, which met an average of 3.6 times per week. Competitive sports were stressed for the older students; relays and informal games were emphasized for the younger students. This points to a deficiency in meeting one of the major national goals recently advocated for the public schools—developing physical skills needed for an active life-style throughout adulthood. Almost half of these students failed to engage in an adequate amount of vigorous physical activity to maintain a healthy cardiovascular system. The NCYFS is a landmark investigation of youth fitness in the 1980s.

Although test development was not one of the purposes of the NCYFS studies, the tests selected are of considerable interest in that they provide updated normative data on the fitness of younger age groups as well as information on

TABLE 16-8 *NCYFS II test*

Item	Component of fitness
Mile Walk/Run or Half-Mile Walk/Run (Ages 6-7)	Cardiorespiratory endurance
Modified Pull-Ups	Upper body strength/endurance
Bent-Knee Sit-Ups	Abdominal strength/endurance
Sit-and-Reach	Low back flexibility
Sum of Skinfolds (Triceps, Subscapular, and Calf)	Body fatness

other factors related to the level of fitness in the school-age population. The tests used in NCYFS II are included in Table 16-8. The NCYFS I test battery differed in that a regular pull-ups test was included and triceps and subscapular skinfold sites were measured. The Half-Mile Walk/Run was not an option in NCYFS I.

Valuable practical information on the administration of physical fitness tests was reported by the NCYFS personnel. This information cannot be found in comparable detail in any other source.

The Presidential Physical Fitness Award Program

The President's Council on Physical Fitness and Sports (PCPFS) is an organization based in Washington, DC. The primary mission of the council is to promote physical fitness and sports throughout the United States. The Presidential Physical Fitness Award Program is sponsored by the PCPFS, which is under the auspices of the Department of Health and Human Services. Two publications deal with the PCPFS program, a manual (President's Council on Physical Fitness and Sports, 1987) for the teacher or other test administrator and a monograph (Reiff et al., 1985) describing the results of a recent survey. Although physical fitness is not defined precisely, the components of fitness are identified as cardiorespiratory endurance, abdominal strength/endurance, arm and shoulder strength/endurance, flexibility of lower back and posterior thighs, and leg strength/endurance/power/agility.

The test items selected to measure each of the components are shown in Table 16-9. No norms tables are included in the manual, but a set of norm-referenced standards is reproduced in Table 16-10.

One award, the Presidential Physical Fitness Award, is designated for children and youth who participate in the program. They must score at or above the 85th percentile on all five items to qualify for the awards. A Presidential Instructor Emblem is available to instructors who qualify students for the award. A state champion program recognizes outstanding school achievement in physical fitness.

TABLE 16-9 *Presidential Physical Fitness Test battery*

Item	Component of fitness
Curl-Ups	Abdominal strength/endurance
Pull-Ups	Arm and shoulder strength/endurance
V-sit Reach or Sit and Reach	Low back and posterior thigh flexibility
One-Mile Run/Walk	Cardiorespiratory endurance
Shuttle Run	Leg strength/endurance/power/agility

TABLE 16-10 *Presidential Physical Fitness Award standards*

Age	Curl-ups	Shuttle run (sec)	V-sit reach or Sit and reach (inches +/−)	One-mile run (min/sec)	Pull-ups
			Boys		
6	33	12.1	+3.5	10:15	2
7	36	11.5	+3.5	9:22	4
8	40	11.1	+3.0	8:48	5
9	41	10.9	+3.0	8:31	5
10	45	10.3	+4.0	7:57	6
11	47	10.0	+4.0	7:32	6
12	50	9.8	+4.0	7:11	7
13	53	9.5	+3.5	6:50	7
14	56	9.1	+4.5	6:26	10
15	57	9.0	+5.0	6:20	11
16	56	8.7	+6.0	6:08	11
17	55	8.7	+7.0	6:06	13
			Girls		
6	32	12.4	+5.5	11:20	2
7	34	12.1	+5.0	10:36	2
8	38	11.8	+4.5	10:02	2
9	39	11.1	+5.5	9:30	2
10	40	10.8	+6.0	9:19	3
11	42	10.5	+6.5	9:02	3
12	45	10.4	+7.0	8:23	2
13	46	10.2	+7.0	8:13	2
14	47	10.1	+8.0	7:59	2
15	48	10.0	+8.0	8:08	2
16	45	10.1	+9.0	8:23	1
17	44	10.0	+8.0	8:15	1

Comparison of Test Batteries

In general, the test batteries are more alike than different with regard to the components of physical fitness they measure. All the batteries include tests of aerobic capacity, flexibility, and abdominal muscular strength and endurance. Body composition was identified as an important component of fitness in four of the six tests, and upper body strength was measured in five test batteries. Agility was measured in two of the batteries but was recommended only for young children in one battery. There is considerable similarity in the tests selected to measure the components of fitness as well. The same sit-ups test is used in all six batteries. However, the tests are given different names, which is likely to be confusing to practitioners. All batteries include distance run tests of one mile or longer, with the exception of shorter distances for young children in two instances. The triceps and calf sites are measured in the sum of skinfold tests in all batteries dealing with body composition. The body mass index is offered as an option to the skinfold measures in two instances. Some variation is noted in the flexibility test. The sit-and-reach test is most frequently used, but the reach is measured in inches in some cases and centimeters in others. The V-sit Reach is recommended in two of the batteries. The greatest variability occurs in the upper body strength measures. Variations include regular pull-ups, a pull-ups/flexed-arm hang option, and a modified pull-ups test.

Instructions for Test Administration

Each test developer may have slight variations in the instructions for administering fitness tests. Instructions for the most popular tests are given below. They are modeled on the instructions given for the Health-Related Physical Fitness Test (AAHPERD, 1980). The Pull-Ups/Flexed-Arm Hang Test options were not included in the Health-Related Test. One or both of these options are now a part of all of the national fitness tests. Descriptions of these tests can be found in Chapter 17.

Distance Runs Distance runs are included in the battery as measures of cardiorespiratory (CR) function. An individual who possesses a satisfactory level of CR function is able to engage in sports or other physical activities that require sustained effort. A number of physiological parameters reflect CR function; however, a person's maximal oxygen uptake is widely accepted as the best single indicator of the function. Maximal oxygen uptake ($\dot{V}o_2$) is the maximal amount of oxygen an individual can transport and use during exercise (Astrand and Rodahl, 1970; see also Chapter 12). When the exercise continues to become more difficult yet the oxygen consumption fails to increase, this is referred to as the point of *maximal oxygen uptake* or *maximal oxygen consumption*. "Maximal oxygen consumption is one of the most important factors that determine a person's ca-

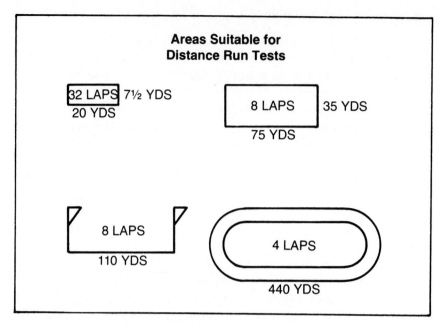

FIGURE 16-2 *Schematic drawing of areas that can be used for distance run tests.* From Health Related Physical Fitness Test Manual.

pacity to sustain high-intensity exercise for longer than 4 to 5 minutes" (Katch and McArdle, 1983, p. 56).

Test Objective The distance runs are used to measure maximal functional capacity and endurance of the CR system.

Description The 1-mile run for time or the 9-minute run for distance may be administered, depending primarily on the teacher's personal preference. In addition, optional distance run tests may be used for students 13 years of age and older. These are the 1½-mile run for time or the 12-minute run for distance. The distance runs can be tested in a variety of settings. Examples of some of these are included in Figure 16-2.

Instructions Regardless of whether the distance or the time of the run is fixed, students are instructed to run with maximal effort.

One-Mile Run Instruct the students to run as fast as possible, beginning on the signal "*Ready, start!*" As the student crosses the finish line, call out the elapsed time, which should be recorded by the student or the student's partner. Walking, although permissible, should be discouraged since the purpose of the test is to measure maximal capacity. These instructions are also appropriate for the 1½ -mile run.

Nine-Minute Run Instruct the students to run as far as possible, beginning on the signal *"Ready, start!"* After 9 minutes, a whistle is blown and the student's partner records the distance run. These instructions are also appropriate for the 12-minute run test.

Test Area The distance run tests can be administered on a 440-yard or 400-meter track or on any other flat, measured surface. Examples of tests areas are displayed in Figure 16-2.

Equipment Stopwatch, scorecards, and pencils.

Scoring The 1-mile and 1½ -mile runs are scored to the nearest second. The 9-minute and 12-minute runs are scored to the nearest 10 yards or 10 meters. Instructions on recording scores are typically included in the test manual.

Validity Generally, the validity of distance run tests has been established by correlating the test scores with **max $\dot{V}_{O_2}$** scores expressed in milliliters of oxygen per kilogram of body weight per minute (ml/kg/min). This expression is used to adjust for individual variations in body size. Validity coefficients of 0.81 for elementary school boys and 0.71 for girls at the same grade levels have been reported by Jackson and Coleman (1976) for the 9-minute run test. For the 12-minute run test, validity coefficients range from 0.65 to 0.90. The lower sizes of some of the coefficients may be attributable to a lack of motivation in the performance of the distance runs, body fatness, or running inefficiency. For example, if a student is not motivated to run as fast as possible, the distance run score will not be highly related to max $\dot{V}_{O_2}$ scores calculated directly from a treadmill test.

Reliability Performance on distance run tests is usually highly reliable, with the reliability coefficients ranging from 0.75 to 0.94. In most cases the reliability estimates fall at the high end of this range. However, most of the reliability studies have been conducted using adults and adolescent children as subjects. Very few reliability coefficients have been reported for children in the lower elementary grades. Factors such as motivation, body fatness, and running efficiency can affect the reliability as well as the validity of distance runs.

Norms Normative data are provided for each distance run test. Tables of norms from the NCYFS I and II are included in Tables 16-11 to 16-13.

Comments Students should be taught to warm up with passive stretches and walking before participating in a distance run and to cool down in the same way afterward. Check to see that no medical reason exists to prevent a student from engaging in strenuous exercise of this nature. Prepare students in advance for the distance run by teaching them how to pace themselves throughout the run. Begin with shorter runs and gradually increase the distance of the run. Most test manuals now include explicit instructions on preparing examinees to be tested. These preparations should begin well in advance of the testing and should evolve out of a fitness education program. It is doubtful that runs shorter than one mile are valid measures of CR function (Jackson and Coleman, 1976). Thus, the use of

TABLE 16-11 *NCYFS II norms by age for the distance walk/run (in minutes and seconds)*

	Age							
	Boys				Girls			
	Half mile		Mile		Half mile		Mile	
Percentile	6	7	8	9	6	7	8	9
99	3:53	3:34	7:42	7:31	4:05	4:03	8:18	8:06
95	4:15	3:56	8:18	7:54	4:29	4:18	9:14	8:41
90	4:27	4:11	8:46	8:10	4:46	4:32	9:39	9:08
85	4:35	4:22	9:02	8:33	4:57	4:38	9:55	9:26
80	4:45	4:28	9:19	8:48	5:07	4:46	10:08	9:40
75	4:52	4:33	9:29	9:00	5:13	4:54	10:23	9:50
70	4:59	4:40	9:40	9:13	5:20	5:00	10:35	10:15
65	5:04	4:46	9:52	9:29	5:25	5:06	10:46	10:31
60	5:10	4:50	10:04	9:44	5:31	5:11	10:59	10:41
55	5:17	4:54	10:16	9:58	5:39	5:18	11:14	10:56
50	5:23	5:00	10:39	10:10	5:44	5:25	11:32	11:13
45	5:28	5:05	11:00	10:27	5:49	5:32	11:46	11:30
40	5:33	5:11	11:14	10:41	5:55	5:39	12:03	11:46
35	5:41	5:17	11:30	10:59	6:00	5:46	12:14	12:09
30	5:50	5:28	11:51	11:16	6:07	5:55	12:37	12:26
25	5:58	5:35	12:14	11:44	6:14	6:01	12:59	12:45
20	6:09	5:46	12:39	12:02	6:27	6:10	13:26	13:13
15	6:21	6:06	13:16	12:46	6:39	6:20	14:18	13:44
10	6:40	6:20	14:05	13:37	6:51	6:38	14:48	14:31
5	7:15	6:50	15:24	15:15	7:16	7:09	16:35	15:40

Reprinted from the National Children and Youth Fitness Study II. Washington, DC: Department of Health and Human Services, 1987.

shorter runs to accommodate young children may be viewed as a necessity from a motivational point of view but questionable as a sound fitness measure.

Several factors affect the distance run performance of children. Children display less economy of gait than adults when walking and running. For this reason, they experience a higher metabolic cost (Wells, 1986). The younger the child, the more difficult it is to predict maximal oxygen uptake. Other factors which can have a negative impact on children's performance are experience, motor efficiency, environmental conditions, and motivation (Krahenbuhl and others, 1978).

TABLE 16-12 *NCYFS norms by age for the one mile walk/run—girls (in minutes and seconds)*

Percentile	10	11	12	13	14	15	16	17	18
99	7:55	7:14	7:20	7:08	7:01	6:59	7:03	6:52	6:58
90	9:09	8:45	8:34	8:27	8:11	8:23	8:28	8:20	8:22
80	9:56	9:35	9:30	9:13	8:49	9:04	9:06	9:10	9:27
75	10:09	9:56	9:52	9:30	9:16	9:28	9:25	9:26	9:31
70	10:27	10:10	10:05	9:48	9:31	9:49	9:41	9:41	9:36
60	10:51	10:35	10:32	10:22	10:04	10:20	10:15	10:16	10:08
50	11:14	11:15	10:58	10:52	10:32	10:46	10:34	10:34	10:51
40	11:54	11:46	11:26	11:22	10:58	11:20	11:08	10:59	11:27
30	12:27	12:33	12:03	11:55	11:35	11:53	11:49	11:43	11:58
25	12:52	12:54	12:33	12:17	11:49	12:18	12:10	12:03	12:14
20	13:12	13:17	12:53	12:43	12:10	12:48	12:32	12:30	12:37
10	14:20	14:35	14:07	13:45	13:13	14:07	13:42	13:46	15:18

Reprinted from the National Children and Youth Fitness Study I. Washington, DC: Department of Health and Human Services, 1985.

TABLE 16-13 *NCYFS norms by age for the one mile walk/run—boys (in minutes and seconds)*

Percentile	10	11	12	13	14	15	16	17	18
99	6:55	6:21	6:21	5:59	5:43	5:40	5:31	5:14	5:33
90	8:13	7:25	7:13	6:48	6:27	6:23	6:13	6:08	6:10
80	8:35	7:52	7:41	7:07	6:58	6:43	6:31	6:31	6:33
75	8:48	8:02	7:53	7:14	7:08	6:52	6:39	6:40	6:42
70	9:02	8:12	8:03	7:24	7:18	7:00	6:50	6:46	6:57
60	9:26	8:38	8:23	6:46	7:34	7:13	7:07	7:10	7:15
50	9:52	9:03	8:48	8:04	7:51	7:30	7:27	7:31	7:35
40	10:15	9:25	9:17	8:26	8:14	7:50	7:48	7:59	7:53
30	10:44	10:17	9:57	8:54	8:46	8:18	8:04	8:24	8:12
25	11:00	10:32	10:13	9:06	9:10	8:30	8:18	8:37	8:34
20	11:25	10:55	10:38	9:20	9:28	8:50	8:34	8:55	9:10
10	12:27	12:07	11:48	10:38	10:34	10:13	9:36	10:43	10:50

Reprinted from the National Children and Youth Fitness Study I. Washington, DC: Department of Health and Human Services, 1985.

Sum of Skinfold Fat   The body composition of a person consists of bone, muscle mass, and fatty tissue. Obesity is the result of an excess of fatty tissue and is associated with a number of disease states such as diabetes, hypertension, heart disease, and heat intolerance. Thus it is appropriate to include a measure of body composition in a health-related fitness battery.

Test Objective   This test is used to assess **body composition,** or more specifically, the level of fatness in an individual.

Description   Two skinfold sites are used to measure body fatness in recent revisions of fitness test batteries—the triceps and calf muscles. The subcutaneous adipose tissue can be lifted with the fingers to form a skinfold. A **skinfold caliper** is used to obtain the skinfold measure by measuring the thickness of a double layer of subcutaneous fat and skin at the designated site.

Instructions   To ensure accuracy and consistency across skinfold measures, the sites should be marked with a grease pencil. To obtain the triceps skinfold, mark the point halfway between the elbow and the acromial process of the scapula. The mark for the skinfold should be made parallel to the longitudinal axis of the upper arm. Mark the calf site "on the inside (medial side) of the right lower leg at the largest part of the calf girth. Grasp and gently lift the skin up slightly above the level of the largest part of the calf with the thumb and index finger so that the calipers may be placed at the level of the largest part of the calf. Have students place their right foot on a bench with the knee slightly flexed when taking the calf measurement" (AAHPERD, 1988, p. 17). Both measurements are

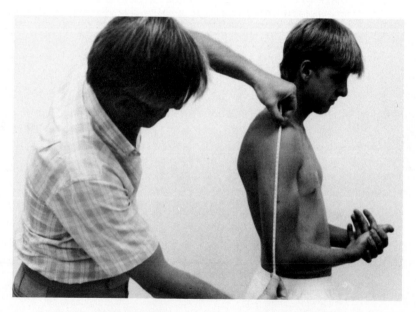

Figures on pp. 358-360 reproduced by permission of Timothy Lohman.

taken on the right side of the body. (Refer to the figures for examples of properly marked sites.)

In one test manual (AAHPERD, 1980, p. 13) the following procedure is recommended for obtaining a skinfold measure:

1. Firmly grasp the skinfold between the thumb and forefinger and lift up.
2. Place the contact surface of the caliper 1 cm (½ inch) above or below the finger.
3. Slowly release the grip on the caliper enabling them (the jaws of the caliper) to exert their full tension on the skinfold.
4. Read skinfold to nearest 0.5 mm after needle stops (1 to 2 seconds after releasing grip on caliper).

Test Area A private testing area should be available for administering this test so that students will not suffer any embarassment resulting from the test.

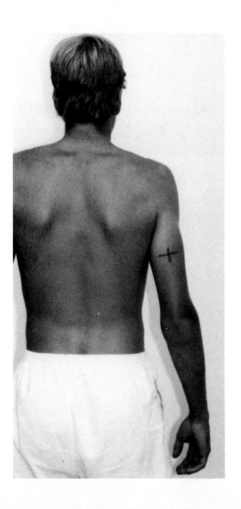
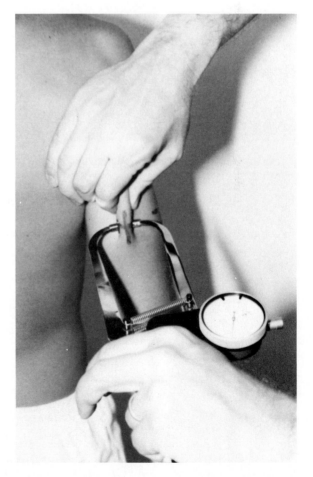

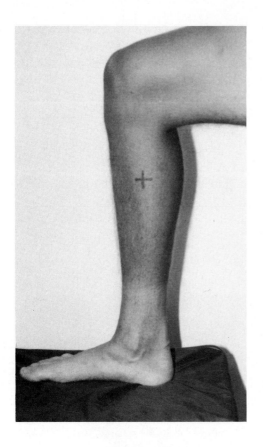

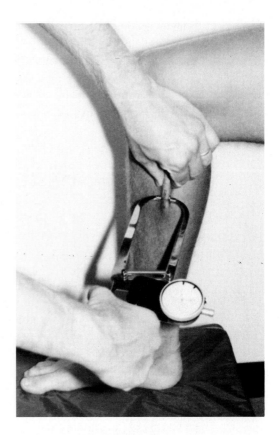

Equipment A better constructed and more expensive caliper, such as the Harpenden or Lange skinfold caliper, is recommended for this test. (See photograph on p. 361.) These calipers are expensive, but they provide a constant pressure of 10 g/mm² throughout the range of skinfold thicknesses. Other less expensive calipers are now on the market and may be suitable for testing in a school setting. However, the pressure may not be constant throughout the lower portion of the range, thus yielding inaccurate measures.

Scoring Three measures are taken at each site, and the median of each set of three measures is recorded to the nearest 0.5 mm. The median scores for the two sites are then summed, as in the following example:

$$\begin{array}{lll} \text{Triceps: 10, 7, 8} & \text{Median} = & 8 \\ \text{Calf: 6, 5, 7} & \text{Median} = & \underline{6} \\ \textsc{total score} & & 14 \end{array}$$

Validity The validity of the sum of skinfold fat is usually determined by correlating this sum with body fatness measured through **hydrostatic weighing,** where

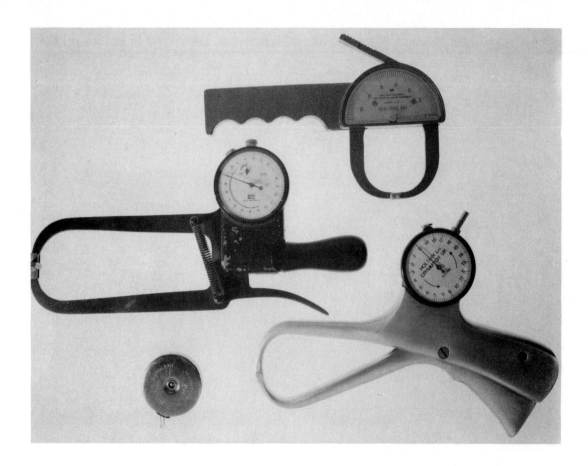

the percent body fat and lean body mass are determined by submerging the individual underwater. The validity coefficients range from 0.70 to 0.90 in both children and adults (Baumgartner and Jackson, 1982), although far fewer studies have been conducted using children as subjects.

Reliability The intertester reliability of skinfold measures is high, over 0.95 when experienced testers measured adult subjects. Similar coefficients were obtained for boys and girls of middle school age.

Norms Norms for the triceps and subscapular skinfold measurements were reported in NCYFS I for 10–17-year-old children. The same sites plus the calf skinfold were measured in NCYFS II, where the subjects were 6–9 years of age. Norms are presented in Tables 16-14 to 16-21.

Comments Be careful to place the caliper properly. The correct location is midway between the crest and base of the skinfold, not *at* the base. Teachers who are inexperienced in using the caliper should practice measuring skinfolds

---

TABLE 16-14 *NCYFS II norms by age for the medial calf skinfold (in millimeters)*

| | Age | | | | | | | |
| | Boys | | | | Girls | | | |
Percentile	6	7	8	9	6	7	8	9
99	4	4	4	4	5	5	5	5
95	5	5	5	5	6	6	6	7
90	5	5	5	5	7	7	7	7
85	6	6	6	6	8	7	8	8
80	6	6	6	7	8	8	8	9
75	6	7	7	7	8	8	9	10
70	7	7	7	8	9	9	10	10
65	7	7	7	8	9	9	10	11
60	7	7	8	9	10	10	11	11
55	7	8	8	10	10	10	11	12
50	8	8	9	10	10	11	12	13
45	8	9	10	11	11	12	13	14
40	9	9	10	11	11	12	13	14
35	9	10	11	12	12	13	14	15
30	10	11	11	13	13	13	15	16
25	10	11	12	14	13	15	16	17
20	11	12	14	15	14	15	18	18
15	12	14	15	17	16	17	19	20
10	13	16	19	20	17	18	21	22
5	17	19	21	24	20	21	24	27

Reprinted from the National Children and Youth Fitness Study II. Washington, DC: Department of Health and Human Services, 1987.

with students as subjects. Measure each site a number of times and try to obtain the same reading within 1 or 2 mm.

Much is still unknown about the relationship of skinfold fat to body fatness in children, since changes occur with gender and with age. A specific skinfold thickness, then, does not represent the same amount of body fat in a young child as it does in an older child.

Skinfold measures can be used to estimate percent body fat and ideal weight. A simple program for calculating these estimates on the Apple IIe microcomputer is included in Appendix E. Three skinfold sites must be measured to use the program—chest, abdomen, and thigh for men; and triceps, thigh, and su-

TABLE 16-15 *NCYFS II norms by age for the triceps skinfold (in millimeters)*

	Age							
	Boys				Girls			
Percentile	6	7	8	9	6	7	8	9
99	5	5	5	5	5	6	6	6
95	6	5	6	6	7	7	7	7
90	6	6	6	6	8	7	8	8
85	7	7	7	7	8	8	8	9
80	7	7	7	7	9	8	9	10
75	7	7	7	8	9	9	9	10
70	7	7	8	8	9	9	10	11
65	8	8	8	9	10	10	10	11
60	8	8	8	10	10	10	11	12
55	8	8	9	10	11	11	12	12
50	8	9	9	10	11	11	12	13
45	9	9	10	11	12	12	13	14
40	9	10	10	12	12	12	14	14
35	10	10	11	13	13	13	15	15
30	10	11	12	14	13	13	16	16
25	10	11	13	15	14	14	17	18
20	11	12	14	16	14	15	18	19
15	12	14	15	18	15	17	19	21
10	13	16	19	21	17	19	21	22
5	16	20	23	23	20	22	25	25

Reprinted from the National Children and Youth Fitness Study II. Washington, DC: Department of Health and Human Services, 1987.

prailium for women. Even more convenient is a set of nomograms developed by Lohman (1987) to convert the sum of triceps plus calf (or triceps plus subscapular) skinfolds to percent body fat merely by reading down the chart. Four of these nomograms, two for boys and two for girls (ages 6–17) are shown in Figure 16-3 on p. 365.

The Body Mass Index (BMI) may be used as an optional item to measure body composition. BMI is defined as the ratio of body weight (measured in kilograms) and the square of height (measured in meters).

$$\text{BMI} = \frac{\text{Body Weight (kg)}}{\text{Height}^2 \text{ (m)}}$$

TABLE 16-16 *NCYFS II norms by age for the subscapular skinfold (in millimeters)*

	Age							
	Boys				Girls			
Percentile	6	7	8	9	6	7	8	9
99	4	4	4	4	4	4	4	4
95	4	4	4	4	4	4	5	5
90	4	4	4	5	5	5	5	5
85	4	5	5	5	5	5	5	5
80	5	5	5	5	5	5	5	6
75	5	5	5	5	5	5	6	6
70	5	5	5	5	5	5	6	6
65	5	5	5	6	6	6	6	6
60	5	5	5	6	6	6	6	7
55	5	5	6	6	6	6	7	7
50	5	5	6	6	6	6	7	8
45	5	6	6	7	6	7	7	8
40	6	6	6	7	7	7	8	9
35	6	6	6	7	7	7	8	9
30	6	6	7	8	7	8	9	10
25	6	7	7	9	8	9	10	12
20	7	7	8	10	8	10	12	15
15	7	8	10	12	10	11	15	17
10	8	10	14	15	12	13	17	21
5	12	16	19	20	16	19	21	25

Reprinted from the National Children and Youth Fitness Study II. Washington, DC: Department of Health and Human Services, 1987.

Modified Sit-Ups Two test items are included in a number of test batteries as measures of musculoskeletal function in the abdominal and low back area. The Modified Sit-Ups Test is characterized by a 1-minute time limit and a positioning of the arms in front of the chest.

Many Americans are affected by low back pain. This dysfunction can lead to a state of extreme discomfort, causing the sufferer to lose work days and preventing him or her from leading a normal life. In a functional health context this syndrome is associated with weak abdominal muscles and excessively contracted muscles in the lower back. Many doctors recommend exercise to reduce low back pain.

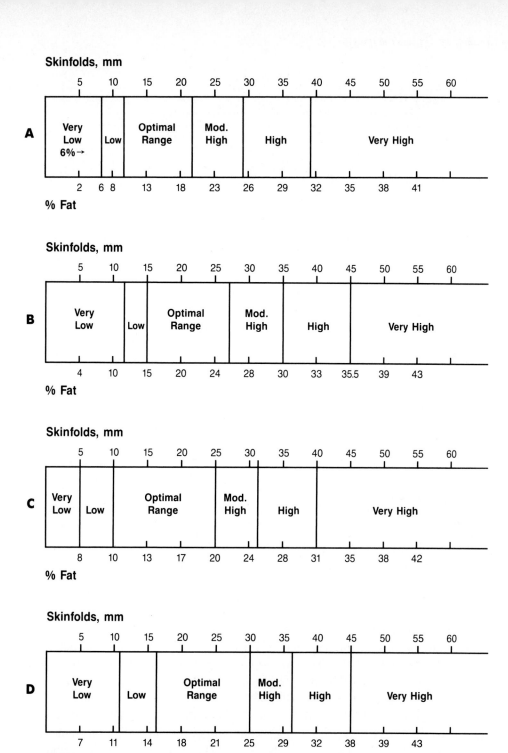

FIGURE 16-3 *Body composition nomograms.* **A,** *Triceps plus subscapular skinfolds (boys).* **B,** *Triceps plus subscapular skinfolds (girls).* **C,** *Triceps plus calf skinfolds (boys).* **D,** *Triceps plus calf skinfolds (girls).*
From Lohman, T.J., 1987.

TABLE 16-17 *NCYFS II norms by age for the sum of triceps and medial calf skinfold (in millimeters)*

	Age							
	Boys				Girls			
Percentile	6	7	8	9	6	7	8	9
99	9	9	9	9	11	11	11	12
95	11	11	11	11	13	13	14	14
90	12	12	12	12	15	15	15	16
85	12	13	13	13	16	16	16	18
80	13	13	13	14	17	17	18	19
75	14	14	14	15	18	18	19	20
70	14	14	15	16	18	18	20	21
65	15	15	15	18	19	19	21	22
60	15	16	17	18	20	20	22	23
55	16	16	17	19	21	21	23	25
50	16	17	18	21	21	22	24	26
45	17	18	19	22	22	23	26	27
40	17	19	20	23	23	24	27	29
35	18	20	21	25	24	25	29	30
30	20	21	23	27	25	26	31	32
25	20	22	24	29	27	28	33	35
20	22	24	27	31	28	31	35	37
15	23	27	31	35	30	33	38	41
10	27	32	37	40	33	37	43	45
5	33	39	44	47	38	43	49	52

Reprinted from the National Children and Youth Fitness Study II. Washington, DC: Department of Health and Human Services, 1987.

Test Objective The Modified Sit-Ups Test is used to measure abdominal strength and endurance.

Description The starting position of the test is a back-lying position with knees flexed, feet on floor, and heels between 12 and 18 inches from the buttocks. The arms are crossed on the chest with the hands on opposite shoulders. A partner holds the examinee's feet to keep them in contact with the testing surface. The examinee curls to a sitting position, maintaining arm contact with the chest. The chin should be tucked on the chest and should remain in this position until the completion of the sit-up. When the elbows touch the thighs, the sit-up is completed. The examinee curls back down to the floor until the midback contacts the testing surface. Another sit-up may then be attempted. (See photographs below.)

Instructions The examinee begins executing consecutive sit-ups on the word "*Go!*", using the signal "*Ready Go!*" At the end of 60 seconds, the test is ended with the word "*Stop!*" The score is the number of sit-ups executed correctly during this time. Pausing between sit-ups is permissible.

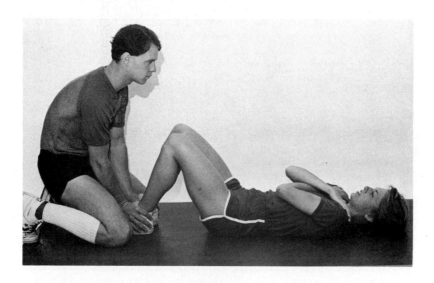

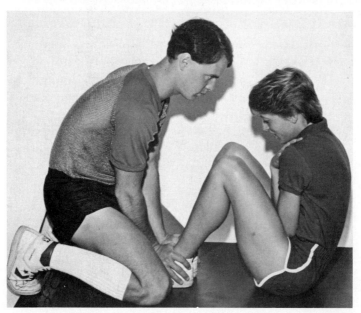

TABLE 16-18 *NCYFS norms by age for the triceps skinfold—boys (in millimeters)*

Percentile	10	11	12	13	14	15	16	17	18
99	5	4	4	4	4	4	4	4	4
90	7	7	6	6	5	5	5	5	5
80	8	7	8	7	6	6	6	6	6
75	8	8	8	7	7	7	6	6	6
70	9	9	9	8	7	7	7	7	7
60	10	10	10	9	8	8	7	7	8
50	11	11	11	10	9	9	8	8	8
40	13	12	12	11	10	10	9	9	10
30	14	14	14	13	11	11	11	11	11
25	15	15	15	14	12	12	11	12	12
20	16	16	17	15	13	13	12	13	13
10	20	20	21	20	18	18	16	15	16

Reprinted from the National Children and Youth Fitness Study I. Washington, DC: Department of Health and Human Services, 1985.

TABLE 16-19 *NCYFS norms by age for the triceps skinfold—girls (in millimeters)*

Percentile	10	11	12	13	14	15	16	17	18
99	5	6	6	6	6	7	7	8	7
90	7	8	9	9	9	10	10	11	10
80	9	9	10	10	11	12	12	12	12
75	10	10	10	11	12	13	12	13	13
70	10	10	11	11	12	13	13	14	13
60	11	12	12	13	14	15	14	15	14
50	12	13	13	14	15	16	15	17	15
40	14	15	14	15	16	17	17	18	17
30	15	16	16	17	18	19	18	20	19
25	16	17	17	18	19	20	19	21	20
20	17	19	18	20	20	21	20	21	21
10	21	23	22	24	23	25	24	24	23

Reprinted from the National Children and Youth Fitness Study I. Washington, DC: Department of Health and Human Services, 1985.

TABLE 16-20 *NCYFS norms by age for the sum of triceps and subscapular skinfolds—boys (in millimeters)*

Percentile	10	11	12	13	14	15	16	17	18
99	9	9	9	9	9	10	10	10	11
90	12	12	12	11	12	12	12	13	13
80	13	13	13	13	13	13	13	14	14
75	14	14	14	13	13	14	14	14	15
70	15	15	15	14	14	14	14	15	15
60	16	16	16	15	15	15	15	15	17
50	17	18	17	17	17	17	17	17	18
40	20	20	20	19	18	18	18	19	19
30	22	23	22	21	21	20	20	21	22
25	24	25	24	23	22	22	22	22	24
20	25	26	28	25	25	24	23	24	25
10	35	36	38	34	33	32	30	30	30

Reprinted from the National Children and Youth Fitness Study I. Washington, DC: Department of Health and Human Services, 1985.

TABLE 16-21 *NCYFS norms by age for the sum of triceps and subscapular skinfolds—girls (in millimeters)*

Percentile	10	11	12	13	14	15	16	17	18
99	10	11	11	12	12	13	13	16	14
90	13	14	15	15	17	19	19	20	19
80	15	16	17	18	19	21	21	22	21
75	16	17	18	19	20	23	22	23	22
70	17	18	18	20	21	24	23	24	23
60	18	19	21	22	24	26	24	26	25
50	20	21	22	24	26	28	26	28	27
40	22	24	24	26	28	30	28	31	28
30	25	28	27	29	31	33	32	34	32
25	27	30	29	31	33	34	33	36	34
20	29	33	31	34	35	37	35	37	36
10	36	40	40	43	40	43	42	42	42

Reprinted from the National Children and Youth Fitness Study I. Washington, DC: Department of Health and Human Services, 1985.

Test Area Any area with sufficient floor space may be used.

Equipment Mats are recommended for safety and comfort and a stopwatch.

Scoring The score is the number of sit-ups executed correctly during 60 seconds. Incorrect execution includes failure to curl up, pulling the arms away from the chest, failure to touch the thighs with the elbows, and failure to touch the midback to the testing surface in the down position.

Validity The validity of the sit-ups test has not been clearly established. Electromyographic studies of sit-ups have shown that the abdominal muscles are active during the execution of a sit-up. However, other muscles are active as well, in particular the hip flexors. No evidence exists to justify a specified number of

TABLE 16-22 *NCYFS II norms by age for the timed bent-knee sit-ups (number in 60 seconds)*

	Age							
	Boys				Girls			
Percentile	6	7	8	9	6	7	8	9
99	36	42	43	48	36	40	44	43
95	31	35	38	42	31	35	37	39
90	28	32	35	39	28	33	34	36
85	26	30	33	36	26	30	32	34
80	25	29	32	35	24	28	30	32
75	24	28	30	33	23	27	29	31
70	22	27	29	32	22	26	28	30
65	21	26	28	31	21	24	27	29
60	20	25	27	30	20	23	26	28
55	19	24	26	29	19	22	25	26
50	19	23	26	28	18	21	25	26
45	18	22	25	27	17	21	24	25
40	17	21	24	26	17	20	23	24
35	16	20	23	25	16	19	21	23
30	15	19	21	24	15	17	20	22
25	14	18	20	23	14	16	19	21
20	12	16	19	22	12	15	17	19
15	11	14	17	19	10	13	16	17
10	9	12	15	16	6	11	13	15
5	4	7	11	13	1	7	9	10

Reprinted from the National Children and Youth Fitness Study II. Washington, DC: Department of Health and Human Services, 1987.

sit-ups as representative of a desirable amount of abdominal strength. Thus, the Modified Sit-Ups Test is validated on the basis of logical validity.

Robertson and Magnusdottir (1987) proposed a partial curl-up test that places the greatest demand on the abdominals and very little on the hip flexors. The test is highly reliable for adult men (.93) and women (.94). It requires a range of motion less than 45°, which has been recommended for maximum involvement of the abdominals. Tests requiring a complete sit-up use a much larger range of motion.

Reliability The reliability of this test is generally satisfactory. The range of test-retest reliability coefficients is 0.68 to 0.94; the lower coefficients are probably attributable to inconsistency in the level of motivation.

Norms Normative data were obtained from NCYFS I and II. Norms tables are presented in Tables 16-22 to 16-24.

Comments The position assumed by the examinee should be carefully checked before and during the execution of the sit-up. The distance between the heels and the buttocks (12 to 18 inches) should be monitored continuously, measuring if necessary. The use of partners to count and record scores is permissible; however, the execution of the sit-ups must be observed by the tester to be sure the partners are counting only correctly executed sit-ups. For example, as an examinee begins to fatigue, sit-ups are often executed with a straight back rather

TABLE 16-23 *NCYFS norms by age for the timed bent-knee sit-ups—girls (number in 60 seconds)*

Percentile	10	11	12	13	14	15	16	17	18
99	50	53	66	58	57	56	59	60	65
90	43	42	46	46	47	45	49	47	47
80	39	39	41	41	42	42	42	41	42
75	37	37	40	40	41	40	40	40	40
70	36	36	39	39	40	39	39	39	40
60	33	34	36	35	37	36	37	37	38
50	31	32	33	33	35	35	35	36	35
40	30	30	31	31	32	32	33	33	33
30	27	28	30	28	30	30	30	31	30
25	25	26	28	27	29	30	30	30	30
20	24	24	27	25	27	28	28	29	28
10	20	20	21	21	23	24	23	24	24

Reprinted from the National Children and Youth Fitness Study I. Washington, DC: Department of Health and Human Services, 1985.

TABLE 16-24 *NCYFS norms by age for the timed bent-knee sit-ups—boys (number in 60 seconds)*

Percentile	10	11	12	13	14	15	16	17	18
99	60	60	61	62	64	65	65	68	67
90	47	48	50	52	52	53	55	56	54
80	43	43	46	48	49	50	51	51	50
75	40	41	44	46	47	48	49	50	50
70	38	40	43	45	45	46	48	49	48
60	36	38	40	41	43	44	45	46	44
50	34	36	38	40	41	42	43	43	43
40	32	34	35	37	39	40	41	41	40
30	30	31	33	34	37	37	39	39	38
25	28	30	32	32	35	36	38	37	36
20	26	28	30	31	34	35	36	35	35
10	22	22	25	28	30	31	32	31	31

Reprinted from the National Children and Youth Fitness Study I. Washington, DC: Department of Health and Human Services, 1985.

than a curl up. Partners should be instructed not to count the straight-back sit-ups.

Sit-and-Reach Test The Sit-and-Reach Test is the second of the two tests often included as measures of abdominal and low back–hamstring musculoskeletal function. The abdominal area is tested by the Modified Sit-Ups Test, and the Sit-and-Reach Test is used to measure the low back–hamstring area.

Test Objective The Sit-and-Reach Test is designed to evaluate the flexibility of the low back and posterior thigh.

Description The examinees must remove their shoes to be tested. To begin the test, the examinee sits in front of the test apparatus with feet flat against the end board. The knees should be fully extended and the feet shoulder-width apart. To perform the test, the examinee extends the arms forward with one hand placed on top of the other.

Instructions In the actual test the examinee reaches forward, palms down, along the measuring scale of the testing apparatus. (See Figures 16-4 and 16-5 for drawings of the initial and final test positions.) The reach is repeated three consecutive times, and, on the fourth trial, the maximum reach is held for 1 second. The distance of the maximum reach is recorded as the test score.

Test Area Any small testing area with adequate floor space would be suitable.

Equipment The test apparatus is a specially constructed box with a measuring scale in which 23 cm is set at the level of the feet. A drawing of one version of the box is presented in Figure 16-6. Refer to the test manual (AAHPERD, 1988)

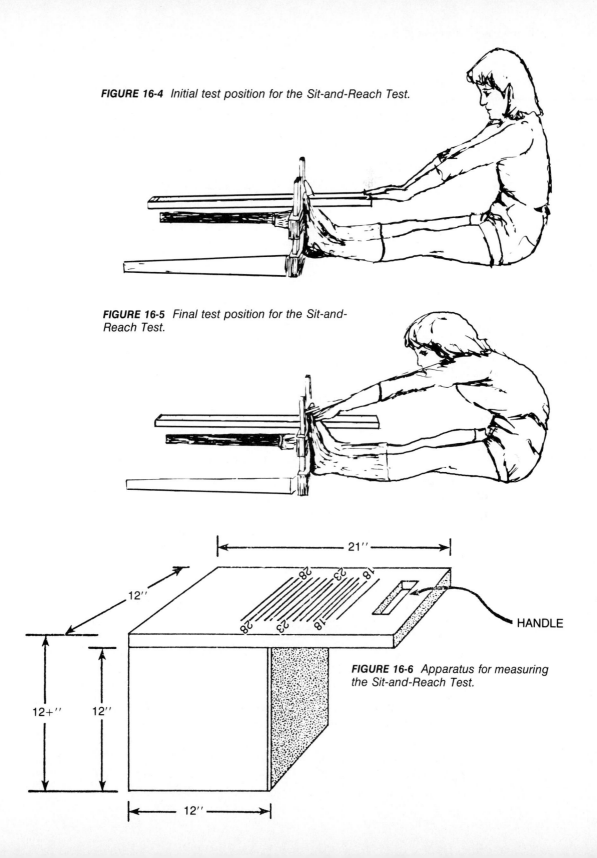

FIGURE 16-4 *Initial test position for the Sit-and-Reach Test.*

FIGURE 16-5 *Final test position for the Sit-and-Reach Test.*

HANDLE

FIGURE 16-6 *Apparatus for measuring the Sit-and-Reach Test.*

for detailed instructions on constructing this version of the apparatus.

Scoring The score, measured to the nearest centimeter, is the most distant point reached on the fourth trial. The fingertips of both hands should reach this point. If the reach of the two hands is uneven, the test should be readministered.

Validity The Sit-and-Reach Test has been validated by comparing it with several other types of flexibility tests, with validity coefficients ranging between

TABLE 16-25 *NCYFS II norms by age for the sit-and-reach (in inches)*

	Age							
	Boys				Girls			
Percentile	6	7	8	9	6	7	8	9
99	17.5	18.0	18.0	17.5	18.5	18.0	19.0	19.0
95	16.5	16.5	16.5	16.0	17.5	17.5	17.5	18.0
90	16.0	16.0	16.0	15.5	16.5	17.5	17.0	17.0
85	15.5	16.0	15.5	15.0	16.0	16.5	16.5	16.5
80	15.0	15.5	15.0	14.5	16.0	16.0	16.0	16.0
75	15.0	15.0	14.5	14.5	15.5	16.0	16.0	16.0
70	14.5	14.5	14.5	14.0	15.0	15.5	15.5	15.5
65	14.0	14.0	14.0	14.0	15.0	15.0	15.0	15.0
60	14.0	14.0	14.0	13.5	15.0	15.0	15.0	15.0
55	13.5	13.5	13.5	13.0	14.5	15.0	14.5	14.5
50	13.5	13.5	13.5	13.0	14.0	14.5	14.0	14.0
45	13.0	13.0	13.0	12.5	14.0	14.5	14.0	14.0
40	12.5	12.5	12.5	12.0	14.0	14.0	13.5	14.0
35	12.5	12.5	12.5	12.0	13.5	14.0	13.5	13.5
30	12.0	12.0	12.0	11.5	13.0	13.5	13.0	13.0
25	12.0	11.5	11.5	11.0	12.5	13.0	12.5	12.5
20	11.5	11.5	11.0	10.5	12.0	12.5	12.0	12.0
15	11.0	11.0	10.5	10.0	12.0	12.0	11.5	11.5
10	10.5	10.0	9.5	9.5	11.5	11.5	11.0	11.0
5	10.0	9.0	8.5	8.0	10.5	10.5	10.0	9.0

NOTE: The NCYFS set the "0" point at 12 inches, whereas the 1980 AAHPERD norms employed a "0" point of 23 cm. To translate the NCYFS inches into cm and to adjust the "0" point to 23 cm, the following formula may be applied to the NCYFS norms: score in cm = (score in inches × 2.54) − 7.48.

Reprinted from the National Children and Youth Fitness Study II. Washington, DC: Department of Health and Human Services, 1987.

0.80 and 0.90. Logical validity has also been claimed for the test, since higher scores reflect better extensibility in the low back, hip, and posterior thigh.

A more recent study by Jackson and Baker (1986) provide a thorough examination of this test. They compare the Sit-and-Reach Test with a test of back flexibility and a test of hamstring flexibility. The Sit-and-Reach Test had moderate validity (.60–.73) when compared with hamstring flexibility but was *not* a valid measure (.27–.30) of low back flexibility.

Reliability This test has acceptable reliability, with reliability coefficients of 0.70 or higher.

Norms Normative data were reported in NCYFS I and II. Tables of norms are presented in Tables 16-25 to 16-27.

Comments The test must be repeated if the knees are flexed during the reach. To ensure that the knees remain extended, the tester should place one hand lightly across the knees. As with all measures of physical fitness, the accuracy and consistency of test scores are increased by adequately warming up before testing. In this case warmups should include passive stretching of the low back–hamstring area. If the recommended test apparatus cannot be secured, a bench with a metric ruler attached may be substituted for the V-sit Reach, with the student seated on the floor. When preadolescent boys and girls as well as

TABLE 16-26 *NCYFS norms by age for the sit-and-reach—boys (in inches)*

Percentile	10	11	12	13	14	15	16	17	18
99	18.0	18.5	18.5	19.5	20.0	21.5	22.0	21.5	22.0
90	16.0	16.5	16.0	16.5	17.5	18.0	19.0	19.5	19.5
80	15.0	15.5	15.0	15.0	16.0	17.0	18.0	18.0	18.0
75	14.5	15.0	15.0	15.0	15.5	16.5	17.0	17.5	17.5
70	14.5	14.5	14.5	14.5	15.0	16.0	17.0	17.0	17.0
60	14.0	14.0	13.5	13.5	14.0	15.0	16.0	16.0	16.0
50	13.5	13.0	13.0	13.0	13.5	14.0	15.0	15.5	15.0
40	12.5	12.5	12.0	12.5	13.0	13.5	14.0	14.5	14.5
30	12.0	12.0	11.5	12.0	12.0	12.5	13.5	13.5	13.5
25	11.5	11.5	11.0	11.0	11.0	12.0	13.0	13.0	13.0
20	11.0	11.0	10.5	10.5	11.0	11.5	12.0	12.5	12.5
10	10.0	9.5	8.5	9.0	9.0	9.5	10.0	10.5	10.0

NOTE: The 1980 AAHPERD norms used a zero point of 23 centimeters, but NCYFS used 12 inches. To adjust the zero point and to change inches to centimeters, use the following formula: Score in centimeters = (Score in inches × 2.54) − 7.48.
Reprinted from the National Children and Youth Fitness Study I. Washington, DC: Department of Health and Human Services, 1985.

TABLE 16-27 *NCYFS norms by age for the sit-and-reach—girls (in inches)*

Percentile	10	11	12	13	14	15	16	17	18
99	20.5	20.5	21.0	22.0	22.0	23.0	23.0	23.0	22.5
90	17.5	18.0	19.0	20.0	19.5	20.0	20.5	20.5	20.5
80	16.5	17.0	18.0	19.0	19.0	19.0	19.5	19.5	19.5
75	16.5	16.5	17.0	18.0	18.5	19.0	19.0	19.0	19.0
70	16.0	16.5	17.0	17.5	18.0	18.5	19.0	19.0	18.5
60	15.0	15.5	16.0	17.0	17.5	18.0	18.0	18.0	18.0
50	14.5	15.0	15.5	16.0	17.0	17.0	17.5	18.0	17.5
40	14.0	14.0	15.0	15.5	16.0	17.0	17.0	17.0	17.0
30	13.0	13.5	14.5	14.5	15.0	16.0	16.5	16.0	16.0
25	13.0	13.0	14.0	14.0	15.0	15.5	16.0	15.5	15.5
20	12.0	13.0	13.5	13.5	14.0	15.0	15.5	15.0	15.0
10	10.5	11.5	12.0	12.0	12.5	13.5	14.0	13.5	13.0

NOTE: The 1980 AAHPERD norms used a zero point of 23 centimeters, but NCYFS used 12 inches. To adjust the zero point and to change inches to centimeters, use the following formula: Score in centimeters = (Score in inches × 2.54) − 7.48.
Reprinted from the National Children and Youth Fitness Study I. Washington, DC: Department of Health and Human Services, 1985.

those in their adolescent growth spurt are tested, it is normal for many of them to be unable to reach 23. During this growth period the legs become proportionally longer than the trunk.

Pull-Ups The pull-ups test and various modifications of this test are discussed in Chapter 17. All the recently revised physical fitness tests include a measure of arm and shoulder girdle strength. NCYFS norms for the pull-ups test and a modified (Vermont) pull-ups tests are presented in Tables 16-28 to 16-30.

Overview of Health-Related Physical Fitness Test Items Although health-related physical fitness tests are widely used, the test items are not without criticism. For example, questions have been raised about the validity of distance run tests as indicators of CR capacity.

Cureton (1982) discusses several factors other than CR capacity that might reflect individual differences in distance running performance—body fatness, running skill or efficiency, motivation, and use of proper pace. Cureton notes that distance run tests have usually been validated by using max $\dot{V}o_2$ expressed as milliliters per kilogram of body weight per minute (ml/kgBW/min) as a criterion measure. However, both variables (distance run score and max $\dot{V}o_2$ as previously expressed) are negatively affected by the percentage of body fat. In other words, as percent fat increases, both distance run performance and max $\dot{V}o_2$ would be more appropriately expressed by milliliters per kilogram of fat-free

TABLE 16-28 *NCYFS II norms by age for the modified pull-ups (number completed)*

	Age							
	Boys				Girls			
Percentile	6	7	8	9	6	7	8	9
99	25	27	38	35	24	27	25	30
95	18	20	21	25	17	20	20	20
90	15	19	20	20	13	16	17	17
85	12	15	17	20	11	14	14	15
80	11	13	15	17	10	12	12	13
75	10	13	14	15	9	11	11	12
70	9	12	13	14	9	10	11	11
65	8	11	12	13	7	9	10	10
60	7	10	11	12	7	8	9	10
55	7	9	10	11	6	8	9	9
50	6	8	10	10	6	7	8	9
45	6	8	9	10	5	7	7	8
40	5	7	8	9	5	6	6	7
35	5	6	8	8	4	5	6	6
30	4	5	7	7	4	4	5	5
25	3	4	6	6	3	4	4	4
20	3	4	5	5	2	3	4	4
15	2	3	4	4	1	2	3	2
10	1	1	3	3	0	1	1	1
5	0	0	1	2	0	0	0	0

Reprinted from the National Children and Youth Fitness Study II. Washington, DC: Department of Health and Human Services, 1987.

weight per minute (ml/kgFFW/min). He then demonstrates the accuracy of his analysis using data from a number of studies of adults and a single study of children. For example, he refers to a 1977 study (Cureton and others, 1977), which showed the following relationships for boys and girls ages 8 to 12.

Distance	$\dot{V}O_2$ max (BW)	$\dot{V}O_2$ max (FFW)
600 yards	−.62	−.32
1 mile	−.66	−.40

In short, between 35% and 45% of the variance in distance runs can be accounted for by $\dot{V}O_2$ max when total body weight is used to adjust the expression, but the percentage of variance accounted for drops to between 9% and 16%

TABLE 16-29 *NCYFS norms by age for the chin-ups—boys (number completed)*

Percentile	10	11	12	13	14	15	16	17	18
99	13	12	13	17	18	18	20	20	21
90	8	8	8	10	12	14	14	15	16
80	5	5	6	8	9	11	12	13	14
75	4	5	5	7	8	10	12	12	13
70	4	4	5	7	8	10	11	12	12
60	2	3	4	5	6	8	10	10	11
50	1	2	3	4	5	7	9	9	10
40	1	1	2	3	4	6	8	8	9
30	0	0	1	1	3	5	6	6	7
25	0	0	0	1	2	4	6	5	6
20	0	0	0	0	1	3	5	4	5
10	0	0	0	0	0	1	2	2	3

Reprinted from the National Children and Youth Fitness Study I. Washington, DC: Department of Health and Human Services, 1985.

TABLE 16-30 *NCYFS norms by age for the chin-ups—girls (number completed)*

Percentile	10	11	12	13	14	15	16	17	18
99	8	8	8	5	8	6	8	7	6
90	3	3	2	2	2	2	2	2	2
80	2	1	1	1	1	1	1	1	1
75	1	1	1	1	1	1	1	1	1
70	1	1	1	0	1	1	1	1	1
60	0	0	0	0	0	0	0	0	0
50	0	0	0	0	0	0	0	0	0
40	0	0	0	0	0	0	0	0	0
30	0	0	0	0	0	0	0	0	0
25	0	0	0	0	0	0	0	0	0
20	0	0	0	0	0	0	0	0	0
10	0	0	0	0	0	0	0	0	0

Reprinted from the National Children and Youth Fitness Study I. Washington, DC: Department of Health and Human Services, 1985.

TABLE 16-31 *Children's heart data*

Age	Average HRrest*	Normal range*	Target HRR 60-85% HRmax	20 sec values
4	100	80-120	170-199	56-66
6	100	75-115	168-197	56-64
8	90	70-110	163-194	54-64
10	90	70-110	162-192	54-64
Girls (225 = max HR)				
12	90	70-110	164-190	52-63
14	85	65-105	161-187	51-62
16	80	60-100	157-185	50-61
18	75	55-95	155-183	49-60
Boys (220 = max HR)				
12	85	65-105	159-190	52-63
14	80	60-100	156-187	51-62
16	75	55-95	152-185	50-61
18	70	50-90	149-182	49-60

*Data from Nelson, W.E. et al. 1987. *Textbook of Pediatrics.* Philadelphia: WB Saunders.
From Siegel, J. 1988. Journal of Physical Education, Recreation and Dance, 59(4):79.

when fat-free weight is used. Thus, variability in body fatness accounts for almost half the relationship between max $\dot{V}o_2$ and distance runs. For this reason, it is inappropriate to suggest that distance run tests measure only one physiological variable. Cureton also notes that changes in distance run performance in children are often not paralleled by similar changes in max $\dot{V}o_2$. Changes are more likely to occur in running efficiency as well as percent fat and anaerobic capacity. Nonetheless, he supports the use of distance run tests in the assessment of physical fitness in children. Such tests evaluate a unique physical ability not tapped in most other tests of physical performance. They reflect "the level of energy expenditure that a person can sustain over an extended period of time, or the physical work capacity in weight-bearing exercise" (Cureton, 1982, p. 66).

As a part of a fitness education program, children should be taught to use heart rate to monitor the intensity of activity. According to Siegel (1988), most children from age nine or ten, grade three, can be taught to accurately count a 10-second carotid heart rate (p. 78). If resting heart rate values are not available for a group of children, average heart rate (shown in Table 16-31) can be used to calculate the target heart rate range.

Problems in measuring the skinfold thicknesses of young children have been summarized by Lohman (1982). In laboratory settings investigators assume children are chemically mature with regard to such elements as potassium and water content. Under these assumptions, a mean fat content of 20% is usually found. In a field setting a different value for body fat is estimated using a regression equation. However, equations for predicting percent body fat of adults are not appropriate for children. Furthermore, the relationship between anthropometric measures and body density varies between ages 8 and 15. For these reasons it is both logical and defensible to use the sum of skinfolds to measure body composition in elementary school children rather than applying invalid prediction equations in an effort to estimate percent body fat.

The expense of the skinfold caliper required to measure body composition has been viewed as problematic by some. The major criterion for a skinfold caliper is that it exert a constant force of 10 g/mm^2 at the skinfold site, regardless of the thickness of the skinfold. Large errors in skinfold measures occur at low pressures, that is, lower than 10 g/mm^2. In a study conducted by Lohman and Pollock (1981), three types of calipers were compared. A plastic caliper with neither spring nor tension required the tester to apply the appropriate amount of tension. A plastic caliper with a spring depended on the spring for the tension exerted. The third instrument was metal with a uniform tension independent of skinfold thickness. Both experienced and inexperienced testers measured a group of children at the triceps and subscapular sites. Differences between the scores of experienced and inexperienced testers occurred except when the expensive metal caliper was used. When the inexperienced testers were trained, the scores obtained using both pairs of calipers were more similar. The less expensive calipers may prove to be suitable for use in a field test setting, providing the tester is well trained. Several inexpensive skinfold calipers are shown in Figure 16-7.

Lohman and Pollock make several suggestions regarding the training of testers. At the very least, inexperienced testers should be trained above and beyond the required reading of the test manual. To attain proficiency in measuring skinfold thicknesses, testers should practice measuring between 50 and 100 people. Initially the sites should be marked with a grease pencil on the skin of the individual being tested. Testers within the same fitness club or school system should train together.

Several articles on the health-related physical fitness testing, which should be useful for the practitioner, have been published in recent years. For the physical education teacher, Pate and Corbin (1981) propose implications for curriculum. Program ideas are presented, including those with cognitive and affective outcomes as well as psychomotor. The article includes excellent suggestions for teachers, which an innovative reader could apply in a nonschool setting as well. Their taxonomy of physical fitness objectives is shown in Table 16-32. The levels of the taxonomy range from the acquisition of a physical fitness vocabulary to the development of physical fitness problem-solving ability. Another excellent article

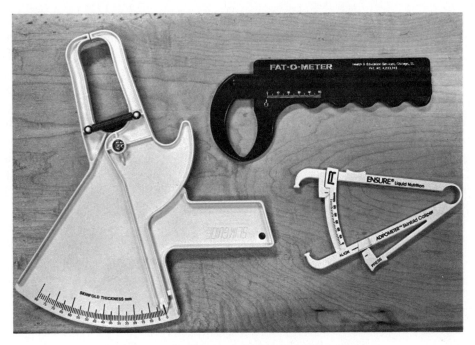

FIGURE 16-7 *Variety of inexpensive skinfold calipers.*

TABLE 16-32 *Physical fitness objectives*

Level	Objective
1	Physical fitness vocabulary (fitness components; distinction between health-related and skill-related components)
2	Exercising (teacher interacts and encourages students to exercise)
3	Achieving physical fitness (help children experience the satisfaction of being fit)
4	Establishing regular exercise patterns (objectives become learner-oriented rather than teacher-oriented)
5	Physical fitness evaluation
6	Physical fitness problem solving (interpret data and modify own exercise program)

From Pate, R., and Corbin, C.

for teachers and exercise specialists is written by Pollock and Blair (1981). An overview of the state of the art of exercise prescription is presented, beginning with a discussion of the physiological and behavioral components of exercise prescription. This is followed by a review of the principles of overload, specificity, warm-up, initial levels of fitness, progressions, and individual differences. Finally, the effect of exercise on CR function is discussed, in particular, frequency, intensity, duration, and mode of exercise. A number of articles of this nature have appeared in the *Journal of Physical Education, Recreation and Dance*, published by the AAHPERD.

Step Tests

Distance run tests, already described as measures of CR function, can be used as a part of a health-related physical fitness test or can be administered separately by physical education teachers and exercise specialists. Another practical test of CR function that can be used in a field setting is the step test. In this section the Harvard Step Test, the best-known step test, is described, followed by a description of several modifications of the Harvard test.

The Harvard Step Test The Harvard Step Test was developed at the Harvard Fatigue Laboratory in 1943. A landmark test in its day, it is no longer widely used because of its strenuousness. However, it still provides the standard for all step tests developed since that time and thus merits a thorough overview.

Test Objective The Harvard Step Test was designed to measure the CR function of adult males.

Description The examinee exercises on a 20-inch bench for as long a period as possible up to 5 minutes.

Instructions The stepping pattern is up with the left foot, up with the right foot, down with the left foot, and down with the right foot. Both of the examinee's legs should be straight when standing on the bench. The steps should be taken at a cadence of 30 steps per minute. The cadence can be easily established using a metronome, although a stopwatch can also be used. The test instructions and cadence can also be recorded on an audio tape for ease of administration. The test ends after the 5-minute period has elapsed, although examinees may stop at any time before the 5-minute limit.

Whenever the examinee stops exercising, a pulse count is taken during three recovery periods—from 1 to 1½ minutes, 2 to 2½ minutes, and 3 to 3½ minutes after exercise ceases. Two scores are recorded: the number of seconds the examinee exercised and the sum of the pulse counts in the three recovery periods.

Test Area One of the desirable features of a step test is that it can be administered in small areas.

Equipment Metronome or stopwatch and 20-inch bench.

Scoring Formula 11-1 is used to determine the index of physical efficiency.

$$\text{Index} = \frac{\text{Duration of exercise in seconds} \times 100}{2 \times \text{sum of 3 recovery pulse counts}} \qquad \text{Formula 11-1}$$

Suppose an examinee stops exercising at the end of 4 minutes (240 seconds) and his recovery pulse rates are 80, 60, and 50, respectively. Using Formula 11-1, determine his index of physical efficiency.

$$\text{Index} = \frac{240 \times 100}{2(80 + 60 + 50)} = 63.2$$

What does a score of 63.2 mean? Is it a good score or a poor score? Mathews (1978, p. 269) at Ohio State developed a set of standards for adult males based on a large data set accumulated over a period of several years.

Harvard Step Test Standards

Above 90	Excellent
80-89	Good
65-79	Average
55-64	Low average
Below 55	Poor

In the hypothetical example the score of 63.2 is interpreted as a low-average score.

Validity The validity of the Harvard Step Test has been determined by correlating it with max $\dot{V}o_2$, based on a maximal stress test, as a criterion measure. Validity coefficients ranging from -0.35 to 0.77 have been reported, indicating that this step test is not a very precise indicator of CR function. Negative validity coefficients were obtained because several investigators used a modified scoring system where lower scores represented better performance on the step test.

Reliability Reliability coefficients ranging from 0.65 to 0.95 have been obtained for the Harvard Step Test of the test in modified form. Most of these coefficients are higher than 0.80. The reproducibility or objectivity of the test, which is the ability to obtain the same heart rate using different testers, is high. Coefficients of 0.992 to 0.995 have been reported by Montoye (1978). Most of the reliability estimates are confounded (probably made lower) by the potential for error in obtaining the pulse rate. Sometimes the pulse rate is counted by a partner. On other occasions the same tester is not used for both testing sessions. Certainly, the lack of objectivity in obtaining a pulse rate is a problem, but the extent to which this problem affects the size of the reliability coefficient is unknown.

Comments The Harvard Step Test has been modified for young women and for boys and girls. Montoye (1978) has recommended specific bench heights, rates of stepping, and maximum durations for various age groups and both genders:

Ages 8 to 10 (Boys and Girls) Use a bench height of 8 inches, a stepping rate of 24 (4 counting cycles per minute), and a maximum duration of 3 minutes.

Ages 10 to 12 (Boys and Girls) Use a bench height of 12 inches, a stepping rate of 24, and a maximum duration of 3 minutes.

Ages 12 to 14 (Boys and Girls) Use a bench height of 18 inches, a stepping rate of 24, and a maximum duration of 3 minutes.

Ages 15 to 22 (Girls) Use a bench height of 18 inches, a stepping rate of 24, and a maximum duration of 3 minutes. (These test specifications can also be used for women, ages 23 to 34.)

Ages 15 to 22 (Boys) Use a bench height of 20 inches, a stepping rate of 30, and a maximum duration of 5 minutes. (These test specifications can also be used for men, ages 23 to 34.)

The Ohio State University Step Test Because of the strenuous nature of the Harvard Step Test, a more practical and less taxing step test was developed at Ohio State University (OSU) in 1969. This test can easily be used in a field setting.

Test Objective The purpose of this test is to measure cardiorespiratory function for males and females.

Description The OSU Step Test is divided into a series of 18 innings of exercise. Each inning is 30 seconds long and is followed by a 20-second rest period. Each 20-second rest period consists of 5 seconds to locate the pulse, 10 seconds to count the pulse, and 5 seconds to prepare for the beginning of the next inning. Therefore a new inning of exercise begins every 50 seconds. The 18 innings are divided into 3 phases:

Phase I—6 innings at 24 steps/minute on a 15-inch bench

Phase II—6 innings at 30 steps/minute on a 15-inch bench

Phase III—6 innings at 30 steps/minute on a 20-inch bench

During the 10-second interval of each rest period, the pulse rate is counted. If the pulse rate is less than 25 beats per 10 seconds, the examinee continues with the next inning. The first rest interval in which the pulse rate reaches or exceeds 25 is the inning that terminates the test. The test can also be terminated by completing all 18 innings without attaining a pulse rate of 25.

Instructions Before beginning the test, the examinee stands in front of the bench and grasps the handbar with both hands. The handbar should be level with the top of the examinee's head. The stepping pattern is initiated at the signal *"Ready, Go!,"* and the examinee proceeds in cadence with the metronome. The up-up-down-down stepping pattern described for the Harvard Step Test is used, except either the left or the right foot can initiate the first step up. The legs must be straight when both feet are on the bench, and the back should also be straight at this point. The examinee should be forewarned when the cadence changes at the beginning of a new phase.

Test Area A relatively small space is sufficient for administering the OSU Step Test.

Equipment A split-level bench with an adjustable handbar (lower level of the bench is 15 inches high; higher level, 20 inches) and a metronome and stopwatch, unless the cadence and time units are recorded on tape.

Scoring The score is the number of innings the individual is able to complete before reaching a heart rate of 25 in 10 seconds. The examinee may be permitted to count his or her own pulse, if able to do so fairly accurately. The tester should make arrangements before administering a step test to have additional help available for those who have difficulty detecting their pulse. Several students in class might assist in this capacity. The entire group of examinees should be informed that this type of assistance is available.

Validity The validity coefficient for the OSU Step Test when compared to a submaximal stress test is 0.94. Max $\dot{V}_{O_2}$ values were estimated from the submaximal test. When the OSU Step Test scores were correlated with max $\dot{V}_{O_2}$ measured directly in a maximum stress test, the validity coefficients were considerably lower, ranging from 0.47 to 0.57. These latter coefficients correspond closely to those obtained for the Harvard Step Test.

Reliability The OSU Step Test has acceptable reliability, with reliability coefficients ranging from 0.69 to 0.94.

Comments The OSU Test has been modified for college women (Witten, 1973) and for elementary school boys (Callan, 1968).

College Women A trilevel bench is used with heights of 14, 17, and 20 inches. Twenty innings, divided into four phases, are used. In innings 1 to 5, a cadence of 24 steps per minute is used with a bench height of 14 inches. In innings 6 to 10, the cadence is 30 steps per minute using a bench height of 14 inches. In innings 11–15, the cadence is 30 steps per minute using a bench height of 17 inches. In the final innings, 16–20, the cadence is 30 steps per minute with a bench height of 20 inches. Otherwise the test is similar to the OSU Test for college males, except that the test is terminated when the pulse rate reaches 28 or higher.

Elementary School Boys This is an adaptation for boys in grades 4 through 6. The test is identical to the one used for college males, with two exceptions — the tester must count the heart rate using a stethoscope and the test is terminated when the heart rate reaches 29 beats during the 10-second period.

The Queens College Step Test A simplified version of the step test, developed at Queens College (Katch and McArdle, 1983), is useful for the quick screening of the CR function of college students. A bench height of 16¼ inches is used. This is the height of a bleacher step at Queens, thus allowing for mass testing. A metronome is used to monitor the stepping cadence, which is 88 steps per minute (22 complete step-ups) for women and 96 steps per minute (24 complete step-ups) for men. After a 15-second practice period, all examinees begin the test and continue for 3 minutes. At the end of 3 minutes the examinees are

TABLE 16-33 *Percentile rankings for recovery heart rate and predicted maximal oxygen consumption for male and female college students*

Percentile ranking	Recovery HR, female	Predicted max $\dot{V}O_2$ (ml/kg· min)	Recovery HR, male	Predicted max $\dot{V}O_2$ (ml/kg· min)
100	128	42.2	120	60.9
95	140	40.0	124	59.3
90	148	38.5	128	57.6
85	152	37.7	136	54.2
80	156	37.0	140	52.5
75	158	36.6	144	50.9
70	160	36.3	148	49.2
65	162	35.9	149	48.8
60	163	35.7	152	47.5
55	164	35.5	154	46.7
50	166	35.1	156	45.8
45	168	34.8	160	44.1
40	170	34.4	162	43.3
35	171	34.2	164	42.5
30	172	34.0	166	41.6
25	176	33.3	168	40.8
20	180	32.6	172	39.1
15	182	32.2	176	37.4
10	184	31.8	178	36.6
5	196	29.6	184	34.1

From Nutrition, Weight Control, and Exercise. By Katch, F.I. and McArdle, W.D., 1983, ed. 2. By permission of Lea and Febiger.

stopped. They are allowed 5 seconds to detect their pulse at the carotid artery. After 5 seconds examinees count their pulse rate for 15 seconds and multiply the value by 4. A table of percentile ranks and predicted maximal oxygen consumption for male and female students is shown in Table 16-33.

To determine test validity, scores on the Queens College Test were correlated with measures of max $\dot{V}O_2$ obtained during treadmill testing. Validity coefficients are $-.75$ for college women and $-.72$ for college men. These coefficients are negative, since lower heart rates are associated with higher max $\dot{V}O_2$ values. The test is highly reliable, with coefficients of 0.92 reported for women and 0.89 for men.

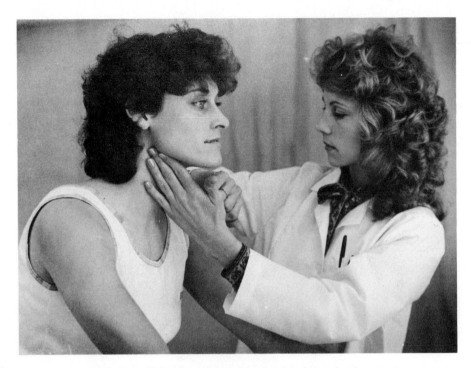

FIGURE 16-8 *Palpation of carotid artery to determine heart rate.*

A number of fitness tests require the determination of heart rate through palpation of the carotid artery in the neck. The correct positioning of the fingers is shown in Figure 16-8. The pressure on the artery should be firm but light. Excessive pressure will distort the heart rate.

MEASURING HEALTH-RELATED FITNESS IN A LABORATORY SETTING
Cardiorespiratory Function

The most desirable approach to determining cardiorespiratory function is to measure it *during* exercise. With this approach, changes in physiological parameters can be monitored throughout the exercise cycle.

Maximal Stress Testing To assess max $\dot{V}o_2$ directly, an individual's expired air is measured during exhaustive physical work. Typically, the examinee exercises on a bicycle ergometer or a motor-driven treadmill, as depicted in Figure 16-9, although a stepping bench can also be used. The workload is gradually increased. On the treadmill this is accomplished by increasing the speed, raising the slope, or both. On the bicycle ergometer the workload is increased by increasing the friction on the flywheel. As the workload increases, oxygen consumption also increases. Throughout the test period exhaled air is collected us-

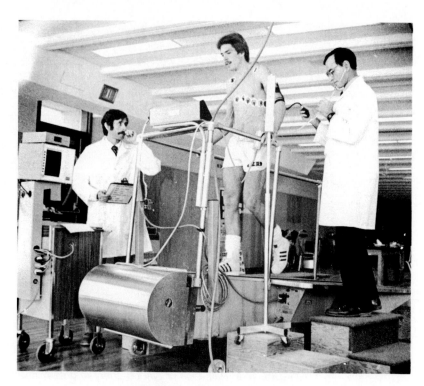

FIGURE 16-9 *Balke Treadmill Test.*

ing a portable spirometer, Douglas bags, or computerized instrumentation. When the examinee can no longer continue, the test is stopped. Maximal oxygen uptake is obtained when the increased workload is no longer accompanied by an increase in oxygen uptake.

Measuring time on the treadmill (between the initiation of the test to the point of exhaustion) can also be used to determine maximal stress. The time score is then used to predict oxygen uptake.

Submaximal Stress Testing Indirect methods of measuring CR function are frequently used in a laboratory setting. Since heart rate and oxygen uptake increase linearly with increases in workload, heart rate can be used to *predict* oxygen uptake. While these tests are not as accurate as a direct measure, they do not require the examinee to exercise to exhaustion.

Balke Treadmill Test Balke (1952) devised a submaximal test that measures the duration of exercise required to produce a heart rate of 180 beats per minute. The examinee walks on a treadmill at a constant speed, approximately 3.5 mph. At the end of each minute, the heart rate is taken and the slope of the treadmill is increased. Blood pressure is usually recorded as well, as shown in Figure 16-9. After the first minute and each succeeding minute of exercise, the slope is increased by a 1% grade. The equipment required to administer the test is a treadmill, stopwatch, and electrocardiograph. The test score is the number of minutes required to attain a heart rate of 180. The test is highly reliable and valid, although an individual's performance can be affected by several possible sources of error, such as time of most recent meal, time of day, temperature and emotional state. One of the notable advantages of the Balke test is its safety. Since the work is increased at a gradual pace, the subject's physiological changes can be monitored on a continual basis and the test can be stopped when appropriate for an individual subject.

A classification scale has been devised to interpret test scores of adult men:

Minutes to HR of 180	Classification
22-above	Excellent
20-21	Very good
18-19	Good
17	Average
15-16	Fair
13-14	Poor
12-below	Very poor

Astrand and Ryhming Test A submaximal stress test on the bicycle ergometer was developed by Astrand and Ryhming (1954). The examinee pedals for 6 or more minutes at a set cadence, with a heart rate between 125 and 170 beats per minute. Baumgartner and Jackson (1987) recommended workloads of 600 kpm/min for college women and 800 kpm/min for college men. The test score must be corrected for subjects 30 years of age or older. Validity coefficients ranging from 0.33 to 0.872 have been reported. In both cases the test scores were compared with a direct measure of CR function.

A maximal stress test can also be conducted on the bicycle ergometer. This procedure, with expired gas collected in Douglas bags, is shown in Figure 16-10.

PWC$_{170}$ Test The PWC$_{170}$ Test is administered on a bicycle ergometer, with 4 to 10 minutes of exercise at each workload. The subject's work capacity is the workload maintained up to a heart rate of 170. Heart rate is measured at each workload. Since PWC$_{170}$ is correlated with body size, a correction of the test score is necessary. The validity coefficients range from 0.57 to 0.88, when PWC$_{170}$ scores are correlated with max $\dot{V}o_2$ values. This test is often recommended for testing the physical work capacity of children.

Recommendations for Testing Cardiorespiratory Function For purposes of mass screening, Montoye (1978) recommends administering some form of a step test to individuals between the ages of 8 and 22. A step test may also be used to test healthy subjects ages 22 to 34. For individuals over 35 years of age, Montoye notes the potential medical risks and recommends that a physician be present when fitness tests are administered.

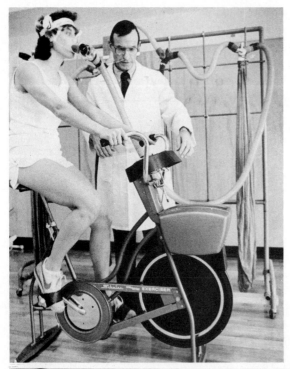

A

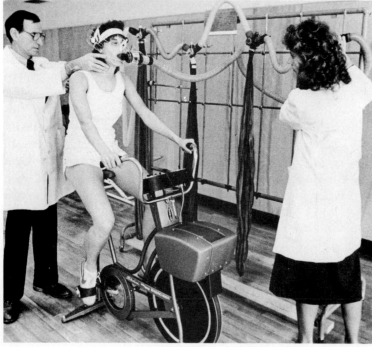

B

FIGURE 16-10 *A, Maximal stress testing on the bicycle ergometer. B, Measuring heart rate and collecting expired gas during maximal stress testing on the bicycle ergometer.*

Body Composition

A direct measure of body composition can be made by chemical analysis. Until recently, making this analysis required a human cadaver. However, a new method of determining body composition using electrical waves passing through the wrists and ankles has now been developed (see photographs on p. 392). The most frequently used indirect measure in a laboratory setting is hydrostatic weighing.

Hydrostatic Weighing Generally the assessment of body composition involves determining the relative percentage of fat and muscle. Specific gravity, which reflects body density, is a better indicator of body composition than weight alone. Specific gravity equals the ratio of the density of a body to that of an equal volume of water. The specific gravity of human beings is usually estimated by weighing the body in water. The subject is immersed up to the neck in a specially built tank of water warmed to a comfortable temperature. The subject is instructed to hold his or her breath for 5 seconds, lower the head underwater, and expire the air forcefully, as depicted in Figure 16-11. At this point the un-

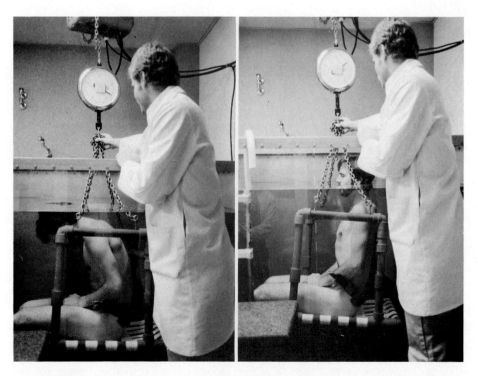

FIGURE 16-11 *Assessment of body composition through underwater weighing.*
From Pollock, M.L., Schmidt, D.H., and Jackson, A.S.

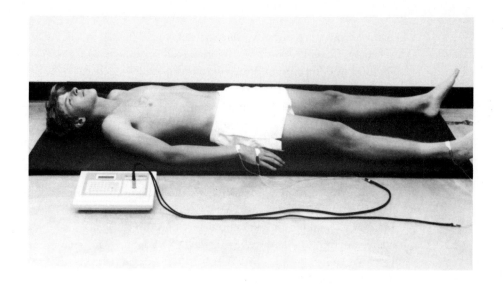

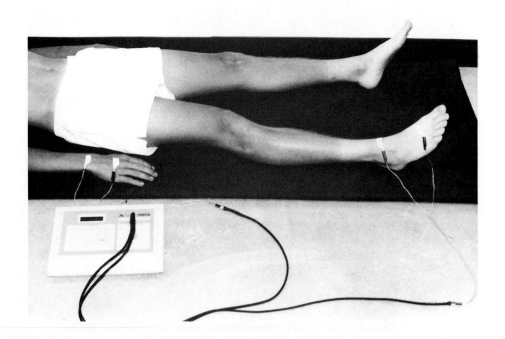

derwater weight of the subject is recorded. To ensure accurate results, 10 to 12 repeated weighings are recommended.

After forceful expiration of air, some air remains in the lungs. This residual lung volume is measured before the underwater weighing; it must be used in calculating body density.

SUMMARY

An emphasis on health-related physical fitness is pervasive in both school and nonschool settings. A distinction should be made between health-related fitness and measures of athletic performance. Although tests of athletic performance are sometimes referred to as health-related physical fitness measures, this label is a misnomer. The 50-yard dash, for example, does not measure health-related physical fitness; rather, it measures a certain fitness for athletic performance, in this case, speed. However, the term *fitness* is used loosely in this context. Health-related physical fitness can be measured in both laboratory and field settings with an acceptable degree of validity and reliability.

LEARNING EXPERIENCES

1. Practice marking the site for triceps skinfold measurement. Use a grease pencil to mark the site. Measure the site five times using a skinfold caliper. Try to obtain the same reading within 1 or 2 mm.
2. Visit a health club or visit a fitness center in your community. Ask the manager or one of the instructors about the tests (if any) they administer to new clients. Request a copy of the form(s) used to record test results to take back to your measurement class. Evaluate the testing program in light of desirable physical fitness objectives.
3. Practice measuring your heart rate by palpating the carotid artery in your neck. Then practice on another person, both before and after exercise.
4. Administer the AAHPERD Physical Best Test or a similar test to several of your fellow students. Study the instructions for test administration carefully before beginning. After you have completed the testing, write a short paper on the problems you encountered in administering the test and how you would alleviate these problems in future administrations of the test.

REFERENCES

American Alliance for Health, Physical Education, Recreation and Dance. 1980. AAHPERD Health-Related Physical Fitness Test Manual. Reston, VA: AAHPERD.

American Alliance for Health, Physical Education, Recreation and Dance. 1988. Physical Best. Reston, VA: AAHPERD.

American Alliance for Health, Physical Education, Recreation and Dance. 1984. Technical Manual. Reston, VA: AAHPERD.

American Association for Health, Physical Education, and Recreation. 1976. AAHPER Youth Fitness Test Manual. Washington, DC: AAHPERD.

American Health and Fitness Foundation. 1988. Fit Youth Today. Austin, TX: American Health and Fitness Foundation.

Astrand, P., and Rodahl, K. 1970. Textbook of Work Physiology. New York: McGraw-Hill.

Astrand, P.O., and Ryhming, I. 1954. A nomogram for calculation of aerobic capacity (physical fitness) from pulse rate during submaximal work. Journal of Applied Physiology, **7**:218-235.

Balke, B. 1952. Correlation of static and physical endurance. I. A test of physical performance based on the cardiovascular and respiratory response to gradually increased work. Air University, USAF School of Aviation Medicine. Project No. 21-32-004, Report No.1, April.

Baumgartner, T.A., and Jackson, A.S. 1987. Measurement for Evaluation in Physical Education, ed. 3. Dubuque, IA: Wm C Brown Group.

Chrysler Fund-Amateur Athletic Union. 1987. Physical Fitness Program. Bloomington, IN: The Chrysler Fund-Amateur Athletic Union.

Cureton, K.J. 1982. Distance running performance tests in children—what do they mean? Journal of Physical Education, Recreation and Dance, **53**: 64-66.

Cureton, K.J., Boileau, R.A., Lohman, T.G., and Misner, J.E. 1977. Determinants of distance running performance in children: analysis of a path model. Research Quarterly **48**: 270-279.

Institute for Aerobics Research. 1987. FITNESSGRAM User's Manual. Dallas, TX: Institute for Aerobics Research.

Jackson, A.E., and Coleman, A.E. 1976. Validation of distance run tests for elementary school children. Research Quarterly, **47**: 86-94.

Jackson, A.W., and Baker, A.A. 1986. The relationship of the Sit and Reach Test to criterion measures of hamstring and back flexibility in young females. Research Quarterly for Exercise and Sport, **57**: 183-186.

Katch, F.I., and McArdle, W.D. 1983. Nutrition, Weight Control, and Exercise, ed. 2. Philadelphia: Lea & Febiger.

Krahenbuhl, G.S., Pangrazi, R.P., Petersen, G.W., Burkett, L.N., and Schneider, M.J. 1978. Field testing of cardiorespiratory fitness in primary school children. Medicine and Science in Sports, **10**: 208-213.

Lohman, T.J. 1982. Measurement of body composition in children. Journal of Physical Education, Recreation and Dance, **53**(7):67-70.

Lohman, T.J. 1987. The use of skinfold to estimate body fatness on children and youth. Journal of Physical Education, Recreation and Dance, **58**: 98-102.

Lohman, T.J., and Pollock, M.L. 1981. Which caliper? How much training? Journal of Physical Education, Recreation and Dance, **52**(1): 27-29.

Montoye, H.J. 1978. An Introduction to Measurement in Physical Education. Boston: Allyn & Bacon, Inc.

Pate, R.R., and Corbin, C. 1981. Implications for curriculum. Journal of Physical Education, Recreation and Dance, **52**(1): 36-38.

Pollock, M.L., and Blair, S.N. 1981. Exercise prescription. Journal of Physical Education, Recreation and Dance, **52**(1): 30-35, 81.

President's Council on Physical Fitness and Sports. 1987. The Presidential Physical Fitness Award Program. Washington, DC: The President's Council on Physical Fitness and Sports.

Reiff, G.G., Dixon, W.R., Jacoby, D., Ye, G.X., Spain, C.G., and Hunsicker, P.A. 1985. National School Population Fitness Survey. The President's Council on Physical Fitness and Sports 1985. Research Project 282-84-0086.

Robertson, L.D., and Magnusdottir, H. 1987. Evaluation of criteria associated with abdominal fitness testing. Research Quarterly for Exercise and Sport, **58**: 355-359.

Ross, J.G., and Gilbert, G.G. 1985. The national children and youth fitness study: a summary of findings. Journal of Physical Education, Recreation and Dance, **56**: 45-50.

Ross, J.G., and Pate, R.R. 1987. The national children and youth fitness study II: a summary of findings. Journal of Physical Education, Recreation and Dance, **58**: 51-61.

Siegel, J. 1988. Children's target heart rate range. Journal of Physical Education, Recreation and Dance, **59**: 78-79.

Wells, C.L. 1986. The effects of physical activity on cardiorespiratory fitness in children. In G. Stull and H. Eckert, Effects of physical activity on children. Champaign, IL: Human Kinetics Publishers, Inc. pp.114-126.

ANNOTATED READINGS

Cooter, G.R. 1976. Who wants to be normal? Journal of Physical Education and Recreation, **47**: 50.

Cites misuse of norms by doctors, physical educators, and weight-conscious people; notes that norms represent average characteristics; in the health-related professions, desirable standards rather than normative standards should be stressed; gives examples of misuse of norms in measuring physical fitness, weight, cholesterol, percent body fat, blood pressure, and other physical parameters.

Fox, K.R., and Biddle, S.J.H. 1988. The use of fitness tests: educational and psychological considerations. Journal of Physical Education, Recreation, and Dance, **59**: 47-53.

Stresses a focus on lifetime fitness, which places greater emphasis on the psychological orientation of students toward physical activity; identifies factors affecting fitness performance and discusses their impact on fitness test scores; encourages an emphasis on the process of regular exercise rather than the product of fitness (e.g., overuse of fitness norms); applies psychological principles to the fitness testing situation.

Koslow, R.E. 1988. Can physical fitness be a primary objective in a balanced PE program? Journal of Physical Education, Recreation and Dance, **59**: 75-77.

Discusses the issue of the development and maintenance of physical fitness as a primary objective in physical education; reviews the principles and concepts pertaining to fitness development; describes the time requirements necessary to meet a fitness objective; points to the importance of setting objectives that are specific, measurable, and attainable within the restraints of the program.

Lacy, E., and Marshall, B. 1984. FITNESSGRAM: an answer to physical fitness improvement for school children. Journal of Physical Education, Recreation and Dance, **55**(1): 18-19.

Describes the pilot program of FITNESSGRAM in Tulsa, Oklahoma; discusses the unique aspects of the FITNESSGRAM program in promoting physical fitness in the community.

Pate, R.R. 1978. Fitness testing with a realistic purpose. Journal of Physical Education and Recreation, **49**: 47.

Notes that fitness testing may be popular for the wrong reasons when teachers fail to consider the purposes of these tests; suggests reassessing current beliefs in the proper role of fitness testing; discusses contributions of fitness testing and five objectives dealing with fitness testing.

Pate, R.R., and Ross, J.G. 1987. Factors associated with health-related fitness. Journal of Physical Education, Recreation and Dance, **58**: 93-95.

Reports on one phase of the National Children and Youth Fitness Study II on the relationship between the physical activity patterns of 6–9-year-old children and their health-related fitness; emphasizes two key components of health-related fitness—cardiorespiratory endurance and body composition; children with higher levels of cardiorespiratory endurance tend to participate in more community-based physical activity, watch less television, and receive higher ratings on being physically active.

Pate, R.R., Ross, J.G., Dotson, C.O., and Gilbert, G.G. 1985. The new norms: a comparison with the 1980 AAHPERD norms. Journal of Physical Education, Recreation and Dance, **56**(1): 70-72.

Compares norms developed from the National Children and Youth Fitness Study I data with the 1980 norms developed for the AAHPERD Health-Related Physical Fitness Test; discusses the sampling approaches used in both studies.

Ross, J.G., Dotson, C.O., Gilbert, G.G., and Katz, S.J. 1985 Maturation and fitness test performance. Journal of Physical Education, Recreation and Dance, **56**(1): 67-69.

Provides a new perspective of developmental trends in fitness by examining test performance on five different dimensions of fitness; the common beliefs about the effects of age on fitness test performance were not verified by the data from the National Children and Youth Fitness Study.

Ross, J.G., Dotson, C.O., Gilbert, G.G., and Katz, S.J. 1985. New standards for fitness measurement. Journal of Physical Education, Recreation and Dance, **56**(1): 62-66.

Discusses the development of fitness norms (included in this chapter) based on data from the National Children and Youth Fitness Study I; includes tables of percentiles by age and sex for five fitness tests, consisting of the Health-Related Physical Fitness Test items and a chin-ups test.

Siegel, J. 1988. Children's target heart rate range. Journal of Physical Education, Recreation and Dance, **59:** 78-79.

Stresses the importance of using heart rate to control the intensity of activity; reviews the standard formula for deriving training heart rate and applies it to children; notes difficulty in obtaining resting heart rate in children; and presents table of average resting heart rate values for same-age children.

17

Tests of Performance-Related Physical Fitness

KEY WORDS *Watch for these words as you read the following chapter:*

50-Yard Dash Test

Flexed-Arm Hang Test

individually based norms

percentile norms

performance-related physical fitness

Pull-Ups Test

Shuttle Run Test

Standing Long Jump Test

systematic decrease in scores

systematic increase in scores

Every physical education teacher and exercise scientist knows that physical fitness necessary to engage in sports and other forms of physical activity encompasses more than health-related physical fitness. (For a discussion of the distinction between health-related physical fitness and performance-related physical fitness, see Chapter 16.) The performance of most motor tasks probably involves some combination of health-related and performance-related fitness. However, some aspects of fitness may be more strongly related to a specific sport or to a general factor found in a cluster of activities than health-related fitness. Fitness specific to a sport is often referred to as **performance-related physical fitness.** One example of this type of fitness is agility. In many situations physical education teachers recognize the need to increase the amount of agility in students. An optimal amount of agility may be needed so that a student can effectively move from one point to another, shifting weight properly and using optimum speed. Agility is highly specific to a task; thus there is no valid measure of overall agility. Furthermore, health-related physical fitness is not strongly reflected in agility. Agility does not meet the definition of this type of fitness (see Chapter 16). A one-to-one relationship between agility, for example, and a positive health state has not been established. Nonetheless, a task-specific measure of agility might be used in a school or nonschool setting as a measure of performance-related physical fitness.

The tests described in this chapter are primarily performance-related items that have been used on a large-scale basis for many years in the physical education field. It bears repeating that the examinee's medical record should be checked before administering any type of fitness test. In a school setting, these

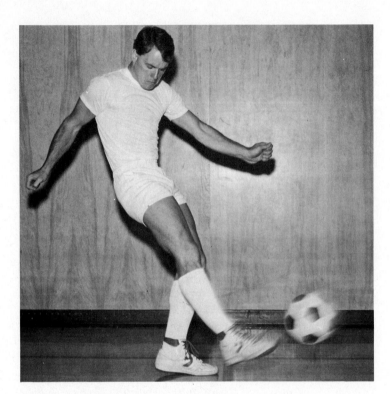

Soccer Test.

checks are usually made before participation in physical education classes. Because of this procedure, little risk exists in administering a fitness test to a school-age child. In a nonschool setting, care must be taken to see that the appropriate medical information is obtained for each client. If the client is over 35 years of age, a physician's permission should be obtained before the client is allowed to participate in vigorous physical activity. General medical information should be secured from a client who joins a health or fitness club.

AAHPER YOUTH FITNESS TEST

Portions of the AAHPER Youth Fitness Test are described in this chapter even though the total test battery is no longer one of the physical fitness tests sponsored by national organizations promoting physical fitness. Its long-standing popularity warrants a brief overview in this chapter, although the test battery as a whole is not recommended as the most valid measure of overall fitness today. Yet, individual items in the test can still be useful to physical educators and exercise scientists. Three of the items measure predominantly athletic performance-related physical fitness: standing long jump, 50-yard dash, and shuttle run. The remaining three items—sit-ups, distance run, and pull-ups (boys) and flexed-arm hang (girls)—measure primarily health-related physical fitness. The Youth Fitness Test was published by the American Alliance for Health, Physical Education, Recreation and Dance (AAHPERD), which is one of the national organizations that has assumed responsibility for fitness test development. The test manual (AAHPER, 1976) contains test instructions, national norms for each item, and information on the award system for the test.

The first version of the youth fitness test was published in 1958. Seven test items were included in the original battery, with each test judged to be a valid component of fitness. Both the age and classification norms were revised (Hunsicker and Reiff, 1966) and were published in the 1965 revision of the test manual. The classification norms were based on a combination of age, height, and weight. The normative data in the 1965 manual showed considerable improvement on most test items for boys and girls at almost every level. In 1975 the battery was revised:

1. The sit-up was changed from a straight-leg to a bent-knee position to provide a more accurate measure of strength of the abdominal muscles.
2. The softball throw was eliminated because it measured a specific skill to a large extent, whereas the primary purpose of the battery was to measure fitness.
3. The 600-yard walk-run was modified to include two optional runs: the 1-mile or 9-minute run for ages 10 to 12 or the 1.5-mile or 12-minute run for children age 13 or older. The optional runs were recommended as valid substitutes in schools where extensive running is a regular part of the physical education program.

In 1976, a revised set of age norms was published, and the use of classification norms was dropped. The organization of the test battery and the development of national norms represented a significant contribution to the physical education field. The test was popular in many parts of the United States for a variety of reasons—the items were motivating to students and the award system enabled them to receive national recognition for their performance on the test. Furthermore, many valued the measurement of a combination of health-related and athletic performance-related physical fitness. However, the test did not reflect a definition of health-related fitness that applies to all individuals, as does the Physical Best Test, the FITNESSGRAM test, and several others. The Youth Fitness Test was not a test that would appeal in its entirety to older age groups in general. Questions have also been raised about the measurement characteristics of the test, in particular, the validity and reliability. In the test manual, no validation procedures were described for the individual test items, except for a general statement of expert opinion regarding the important components of fitness. Reliability estimates for the various age groups on the battery items were not reported in the manual. However, studies of the Youth Fitness Test have been published in a variety of journals, and an effort has been made to incorporate this information into the test descriptions presented in the next section. Generally, these studies have reported that the items in the Youth Fitness Test have satisfactory reliability.

The following test items are popular performance-related physical fitness items. The first item (Pull-Ups or Flexed-Arm Hang) is also viewed as a health-related physical fitness item, especially for female examinees. However, it is often used as a performance-related item in activities with high upper body strength/endurance demands. Note that this test has been included in several of the recently revised national fitness tests described in the last chapter.

Pull-Ups (Boys) and Flexed-Arm Hang (Girls) (AAHPER Youth Fitness Test, 1976)

Test Objective To measure arm and shoulder girdle strength.

Description To perform the **Pull-Ups Test,** the student begins by hanging from the bar by using an overhand (palms outward) grip (see Figures 17-1 and 17-2) with his legs and arms fully extended. The feet should not contact the floor. From the hanging position, the student raises his body using his arms until his chin is positioned over the bar. He then lowers his body to a full hang, the starting position. This task is repeated as many times as possible. One trial is allowed.

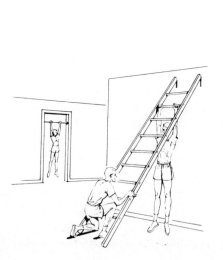

FIGURE 17-1 *Equipment options for Pull-Ups Test.*
From Youth Fitness Test Manual.

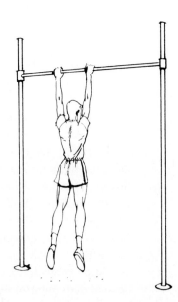

FIGURE 17-2 *Starting position for Pull-Ups Test.*
From Youth Fitness Test Manual.

In the **Flexed-Arm Hang Test,** two spotters should assist in administering the test, one in front and one in back of the girl. The height of the bar should be adjusted so that it is approximately equal to the standing height of the examinee. The correct position of the hands is depicted in Figures 17-3 and 17-4. With the assistance of both spotters, the examinee lifts the girl's body off the floor until her chin is positioned above the bar, elbows flexed, and the chest close to the bar. This position should be held as long as possible. One trial is allowed.

Test Area For the Pull-Ups Test, the manual suggests that only space adequate for the equipment is needed. A doorway, a small area for an inclined ladder, or a separate bar unit would suffice. The Flexed-Arm Hang Test can be administered in the same space.

Equipment Metal or wooden bar roughly 1½ inches in diameter (alternatives are a doorway gym bar, a piece of pipe, or an inclined ladder).

Scoring The score for the Pull-Ups Test is the number of completed pull-ups to the nearest whole number. For the Flexed-Arm Hang Test, the score is the number of seconds to the nearest second the student holds the hanging position. There is no criterion time after which the test should be terminated. The student should maintain the position as long as possible.

Validity No evidence of validity for either the Pull-Ups Test or the Flexed-Arm Hang Test is reported in the manual. Several educators and therapists have suggested that pull-ups might not be an adequate measure of arm strength. The

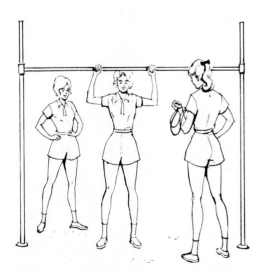

FIGURE 17-3 *Starting position for Flexed-Arm Hang Test.*
From Youth Fitness Test Manual.

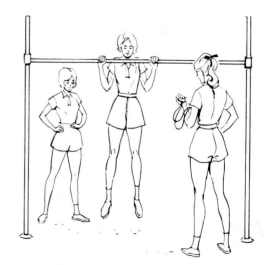

FIGURE 17-4 *Flexed-Arm Hang.*
From Youth Fitness Test Manual.

criterion measure was an isokinetic dynamometer pull, designed to determine the amount of force exerted in foot-pounds at any given point throughout the range of motion. The correlations between this measure and both the flexed-arm hang and pull-ups were low, as were the relationship between the latter two measures and lean body mass. The isokinetic measure, however, was related to lean body mass. This analysis demonstrated the inability of pull-ups and the flexed-arm hang to provide an indicator of the full range of arm and shoulder girdle strength. It is also suggested that fatness, not total body weight, affected performance on both these test items.

The muscular strength and endurance of the arms and shoulder girdle involve the ability to move or support one's weight with the arms. Both strength and endurance are needed to execute the flexed-arm hang/pull-up, but in varying degrees for different people. Performance on these tests is negatively correlated with body weight, presumably because of the relationship between the tests and body fatness. Verifying that either test measures strength and endurance is difficult. When the endurance tests dips and bench press were used to

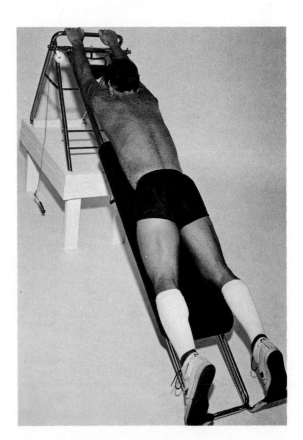

Starting position for the Modified Pull-Ups Test.

evaluate performance in body conditioning courses at the University of Houston, the correlation between the two tests was low, only 0.32. This indicates that the two tests measure different abilities. When a repetition bench press was correlated with the maximum weight a student could lift (strength), the correlation was over 0.90 (Jackson and Smith, 1974).

Modified Pull-Ups Tests Baumgartner (1978) devised a Modified Pull-Ups Test for all ages and both sexes. This test appears to resolve many of the difficulties associated with other measures of arm and shoulder girdle strength-endurance, such as pull-ups and the flexed arm-hang. A special piece of equipment now available commercially is used. Baumgartner suggests that the parts required to construct the equipment can be purchased for approximately $50.

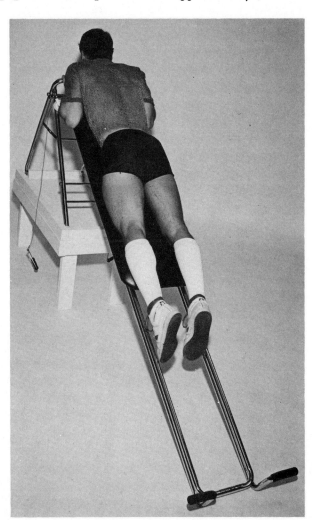

Up position for the Modified Pull-Ups Test.

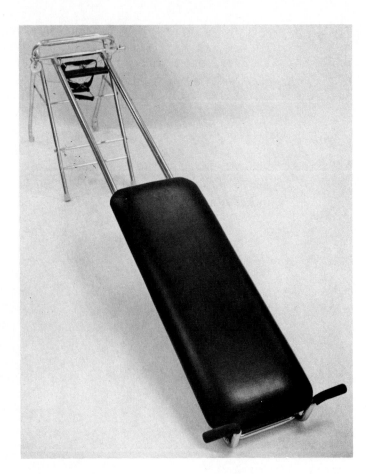

Equipment for Modified Pull-Ups Test.

In the modified test, the examinee performs pull-ups on an inclined board. An overhand grip is used, with hands placed shoulder-width apart. Otherwise, the test is performed like the regular pull-ups test. All examinees, including elementary schools girls and college women, were able to execute at least one pull-up; most performed four or more. Logical validity was claimed for the test. Only the data set for the college women was substantial enough to estimate reliability and calculate norms. The intraclass correlation coefficient for one trial over 2 days was 0.91, reflecting highly acceptable test reliability.

The equipment for the Modified Pull-Ups Test has recently been improved to make it safer (Baumgartner and others, 1984). Additional norms have also been developed for the test. For example, the 50th percentile for college males is 30 modified pull-ups; for college females, 11 modified pull-ups. Scores below 2 and above 60 are rare.

Another modification of the pull-ups test was used in the National Children and Youth Fitness Study II (Pate and others, 1987). This test is similar to an item in the Vermont Physical Fitness Test.

Modified Pull-Up Test (NCYFS II)

Test Objective To measure upper body muscular strength and endurance.

Description The examinee is positioned on his/her back with the shoulders directly below a bar that is set at a height 1 or 2 inches beyond the child's reach. An elastic band is suspended across the uprights parallel to and about 7 to 8 inches below the bar. The examinee grasps the bar, which raises the buttocks off the floor. The arms and legs are straight, and only the heels are in contact with the floor. An overhand grip (palm away from body) is used, and thumbs are placed around the bar (see Figure 17-5). To execute the pull-up, the examinee lifts the extended body until the chin is hooked over the elastic band (see Figure 17-6). The movement should be accomplished using only the arms, and the body must be kept straight. The examinee executes as many pull-ups as possible (no time limit), keeping the hips and knees extended through each attempt (Pate and others, 1987, pp. 71-72).

Test Area Only a small area is required for this test. A corner of the gymnasium would suffice.

Equipment A specially constructed device, depicted in Figures 17-7 and 17-8, was used in the NCYFS II study. However, the NCYFS staff suggest that any low pull-up bar that can be adjusted for height would suffice. The apparatus

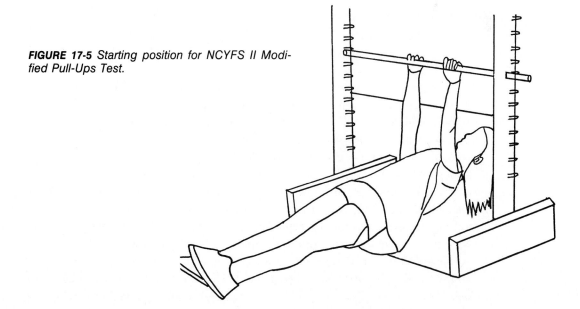

FIGURE 17-5 *Starting position for NCYFS II Modified Pull-Ups Test.*

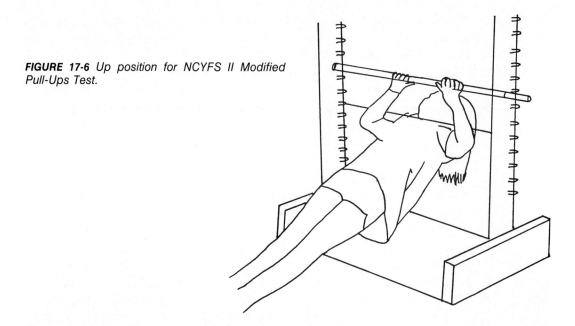

FIGURE 17-6 *Up position for NCYFS II Modified Pull-Ups Test.*

could be constructed for a minimal amount of money ($15–$35). The specifications can be obtained from Macro Systems.

Scoring Each complete pull-up is given a score of 1. Partial pull-ups are not scored. The total score is the number of complete pull-ups executed by the examinee.

Validity At the time this test was used in NCYFS II, it was validated on the basis of logical validity. Since then, Pate (1988) has conducted a validity study of the modified test. Satisfactory validity was established when the test was compared with tests of arm and shoulder girdle strength using weight machines.

Reliability Pate (1988) has reported a reliability coefficient of .80 for 94 elementary school children. Kollath (1989) found a higher reliability, .98, for high school students.

Comments The modified test is viewed as an improvement over the more traditional tests of upper body strength. Almost every child (boy or girl) can perform several pull-ups using the modified version of the test. On the other hand, it is not an easy test to administer. Some examinees experience difficulty in maintaining the hips in an extended position throughout the execution of the pull-up. According to the NCYFS II staff, this problem can be alleviated somewhat by orienting the child properly prior to administering the test.

Flexed-Arm Hang Cotten and Marwitz (1969) studied the validity of the flexed-arm hang for girls by comparing performance on the AAHPER Youth Fitness Test with a pull-ups test and a modified flexed-arm hang test. Pull-ups were

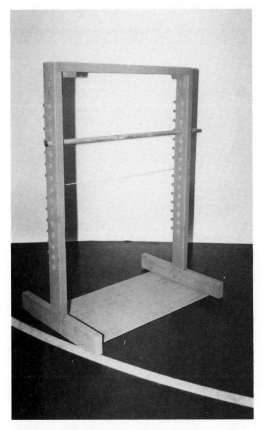

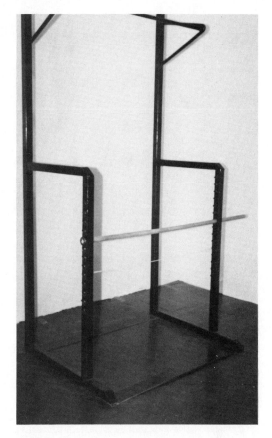

FIGURE 17-7 *Wood version of equipment for NCYFS II Modified Pull-Ups Test.*

FIGURE 17-8 *Metal version of equipment for NCYFS II Modified Pull-Ups Test.*

measured using the overhand grip and partial scores were given, up to 1 (0.25, 0.50, 0.75). The reliability of the pull-ups test was 0.89. The correlation between this test and the AAHPER Flexed-Arm Hang was 0.72. In the modified Flexed-Arm Hang Test developed by Cotten and Marwitz, the hanging position was identical to the AAHPER Test, but the stopwatch was allowed to run until the angle at the elbow became greater than 90 degrees. The reliability for the modified test was 0.83. The correlation between the modified hang and the pull-ups was 0.93. The results of this study indicate that the modified flexed-arm hang may be a better measure of the kind of arm strength measured by the pull-ups than the standard flexed-arm hang test. However, this conclusion must be viewed with caution, since the results were based on test scores of only 14 college women.

TABLE 17-1 *Reliabilities for AAHPER Youth Fitness Test items*

Item	Source	Sample	Trials (t) and days (d)	Reliability coefficient
Pull-ups	Klesius (1968)	150 tenth-grade males	1t 2d	0.89, 0.82
Flexed-arm hang	Cotten and Marwitz (1969)	14 female P.E. majors	2t 1d	0.74
Standing long jump	Klesius (1968)	150 tenth-grade males	2t 1d	0.94, 0.93
	Fleishman (1964)	Adult males	2t	0.90
	Kane and Meredith (1952)	100 males, age 7	12t[a], 1d	0.97
		100 females, age 7	12t[a], 1d	0.98
		100 males, age 8	12t[a], 1d	0.98
		100 females, age 8	12t[a], 1d	0.98
		100 males, age 9	12t[a], 1d	0.99
		100 females, age 9	12t[a], 1d	0.98
		75 males, age 7	12t 2d[b]	0.83
		75 females, age 7	12t 2d[b]	0.86

[a]Best of 12 correlated with second-best.
[b]Best of 12 on one day correlated with best of 12 on second day.
[c]Intraclass correlation coefficient.

Reliability Reliability estimates ranging from 0.74 to 0.89 have been reported for pull-ups and the flexed-arm hang. A summary of the reliabilities of AAHPER Youth Fitness items is presented in Table 17-1.

Norms Norms are published in the test manual for ages 9 through 17+ and both genders. An abbreviated form of the tables is presented in Tables 17-2 and 17-3.

Comments When administering the Pull-Ups Test, carefully monitor the alignment and positioning of the student's body. When the youth performs the Pull-Ups Test, the body must not swing during the execution of the movement. If the student begins swinging, the tester should check this by extending the arm across the front of the thighs. The examinee's body should remain vertical during the pull-up. Neither raising the knees nor kicking the legs is permitted. In the

TABLE 17-1 *Reliabilities for AAHPER Youth Fitness Test items—cont'd*

Item	Source	Sample	Trials (t) and days (d)	Reliability coefficient
50-yard dash	Baumgartner and Jackson (1970)	76 male P.E. majors	2t 1d	0.949[c]
	Klesius (1968)	150 tenth-grade males	2t 1d	0.86, 0.83
Softball throw	Klesius (1968)	150 tenth-grade males	2t 1d	0.93, 0.90
	Fleishman (1964)	adult males	2t	0.93
600-yard run-walk	Klesius (1968)	150 tenth-grade males	1t 2d	0.80, 0.80
	Wilgoose and others (1961)	70 junior high males	1t 2d	0.92
		70 junior high females	1t 2d	0.92
	Askew (1966)	71 senior high males	1t 2d	0.762
		46 senior high females	1t 2d	0.653
	Doolittle and Bigbee (1968)	9 ninth-grade males		0.92
Sit-ups	Klesius (1968)	150 tenth-grade males	1t 2d	0.57, 0.68
Shuttle run	Klesius (1968)	150 tenth-grade males	1t 2d	0.68, 0.75

Flexed-Arm Hang Test, the stopwatch should be started as soon as the student is fully supporting herself in the hanging position. Stop the watch when the chin touches the bar or falls below the level of the bar.

Gabbard and his associates (1983) studied the effects of grip and forearm position on flexed-arm hang performance. Superior performance on the hang was obtained with the forearm supinated (palms turned inward) and the thumb over the bar. Their work demonstrates the need for standardizing both the thumb and forearm positions in the flexed-arm hang test.

Shuttle Run Test (AAHPER Youth Fitness Test, 1976)

Test Objective To measure speed and change of direction.

Description For the **Shuttle Run Test** place two parallel lines on the floor 30 feet apart. Place two wooden blocks behind one of the lines as shown in Figure

TABLE 17-2 *Percentile rank norms for girls on the AAHPER flexed-arm hang test (in seconds)*

Percentile	Age							
	9-10	11	12	13	14	15	16	17+
95	42	39	33	34	35	36	31	34
75	18	20	18	16	21	18	15	17
50	9	10	9	8	9	9	7	8
25	3	3	3	3	3	4	3	3
5	0	0	0	0	0	0	0	0

Modified from Youth Fitness Test Manual.

TABLE 17-3 *Percentile rank norms for boys on the AAHPER pull-ups test (number)*

Percentile	Age							
	9-10	11	12	13	14	15	16	17+
95	9	8	9	10	12	15	14	15
75	3	4	4	5	7	9	10	10
50	1	2	2	3	4	6	7	7
25	0	0	0	1	2	3	4	4
5	0	0	0	0	0	0	1	0

Modified from Youth Fitness Test Manual.

17-9. The student starts from behind the other line. To start the test, use the signal *Ready, Go!* On the word *Go!* the student runs to the blocks, picks one up, runs back to the starting line, and places the block on the floor beyond the line. The student runs back, picks up the other block, and runs across the finish line as fast as possible. Start the stopwatch on the signal Go and stop it as the student crosses the starting line. Two trials are administered, with a rest in between.

Test Area An area equivalent to the width of a volleyball court is suitable.

Equipment Two blocks of wood, 2 inches by 2 inches by 4 inches, and a stopwatch. If two stopwatches are available, or one with a split second timer, two students can be tested at the same time.

Score The time of the better of two trials, recorded to the nearest tenth of a second, is the score.

Validity No studies have been conducted on the validity of the shuttle run test; however, the nature of agility has been studied. Several investigators (Hilsendager, Strow, and Ackerman, 1969) attempted to improve agility by in-

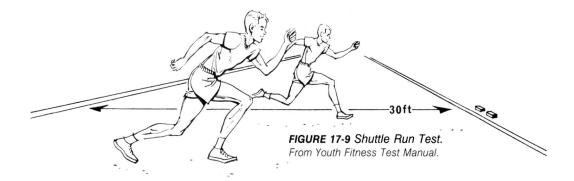

FIGURE 17-9 Shuttle Run Test.
From Youth Fitness Test Manual.

creasing speed and strength. They found that students who practiced specific agility items increased agility more than those who practiced either speed or strength. Their study also showed that the so-called agility tests that have been published do not measure the same underlying ability. The test directions for the shuttle run are more complex than for those of other items in the battery. Furthermore, the test tends to be less familiar to students. If the student has not had sufficient practice on this test, the score may represent performance on a novel task, rather than a test of agility.

Reliability Reliability estimates, based on test data, range from 0.68 to 0.75.

Norms Normative data have been published for boys and girls ages 9 to 10 through age 17+ in the AAHPER Youth Fitness Test Manual (AAHPER, 1976). An abbreviated form of the tables of norms is shown in Tables 17-4 and 17-5.

Comments To eliminate the necessity of returning the blocks after each trial, start the trials alternately, first from behind one line then from behind the other. Students should wear sneakers or run barefooted. Marmis and colleagues (1969) studied the number of trials needed for a reliable test and concluded that three instead of two trials of the shuttle run test should be administered.

Standing Long Jump (AAHPER Youth Fitness Test, 1976)

Test Objective To measure explosive leg power.

Description In the **Standing Long Jump Test** the student stands behind the restraining line, with feet several inches apart and the toes pointed straight ahead, as shown in Figure 17-10. To get ready for the jump, the examinee should swing the arms backward and bend the knees. To execute the jump, the student should swing the arms forward, extend the knees, and jump forward as far as possible, attempting to land on the feet and fall forward instead of backward if balance is lost. Three trials are taken.

Test Area The jump may be tested in an outdoor jumping pit or on a flat surface indoors or outdoors, with a clearance of 25 feet.

Equipment If testing takes place on a flat surface as opposed to a jumping pit, a mat is preferred; use a tape measure to determine the distance of the jump.

TABLE 17-4 *Percentile rank norms for girls on the shuttle run (in seconds and tenths)*

Percentile	Age							
	9-10	11	12	13	14	15	16	17+
95	10.2	10.0	9.9	9.9	9.7	9.9	10.0	9.6
75	11.1	10.8	10.8	10.5	10.3	10.4	10.6	10.4
50	11.8	11.5	11.4	11.2	11.0	11.0	11.2	11.1
25	12.5	12.1	12.0	12.0	12.0	11.8	12.0	12.0
5	14.3	14.0	13.3	13.2	13.1	13.3	13.7	14.0

Modified from Youth Fitness Test Manual.

TABLE 17-5 *Percentile rank norms for boys on the shuttle run (in seconds and tenths)*

Percentile	Age							
	9-10	11	12	13	14	15	16	17+
95	10.0	9.7	9.6	9.3	8.9	8.9	8.6	8.6
75	10.6	10.4	10.2	10.0	9.6	9.4	9.3	9.2
50	11.2	10.9	10.7	10.4	10.1	9.9	9.9	9.8
25	12.0	11.5	11.4	11.0	10.7	10.4	10.5	10.4
5	13.1	12.9	12.4	12.4	11.9	11.7	11.9	11.7

Modified from Youth Fitness Test Manual.

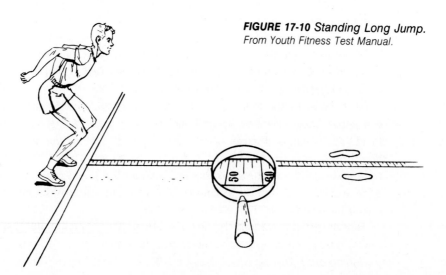

FIGURE 17-10 *Standing Long Jump.*
From Youth Fitness Test Manual.

TABLE 17-6 *Percentile rank norms for boys on the standing long jump (in feet and inches)*

	Age							
Percentile	9-10	11	12	13	14	15	16	17+
95	6' 0"	6'2"	6' 6"	7'1"	7'6"	8'0"	8'2"	8'5"
75	5' 4"	5'7"	5'11"	6'3"	6'8"	7'2"	7'6"	7'9"
50	4'11"	5'2"	5' 5"	5'9"	6'2"	6'8"	7'0"	7'2"
25	4' 6"	4'8"	5' 0"	5'2"	5'6"	6'1"	6'6"	6'6"
5	3'10"	4'0"	4' 2"	4'4"	4'8"	5'2"	5'5"	5'3"

Modified from Youth Fitness Test Manual.

TABLE 17-7 *Percentile rank norms for girls on the standing long jump (in feet and inches)*

	Age							
Percentile	9-10	11	12	13	14	15	16	17+
95	5'10"	6' 0"	6' 2"	6'5"	6' 8"	6' 7"	6'6"	6' 9"
75	5' 2"	5' 4"	5' 6"	5'9"	5'11"	5'10"	5'9"	6' 0"
50	4' 8"	4'11"	5' 0"	5'3"	5' 4"	5' 5"	5'3"	5' 5"
25	4' 1"	4' 4"	4' 6"	4'9"	4'10"	4'11"	4'9"	4'11"
5	3' 5"	3' 8"	3'10"	4'0"	4' 0"	4' 2"	4'0"	4' 1"

Modified from Youth Fitness Test Manual.

Scoring Measure the distance from the restraining line to the heel or other part of the body that touched the floor closest to the restraining line. If the student falls backward and touches the testing surface with the hand, the distance is measured from the part of the hand closest to the restraining line to the line itself. Record the best of three trials in feet and inches to the nearest inch.

Validity The standing long jump is generally accepted as an adequate measure of explosive power, although an element of timing exists in executing the jump that does not exist to the same extent for other measures of explosive power such as the vertical jump. The validity of this test might be improved by standardizing the directions for executing the jump.

Reliability This item tends to be highly reliable, with reliability coefficients ranging from 0.83 to 0.99 in various studies.

Norms National norms have been published for boys and girls, ages 9 to 10 through 17+. An abbreviated form of the tables of norms is shown in Tables 17-6 and 17-7.

Comments Be sure the student knows how to perform a jump off both feet, landing on both feet. Children who are not familiar with this procedure have been tested, and their natural tendency is to jump off one foot. Of course, this invalidates the trial, and valuable time must be spent in teaching the student how to execute the jump properly. If the test is administered indoors, tape the tape measure to the floor and stand to the side, noting the distance to the nearest inch after each jump. Marmis and colleagues (1969) studied the number of trials recommended by the test manual and concluded that only two trials of the standing long jump are needed.

50-Yard Dash (AAHPER Youth Fitness Test, 1976)

Test Objective To measure speed.

Description For the **50-Yard Dash Test** the student assumes a standing start behind the restraining line. Use the commands Are you ready? and Go!, timing the latter signal with a downward sweep of the arm. The student runs as fast as possible, without slowing down until he or she crosses the finish line (see Figure 17-11). The stopwatch is started as the starter's arm reaches the downward position and is stopped as the finish line is crossed. Two trials are taken.

Test Area Usually administered outdoors, using any open area.

Equipment One stopwatch is essential; using two watches or a split-second timer for simultaneous testing of two students is recommended.

Scoring Record the time in seconds to the nearest tenth of a second.

Validity Performance in the 50-yard dash is a function of running efficiency as well as pure speed. The student must clearly understand that slowing down before reaching the finish line will invalidate the test.

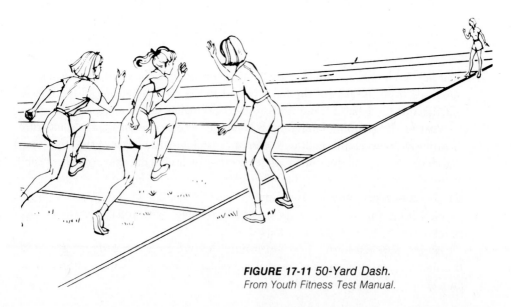

FIGURE 17-11 *50-Yard Dash.*
From Youth Fitness Test Manual.

Reliability Reliability coefficients ranging from 0.83 to 0.95 have been reported. The 50-yard dash is a very reliable measure, but the greatest source of error occurs during the first 20 yards. The student requires time to build up maximum speed. However, the test as a whole has satisfactory reliability. Only if finer discrimination is desired might the teacher consider timing only the last 30 yards of the dash test as the student's score. Norms must then be developed for the modified test.

Norms Norms have been published for boys and girls, ages 9 to 10 through 17+. An abbreviated form of the tables of norms is presented in Tables 17-8 and 17-9.

Comments Require the students to practice starting the test with the maximum possible speed and continuing at the fastest speed possible until past the finish line. Motivation is always important in test administration but especially in tests of short duration.

TABLE 17-8 *Percentile rank norms for girls on the 50-yard dash (in seconds and tenths of seconds)*

	Age							
Percentile	9-10	11	12	13	14	15	16	17+
95	7.4	7.3	7.0	6.9	6.8	6.9	7.0	6.8
75	8.0	7.9	7.6	7.4	7.3	7.4	7.5	7.4
50	8.6	8.3	8.1	8.0	7.8	7.8	7.9	7.9
25	9.1	9.0	8.7	8.5	8.3	8.2	8.3	8.4
5	10.3	10.0	10.0	10.0	9.6	9.2	9.3	9.5

Modified from Youth Fitness Test Manual.

TABLE 17-9 *Percentile rank norms for boys on the 50-yard dash (in seconds and tenths of second)*

	Age							
Percentile	9-10	11	12	13	14	15	16	17+
95	7.3	7.1	6.8	6.5	6.2	6.0	6.0	5.9
75	7.8	7.6	7.4	7.0	6.8	6.5	6.5	6.3
50	8.2	8.0	7.8	7.5	7.2	6.9	6.7	6.6
25	8.9	8.6	8.3	8.0	7.7	7.3	7.0	7.0
5	9.9	9.5	9.5	9.0	8.8	8.0	7.7	7.9

Modified from Youth Fitness Test Manual.

600-Yard Run (AAHPER Youth Fitness Test, 1976)

Test Objective To measure cardiorespiratory (CR) function.

Description Instruct the student to use a standing start. Give the signal Ready, Go!, and start the stopwatch on the signal Go!. The student begins running and continues running as fast as possible until he or she crosses the finish line. Although the examinee may walk during the test, it is not encouraged. One trial is taken.

Test Area A variety of open spaces is suitable. See the examples presented in Figures 17-12 to 17-14.

Equipment A stopwatch.

Scoring The time is recorded in minutes and seconds. A partner should be identified for each runner. The partner either records the time or remembers it and reports it to the scorer.

Validity When the 600-Yard Run has been correlated with a measure of max $\dot{V}O_2$, moderate correlations have resulted, ranging from -0.27 to -0.71. This re-

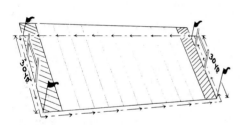

FIGURE 17-12 *Using football field for 600-Yard Run Test.*
From Youth Fitness Test Manual.

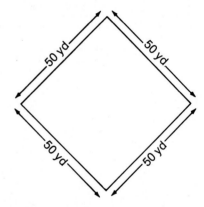

FIGURE 17-13 *Using any open area for 600-Yard Run Test.*
From Youth Fitness Test Manual.

FIGURE 17-14 *Using inside track for 600-Yard Run Test.*
From Youth Fitness Test Manual.

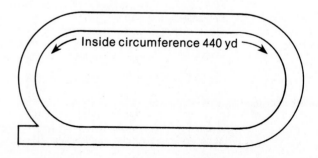

sult means that there is some relationship between the test and criterion measure, but the relationship is not substantial. As the walk-run scores improve (i.e., distance is run in a shorter time), the max $\dot{V}_{O_2}$ scores also get better (i.e., scores are higher) for some subjects. However, this does not happen in all cases; thus the relationship is not very strong. The 600-yard run, then, may not be an adequate predictor of CR endurance. (See Chapter 16 for a more detailed treatment of this topic.) The options available for this test (1 mile or 9 minutes; 1½ mile or 12 minutes) have greater validity.

Reliability Reliability coefficients ranging from 0.65 to 0.92 have been reported. In general, the estimates are high, suggesting that with proper motivation, the test can be properly administered.

Norms Norms have been published for boys and girls, ages 9 to 10 through 17+. An abbreviated form of the tables is shown in Tables 17-10 and 17-11.

TABLE 17-10 *Percentile rank norms for boys on the AAHPER 600-yard run (in minutes and seconds)*

Percentile	Age							
	9-10	11	12	13	14	15	16	17+
95	2:05	2:02	1:52	1:45	1:39	1:36	1:34	1:32
75	2:17	2:15	2:06	1:59	1:52	1:46	1:44	1:43
50	2:33	2:27	2:19	2:10	2:03	1:56	1:52	1:52
25	2:53	2:47	2:37	2:27	2:16	2:08	2:01	2:02
5	3:22	3:29	3:06	3:00	2:51	2:30	2:31	2:38

Modified from Youth Fitness Test Manual.

TABLE 17-11 *Percentile rank norms for girls on the AAHPER 600-yard run (in minutes and seconds)*

Percentile	Age							
	9-10	11	12	13	14	15	16	17+
95	2:20	2:14	2:06	2:04	2:02	2:00	2:08	2:02
75	2:39	2:35	2:26	2:23	2:19	2:22	2:26	2:24
50	2:56	2:53	2:47	2:41	2:40	2:37	2:43	2:41
25	3:15	3:16	3:13	3:06	3:01	3:00	3:03	3:02
5	4:00	4:15	3:59	3:49	3:49	3:28	3:49	3:45

Modified from Youth Fitness Test Manual.

Comments Before administering any of the distance run tests, warm-up preparatory training is essential. The student should be instructed about proper pacing and running efficiency. A group of students may be tested at one time, each working with a partner. The student should not attempt to run as fast as possible but should run at a pace that can be maintained throughout the entire distance. However, this pace should be maintained at as fast a rate as possible during the test. As discussed previously, the 600-yard run is not the best field test of CR function. The optional tests, which consist of the longer distance runs, are strongly recommended, even for young children. This test was included, nonetheless, for the benefit of those physical educators who believe that the only feasible distance runs for children should be shorter than a mile. Abbreviated forms of the tables for longer distances are included in Chapter 16.

EXAMPLES OF OTHER TESTS

There are many versions of the tests designed to measure physical fitness. In general, the older tests do not differentiate between health-related physical fitness and athletic performance-related physical fitness. Many of these tests include both types of items. As long as it is understood that both types of fitness are being measured, the tests can provide useful information on the fitness state of the individual.

Manitoba Physical Fitness Performance Test

The province of Manitoba has taken leadership in Canada by developing the Manitoba Physical Fitness Performance Test, which identifies desirable fitness and life-style objectives for Canadian school children and teachers. The test measures primarily the health-related fitness of youths ages 5 through 19. However, an agility item is included, which is a questionable measure of health-related fitness, according to the manual. Six items are included in the test battery:

1. One-Minute Speed Sit-Ups—to measure abdominal endurance
2. Sit and Reach—to measure flexibility
3. Flexed-Arm Hang—to measure upper body muscular endurance
4. Agility Run—to measure agility
5. Meter Run—to measure CR endurance
6. Skinfold Measurement—to measure subcutaneous body fat (biceps, triceps, subscapular, and suprailiac)

A fine test manual has been published for this battery. Although extensive technical material on reliability and validity is not included, the test descriptions are excellent. The manual also includes general guidelines for test administration, suggestions to improve performance, tables of percentile norms for students, and an excellent section on criterion-referenced standards for students, ages 5 through 19, and teachers, ages 20 to 60+! While the standards may be tentative and need further study, the Canadian test presents the first large-scale effort to identify performance standards in the fitness area for a large population of individuals.

ADMINISTRATION OF PHYSICAL FITNESS TESTS

Tests of motor performance are more complex to administer than most written tests. First, the examinee must understand the test instructions. Then he or she must be able to translate these instructions into the movements required by the test. Assume, for example, that John is taking a shuttle run test for the first time. On the first attempt he makes several errors. Perhaps he threw the block across the line, instead of placing it on the floor, or maybe he forgot the number of times he should change directions. Did the errors occur because he did not understand the instructions or because he was unable to follow them? Before actual testing, John should see a demonstration of the test, first in slow motion and then at full speed. Then he should be allowed to move through the test slowly

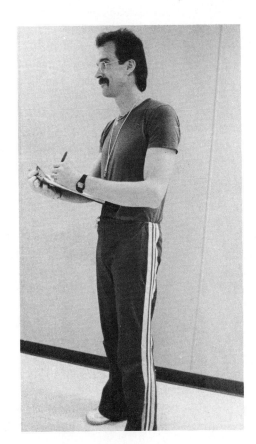

Test administrator.

while the test administrator gives him cues on his movements. The test instructions can also be written on an index card and posted on a bulletin board in the gym. If a student has difficulty with the instructions, a review of the written instructions might be helpful. Finally, John should have the opportunity to practice the test at maximum speed. Now John is ready to be tested. Remember that if John cannot perform the test properly, the trial must be thrown out and another taken. This is time-consuming and inefficient. The time taken in preparing examinees for the test is time well spent.

Preparation for Testing

When fitness tests are administered, test users expect the student to perform at his or her maximum ability. If John had not received the preparation described previously, his agility would not be tested; rather, his ability to perform a novel task would be measured. This really is not the purpose of administering the shuttle run test. Although proper preparation for testing should be emphasized, it can, on the other hand, be carried to extremes. Requiring the student to practice the shuttle run test day after day as part of the regular physical education program makes no sense. If practicing the shuttle run increases the student's agility, some practice is justifiable. However, other means of improving the student's agility are probably incorporated into the physical education program. This is an assumption, since no valid measure of overall agility has been developed. Furthermore, it is more likely that agility is highly task-specific. This means that one's performance on the AAHPER Shuttle Run Test might not reflect how well (or poorly) one would perform on another agility test. Yet it is still very popular in the physical education field to select a single test, such as the shuttle run, as a measure of a component of fitness (agility), assuming that this test measures one's "general" agility. This is not a fault of the test but rather of the test user who is making an erroneous assumption about the test.

Many practical matters should be considered in preparing examinees for a test. One such matter is the clothing worn for the test. In junior and senior high, where students are often expected to bring appropriate clothes for their physical education class, this is not a problem. In the elementary school where special gym wear may not be required, the clothes worn on the day that fitness tests are to be administered can create problems. A wide variety of clothing is satisfactory, however, if the student can move freely. Athletic shoes should always be worn, whether testing takes place indoors or outdoors. Without them it is unlikely that maximum performance can be achieved. No matter how hard one may try, running as fast as possible in leather soled shoes is difficult, if not impossible. Although wearing various types of sport shoes is now quite common for students, these should not be worn in a gym because of the dirt collected on the soles. Even for outdoor testing, the sport shoes worn on a daily basis may not be preferred, especially if the shoes are in poor condition. Removing the shoes during testing does not solve the problem; it merely creates a new one. For example, if a shuttle run test is performed indoors with bare feet, the quick shift of direction can create enough friction between the floor and the bottoms of the feet to be painful and cause blisters. Simply be firm about having students bring proper shoes, instructing them well in advance of the testing day.

Because fitness testing is usually conducted on a mass testing basis, assistants are often needed. Students, teachers, parents, or other members of the community can be recruited as assistants. They should be thoroughly familiarized with the tests they will administer, which will not occur if they are simply given the test instructions to read. The following is a good rule of thumb to follow: Preparing properly for testing always takes longer than you think it will! Do not assume anything. Bring assistants together for a practice session. Review and demonstrate the tests, giving each assistant experience in administering the tests or performing the assigned administrative task. Even when a test is administered year after year in a school, a brief review of procedures is essential. This is equally important in a nonschool setting where new clients are continually coming into the program and the same tests are administered frequently. A periodic check of testing procedures should take place. Provide all materials needed to administer and score the test, and be sure the assistants know how to use them.

In addition to training assistants, frequently equipment must be gathered or lines and targets must be placed for testing. Adequate time must be allowed for setting up the test, which can be very time-consuming. In fact the amount of time required to set up for the test is often the primary factor in deciding to use the test. This factor alone has prevented teachers from using some well-designed tests in physical education classes. If tape will be used for the lines or the target, take care of the taping ahead of time. If good quality tape is used, it will not damage the gym floor and is durable enough that it can remain on the floor for several weeks. If a wall target is to be formed with tape, be sure that the texture of the wall will support the tape. Little problems like adhesive tape can ruin an entire testing session. Plan carefully for the testing session, and have an alternate strategy ready to put into operation for each possible problem.

Data Processing of Physical Fitness Test Results

The process of administering fitness tests to a large group of people is itself an enormous task. Once test scores have been recorded, the test user is faced with the job of analyzing them. There is no point administering the tests if you do not use the results. Many school districts own a mainframe computer or a minicomputer or have access to one. Until recently, this provided the best mechanism for analyzing fitness data. It is still preferred when dealing with large data sets. For example, physical fitness teachers in Illinois have access to a computerized system for analyzing scores on a national physical fitness test. The results can be sent to Northern Illinois University, where the scores are fed into a computer and analyzed descriptively. The computer output containing the results of the analysis is then sent back to the school system. This procedure is also handled locally within a number of school systems around the country, generally when the system has access to a mainframe or a minicomputer. Now the availability of the microcomputer opens up these services to virtually any professional in the country. In Chapter 5, a sample program to convert raw scores to T-scores is included. This is written more as an example for students than a program to be used by teachers, but it serves to exemplify the ease with which these types of programs can be made available to the teacher. Every teacher need not learn how to write programs; however, properly written programs can easily be used by any teacher. (See Chapters 4 and 5 for more information on microcomputers.)

Several microcomputer programs are available for summarizing data from fitness tests and for determining norms. The following programs can be purchased at modest prices:

To be used with the AAHPERD Physical Best Fitness Test for ages 7 through 17+:

AAHPERD
1900 Association Drive
Reston, VA 22091

To be used with the FITNESSGRAM Program:

FITNESSGRAM
Institute for Aerobics Research
12330 Preston Road
Dallas, TX 75230

Number of Trials

When a test is developed, information is always included on the number of trials to be administered. In this way the motor performance test differs significantly from the written test. The written test contains a number of test items, each different from the other. The motor performance test consists of one or more trials, each one exactly the same. There are reasons for this difference, of course. Repeating the same test item in a written test would make no sense. On the other hand, attempting to vary each trial on a motor performance test is nonsensical. Even though the examinee knows the next trial will be the same as the previous one, mental memory differs from motor memory in this context. This knowledge does not mean the trial will be performed in the same way as the previous one, despite the examinee's effort to do so (or change it if the previous performance was not satisfactory).

How, then, is the number of trials determined? The number is usually determined by finding out how many trials are needed for a reliable performance.

Let's suppose you are interested in developing a bowling test. You decide in advance that the test ought to have a reliability of at least 0.80. After completing the test, you decide to work with 10 trials as a starter. You administer the test to a group of students and determine that the reliability of the test is 0.92. This is above the target reliability, but you may decide to use the 10-trial test. However, maybe you could use fewer trials and still reach your target reliability. This has significant practical advantage in that the test would take less time to administer. After experimenting with different numbers of trials, which can be done with a formula (see the discussion of the Spearman-Brown Prophecy formula in Chapter 6), you find that a 5-test trial yields a reliability of 0.82. The test has been reduced in half, and it still has acceptable reliability! The main point is that the number of trials of a test is not determined arbitrarily. One cannot casually decide to use a different number of trials than the number recommended by the test developer. Let's say you are interested in a batting test for elementary school children. You find a test you like, but it requires 20 trials. You decide there is not sufficient time to administer a 20-trial test in class, but a 10-trial test could be administered. Stop right here! You cannot simply drop 10 trials because you have no idea whether a 10-trial test is reliable. Unless you have time to determine the reliability of the shorter version of the test, you should not use it.

A lot of time and effort goes into determining the number of trials to include in a test. Surprisingly, many test users record the best trial out of the total number for an examinee's score. This practice is acceptable in a competitive situation or when the individual's best performance is of primary interest. In most physical education classes, test users are interested in the student's true ability rather than the student's day-to-day fluctuations. In other words, teachers would like to assume that there is some stability (or reliability) to the student's level of ability. Except for a few tests measuring maximum performance, one trial of a test is usually not adequate to reflect reliable performance.

To obtain a stable representation of performance, the effects of practice, learning, and fatigue must be eliminated. One way practice and learning are eliminated is to prepare the examinee properly, as described in the previous section. Practice trials are usually administered before the actual test for this reason. A good test developer will also plot the trial scores and examine them closely. If the trial scores systematically increase or decrease, obviously a reliable performance has not been obtained. Note the example presented in Figure 17-15. Six trials of a test were plotted in this figure. Notice that the scores increase from Trials 1 to 2, 2 to 3, and 3 to 4; then the performance stabilizes. If this test were administered to a student, the test developer might recommend that six trials actually be administered but the average of only the last three trials be used for the student's score.

Baumgartner and Jackson (1970) computed reliabilities for tests having **systematic increases** or **systematic decreases** in trial scores. The trials causing the

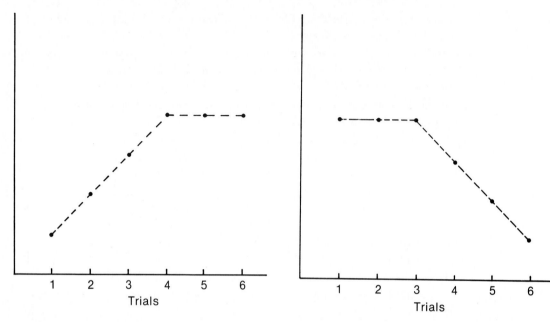

FIGURE 17-15 *Systematic increase in the scores of trials 1 to 4.*

FIGURE 17-16 *Systematic decrease in the scores of trials 4 to 6.*

systematic changes were then dropped, and reliabilities were estimated for the remaining trials. The standing long jump was one of the tests they studied. When six trials were administered to junior high school boys, their performance was stable on the first three trials but dropped off systematically over the last three trials. Presumably, the boys in this age group began to fatigue after the third trial, as depicted in Figure 17-16. Baumgartner and Jackson recommend that the test score be represented by the average of the first three trials. In this case only three trials must be administered. The reliability of the test under these conditions was reported as 0.96. When six trials of the same test were administered to high school boys, the scores increased systematically up to trial 4 (as in Figure 17-15) and then leveled off. Apparently a practice effect caused the change in scores. In this case, administration of a six-trial test was recommended, using the average of the last three trials as the test score. The reliability of the three-trial test was 0.97. Of course, it would be best if enough practice trials could be administered before the test to obtain stable test trials. At the very least, when administering a test with more than one trial, plot the trials on a piece of paper. Examine the plot for systematic changes. If they exist, you will have some evidence that performance is being affected by practice, learning, or fatigue. Nothing can be done about the test scores at that point, but the test user may decide not to place much weight on the results.

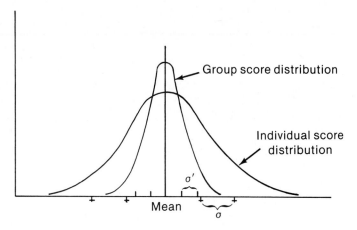

FIGURE 17-17 *Distribution of individual scores versus mean scores (σ = one standard deviation unit for individual score distribution; σ′ = one standard deviation unit for group score distribution).*
From Spray, J.A.

Use of Norms

It is very helpful if norms have been published for the test you have administered, especially if you wish to determine the effectiveness of your program. To be used properly, norms should be available for the same age and gender as the individuals tested. Then any score can be compared with the same score in the table of **individually based norms.** For example, the AAHPER Youth Fitness Test Manual includes tables of **percentile norms.** A test score can be matched with the same score on the appropriate norms table, and the percentile corresponding with this score can be read from this table.

The norms should be used to determine the percentile scores of individual students only. Using tables of norms to interpret group data, although appealing, is not appropriate. For example, assume a physical educator has administered the Youth Fitness Test to a group of students. A mean and a standard deviation is calculated for each test. The teacher refers to the tables of norms and matches each mean with a score in the appropriate table. The percentile for each mean is then read from the table. The teacher would like to be able to say, for example, that performance in the long jump for a group of students falls at the 70th (or some other) percentile. This procedure is incorrect! The norms tables were developed on the basis of individually based norms. As Spray (1977) demonstrates, a group mean should not be compared with individually based norms, since the variability of individually based norms differs from the variability of group means. Thus as is shown in Figure 17-17, the norm for the group mean is an underestimate if the class is above average and an overestimate if the class is below average. The same situation applies if the median is used.

TABLE 17-12 *Seventh- and eighth-grade boys' AAHPER Fitness Test results*

	Percent of students above the national 50th percentile
Eighth grade	
Shuttle run	88.6
600-yard run	77.5
Standing broad jump	72.3
Pull-ups	66.3
Sit-ups	65.2
50-yard dash	50.0
Seventh grade	
Shuttle run	87.6
Sit-ups	85.0
600-yard run	80.9
Standing broad jump	62.4
Pull-ups	58.0
50-yard dash	33.9

From Table 1 in Spray, J.A.

Spray (1977) describes several ways of interpreting group averages when only individually based norms tables are available. In one approach, the percentage of students receiving scores above the 50th percentile for the national norm group is identified for each test item. (For an example of this method, see Table 17-12.) This information could be very useful in evaluating a physical education program. Data for boys in all classes at each grade level were used in determining the percentages for the Waunakee group. Find the percentage of seventh-grade boys scoring at or above the 50th percentile on the Sit-ups test in Table 17-12. Since 85% of the boys performed more than 38 sit-ups, the number representing the 50th percentile for the national group norm, one could conclude that they have above-average abdominal and leg flexor strength. On the other hand, only 33.9% performed above the 50th percentile on the 50-yard dash, suggesting a need for modifications in the physical education program.

A second alternative is to compare the distribution for the national norm group to the distribution of scores for a class. In Figure 17-18, the distribution of scores on the Shuttle Run Test for all seventh-grade boys in a junior high school is compared with the distribution for the national norm group. A large portion of the distribution for the local group falls above the 50th percentile for the national group. In this case, lower times on the shuttle run reflect better performance;

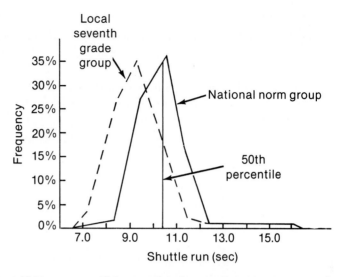

FIGURE 17-18 *Thirteen-year-old boys national norm group versus seventh-grade boys (Waunakee Jr. High School): shuttle run. The distributions appear to be positively skewed since a lower time implies a better performance on the shuttle run.*
From Spray, J.A.

therefore, the higher percentiles are located to the left of the 50th percentile. The same information is shown in Table 17-12 in tabular form.

TESTS OF PHYSICAL FITNESS KNOWLEDGE

Few tests of physical fitness knowledge are available to the physical fitness teacher. Mood (1971) prepared an extensively developed written test; two forms of this 60-item test are available. Ten content areas, including the physiological aspects of physical fitness, physical fitness programs, and nutritional aspects of fitness, are identified to describe the universe of content associated with physical fitness knowledge. Each area is weighted according to its degree of importance in the body of knowledge. In addition to describing the content validity of the test, Mood provides evidence of validity by examining the physical education grade point averages of high and low scorers on the fitness test. High scorers tended to have higher grades in physical education courses. Furthermore, physical education majors obtained higher scores on the knowledge test than non-majors, and students with a background in exercise physiology tended to score higher than those with no background. Test reliabilities ranged from 0.74 to 0.77. Since the test was developed over 10 years ago, a revision and update of the items would be appropriate.

SUMMARY

In this chapter, tests of performance-related physical fitness are discussed and differentiated from tests of health-related physical fitness, which are described in Chapter 16. A certain type of fitness only minimally related to the performer's positive health state is required for participation in athletic events. This does not mean health-related fitness is unimportant to the athlete, but rather that another type of fitness is required as well. However, while health-related physical fitness applies to the entire population of healthy individuals, athletic performance-related fitness is relevant primarily to persons performing in athletic events, including recreational participation as well as organized teams.

LEARNING EXPERIENCES

1. Administer several performance-related fitness items in your class or to a class of children in a neighborhood school. Average the scores for each test. (If you are a female, use the test scores for the females in class. If you are a male, use only the male test scores. Do not combine male and female data.) Since you cannot convert the class averages to percentiles using the tables of norms (Why can't you do this?) that have been published, how can you use the information in the tables to interpret your results? Interpret the results for all six tests.
2. Using one of the above data sets, calculate the z-score and T-score for each raw score in the group. If you need to review the formulas, see Chapter 3.
3. Write a short paper on the problems you encountered in administering the Youth Fitness Test. How could these problems be avoided in the future?

REFERENCES

American Alliance for Health, Physical Education and Recreation. 1976. Youth Fitness Test Manual. Washington, DC:AAHPER.

Askew, N.R. 1966. Reliability of the 600-yard run-walk at the secondary school level. Research Quarterly, **37**:451-454.

Baumgartner, T.A. 1978. Modified pull-up test. Research Quarterly, **49**:80-84.

Baumgartner, T.A. and others. 1984. Equipment improvements and additional norms for the modified pull-up test. Research Quarterly for Exercise and Sport, **55**(1):64-68.

Baumgartner, T.A., and Jackson, A.S. 1970. Measurement schedules for tests of motor performance. Research Quarterly, **41**:10-14.

Berger, R.A., and Medlin, R.L. 1969. Evaluation of Berger's 1-RM chin test for junior high males. Research Quarterly, **40**:460-463.

Burke, E.J. 1976. Validity of selected laboratory and field tests of physical working capacity. Research Quarterly, **47**:95-104.

Considine, W.J. 1973. An analysis of selected upper body tasks as measures of strength (abstract). AAHPER Research Section.

Cotten, D.J., and Marwitz, B. 1971. Relationship between two flexed arm hangs and pull-ups for college women. Research Quarterly, **40**:415-416.

Doolittle, T.L., and Bigbee, R. 1968. The twelve minute run-walk: a test of cardiorespiratory fitness of adolescent boys. Research Quarterly, **39**:491-495.

Falls, H.B., Ismail, A.H., and McCleod, D.F. 1966. Estimation of maximum oxygen uptake in adults from AAHPER Youth Fitness Test items. Research Quarterly, **37**:192-201.

Fleishman, E.A. 1964. The structure and measurement of physical fitness. Englewood Cliffs, NJ: Prentice-Hall, Inc.

Gabbard, C., Gibbons, E., and Elledge, J. 1983. Effects of grip and forearm position on flexed arm hang performance. Research Quarterly for Exercise and Sport, 54(2):198-199.

Hilsendager, D.R., Strow, M.H., and Ackerman, K.J. 1969. Comparison of speed, strength, and agility exercises in the development of agility. Research Quarterly, 37:71-75.

Hunsicker, P., and Reiff, G. 1966. A survey and comparison of youth fitness 1958-1965. Journal of Health, Physical Education and Recreation, 37:22-25.

Jackson, A.S., and Baumgartner, T.A. 1969. Measurement schedules of sprint running. Research Quarterly, 40:708-711.

Jackson, A.S., and Smith, L. March, 1974. The validation of an evaluation system for weight training. Unpublished study presented at the AAHPER Convention, Anaheim, California.

Kendall, F.P. 1965. A criticism of current tests and exercises for physical fitness. Journal of the American Physical Therapy Association, 45:187-197.

Klesius, S.E. 1968. Reliability of the AAHPER Youth Fitness items and relative efficiency of the performance measures. Research Quarterly, 39:801-811.

Kollath, J. 1989. Reliability of the Modified Pull-ups Test. Unpublished Master's Thesis, University of Wisconsin, Madison.

Manitoba Department of Education. 1977. Manitoba Physical Fitness Performance Test and fitness objectives. Manitoba:Department of Education.

Marmis, C. and others. 1969. Reliability of the multi-trial items of the AAHPER Youth Fitness Test. Research Quarterly, 40:240-245.

Metz, K.F., and Alexander, J.F. 1970. An investigation of the relationship between maximum aerobic work capacity and physical fitness in twelve to fifteen year old boys. Research Quarterly, 41:75-81.

Mood, D. 1971. Test of physical fitness knowledge: construction, administration, and norms. Research Quarterly, 42:423-430.

Olree, H. and others. 1965. Evaluation of the AAHPER Youth Fitness Test. Journal of Sports Medicine and Physical Fitness, 5:67-71.

Pate, R.R., and Lonnett, M. 1988. Validity of field tests of upper body muscular strength. Unpublished manuscript.

Pate, R.R. and others. 1987. The modified pull-up test. Journal of Physical Education, Recreation and Dance, 58(9):71-73.

Ponthieux, N.A., and Barker, D.G. 1963. An analysis of the AAHPER Youth Fitness Test. Research Quarterly, 34:525-526.

Safrit, M.J. 1969. The physical performance of inner city children in Milwaukee, Wisconsin, Tech. Report. May 1969. University of Wisconsin, Milwaukee, Department of Physical Education.

Sigerseth, P.O. 1978. Flexibility. In H.J. Montoye, editor. An introduction to measurement in physical education. Boston: Allyn & Bacon, Inc.

Spray, J.A. 1977. Interpreting group or class performances using AAHPER Youth Fitness Test norms. Journal of Physical Education and Recreation, 48:56-57.

Wilgoose, C.E., Askew, N.R., and Askew, M.P. 1961. Reliability of the 600-yard run at the junior high school level. Research Quarterly, 32, 264-266.

ANNOTATED READINGS

Fragione, F.J. 1977. Integrating the why in measurement and evaluation. Journal of Physical Education and Recreation, **48**:56.

Stresses the need for physical education teachers to emphasize the "why" of physical activity in their classes; demonstrates the point using an agility test, a step test, and a hand-weight chart; adheres to the belief that students must understand the reason for participating in various forms of activity to become physically educated.

Hunsicker, P., and Reiff, G. 1977. Youth Fitness Report: 1958-1965-1975. Journal of Physical Education and Recreation, **48**:31-33.

Describes the large-scale studies of physical fitness using the Youth Fitness Test; reveals that little or no improvement took place from 1965 to 1975; compares both boys and girls in grades 5 through 12; samples selected from homerooms rather than physical education classes.

Plowman, S.A., and Falls, H.B. 1978. AAHPER Youth Fitness Test revision. Journal of Physical Education and Recreation, **49**:22-24.

Analyzes the Youth Fitness Test; discusses the rationale for revising the test; recommends a test that includes three components of health-related physical fitness—cardiorespiratory function, body composition, and musculoskeletal function.

Smith, C.D. 1972. Fitness testing: questions about how, why and with what. Journal of Health, Physical Education and Recreation, **43**:37-38.

Suggests ways to approach physical fitness testing; stresses the importance of being open to evolving new ideas about fitness testing; includes an analysis of AAHPER Youth Fitness Test and what it measures; discusses the value of each test item.

Vincent, W.J., and Britten, S.D. 1980. Evaluation of the curl-up. Journal of Physical Education and Recreation, **51**(2):74-75.

Discusses the inappropriateness of the straight leg sit-up based on scientific evidence; suggests that the bent knee sit-up is also unacceptable and provides a rationale for this conclusion; reports low reliabilities for the curl-up test; and notes several possible reasons for this unreliability.

Part Nine

Other Measures of Physical Performance

18

Tests of Sports Skills

Many examples of sports skills tests can be found in the literature. Collins and Hodges (1978) provide an excellent overview of a variety of these tests. The entire book is devoted to tests of skill in a variety of sports. A sampling of sports skills tests is included here to exemplify the types of tests that have been developed in the field of physical education. Describing all tests in each sport is unrealistic in a measurement and evaluation textbook. (See Chapter 10 for examples of skills tests for elementary school children. For information on other tests, refer to Collins and Hodges text and the AAHPERD skills test series, which is undergoing revision.)

Although key words have been included at the beginning of all other chapters in this book, they are omitted here, since the primary purpose of this material is to provide examples of sports skills tests for 13 sports: archery, badminton, baseball, basketball, field hockey, football, golf, racquetball, soccer, softball, swimming, tennis, and volleyball.

One precaution should be kept in mind when reviewing the test set-ups. Many tests of sports skills require the use of a target on the floor or the wall of the gymnasium. The use of masking tape and fiber tape should be avoided, since they can pull the seal off the floor. Special tape can be purchased that does not damage the floor. Water paints can also be used on some floors.

TYPES OF TESTS

Several types of measures can be used in testing a skill. These include time, distance, accuracy, and force. Measures of form (process) can also be included in skill assessment.

Measures of Time

When a time measure is used to measure a skill, the product rather than the process of skill execution is measured. The difference between process and product can be described using the example of measuring the speed of an ice hockey puck hit over a given distance. The *product*, the action of the puck, is being measured. The *process*, the force-producing actions of the player, is of indirect concern but is not directly measured. Time measures have also been used to measure the repeated executions of a skill.

Time measures are appropriate for speed events in such activities as swimming or track and for skills in which the projectile remains on the ground or floor, such as in ice hockey or bowling. (The assumption is that minimal resistance will result from the object contacting the ground or floor.) If the object is projected into the air, a velocity rather than a time measure should be used to measure force.

When a given number of executions of a skill is timed, the use of time as a measure has questionable validity. First, the examinee is encouraged to hurry at the expense of accuracy. Second, when measuring ball skills in this way, the ball rebounds off the wall continuously. There are very few sports in which the player is required to receive his or her own rebound. Thus, handling the rebound may add an unrealistic element of skill to the test. Third, the use of a single score in measuring repeated executions of a skill provides little diagnostic information on the skill itself. If throwing is being measured, for example, a ball rebounding off the wall may be poorly caught, resulting in a poor score. Thus the examinee's skill in catching affects the final score. Furthermore, this error might not occur on every execution of the skill. Measuring a single execution of a skill over several trials is preferable to measuring repeated executions within one trial.

Measures of Distance

Distance measures are frequently used to measure jumps and throws. A distance measure is probably adequate for measuring skill in jumping. However, when measuring skill in throwing, the distance measure is often inappropriate. Skill in throwing requires a combination of force and accuracy. If two objects are thrown, both might land at the same point, and yet the trajectories of the two objects might be quite different. In this case, both throws would be considered equally good if distance was used as the measure. However, only the accuracy of the two throws is identical; the force applied to each differs. Or, conversely, two objects might be projected with the same force and yet the distances of the two throws could vary, due to differences in the angle at which the ball is thrown. Thus skill in throwing should be measured by taking both the accuracy and force components of skill into account. This can best be done by utilizing both velocity and accuracy measures. The concept of measuring both force and accuracy does not apply to competitive situations in field events, where the skill is not a sport skill but rather is a specific skill involving coordination and power. The latter skill requires *maximum* force and *limited* accuracy as opposed to a throw in softball, where the accuracy demands are *high* and an *optimal* force is required.

Measures of Number of Executions in a Given Time

Another variety of motor skills tests measures the number of executions of a given skill that can be performed in a specified time period. A common example of this type of measure is a test of the number of repeated wall volleys executed in 30 seconds. The problems inherent in this type of test are similar to those described for measures of time: The examinee is required to receive his or her own rebound, the time limit stresses speed rather than accuracy, and the test has limited diagnostic value for the skill in question.

Measures of Velocity

Velocity measures take the speed, angle of projection, and distance components of the projectile skill into account. Thus, the force aspect of the skill is measured with a great deal of precision. Velocity is determined by dividing distance by time and is recorded in feet per second. Velocity should be used to measure any skill in which an object is projected into the air. The velocity score reflects the amount of force applied and should be accompanied by an accuracy measure.

Measures of velocity can be approximated in several ways. One method is to use ropes to measure the height of the trajectory. An early test in which a rope was used to measure force was the Tennis Drive Test, developed by Broer and Miller (1950). In this test a rope was placed 4 feet above the net, and any drive where the ball passed between the net and the rope was given a higher score than an equally accurate drive in which the ball passed over the rope. By giving more points for a ball that passes between the rope and the net, the velocity (or force) of the ball is taken into account in a rough fashion. However, Glassow (1957) showed that a wide range of velocities could be obtained within any given scoring area for this particular test and suggested the need for reducing the area between the rope and the net. A refinement of this method was developed by Liba and Stauff (1963) in the Volleyball Pass Test. Three ropes were used instead of one. The top rope was placed so that the trajectory of the volleyball would have a minimum high point of 15 feet in accordance with the definition of good performance. The remaining ropes defined scoring areas at lesser heights. Ropes are useful measures of force as long as their placement is such that the velocity scores within a given target area do not vary to a great extent. A 4-foot range in velocities within a given area should be acceptable. However, the use of the ropes will provide only an approximation of the force applied to the ball.

Another method of roughly assessing a component of velocity (vertical angle of projection) has been described by West and Thorpe (1968). In measuring the short shot in golf using the eight-iron, the authors used ratings of the vertical angle of projection to categorize the height of the trajectory. If the ball was hit at an angle of 29° or more, three points were given for the flight score. If the angle was judged to be less than 29°, two points were given. A topped ball received one point. Because of the subjectivity involved in making these judgments, the interjudge objectivity should be determined. (Intrarater objectivity was satisfactorily established for the West and Thorpe test.)

The most precise measure of velocity is electronic equipment such as the velocimeter currently in use at the University of Wisconsin. Less accurate but usable velocity scores can be obtained using a stopwatch and a wall target. This procedure was described by Safrit and Pavis (1969) for a measure of the force of the overarm softball throw. The velocity scores can be calculated using the method described in Cooper and Glassow (1976). This process is extremely time-consuming, and the use of velocity tables is recommended as a more expedient method. A velocity table for objects projected from a distance of 30 feet is presented in the appendix of the Cooper and Glassow (1963) book. Such tables can easily be developed through the use of a simple computer program.

Measures of Accuracy

Accuracy is one of the most frequently measured components of a skill and is generally measured using a target of some sort, which can range from the simple to the complex. In beginning badminton, for example, a useful target to aid in measuring the accuracy of the long serve might be a simple division of the long service court into three sections. Beginners should learn to hit the shuttlecock to the back section of the court.

It is assumed that the height of the trajectory is also being measured, as this is an important component of the badminton serve. The measurement of accuracy alone is insufficient for the assessment of this skill. Two shuttlecocks might land on the same section of the target and yet have different trajectories.

A more complicated target can be designed using arcs and rays for a more refined measure of accuracy. Deviations from the area with the greatest point value as well as distances from the net can be measured with this approach. Such a test would be diagnostic in that both an accuracy and a deviation score can be obtained. Almost all attempted serves will be scored, which is advantageous, because when many zero scores are obtained, no information is provided about the examinee's weaknesses.

Measures of Form

Often it is useful to measure form, the process by which the skill is executed. Measures of form are frequently carried out by means of a checklist or a rating scale. Both of these methods are discussed in later sections.

If the product is satisfactory, there is some question regarding the need to measure the process. For example, if a player can execute a good place-kick, does it matter if his form does not fit a typical pattern? Certainly a professional football coach would not consider changing a successful soccer-style place-kicker to the more traditional method of kicking off the toe. However, it may be desirable to measure beginners on some aspects of form, especially when deviations from the typical pattern of form are likely to hinder further development of the skill. As the learner develops a skill that is consistently satisfactory in terms of product, the instructor should no longer attempt to change idiosyncrasies in style. The measurement of form should probably be deemphasized after the players have advanced beyond the beginner's level in most sports activities, although this may not be true in such areas as movement education, dance, gymnastics, and swimming.

EXAMPLES OF TESTS
Archery Tests

AAHPER Archery Test (AAHPER, 1967)

Test Objective To measure skill in archery.

Description No more than four archers should be placed at each target. Two ends of six arrows each are shot at distances of 10, 20, and 30 yards for boys and 10 and 20 yards for girls. The test is started at the 10-yard distance. When all archers have completed two ends, the group moves back to the 20-yard line, and so forth. Any examinee not scoring at least 10 points at one distance is not permitted to shoot at the next distance.

Test Area Archery range adequate to test a group of archers at distances of 10, 20, and 30 yards or a standard-size gymnasium with proper backstops.

Equipment Standard 48-inch target faces; bows ranging from 15 to 40 pounds in pull; matched arrows 24 to 28 inches long.

Scoring Standard target scoring is used, with gold = 9, red = 7, blue = 5, black = 3, and white = 1. Arrows falling outside the white area are scored 0. Arrows bouncing off the target or passing completely through are awarded 7 points. The total test score is the sum of the total points at each distance.

Validity Face validity (a test that appears to be valid but has not been formally validated).

Reliability No reliability estimate given in test manual; manual includes statement that no test in the battery has a reliability less than .70, the AAHPER minimum standard.

Comments Abbreviated tables of norms for this test are included in Tables 18-1 and 18-2. Full-length tables are available in the manual. Four practice arrows are permitted at each distance. Generally, two class periods are required to administer the test to girls and three periods for boys.

Criterion-Referenced Archery Test (Shifflett and Shuman, 1982)

Test Objective To measure ability in archery using the criterion-referenced testing approach.

Description Examinees stand at a target line 20 yards from the target. Two ends (12 arrows) are shot at a 48-inch target face.

Test Area Indoor or outdoor archery range.

Equipment Bows (variety of weights), arrows (variety of lengths), targets, target faces, tripods, and scorecards.

TABLE 18-1 *Percentile ranks for AAHPER Archery Test; 20 yards—12 arrows; girls*

Percentile	Age				
	12-13	14	15	16	17-18
95	40	47	55	58	71
75	17	28	34	36	42
50	9	18	23	22	26
25	0	8	13	12	16
5	0	0	0	0	0

Abbreviated form of Table 6 of AAHPER.

TABLE 18-2 *Percentile ranks for AAHPER Archery Test; 20 yards—12 arrows; boys*

Percentile	Age				
	12-13	14	15	16	17-18
95	53	61	77	78	78
75	31	38	58	59	59
50	22	26	39	46	43
25	12	16	24	33	29
5	3	6	9	14	11

Abbreviated form of Table 2 of AAHPER.

Scoring Target scores of 1, 3, and 5 are converted to 0; scores of 7 and 9, to 1. The total test score is the sum of the converted scores for all 12 trials. A student with a test score of 5 or greater is classified as a *master* and with a test score of less than 5, a *nonmaster*.

Validity The validity coefficient is .73, based on test scores of college men and women using the instructed/uninstructed approach to validation.

Reliability $P = 0.87$, where P is the proportion of agreement between two administrations of the test; subjects—college women.

Comments The same test standard is used for both males and females. The test developers suggest that this test could be used to exempt students from a beginning archery class or to grade students in physical education where a pass-fail grading system is used.

Badminton Tests

Poole Long Serve Test (Poole and Nelson, 1970)

Test Objective To measure the ability to serve high and deep into the opponent's backcourt.

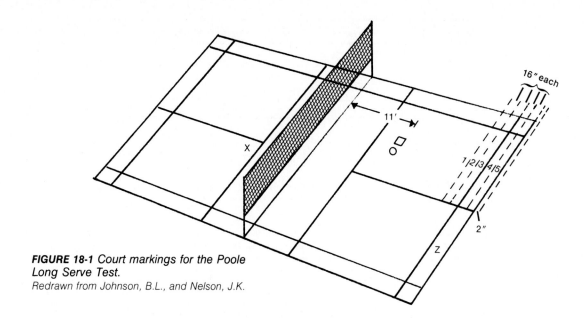

FIGURE 18-1 *Court markings for the Poole Long Serve Test.*
Redrawn from Johnson, B.L., and Nelson, J.K.

Description The examinee stands behind the short service line, anywhere in the service court diagonally opposite the target area. Twelve consecutive trials are taken, in which the examinee attempts to serve the shuttle over the extended racket of an assistant standing in a square 11 feet from the net, as shown in Figure 18-1.

Test Area Regulation-size badminton court.

Equipment Badminton rackets, 12 shuttlecocks, floor tape, and scorecards.

Scoring The scorer stands in the court adjacent to the target area. If the shuttlecock passes over the extended racket of the assistant, a check is recorded for height. The point value of the target area in which the shuttle lands is rescored for accuracy. If the shuttle does not pass over the racket, verified by the assistant calling "low," an X is recorded under "height" and one point is subtracted from the point value of the target area. The total test score is the sum of the best 10 of 12 trials.

Validity $r_{xy} = 0.51$, using the results of tournament play as a criterion measure.

Reliability $R_{xx'} = 0.81$, using the test-retest method; subjects—college men and women.

Comments Although this test is simpler to set up than the Scott-Fox Test (Scott and French, 1959), it is not as objective because an assistant with an extended racket is substituted for a rope. Poole and Nelson believe the use of an assistant is more realistic, but they agree that a rope could also be used to judge

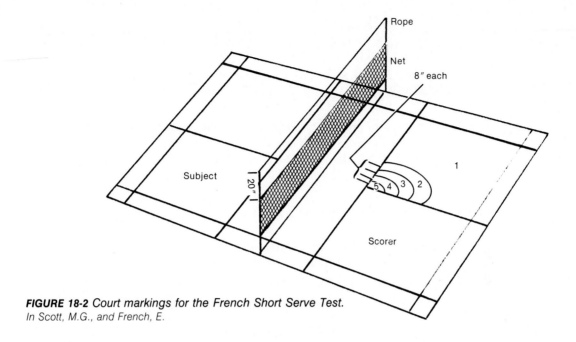

FIGURE 18-2 *Court markings for the French Short Serve Test.*
In Scott, M.G., and French, E.

the height of the serve. The test developers suggest that the height of the assistant is immaterial, except in extreme cases. The target area is more appropriate, compared with the Scott-Fox target, for examinees of average ability. Note that the target extends beyond the baseline by a few inches. Generally, a shuttle dropping into this area would be returned by the receiver. If this test cannot be used because of its length requirements, the authors recommend shortening it to the best 6 of 8 trials.

French Short Serve Test (Scott and Others, 1941)

Test Objective To measure the examinee's ability to serve accurately with a low and short placement.

Description The examinee stands behind the short service line, anywhere in the right service area, and takes 20 short serves. Each serve that passes between the net and the rope and lands in the target area shown in Figure 18-2 is scored. The serve must be executed legally; for example, the examinee may not take a step while performing the serve.

Test Area Regulation-size badminton court.

Equipment Badminton rackets, 25 shuttlecocks, rope to stretch above net, tape, and scorecards.

Scoring A scorer stands in the court adjacent to the target area and records a check if the shuttle passes between the rope and net and an X if it does not. The target score (5, 4, 3, 2, or 1) is also recorded if the height was acceptable; otherwise, a 0 is recorded for the target score. If the shuttle lands on a target line, the score value of the higher area is given. If it hits the rope, the trial is retaken. The total test score is the sum of 20 trials.

Validity r_{xy} = 0.66, using a criterion measure of ladder tournament rankings.

Reliability $R_{xx'}$ = 0.51 to 0.89; subjects—college women (physical education majors).

Comments Two practice trials are permitted. Approximately 20 students can be tested in a 60-minute period at a single testing station. This test is also appropriate for junior high and high school students. A version of the test adopted by the University of Wisconsin uses the same rope height but an easier target. Instead of a fan-shaped target, the Wisconsin version is a series of lines parallel to the short service line, with the highest point value given to the area closest to the service line.

Poole Forehand Clear Test (Poole and Nelson, 1970)

Test Objective To measure the ability to hit a forehand clear from the backcourt high and deep into the opponent's backcourt.

Description The examinee stands with one foot in the square marked X as in Figure 18-3. If the examinee is righthanded, the right foot should be in the square, and vice versa. Place the shuttle with the feather end down on the forehand side of the racket. The shuttle is tossed into the air by the examinee, who then hits an overhead forehand clear so that the shuttle passes over the extended racket of an assistant standing at point 0 as in Figure 18-3. The foot in contact with the square should remain so until the shuttle is hit; 12 trials are taken.

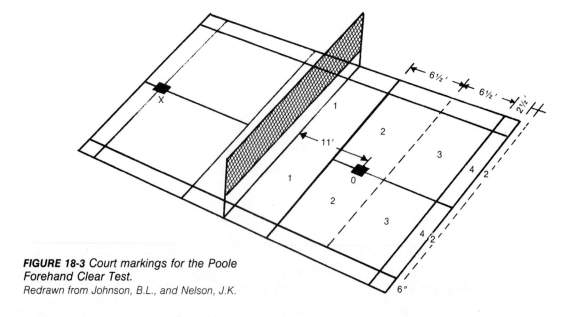

FIGURE 18-3 *Court markings for the Poole Forehand Clear Test.*
Redrawn from Johnson, B.L., and Nelson, J.K.

Test Area Regulation-size badminton court.

Equipment Badminton rackets, 12 shuttlecocks, floor tape, and scorecards.

Scoring Same as Poole Long Serve Test.

Validity $r_{xy} = 0.70$, using tournament play as a criterion measure.

Reliability $R_{xx'} = 0.90$, using test-retest method; subjects—college men and women.

Comments The test developers note that tossing the shuttle in the prescribed manner should be practiced on several occasions before actual testing. This test can also be used to measure the backhand clear, althought it is not quite as valid and reliable as the forehand clear test. A shortened version of the test, consisting of the best 6 of 8 trials, can be used.

Lockhart-McPherson Badminton Test (Lockhart and McPherson, 1949)

Test Objective To measure badminton playing ability.

Description The examinee assumes a service stance in back of the starting line on the floor 6½ feet from and parallel to the base of the wall. On the signal Ready Go! the examinee serves the shuttle against the wall. The shuttle is then hit as many times as possible during a 30-second time period, as long as it is hit from behind the restraining line, which is 3 feet from and parallel to the base of the wall and above a 5-foot line on the wall. Three 30-second trials are taken. A 15-second practice session is permitted before testing.

Test Area Smooth wall at least 10 feet by 10 feet and floor space of equal dimensions.

Equipment Racket, six shuttlecocks, stopwatch, tape measure, floor and wall tape, and scorecards.

Scoring A point is scored each time the shuttle is hit from behind the restraining line and strikes the wall on or above the 5-foot wall line. If the shuttle falls to the floor during a trial, the examinee must pick it up and restart the wall volley with a legal serve. If, while taking consecutive hits, the examinee steps on or across the restraining line or strikes under the wall line, the trial continues, but no points are scored. The total test score is the sum of the legal hits in three 30-second trials.

Validity $r_{xy} = 0.71$ to 0.90, using criterion measures of judges' ratings and round robin tournament rankings.

Reliability $R_{xx'} = 0.90$ (test-retest); subjects—college women.

Comments This test is appropriate for both males and females as young as junior high school age. It is easy to administer, and several testing stations can often be used with ease. However, the volleys are sometimes executed with poor form. In these cases proper form should immediately be stressed.

The Miller Wall Volley Test (Miller, 1951) is another version of this test. The lines are set higher and farther from the wall so that the performer must use an overhead clear to perform well on the test. The restraining line is 10 feet from the wall, and the wall height is 7½ feet from the floor. Although any type of stroke can be used in the Miller test, a definitive advantage exists for the player who is able to hit repeated clears against the wall.

Baseball Tests

Kelson Baseball Classification Plan (Kelson, 1953)

Test Objective To classify boys for baseball participation at the elementary school and Little League levels.

Description This is a simple baseball throw for distance. The testing takes place out-of-doors. The examinee, holding a baseball, either stands behind the restraining line or runs up to the line, as long as the line is not stepped on or over. Three trials are taken, with instructions to throw the ball as far as possible.

Test Area Level field 250 feet long and 50 feet wide; the throwing area is marked off from 50 to 200 feet with lines 5 feet apart.

Equipment Baseballs, field marking materials, tape measure, and scorecards.

Scoring The best of the three throws is the test score. Each of the three trial scores is recorded by the scorers. For the most effective scoring, it is recommended that scorers be positioned every 25 feet of the throwing area.

Validity $r_{xy} = 0.85$, using a criterion measure of a composite of baseball skills including batting averages and judges' ratings of throwing, catching, and fielding.

Reliability Not reported for this specific test.

Comments The strength of this test is purported to be its ability to classify boys in baseball quickly and easily. Kelson developed a classification chart that can be obtained from the original source (Kelson, 1953).

Basketball Tests

Speed Spot Shooting (Hopkins, Shick, and Plack, 1984)*

Test Objective "To measure skill in rapidly shooting from specific positions and, to a certain extent, agility and ball handling" (p. 9).

Description The player begins the test with one foot behind any one of five markers, as shown in Figure 18-4. The 15-foot markers are appropriate for grades 10, 11, and 12 and college. For upper elementary grades 5 and 6, the markers are placed 9 feet from the target; for grades 7, 8, and 9, markers are placed 12 feet from the target. On the signal Ready, Go! the examinee takes the first of three 60-second trials. The ball is shot, retrieved, dribbled to the next

---

*The next four tests—speed spot shooting, passing, control dribble, and defensive movement—are part of a battery of basketball skills tests published by AAHPERD (Hopkins, Shick, and Plack, 1984). Refer to the test manual for detailed information on this test battery. All four tests can be administered in two class periods.

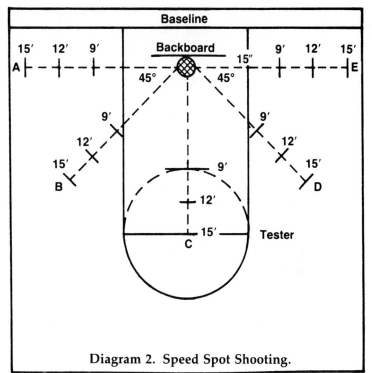

FIGURE *18-4 Court markings for the Speed Spot Shooting Test.*
From Hopkins, D.R., Shick, J., and Plack, J.J.

Diagram 2. Speed Spot Shooting.

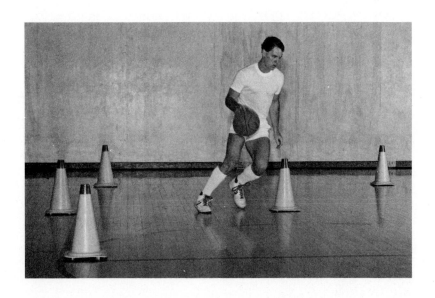

marker, and shot again. At least one shot must be taken from each of the five markers. Although most shots must be taken from the marker, four lay-ups are permitted during the testing period, but no two may be taken in succession.

Test Area Half of a regulation-size basketball court.

Equipment Basketballs, stopwatch, floor tape, tape measure, and scorecards.

Scoring The first trial is a practice trial; the next two are recorded. Two points are awarded for each shot made. One point is given for each unsuccessful shot that hits the rim. The total test score is the sum of scores for the two trials.

Validity r_{xy} = 0.37 to 0.91 for all ages on individual test items, using a criterion measure of two subjective ratings of skill in shooting and game performance; r_{xy} = 0.65 to 0.95 for test battery as a whole.

Reliability $R_{xx'}$ = 0.87 to 0.95 for females (test-retest); $R_{xx'}$ = 0.84 to 0.95 for males (test-retest).

Comments Abbreviated tables of norms are shown in Tables 18-3 and 18-4. Full-length tables are provided in the test manual. The scoring is somewhat complicated, since the scorer must record the following: whether the examinee

TABLE 18-3 *Percentile norms—Speed spot shooting; males*

Percentile	Age							
	10	11	12	13	14	15	16-17	College
95	23	25	27	28	30	27	28	30
75	17	18	19	19	23	20	22	25
50	13	14	15	15	18	16	16	22
25	10	10	11	12	13	11	12	19
5	7	6	7	7	9	6	7	14

Abbreviated form of Table 6, p. 18, from Hopkins, D.R., Shick, J., and Plack, J.J.

TABLE 18-4 *Percentile norms—Speed spot shooting; females*

Percentile	Age							
	10	11	12	13	14	15	16-17	College
95	18	19	22	22	25	23	23	35
75	11	11	13	13	15	15	14	21
50	8	8	10	10	11	11	11	17
25	5	5	7	8	9	8	7	13
5	2	2	3	4	4	4	3	8

Abbreviated form of Table 5, p. 18, from Hopkins, D.R., Shick, J., and Plack, J.J.

took at least one shot from each of the five markers (A, B, C, D, E); the number of lay-ups the student took; and the point value for each legal shot. Refer to the test manual for assistance in setting up a scorecard.

No score is given when ball-handling infractions occur, more than four lay-ups are attempted, or a lay-up is taken immediately following another one. If the examinee does not take a shot from each of the five markers, the trial must be retaken. Each floor marker should be 2 feet long and 1 inch wide.

Passing Test

Test Objective "To measure skill in passing and recovering the ball accurately while moving" (Hopkins, Shick and Plack, p. 11).

Description The examinee, holding a basketball, assumes a ready position behind the restraining line opposite the A target, as shown in Figure 18-5. On the signal Ready, Go! the ball is passed to the first target (A), rebounds, and is recovered while moving in line with the second target (B). This sequence continues until the last target (F) is reached. The ball is passed twice to target F, and the examinee moves back toward target A, attempting to hit each target in succession. The trial is terminated at the end of 30 seconds. Three trials are taken, with the first used as a practice trial. Only the chest pass may be used throughout this test.

Test Area Smooth wall surface of 30 feet.

Equipment Basketballs, stopwatch, floor tape, wall tape or chalk, tape measure, and scorecards.

Scoring Each pass landing within the target or on a target line scores 2 points. Each pass hitting the wall between targets scores 1 point. The total test score is the sum of scores for the two trials.

Validity r_{xy} = 0.37 to 0.91, for individual tests and both sexes; r_{xy} = 0.65 to 0.95, for total test battery.

Reliability $R_{xx'}$ = 0.82 to 0.91, for females (test-retest); $R_{xx'}$ = 0.88 to 0.96, for males (test-retest).

FIGURE 18-5 *Wall markings for the Passing Test.*
From Hopkins, D.R., Shick, J., and Plack, J.J.

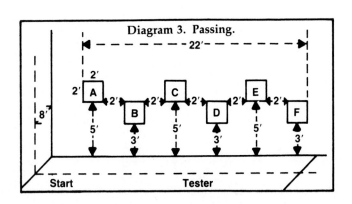

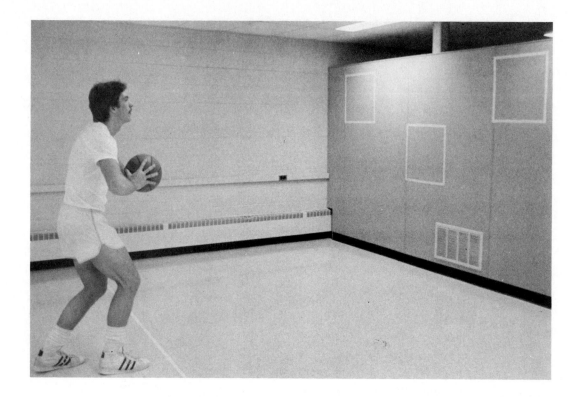

Comments Each pass must be taken from behind the restraining line. It is recommended that a student assistant be used to call out foot faults. No points are awarded if the examinee's foot is on or over the line, a second pass is taken at the same target (except *A* and *F* when appropriate), or a chest pass is not used. Abbreviated norms tables for males and females are given in Tables 18-5 and 18-6. Refer to the test manual for full-length norms tables.

TABLE 18-5 *Percentile norms—passing; females*

| | Age | | | | | | | |
Percentile	10	11	12	13	14	15	16-17	College
95	36	38	43	44	46	47	48	54
75	30	31	35	37	39	40	39	47
50	25	27	31	32	34	35	34	42
25	21	23	26	29	29	28	24	37
5	7	13	20	23	24	19	18	21

Abbreviated form of Table 7, p. 19, from Hopkins, D.R., Shick, J., and Plack, J.J.

TABLE 18-6 *Percentile norms—passing; males*

Percentile	Age							
	10	11	12	13	14	15	16-17	College
95	41	43	48	54	55	55	57	70
75	35	36	40	43	45	48	49	58
50	31	32	35	39	40	39	41	53
25	25	28	30	35	35	23	25	47
5	8	18	22	23	23	18	21	35

Abbreviated form of Table 8, p. 19, from Hopkins, D.R., Shick, J., and Plack, J.J.

Control Dribble Test

Test Objective "To measure skill in handling the ball while the body is moving" (Hopkins, Shick, and Plack, p. 13).

Description The player begins the test at cone A in Figure 18-6. Use the upper diagram for right-handed examinees and the lower one for left-handed individuals. On the signal Ready, Go! the ball is dribbled with the nondominant hand to the nondominant side of cone B. Thereafter the preferred hand may be used to dribble, and hands may be changed whenever appropriate. The watch is stopped as the examinee crosses the finish line. One practice and two test trials are administered.

Test Area Half a regulation-size basketball court.

Equipment Basketballs, six cones, stopwatch, and scorecards.

Scoring The trial score is the time required to complete the course legally. Record each trial score to the nearest tenth of a second. The total test score is the sum of the times for two trials.

Validity $r_{xy} = 0.37$ to 0.91, for individual tests and both sexes; $r_{xy} = 0.65$ to 0.95, for total test battery.

Reliability $R_{xx'} = 0.93$ to 0.97, for females (test-retest); $R_{xx'} = 0.88$ to 0.95, for males (test-retest).

Comments The trial must be retaken in the event of ball-handling infractions, failure to remain outside the cone (by either player or ball), and failure to continue the test from the proper spot when control has been lost. For abbreviated norms tables, see Tables 18-7 and 18-8. For the full-length tables, refer to the test manual.

Defensive Movement Test

Test Objective "To measure performance of basic defensive movements" (Hopkins, Shick, and Plack, p. 15).

Description Three trials are administered—one practice and two test. The test is begun at point A, as shown in Figure 18-7. The examinee faces away from

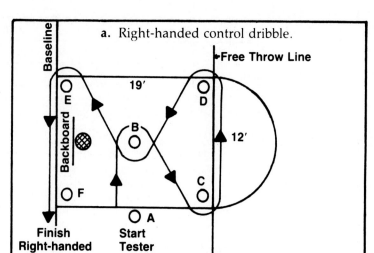

FIGURE 18-6 *Court markings for the Control Dribble Test.*
From Hopkins, D.R., Shick, J., and Plack, J.J.

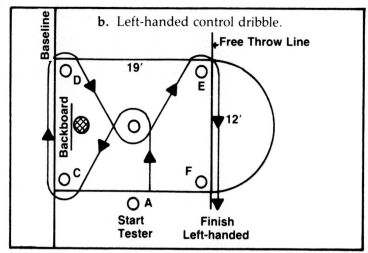

TABLE 18-7 *Percentile norms—Control dribble; males*

Percentile	Age							
	10	11	12	13	14	15	16-17	College
95	9.2	9.0	8.7	7.8	7.5	7.0	7.0	6.7
75	10.4	10.1	9.5	9.0	8.5	8.1	8.1	7.3
50	11.7	11.1	10.5	9.8	9.3	8.9	9.0	7.8
25	13.7	12.6	11.7	10.7	10.3	10.0	10.0	8.5
5	23.0	16.8	16.0	14.4	13.5	12.0	12.4	10.0

Abbreviated form of Table 10, p. 20, from Hopkins, D.R., Shick, J., and Plack, J.J.

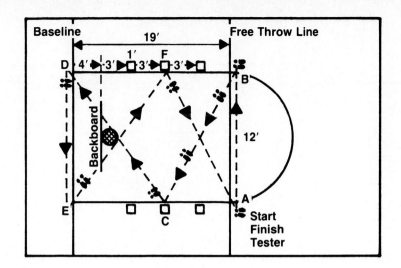

FIGURE 18-7 *Court markings and foot positions for the Defensive Movement Test.*

From Hopkins, D.R., Shick, J., and Plack, J.J.

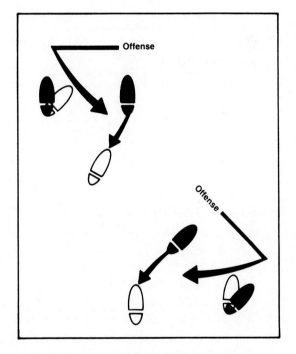

TABLE 18-8 *Percentile norms—Control dribble; females*

Percentile	Age							
	10	11	12	13	14	15	16-17	College
95	10.8	10.3	8.8	8.7	8.4	8.2	8.2	7.6
75	12.3	11.8	10.6	10.0	9.6	9.7	9.8	8.5
50	14.3	13.2	11.9	11.0	10.7	10.7	10.7	9.3
25	16.6	15.0	13.3	12.4	12.0	12.0	12.2	10.4
5	21.7	20.5	19.0	17.8	18.1	15.8	15.0	13.8

Abbreviated form of Table 9, p. 20, from Hopkins, D.R., Shick, J., and Plack, J.J.

TABLE 18-9 *Percentile norms—defensive movement; females*

Percentile	Age							
	10	11	12	13	14	15	16-17	College
95	10.5	10.3	9.5	10.0	9.6	9.7	9.6	8.7
75	11.8	11.8	11.5	11.5	11.0	11.0	11.1	10.3
50	13.2	13.0	12.8	12.5	12.0	12.0	12.0	11.0
25	14.6	14.3	14.1	13.6	13.2	13.4	13.2	12.0
5	19.6	17.4	17.0	16.8	16.4	16.4	16.4	14.5

Abbreviated form of Table 11, p. 21, from Hopkins, D.R., Shick, J., and Plack, J.J.

TABLE 18-10 *Percentile norms—defensive movement; males*

Percentile	Age							
	10	11	12	13	14	15	16-17	College
95	10.0	9.0	8.9	8.9	8.7	7.9	7.3	8.4
75	11.5	10.9	10.7	10.3	10.1	9.3	9.6	9.4
50	12.7	12.0	11.9	11.4	11.3	10.3	10.3	10.3
25	13.9	13.7	13.0	12.8	12.4	11.3	11.5	11.2
5	18.7	17.2	17.0	16.6	15.8	14.0	15.2	12.9

Abbreviated form of Table 12, p. 21, from Hopkins, D.R., Shick, J., and Plack, J.J.

the basket, slides to the left without crossing over the left foot, reaches point B, and touches the floor outside the lane with the left hand. The examinee then executes a dropstep (see Figure 18-7), slides to point C, and touches the floor outside the lane with the right hand. This continues until the course is completed back at point A. The stopwatch is started on the signal Ready, Go! and stopped as the examinee crosses the finish line (A) with both feet.

Test Area Half of a regulation-size basketball court.

Equipment Basketballs, stopwatch, floor tape, tape measure, and scorecards.

Scoring A trial score is the time required to complete the course, measured to the nearest tenth of a second. The total test score is the sum of two trials.

Validity $r_{xy} = 0.37$ to 0.91, for individual tests, males and females; $r_{xy} = 0.65$ to 0.95, for total test battery, males and females.

Reliability $R_{xx'} = 0.95$ to 0.96, for females (test-retest); $R_{xx'} = 0.90$ to 0.97, for males (test-retest).

Comments The trial is retaken if the feet cross during the slide or turn, the examinee runs, or the dropstep occurs before the hand touches the floor. Abbreviated tables of norms are presented in Tables 18-9 and 18-10. Refer to the test manual for the full-length norms tables.

Field Hockey Tests

Chapman Ball Control Test (Chapman, 1982)

Test Objective To measure "the subject's ability to combine quickness in wrist and hand movements needed to manipulate the stick with ability to control the force element when contacting the ball" (p. 239).

Description The ball is placed just beyond the outer circle of the target. On the signal Ready Go! the examinee taps the ball in and out of the center circle with a hockey stick. Three 15-second trials are administered. The two lower examples in Figure 18-8 depict legal hits. Before actual testing, the tester should demonstrate the procedures, and the examinees should be allowed to practice.

Test Area Small indoor testing area; target on floor according to the dimensions shown in upper portion of Figure 18-8; outer circle of target should be colored so that it contrasts with gymnasium floor (orange is suggested).

Equipment Hockey sticks, several hockey balls, floor tape, stopwatch, and scorecards.

FIGURE 18-8 *Target for the Chapman Ball Control Test.*
From Chapman, N.L.

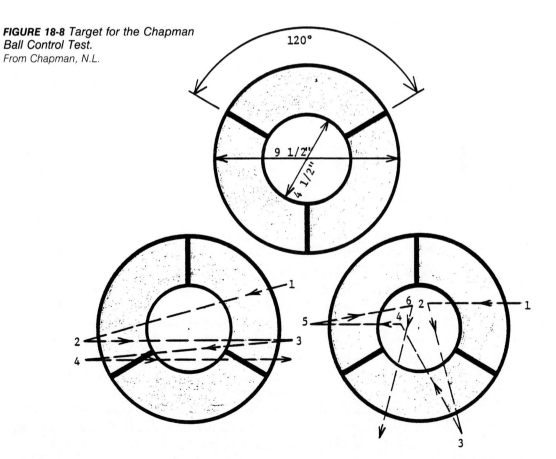

Scoring Score 1 point whenever the ball is tapped (not pushed) either into or through the center circle. A point may also be scored when the ball is tapped from the center of the circle to the outside of the target area, if it passes through a different segment from the one it entered (see the lower right side of Figure 18-8). To score a point, the ball must be tapped from either within the center circle or outside the outer circle. No points are scored when the ball is tapped on the orange area or with the rounded side of the stick. The total test score is the sum of points made on the three 15-second trials.

Validity Logical validity; construct validity on the basis of significant differences between varsity and junior varsity teams' performances on the test; and concurrent validity (r_{xy} = 0.63 and 0.64), using a criterion measure of ratings of stickwork skills.

Reliability $R_{xx'}$ = 0.89, single test administration.

Comments The use of three targets is recommended—two practice and one test. While two examinees practice, a third person can be tested. If only one test administrator is available, the test can be timed using an audio tape of Ready, Go! and Stop! recorded at 15-second intervals.

Football Tests

Ball Changing Zigzag Run (AAHPER, 1966)

Test Objective To measure speed of execution of zigzag movement as the football is changed from arm to arm.

Description Place five chairs in a line 10 feet apart. The first chair is 10 feet from the starting line. To begin the test, the player assumes a ready position behind the starting line, with a football under his right arm. On the signal Go! he runs to the right of the first chair, shifts the ball to his left arm as he passes to the left of the second chair, and continues in this manner, as shown in Figure 18-9. The ball must be under the outside arm each time a chair is passed, and the inside arm must be extended (as in a stiff arm in football) toward the chair being passed. Two trials are taken.

Test Area Football field or any grass field.

Equipment Five chairs, footballs, stopwatch, and measuring tape.

Scoring Each trial is timed to the nearest tenth of a second, starting with the signal Go! and stopping when the player crosses the starting line at the end of the run. The trial with the best time is the test score.

Validity Not reported for this specific test.

Reliability Not reported for this specific test.

Norms An abbreviated table of norms is presented in Table 18-11. The full-length norms table can be found in the test manual.

Comments One practice run is allowed before being tested. The prescribed position (ball under outside arm, inside arm extended) must be maintained when running to the side of a chair throughout the test. Touching a chair is illegal.

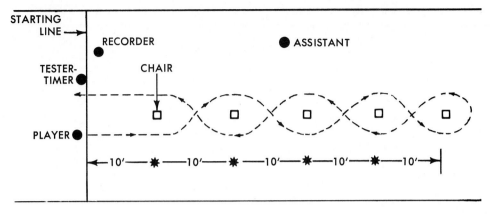

FIGURE 18-9 *Field markings for the Ball Changing Zigzag Run.*
From AAHPER.

TABLE 18-11 *Ball Changing Zigzag Run (test scores in seconds and tenths)*

	Age							
Percentile	10	11	12	13	14	15	16	17-18
95th	9.9	7.7	7.8	8.0	8.7	7.7	7.7	8.4
75th	10.7	9.3	8.8	9.0	9.5	8.6	8.7	9.0
50th	11.5	10.3	9.6	9.7	10.0	9.1	9.3	9.6
25th	12.5	11.3	10.5	10.3	10.7	9.9	10.1	10.3
5th	15.8	14.2	12.3	12.1	12.0	11.5	12.2	12.1

From AAHPER.

Golf Tests

Indoor Golf Skill Test for Junior High School Boys (Shick and Berg, 1983)

Test Objective To measure golf skills, either indoors or outdoors, performed by junior high school boys.

Description A target is placed on the floor of the testing area, as shown in Figure 18-10. Colored markers are recommended to identify the scoring areas. A mat is placed at the front edge of the target, where the student stands. A driving mat is placed 1 foot from the target line. The student hits a plastic ball off the driving mat with a 5-iron as far as possible, aiming for an orange cone. Two practice and 20 test trials are taken.

Test Area Small gymnasium or multipurpose room.

Equipment At least two 5-iron clubs, one right-handed and one left-handed;

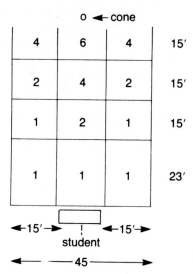

FIGURE 18-10 *Target for Indoor Golf Skill Test for Junior High School Boys.*
From Shick, J., and Berg, N.G.

25 plastic balls; orange cone; floor tape; tape measure; scorecards; mat for examinee; and driving mat.

Scoring Each trial score is the landing point of the ball on the target. If a ball lands beyond the target but is in line with the farthermost target areas (see 4, 6, 4 of Fig. 18-10), the ball is assigned the point value of the closest area. In this case, assume the target lines are extended by imaginary lines. A topped ball that passes through the scoring area is given 1 point. A missed ball is given a score of 0. A ball landing on a target line is given the score of the highest adjacent target area. The total test score is the sum of the trial scores.

Validity $r_{xy} = -0.84$, using a criterion measure of the best of three scores on a par - 3, nine-hole golf course.

Reliability $R_{xx'} = 0.97$, for single test administration; $R_{xx'} = 0.91$, for test-retest administration.

Comments This is a modification of a test developed for older examinees (Cotten, Thomas, and Plaster, 1972). With two testing stations, 20 students can be tested in one 45-minute class period. Since test validity ($r_{xy} = -0.80$) and reliability ($R_{xx'} = 0.90$) were also acceptable for 10 trials administered on one day, using a shortened (10-trial) version of the test would be appropriate.

Racquetball Tests

Racquetball Skills Test (Hensley, East, and Stillwell, 1979)
Test Objective To measure two fundamental components of racquetball—speed and power; although accuracy is not emphasized, a gross accuracy component is measured.

Description Two measures are administered—a short wall volley test and a long wall volley test. In the short wall volley test, the examinee, holding two racquetballs, stands behind the short line, drops a ball, and volleys it against the front wall for 30 seconds. All strokes must occur from behind the short line. The ball may be hit in the air or after taking one or more bounces. If the ball does not return to the short line or if the examinee misses it, the ball may be retrieved or a new ball may be obtained from the scorer. The test consists of two 30-second trials, preceded by a 30-second practice period.

The testing procedures for the long wall volley test are essentially the same except that the ball is volleyed from behind a restraining line located 12 feet behind and parallel to the short line. In both tests any stroke may be used to keep the ball in play.

Test Area Regulation-size racquetball court.

Equipment Racquets, four new racquetballs, colored floor tape, stopwatch, scorecards, and tape measure.

Scoring The stopwatch should be started when the examinee releases the ball on the initial drop. The score in each test is the number of legal hits for two 30-second periods. In scoring the short wall volley test, it is recommended that the scorer stand inside the court; for the long wall volley test, standing outside the court, if possible, is recommended. No points are scored when the student steps on or over the restraining line or when the ball hits the floor or a side wall before reaching the front wall.

Validity Content validity; concurrent validity: $r_{xy} = 0.79$ for the short test, and $r_{xy} = 0.86$ for the long test, using a criterion measure of instructor ratings of ability to sustain a rally.

Reliability The following are test-retest coefficients:

$R_{xx'} = 0.82$ for the long test, college women;

$R_{xx'} = 0.85$ for the long test, college men;

$R_{xx'} = 0.86$ for the short test, college women; and

$R_{xx'} = 0.76$ for the short test, college men.

Comments Refer to the original source for norms for college men and women. This test is easy to administer and requires about 3 minutes of testing time per student. Two extra balls should be available at all times during both tests. If the scorer is able to stand outside the court to score the long wall volley test, place the two extra balls in the crease at the back corner of the court.

Soccer Tests

McDonald Volleying Soccer Test (McDonald, 1951)

Test Objective To measure general soccer ability.

Description The soccer ball is kicked against the wall as many times as possible in 30 seconds. Any type of kick may be used. Both ground balls and fly balls hitting the target count, if the ball is kicked from the ground behind the restraining line. Any part of the body, including the hands, may be used for retrieving a ball. If the player loses control of the ball, a spare ball may be used. This ball must be positioned behind the restraining line before being kicked. Four trials are taken.

Test Area Wall 30 feet wide and 11½ feet high, with a restraining line 9 feet from the wall and parallel to it.

Equipment Three soccer balls (the two spares are placed 9 feet behind the restraining line in the center of the area), stopwatch, and tape measure.

Scoring The score is the number of legal kicks in a 30-second period.

Validity The test scores were correlated with coaches' ratings of playing ability.

$r_{xy} = 0.94$ varsity players;

$r_{xy} = 0.63$ junior varsity players;

$r_{xy} = 0.76$ freshman varsity players; and

$r_{xy} = 0.85$ combined group.

Reliability Not reported for this specific test.

Comments This test can be used with younger age groups by reducing the size of the target and moving the restraining line closer to the wall.

Softball Tests

Shick Softball Test Battery (Shick, 1970)

Test Objective To measure defensive softball skills in college women.

Description Three tests are included in the test battery—repeated throws, fielding test, and target test. They can be used as a battery or as individual tests.

Repeated Throws The examinee stands behind a restraining line placed on the floor 23 feet from the wall. On the signal Ready, Go! the examinee throws a softball at the wall and attempts to hit the wall above the 10-foot line, which is on the wall parallel to the floor. Either an overarm or a sidearm throw may be used. The rebounding ball may either be caught in the air or fielded from the floor. This is repeated as many times as possible in 30 seconds. Four trials are allowed. No penalty is given for a fumbled rebound, since this results in a loss of time. One practice throw is permitted before each trial.

The total test score is the sum of the number of times that the ball hit the wall in four trials. If the examinee steps on or over the restraining line or if the ball is thrown below the wall line, no hit is recorded. The validity of this test is $r_{xy} = 0.69$, using a criterion measure of judges' ratings of individual performance in game situations. Test reliability is $R_{xx'} = 0.86$.

Fielding Test This test is similar to the repeated throws measure except that the primary objective is to field the ball on a bounce or from the floor rather than catching it in the air. The wall line is 4 feet from the floor, and the restraining line is 15 feet from the wall. Otherwise, the test is the same as the repeated throws measure in all respects but two: any type throw may be used, and the ball should be thrown so that it hits the wall below the wall line.

The total test score is the sum of the number of times the ball is legally thrown and hits the wall below the line in four trials. Test validity is 0.48, using the same criterion measure. Test reliability is 0.89.

Target Test Wall and floor targets must be set up as shown in Figure 18-11. The wall target is 66 inches square with the center of the target 36 inches from the floor. The restraining line is 40 feet from the wall. It is recommended that the target areas be color coded. The test consists of two trials of 10 throws each. The examinee stands behind the restraining line with a softball in hand. Two practice throws are permitted. Two scores are given for each test throw: the point value of the wall target area in which the ball is hit and the section of the floor target where the ball lands on its first bounce. No points are given for hits outside the two target areas. The scores are then summed across target areas and trials. Test validity is 0.63, using the same criterion measure. Test reliability is 0.88.

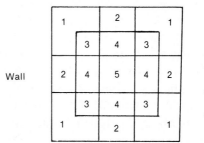

FIGURE 18-11 *Wall and floor targets for the Target Test.*
From Shick, J.

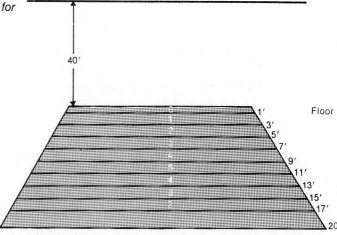

Test Area Regulation-size gymnasium.

Equipment Softballs, stopwatches, floor tape, tape measure, scorecards, and softball gloves.

Comments For the total test battery, test validity is 0.75 and test reliability is 0.88. The entire battery can be administered in two 40-minute class periods.

Swimming Tests

12-Minute Swim Test (Jackson, Jackson, and Frankiewicz, 1979)

Test Objective To provide a practical field test of swimming endurance using the crawl stroke.

Description Each examinee is assigned to swim in an individual lane. The poolside should be marked in 5-yard distances. The swimmer is instructed to start in the water with a pushoff from the side and to swim the crawl stroke for 12 minutes, attempting to cover as much distance as possible. At the signal Ready, Go! the stopwatch is started and the swimmers push off. A partner assigned to each swimmer counts the number of laps. On the signal Stop! the partner records the yardage closest to the swimmer's hand and the number of full laps the swimmer completes. The swimmer should continue swimming at a leisurely pace for another 2 to 3 minutes to unwind from the all out effort.

Test Area Pool of 25 yards or longer, with lane dividers.

Equipment Stopwatch or other suitable timing device in pool and scorecards.

Validity $r_{xy} = 0.89$, using criterion measure of tethered swim, where the heart rate reached at least 172 beats per minute (concurrent validity); significant difference in test scores of competitive swimmers and noncompetitors (construct validity).

Reliability $R_{xx'}$ (alpha coefficient) = 0.99 for single administration of the test; subjects—college males; $R_{xx'} = 0.98$ for test-retest; subjects—college men and women (Fried, 1983).

Comments Before taking the test, swimmers should take a 5- to 10-minute warm-up in the water. It is assumed that the swimmers have had previous instruction and practice in pacing and stroke efficiency. If the swimmers are below average in swimming skills, it might be desirable to remove the effect of swimming skill using the residual score method described in Jackson, Jackson, and Frankiewicz (1979).

Tennis Tests

Hewitt Tennis Achievement Test (Hewitt, 1966)

Test Objective To measure three basic tennis skills—forehand drive, backhand drive, and service; the service placement test, speed of service test, and forehand/backhand drive tests are used.

Test Area Regulation-size tennis court.

Equipment Tennis racquets, 25 tennis balls, and scorecards.

Service Placement Test A 10-minute warm-up is permitted. The examinee stands behind the baseline and serves 10 balls into the marked service court, as shown in Figure 18-12. The ball should pass between the net and the 7-foot high rope. If this occurs, the trial score is the point value of the target area in which the ball lands. A ball traveling over the rope is scored 0.

The test score is the sum of 10 trials. The validity of test ranges from 0.625 to 0.93, using a criterion measure of round robin tournament rankings. Test-retest reliability is 0.94.

Speed of Service Test The court is divided into zones (see Figure 18-13). The examinee serves the ball into the designated court, and the score is based on the zone in which the second bounce lands. The underlying assumption is that the distance the ball travels between the first and second bounce is a valid indicator of the speed of service. The zone number is the score for the trial.

The total test score is the sum of 10 trials. Test validity ranges from 0.723 to 0.89, using a criterion measure of round robin tournament rankings. Test-retest reliability is 0.84. This test can be given at the same time as the service placement test. Place both targets on the same side of the court; the placement score is the target value on the service court, and the speed score is the zone value.

Forehand and Backhand Drive Tests The examinee stands at the center of the baseline, as shown in Figure 18-14. Five practice trials are allowed. The ball is hit to the examinee by the instructor or propelled by a ball machine and lands just beyond the service line. Using either a forehand or backhand drive, the examinee returns the ball. Then 20 test trials are administered in the same way.

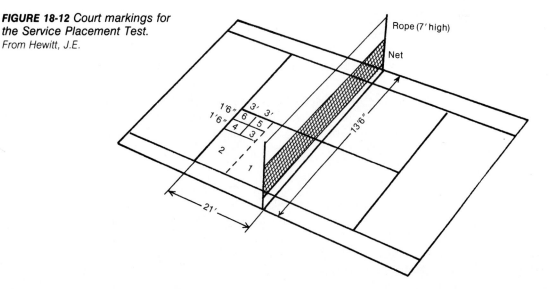

FIGURE 18-12 *Court markings for the Service Placement Test.*
From Hewitt, J.E.

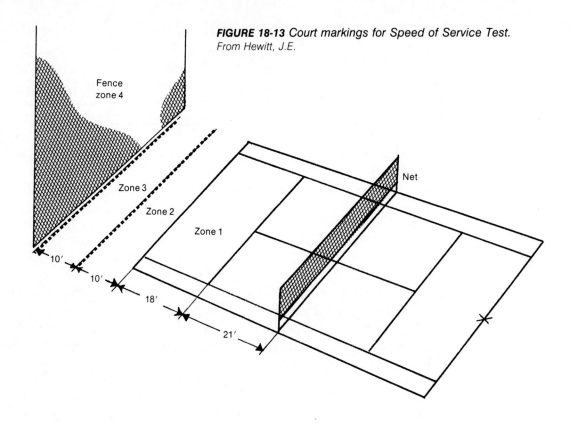

FIGURE 18-13 *Court markings for Speed of Service Test.*
From Hewitt, J.E.

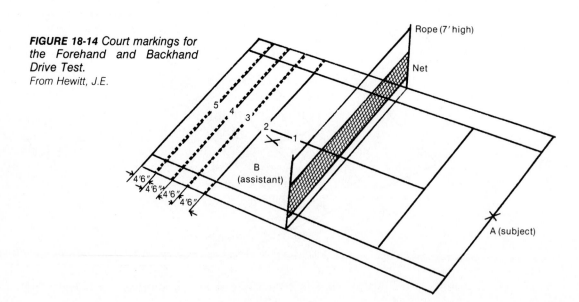

FIGURE 18-14 *Court markings for the Forehand and Backhand Drive Test.*
From Hewitt, J.E.

Although 10 test trials are given for each drive, the examinee is allowed to choose which 10 balls to hit forehand and backhand.

The ball should travel between the rope and the net to maximize the target score. If the ball passes over the rope, half the value of the regular target is awarded. The validity estimates range from 0.57 to 0.67 for the forehand trials and 0.52 to 0.62 for the backhand trials, using a criterion measure of round robin tournament rankings. The test-retest reliability is 0.75 for the forehand drive and 0.78 for the backhand.

Comments A ball machine should be used whenever possible to test the drive. No information is given on recommended settings for the machine. A composite score for the three test items is not recommended. Each test item is scored separately.

Hewitt Revision of the Dyer Backboard Test (Hewitt, 1965)

Test Objective To classify students by measuring rallying and serving ability.

Description With two new tennis balls in hand, the examinee serves the ball against the wall from a restraining line 20 feet from the wall. The stopwatch is started when the ball hits the wall. On the rebound the player begins a rally by hitting the ball continuously against the wall so that the ball hits on or above a wall line placed 3 feet above the testing surface. Three trials of 30 seconds each are taken.

Test Area Smooth gymnasium wall or indoor/outdoor backboard of 20 feet high and 20 feet wide and a 20-foot by 20-foot floor space.

Equipment Tennis racket, two dozen balls, stopwatch (records to the nearest tenth of a second), tape measure, floor and wall tape, and scorecards.

Scoring One point is scored each time the ball hits on or above the wall line. If the examinee steps on or over the restraining line, the rally is continued, but no point is scored and the player should be warned. The total score is the sum of three trials.

Validity $r_{xy} = 0.68$ to 0.73, for beginners;

$r_{xy} = 0.84$ to 0.89, for intermediates.

Reliability $R_{xx'} = 0.82$, for beginners (test-retest);

$R_{xx'} = 0.93$, for intermediates (test-retest).

Comments All lines should be 1 inch wide. Approximately 15 students can be tested at each station in 40 minutes. If the ball does not return to the examinee, another one can be taken from the basket and served against the wall to initiate the rally again. No points are scored on the serve. The count should begin with the first wall hit after the serve.

Tennis Forehand/Backhand Drive Test (Purcell, 1981)

Test Objective To measure the forehand and backhand drives in a setting that closely resembles the actual game situation; to evaluate depth, direction, and speed of the drive by rewarding shots directed deep to the center of the court with sufficient speed.

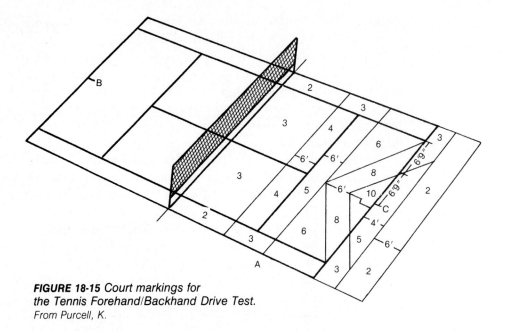

FIGURE 18-15 *Court markings for the Tennis Forehand/Backhand Drive Test.*
From Purcell, K.

Description The test examinee stands within 3 to 6 feet of the baseline of the court, facing the target area, as shown in Figure 18-15. A pneumatic ball-pitching machine is used to project the tennis ball to the examinee, who attempts to return the ball over the net and into the target area. Three practice and 10 test trials are administered for each drive, forehand and backhand. The ball flight is timed from the point of contact to the landing point.

The speed and angle of the ball machine are set so that the ball will pass approximately 2½ feet above the center of the net, land on or close to the service line, and bounce to its highest point about 3 feet from the baseline. With these settings the maximum height of the bounce should be roughly 3 feet; the horizontal velocity should be approximately 59 feet per second. The time of flight of the machine-projected ball should be approximately 1.02 seconds.

Test Area Regulation-size tennis court, with target areas marked on the court using ordinary chalk.

Equipment Ball machine, 40 balls, tennis racket, stopwatch, scorecards, and tape measure.

Scoring The target values for each set of 10 trials are summed, as well as the times for 10 trials. To determine the correction factor for the total time score, see Table 18-12. The total target score is multiplied by the correction factor to yield the test score. This is done for both the forehand and backhand drives. When a ball is clearly deflected by the net, the trial should be retaken. A typical "let" ball is scored in the regular manner.

TABLE 18-12 *Correction factors for converting target value totals into skill test scores using time in flight (TF)*

TF for 10 trials	Correction factor
5 sec.	1.35
6	1.30
7	1.25
8	1.20
9	1.15
10	1.10
11	1.05
12	1.00
13	.95
14	.90
15	.85
16	.80
17	.75
18	.70

From Purcell, K.

Validity $r_{xy} = 0.83$, using a criterion measure of judges' ratings of the forehand and backhand stroke:

$r_{xy} = 0.70$, for forehand trials alone; and

$r_{xy} = 0.83$, for backhand trials alone.

Reliability The following test-retest coefficients were calculated for college women:

$R_{xx'} = 0.84$ total test;

$R_{xx'} = 0.86$ forehand trials alone; and

$R_{xx'} = 0.83$ backhand trials alone.

For the criterion measure, the interjudge objectivity was $R_{j1j2} = 0.87$.

Comments Total testing time per examinee, including practice trials, is about 3½ minutes. Little time is lost between tests if the next examinee is ready to step up to the line as soon as the previous examinee has completed testing. For the group tested in the original study, the following descriptive statistics were reported for college women:

	Mean	Standard deviation
Forehand	30.3	9.4
Backhand	23.6	9.5
TOTAL	53.9	17.7

Once the target lines have been marked on the court, the test should be relatively easy to administer, assuming that a ball machine is available.

Volleyball Tests

Brady Volleyball Test (Brady, 1945)

Test Objective To measure general volleyball-playing ability.

Description No restraining line is used. The examinee begins the test by throwing the ball against the wall and attempting to hit the ball into the target area on the wall repeatedly (see Figure 18-16). One 60-second trial is administered. Only legal hits are allowed. If the examinee catches the ball or loses control of the ball, the test must be restarted by throwing the ball against the wall.

Test Area Smooth wall space, 15 feet by 15 feet.

Equipment Volleyballs, stopwatch, wall tape or chalk, tape measure, and scorecards.

Scoring The test score is the number of legal hits in 1 minute. Thrown balls are not scored, but balls landing on the target line are scored.

Validity $r_{xy} = 0.86$, using a criterion measure of subjective ratings of playing ability.

Reliability $r_{xx'} = 0.93$ (test-retest).

Comments Allow practice time before taking the test. Several students may be tested at the same time. Approximately 2 minutes per person are required to administer the test. This test is especially useful for making quick classifications of students in a class setting. The height of the target might be lowered for younger age groups, especially junior high or grade school students.

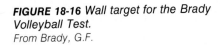

FIGURE 18-16 *Wall target for the Brady Volleyball Test.*
From Brady, G.F.

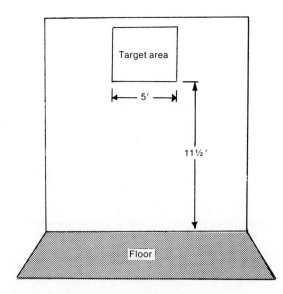

Brumbach Volleyball Service Test (Brumbach, 1967)

Test Objective To measure the ability to serve the volleyball low and deep into the opponent's court.

Description The examinee stands behind the baseline and serves the ball, attempting to hit it between the net and the rope and deep into the backcourt on the opposite side (see Figure 18-17). The test consists of 12 trials, in two sets of six.

Test Area Regulation-size volleyball court.

Equipment Volleyballs, standard extensions, rope, floor tape or chalk, tape measure, and scorecards.

Scoring A ball hit between the net and the rope and landing in the target area receives the higher of the two scores assigned to the target area. A ball passing over the rope and landing in the target area is given the lower of the two scores. The total test score is the sum of the 10 best trials. Foot faults, balls hitting the net, and balls landing outside the target area are scored 0.

Validity Not reported for this specific test.

Reliability Not reported for this specific test.

Comments In one court 20 students can be tested in less than an hour. Only legal serves should be scored. Although this test may be viewed as logically valid, the validity and reliability should be systematically studied. It appears to be appropriate for junior high, high school, and college students.

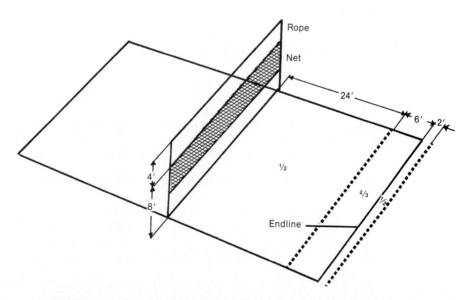

FIGURE 18-17 *Court markings for the Brumbach Volleyball Service Test.*
From Brumbach, W.B.

SUMMARY

This chapter was designed to present a broad overview of the skills tests available in the physical education field. Other than the references already mentioned, the *Research Quarterly for Exercise and Sport* usually publishes the best of the recently developed tests.

LEARNING EXPERIENCES

1. This exercise will be most valuable for students who plan to teach physical education but will also be useful for those who may work in a private sports club. Select one of the tests described in this chapter and administer it to the other students in class. Prepare carefully and well ahead of time for the testing. Plan how you will organize the group during the test administration. Take care of any court markings or targets before the actual testing session. Develop a score sheet or scorecard for each examinee. Sometime after the testing has been completed, discuss the results with the examinees, telling them their scores and the summary data for the class.

2. Select one of the tests in this chapter in which a floor target is used. Determine two ways this target could be safely marked on a gymnasium floor. Experiment with both methods. Write a brief report of the two approaches, comparing them in terms of efficiency, cost, practicality, and so forth. Discuss your preference and give a rationale for your choice.

REFERENCES

American Association for Health, Physical Education and Recreation. 1967. Archery for boys and girls: skills test manual. Washington, DC: AAHPER.

American Association for Health, Physical Education and Recreation. 1966. Football: skills test manual. Washington, DC: AAHPER.

Brady, G.F. 1945. Preliminary investigations of volleyball playing ability. Research Quarterly, **16**:14-17.

Broer, M.R., and Miller. D.M. 1950. Achievement tests for beginning and intermediate tennis. Research Quarterly, **21**:303-313.

Brumbach, W. 1967. Beginning volleyball, a syllabus for teachers, revised edition. Eugene, OR: Wayne Baker Brumbach (Distributed by the University of Oregon).

Chapman, N.L. 1982. Chapman Ball Control Test—field hockey. Research Quarterly for Exercise and Sport, **53**(3):239-242.

Collins, D.R., and Hodges, P.B. 1978. A comprehensive guide to sports skills tests and measurement. Springfield, IL: Charles C Thomas, Publisher.

Cooper, J.M., and Glassow, R.B. 1963, 1976. Kinesiology. St. Louis: The CV Mosby Company.

Cotten, D., Thomas, J.R., and Plaster, T. A plastic ball test for golf iron skill, Unpublished study presented at the American Alliance for Health, Physical Education, Recreation and Dance National Convention, Houston, March 1972.

Fried, C.R. 1983. An examination of the test characteristics of the 12-Minute Swim Test, Unpublished Master's thesis, University of Wisconsin—Madison.

Glassow, R.B. 1957. Comments on the Miller-Broer tennis test. Unpublished paper, The University of Wisconsin—Madison.

Hensley, L.D., East, W.B., and Stillwell, J.L. 1979. A racquetball skills test. Research Quarterly for Exercise and Sport, **50**(1):114-118.

Hewitt, J.E. 1966. Hewitt's tennis achievement test. Research Quarterly, **37**:231-237.

Hewitt, J.E. 1965. Revision of the Dyer Backboard Tennis Test. Research Quarterly, **37**:231-240.

Hopkins, D.R., Shick, J., and Plack, J.J. 1984. Basketball for boys and girls: skills test manual. Reston, VA: American Alliance for Health, Physical Education, Recreation and Dance.

Jackson, A., Jackson, A.S., and Frankiewicz, R.G. 1979. The construct and concurrent validity of a 12-minute crawl stroke swim as a field test of swimming endurance. Research Quarterly for Exercise and Sport, **50**(4):641-648.

Johnson, B.L., and Nelson, J.K. 1979. Practical measurements for evaluation in physical education. Minneapolis:Burgess Publishing Co.

Kelson, R.E. 1953. Baseball classification plan for boys. Research Quarterly, **24**:304-307.

Liba, M.R., and Stauff, M. 1963. A test for the volleyball pass. Research Quarterly, **34**:56-63.

Lockhart, A., and McPherson, F.A. 1949. The development of a test of badminton playing ability. Research Quarterly, **20**:402-405.

McDonald, L.G. 1951. The construction of a kicking skill test as an index of general soccer ability. Unpublished Master's Thesis. Springfield College, MA.

Miller, F.A. 1951. A badminton wall volley test. Research Quarterly, **22**:208-213.

Poole, J., and Nelson, J.K. 1970. Construction of a badminton skills test battery, Unpublished study. Louisiana State University, Baton Rouge.

Purcell, K. 1981. A tennis forehand-backhand drive skill test which measures ball control and stroke firmness. Research Quarterly for Exercise and Sport, **52**(2):238-245.

Safrit, M.J., and Pavis, A. (1969). Overarm throw skill testing. In J. Felshin & C. O'Brien, Eds., Selected softball articles. Washington, DC: American Association of Health, Physical Education and Recreation.

Scott, M.G., and French, E. 1959. Measurement and evaluation in physical education. Dubuque, IA: Wm C Brown Group.

Scott, M.G., and others. 1941. Achievement examinations in badminton. Research Quarterly, **12**:242-253.

Shick, J. 1970. Battery of defensive softball skills tests for college women. Research Quarterly, **41**:82-87.

Shick, J., and Berg, N.G. 1983. Indoor golf skill test for junior high school boys. Research Quarterly for Exercise and Sport, **54**(1):75-78.

Shifflett, B., and Shuman, B.J. 1982. A criterion-referenced test for archery. Research Quarterly for Exercise and Sport, **53**(4):330-335.

West, C., and Thorpe, J. 1968. Construction and validation of eight-iron approach test. Research Quarterly, **39**:1115-1120.

ANNOTATED READINGS

American Association for Health, Physical Education, and Recreation. 1966-1967. Skills test series. Washington, DC: AAHPER.

Separate manual of skills tests for a variety of sports, including archery, basketball, football, softball, and volleyball; revision now available for basketball skills tests, and underway for soccer, tennis, and volleyball tests; although many tests are outdated, can be modified by the teacher to provide valuable learning experiences.

Avery, C.A., Richardson, P.A., and Jackson, A.W. 1979. A practical tennis serve test: measurement of a skill under simulated game conditions. Research Quarterly for Exercise and Sport, **50**(4):554-564.

Good example of more complex type of test that can be used in a class setting; describes a tennis serve test with a high degree of logical as well as statistical validity; excellent test for intermediate and advanced players.

Collins, D.R., and Hodges, P.B. 1978. A comprehensive guide to sports skills tests and measurement. Springfield, IL: Charles C Thomas, Publisher.

A valuable reference for every physical education teacher; presents a wide variety of published and unpublished tests of sports skills; provides thorough descriptions of tests; includes more tests than can be found in any measurement and evaluation textbook in physical education.

Hopkins, D.R. 1979. Using the AAHPERD basketball skills test for women. Journal of Physical Education and Recreation, **50**:72-73.

Describes use of test by coaches in selecting team members; evaluates nine-item test battery primarily designed for instructional purposes; presents descriptive statistics; lists resources for other skills tests.

19

Tests of Muscular Strength and Endurance

KEY WORDS *Watch for these words as you read the following chapter:*

cable tensiometer

dynamic strength

dynamometer

electromechanical instrument

muscular endurance

muscular strength

power

static strength

vertical jump

weight-training machine

Muscular strength and endurance can be measured in many ways, ranging from practical tests requiring little or no equipment to expensive machines. Practical tests can be used in settings that have neither the space nor the money for gym machines. On the other hand, an isokinetic machine such as Cybex is expensive but provides the most accurate information about the strength of a particular muscle group. In this chapter the most expensive alternatives are dealt with only briefly. Examples of tests requiring use of the weight training machines such as Nautilus or Universal Gym equipment are included, as well as tests requiring the use of free weights or gymnastics equipment available in many schools.

Muscular strength is defined as "the maximum force or tension level that can be produced by a muscle group"; **muscular endurance** is "the ability of the muscle to maintain submaximal force levels for extended periods" (Heyward, 1984, pp. 4-5). Tests requiring continuous repetitions of a movement measure endurance, not strength. A true measure of strength determines the maximum amount of weight that can be moved in a single effort. However, a high relationship does exist between strength and endurance measures. Correlations of 0.90 and higher have been reported between one maximum effort and the number of submaximal repetitions (Baumgartner and Jackson, 1982). In this chapter, examples of both strength and endurance tests are presented. Since the same tests are included under both topics in several cases, keep in mind the distinguishing factor between strength and endurance tests. When the test is used as a measure of strength, one repetition to maximum is executed. When it is used to measure endurance, a number of submaximum repetitions are performed.

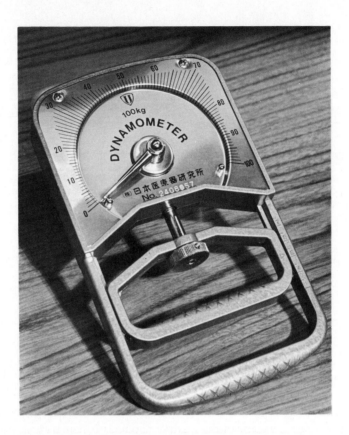

There is no individual test of overall body strength or endurance. Both strength and endurance are specific to a muscle group. Thus a person may have strong legs and weak arms or strong abdominal muscles and a weak grip. Since muscle groups must be tested separately, choices about the most important muscle groups to be tested in a given setting must be made.

Body weight is often a factor in strength and endurance testing. When an examinee must move (lift or lower) his or her body in executing a strength or endurance test, standards are varied according to weight. For instance, a higher score would be given to a lighter person who executes a given number of repetitions than to a heavier person executing the same number.

Several practical tests of strength and endurance can be found in Chapters 16 and 17. For example, the Sit-ups Test is a test of endurance of the abdominal muscles; the Pull-ups Test measures endurance of the arm and shoulder girdle; and the Standing Long Jump Test is a measure of explosive leg power.

TECHNIQUES FOR MEASURING MUSCULAR STRENGTH AND ENDURANCE

When special equipment is required for strength and endurance testing, it is usually one of four types—dynamometers, cable tensiometers, weight-training machines, and electromechanical instruments. Many colleges and universities have all four types, but some public school systems do not have any. Weight training machines are becoming common, however, in health and fitness clubs.

Dynamometers

A **dynamometer** is used to measure static strength and endurance. Strength and endurance may be referred to as static or dynamic. *Isometric strength* is the force exerted against an immovable resistance; *isotonic strength* is force exerted by a muscle group as a body part moves through space. Isometric strength is often called **static strength;** isotonic strength is often called **dynamic strength.**

Two types of dynamometers are available, one for handgrip and one for back and leg strength. The most common type is the hand or grip dynamometer shown in Figure 19-1.

To use the hand dynamometer, adjust the handgrip to fit the examinee's hand. The subject should stand, holding the dynamometer parallel to the side of the dial facing away from the body. To measure grip strength, the dynamometer should be squeezed as hard as possible without moving the arm. Three trials are recommended with a 1-minute rest between trials (Heyward, 1984).

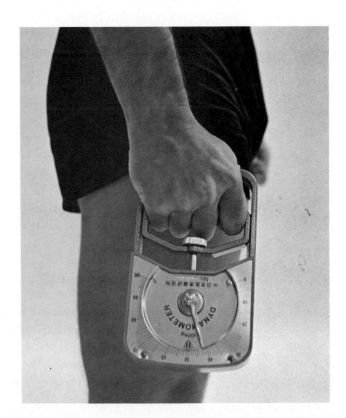

FIGURE 19-1 *Hand dynamometer.*

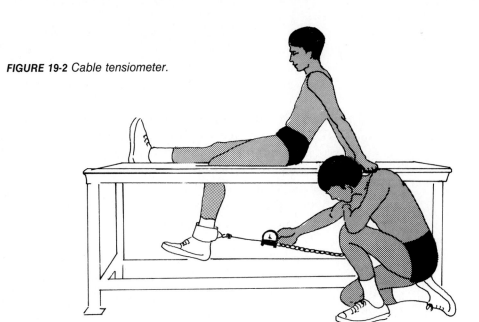

FIGURE 19-2 *Cable tensiometer.*

When measuring grip endurance, the examinee should squeeze as hard as possible and continue squeezing for 60 seconds. Record the force in kilograms (kg) every 10 seconds. Relative endurance can be determined by dividing the final force by the initial force times 100. Instead of an allout force, a submaximal force can be used, such as 50% of maximum. This is scored by the amount of time the submaximal force can be maintained.

Cable Tensiometer

A **cable tensiometer** is used to assess isometric strength. This technique that was developed and refined by Harrison Clarke (1966) at the University of Oregon can be used to test 38 different muscle groups. A goniometer is used to position the cable at the proper angle. The tensiometer yields a score in pounds, with possible scores ranging from 0 to 400. An example of the cable tensiometer is shown in Figure 19-2.

Weight-Training Machines

Weight-training machines are designed to measure isotonic muscle strength and endurance. The most useful of these machines offers both constant and variable resistance. The force varies throughout the movement, which is better for overall strength and endurance. Many tests of dynamic strength measure maximum strength at one point during the motion. A variable resistance machine can adjust load so that maximum strength is being measured during several phases of

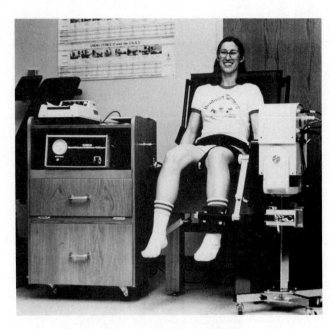

FIGURE 19-3 *Cybex II.*

the movement; however, measuring maximum contraction throughout the movement on these machines is not possible.

Electromechanical Instruments

Electromechanical instruments measure isometric and isotonic strength, endurance, and power. A well-known example is the Cybex II, depicted in Figure 19-3. When this machine is used, the maximum contraction of a muscle group is measured at a constant speed throughout the entire range of motion.

EXAMPLES OF STRENGTH TESTS

When strength measurement is being discussed, the term *1-RM* is often used, meaning one repetition maximum. This method, used to test a variety of muscle groups—such as those used in the bench press, standing press, arm curl, and leg press—is described first, followed by other techniques requiring less expensive equipment.

The 1-RM Test

Test Objective To measure dynamic strength; to measure the maximum weight lifted in 1-RM.

Description Determine the 1-RM value by trial and error. Start with a weight the examinee can lift. After a successful trial, allow the examinee to rest for 3 minutes. Increase the weight by 5 to 10 pounds and take another trial. Allow for

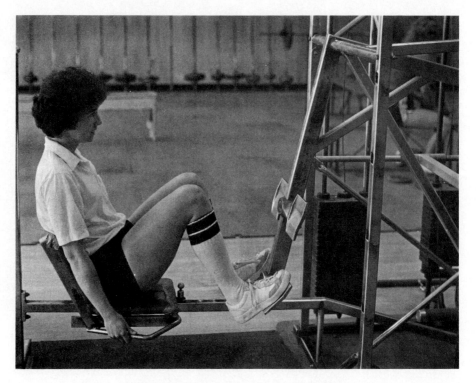

FIGURE 19-4 Leg press with knees flexed.

resting, then continue with the same pattern until the examinee can no longer execute a successful trial.

As an example, to test the leg extensors, seat the subject with hips and knees flexed, holding onto the chair rung with the hands. (See Figures 19-4 and 19-5.) Adjust the seat to standardize the knee angle at approximately 120 degrees. The weights are lifted by fully extending the legs. To determine the maximum weight, refer to the previous paragraph.

Test Area A small, multipurpose room.

Equipment A weight-training machine and scorecards.

Scoring A direct relationship exists between body weight and weight lifted. All other factors being equal, heavier people can lift heavier weights. Thus the test score—the maximum weight that can be lifted—should be interpreted considering the person's weight.

Validity Logical and construct validity.

Reliability Can be expected to be very high, since an allout effort is being measured; verified by Jackson and others (1980).

Norms See Table 19-1 for norms on gender and body weight.

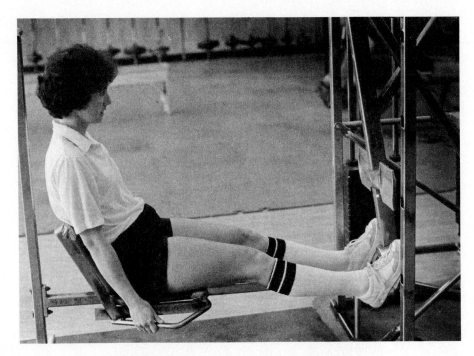

FIGURE 19-5 *Leg press with legs fully extended.*

TABLE 19-1 *Optimal strength values for various body weights (based on the 1-RM Test)*

	Bench press		Standing press		Curl		Leg press	
Body weight	Men	Women	Men	Women	Men	Women	Men	Women
80	80	56	53	37	40	28	160	112
100	100	70	67	47	50	35	200	140
120	120	84	80	56	60	42	240	168
140	140	98	93	65	70	49	280	196
160	160	112	107	75	80	56	320	224
180	180	126	120	84	90	63	360	252
200	200	140	133	93	100	70	400	280
220	220	154	147	103	110	77	440	308
240	240	168	160	112	120	84	480	336

From Pollock, M.L., and others.
Data collected on Universal Gym apparatus. Information collected on other apparatus could modify results.
Data expressed in pounds.

Comments Several measurement experts (e.g., Jackson, 1986) have correctly noted that the assessment of isotonic strength is more accurate when individual differences are taken into account. Individual differences due to body weight are of particular concern because body weight and 1-RM performance are moderately correlated. Several methods have been proposed for evaluating isotonic strength while controlling individual differences in body weight.

One of these methods is to express 1-RM as a percentage of body weight. Table 19-2 is used to determine the score. For example, a 140-pound woman who bench presses 100 pounds has a strength to body weight of 0.71 (see Figures 19-6 and 19-7). Referring to the closest ratio (0.70) in Table 19-2, the score on the bench test is 7.

If no weight-training machine is available, free weights can be used (see Figures 19-8 and 19-9). Select a 5- to 6-foot-long weight bar and a variety of weight plates. A test-retest reliability coefficient of 0.93 was reported for the free weight version of the test (Johnson, 1966).

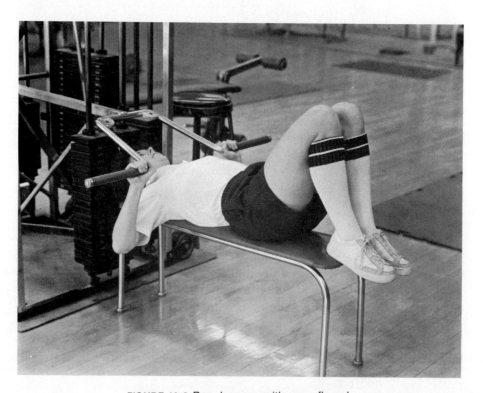

FIGURE 19-6 *Bench press with arms flexed.*

TABLE 19-2 *Strength-to-body weight ratios for selected dynamic strength tests*

			Men			
Bench press	Arm curl	Lateral pull-down	Leg press	Leg extension	Leg curl	Points
1.50	0.70	1.20	3.00	0.80	0.70	10
1.40	0.65	1.15	2.80	0.75	0.65	9
1.30	0.60	1.10	2.60	0.70	0.60	8
1.20	0.55	1.05	2.40	0.65	0.55	7
1.10	0.50	1.00	2.20	0.60	0.50	6
1.00	0.45	0.95	2.00	0.55	0.45	5
0.90	0.40	0.90	1.80	0.50	0.40	4
0.80	0.35	0.85	1.60	0.45	0.35	3
0.70	0.30	0.80	1.40	0.40	0.30	2
0.60	0.25	0.75	1.20	0.35	0.25	1
			Women			
0.90	0.50	0.85	2.70	0.70	0.60	10
0.85	0.45	0.80	2.50	0.65	0.55	9
0.80	0.42	0.75	2.30	0.60	0.52	8
0.70	0.38	0.73	2.10	0.55	0.50	7
0.65	0.35	0.70	2.00	0.52	0.45	6
0.60	0.32	0.65	1.80	0.50	0.40	5
0.55	0.28	0.63	1.60	0.45	0.35	4
0.50	0.25	0.60	1.40	0.40	0.30	3
0.45	0.21	0.55	1.20	0.35	0.25	2
0.35	0.18	0.50	1.00	0.30	0.20	1

Total points	Strength fitness category
48-60	Excellent
37-47	Good
25-36	Average
13-24	Fair
0-12	Poor

From Heyward, V.H.
Based on data compiled by author for 250 college-age men and women.

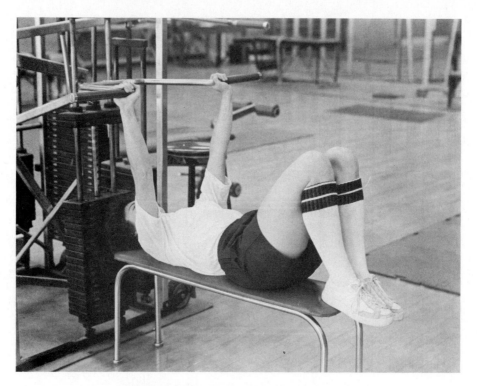

FIGURE 19-7 *Bench press with arms extended.*

Bench Squat Test (Johnson, 1966)

Test Objective To measure leg and back strength.

Description Use two assistants to handle the weight bar. The examinee should sit near the edge of the chair or bench. The assistants should place the bar on the shoulders and behind the neck of the subject. With feet a comfortable distance apart, the examinee should grasp the bar firmly and lower the body to a sitting position on the chair or bench. Using a smooth movement, the examinee stands again. Two trials may be taken. The weight can be adjusted before the second trial.

Test Area A small, multipurpose room.

Equipment Bench or chair, 15 to 17 inches in height; weight bar 5 to 6 feet long; sufficient assortment of weight plates; and a thick towel to provide padding at the base of the neck where the bar will be placed.

Scoring Total weight of the barbell lifted in the maximum repetition divided by body weight.

Validity Face validity.

Reliability $r_{xx'} = 0.95$, test-retest.

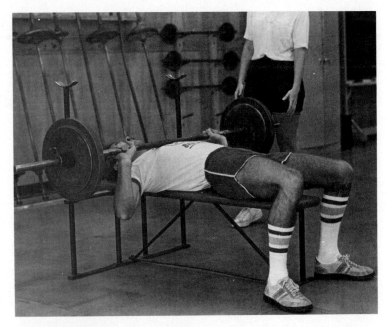

FIGURE 19-8 *Bench press using free weights, with arms flexed.*

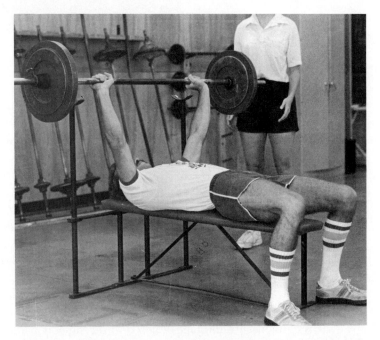

FIGURE 19-9 *Bench press using free weights, with arms extended.*

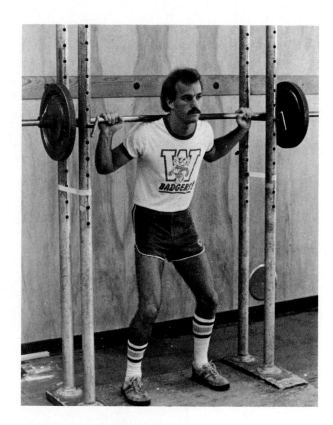

FIGURE 19-10 *Squat test—bar lifted off pins.*

Norms Norms have been developed for college men (see Johnson and Nelson, 1974).

Comments This test can be used with females as well as males. Careful spotting is required by the two assistants in case the examinee loses control of the bar or begins to fall. Be sure the examinee sits on the edge of the chair or bench rather than farther back. Adjusting the height of the bench or chair may improve the testing conditions.

Although strength and endurance are highly correlated, the use of continuous repetitions of a leg movement is not recommended (Baumgartner and Jackson, 1987). Some subjects can continue indefinitely; thus, the development of a valid table of norms is a problem.

Because of the potential danger to the spine in executing a squat test requiring the examinee to sit down on a bench, use of the standard equipment shown in Figures 19-10 and 19-11 is recommended. The subject lifts the bar off the pins in the support poles, rests the bar on the shoulders, and lowers the body in the squat position until the tape adhered to the support poles is broken. The lower pins are a safety feature, in case the subject drops the bar.

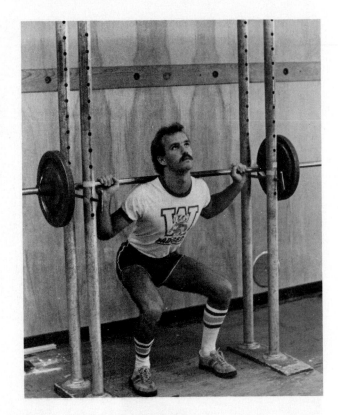

FIGURE 19-11 *Squat test—body lowered.*

Pull-Ups Test The Pull-Ups Test (see Figures 19-12 and 19-13) is used to measure arm and shoulder girdle endurance. (See Chapter 17.) It is recommended for males age 10 and older. Although it is often referred to as a strength test, it is more accurately classified as an endurance test.

Johnson (1966) developed a version of the pull-ups test measuring maximum effort on one repetition. In addition to the usual equipment, weight plates of 2½, 5, 10, and 25 pounds must be available. A rope or strap should be used to secure the weight to the waist of the subject. Actually, the weight can hang in back of the subject, secured to a strap around the waist.

The examinee stands on a chair and grasps the chinning bar. The chair is removed, and the subject assumes a straight-arm hang. One pull-up is performed; the chair is replaced, and he lowers himself to the chair. A second trial is taken if desired. The weight may be adjusted before the second trial. The score is the amount of extra weight lifted in the best of two trials divided by the body weight. A score of 0 is given to any subject who cannot complete the pull-up with more than his own body weight.

A reliability coefficient of 0.99 was reported (Johnson, 1966); otherwise, the test description is similar to that in Chapter 17.

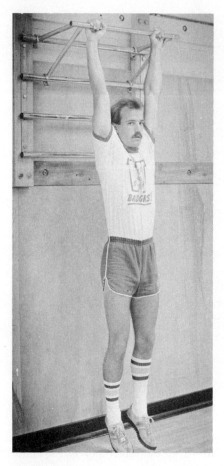

FIGURE 19-12 *Pull-Ups Test—body extended.*

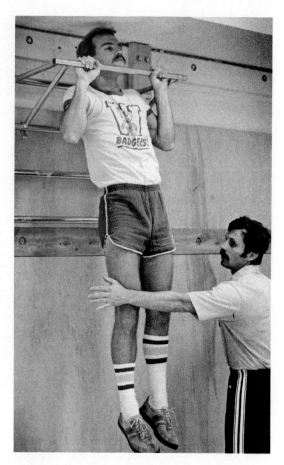

FIGURE 19-13 *Pull-Ups Test—elbows flexed.*

Sit-Ups Test This test is almost identical to a repeated sit-ups test, except only one repetition is executed. A weight plate should be held behind the neck. A dumbbell or barbell can also be used. The score is the maximum number of pounds lifted in a single repetition.

Examples of Endurance Tests

Lateral Pull-Down (Jackson and Smith, 1974)

Test Objective To measure arm strength; to execute repeated lifts using arm flexors.

Description Select a weight that can be pulled down at least once by everyone in the group. The examinee assumes a kneeling position on the floor, grasping the bar on the handle grips, as shown in Figure 19-14. For one repetition,

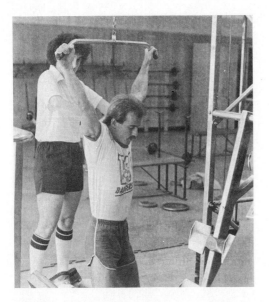

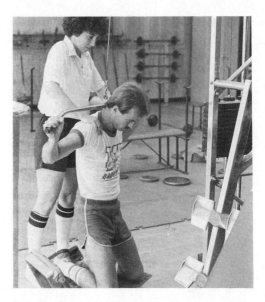

FIGURE 19-14 *Lateral pull-down—bar properly grasped.*

FIGURE 19-15 *Lateral pull-down—bar touching upper back.*

the examinee pulls the bar down behind the head until it touches the upper back at the shoulder level (see Figure 19-15). The weight is then returned to the starting position, avoiding jerky movements. The knees and lower legs must remain on the floor during the return movements. Use a 3-second cadence for each repetition. Note the way in which a spotter is used in this test. The examinee can be asked to touch the spotter's hands with the bar to complete the pulldown. The use of a spotter is especially important if a 1-RM test is being administered.

Test Area and Equipment Identical to those described in the Bench Press Test.

Scoring, Validity, Reliability, and Norms Identical to those described in the Bench Press Test.

The bar can also be pulled down to the front of the body, as shown in Figures 19-16 and 19-17. Note the hands are placed much closer together on the bar. A different muscle group is used in this pull-down action.

Comments Instead of using the same weight for everyone, the test can be individualized by using a weight that requires a percentage of maximum strength to be lifted. Pollock and associates (1978) recommended using a weight that is 70% of the 1-RM value for each exercise.

Bench Press (Jackson and Smith, 1974)

Test Objective To measure arm strength by lifting a constant weight load repeatedly until exhausted.

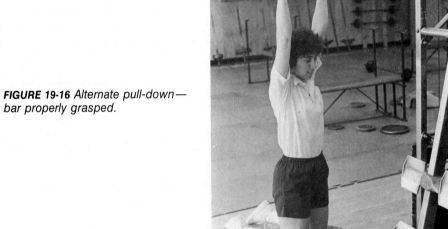

FIGURE 19-16 Alternate pull-down— bar properly grasped.

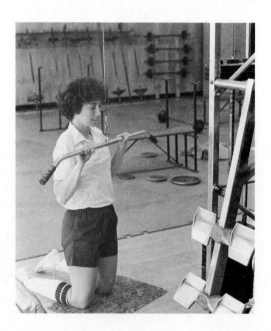

FIGURE 19-17 Alternate pull-down— bar pulled in front of body.

Description The weight load is constant for everyone in the group. The examinee assumes a back-lying position on the bench, similar to the position shown in Figures 19-6 and 19-7, except that the feet must be flat on the floor. Use a weight load that can be lifted at least once by all examinees in the group. For example, a weight of 110 pounds is recommended for male college freshmen.

The back should rest flat on the bench. The handles are grasped with both hands, placed farther apart than the shoulders. The weight is lifted upward until the arms are fully extended, then lowered until the weights touch the weights beneath them. The weights should not be dropped or slammed. If free weights are used, the bar should be lowered to the chest.

Continue with repetitions of the same movement on a 3-second cadence. The examinee should not be allowed to begin a new repetition until the beginning of a new 3-second interval.

Test Area A small, multipurpose room.

Equipment A weight-training machine or free weights, metronome or tape of recording of cadence, and scorecards.

Scoring The score is the number of repetitions completed. The test is ended when an examinee can no longer execute a repetition correctly or maintain the proper cadence.

Validity Logical, as an endurance measure; concurrent as a strength measure—high correlation with the maximum weight lifted with one repetition ($r_{xy} > 0.90$).

Reliability None reported, but can be expected to be high if examinees are motivated to maximum performance.

Norms Available for college men in original source.

Comments Although this is a measure of muscular endurance, the authors believe the test can be used as a measure of strength since it is highly correlated with 1-RM.

Arm Curl (Jackson and Smith, 1974)

Test Objective To measure arm strength; to execute repeated curls using arm flexors.

Description Before beginning the test, the examinee must first be stabilized by standing with head, shoulders, and buttocks against a wall. The feet, placed 12 to 15 inches from the wall, are used to brace the back. To ensure that this position is maintained during exercise, the test developers recommend placing a sheet of paper behind the buttocks. The paper must remain pinned against the wall throughout the test. When the paper falls, the test is terminated.

To administer this test as described, the weight-training unit must be positioned close to a wall. Obviously, this may not be possible in many settings. If this is not possible, the standard curl shown in Figures 19-18 and 19-19 may be used. If the hips are thrust forward during the repetitions, the test should be terminated. Only the arms should move during this test.

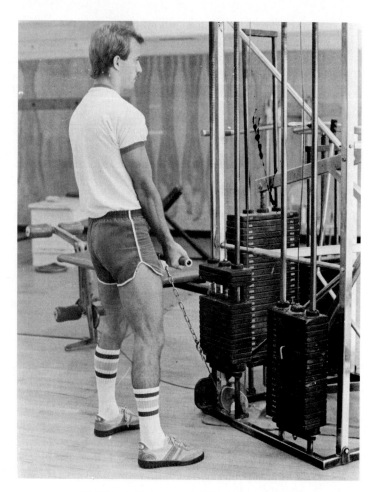

FIGURE 19-18 *Arm curl with arms extended.*

The examinee should begin with arms fully extended. In this position, the exercise weight should be suspended slightly above the remaining weights. The examinee should flex the arms fully, touch the bar to the chin, and fully extend the arms again. A 3-second cadence for each repetition is used.

This test can also be administered using free weights, as shown in Figures 19-20 and 19-21. Note the equipment used to stabilize the examinee. This prevents any other body part from being used to assist in executing the curl.

Test Area and Equipment Identical to those described in the Bench Press Test.

Scoring, Validity, Reliability, and Norms Identical to those described in the Bench Press Test.

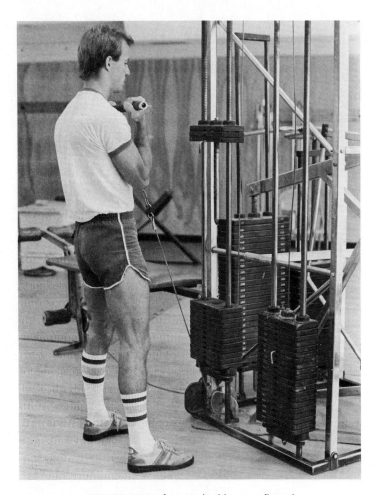

FIGURE 19-19 *Arm curl with arms flexed.*

Squat Thrust Test (Burpee, R.H., in Clark, 1976.)

Test Objective To measure the general muscular endurance of the body.

Description The examinee stands erect, with arms hanging at the side. At the signal Ready, Go! a squat position is assumed with the hands on the floor. Then the body is extended fully, as shown in Figure 19-22. The examinee returns to the squat position and then to the standing position. The procedure is repeated as rapidly as possible for 10 seconds. On the signal Stop! the test ends. Three trials are taken.

Test Area A small room with smooth floor surface.

Equipment Stopwatch and scorecards.

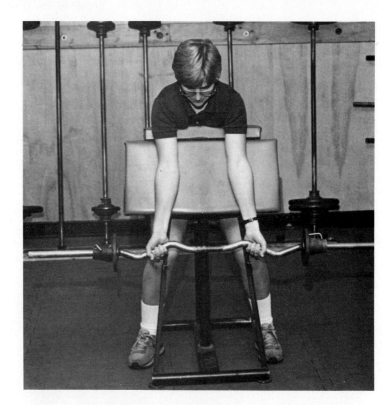

FIGURE 19-20 *Arm curl using free weights, arms extended.*

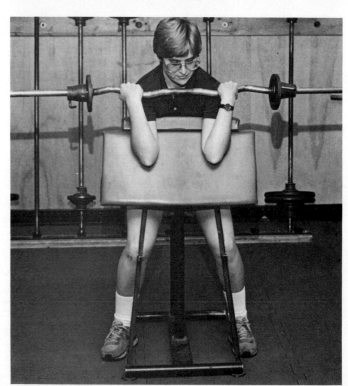

FIGURE 19-21 *Arm curl using free weights, arms flexed.*

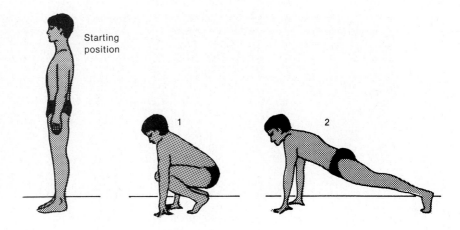

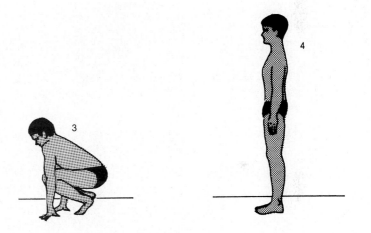

FIGURE 19-22 *Squat thrust.*

Scoring Score 1 point for each completed squat thrust. Each quarter movement is given ¼ point. The test score is the best of three trials.

Validity r_{xy} = 0.55, reported by C.H. McCloy.

Reliability $r_{xx'}$ = 0.92, reported by C.H. McCloy.

Comments A large group of examinees can be tested at the same time. Each examinee should work with a partner, who counts the number of squat thrusts. Careful attention should be paid to the positions assumed in the squat thrusts. In particular, be sure that the body is fully extended at position No. 2. Instruct the examinees on the correct procedure for executing this movement before the actual test.

Other Approaches to Endurance Testing A number of other practical approaches to endurance training have been reported in the literature. Among the

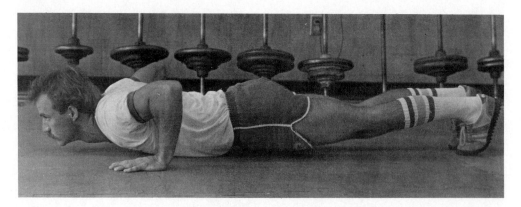

FIGURE 19-23 *Push-up with arms flexed.*

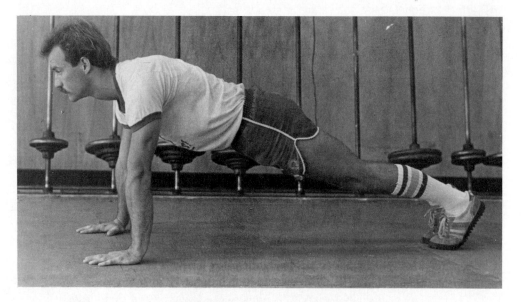

FIGURE 19-24 *Push-up with arms extended.*

more popular items are push-ups, used to measure arm and shoulder girdle endurance (see Figures 19-23 and 19-24). The problem with this test is that as with
pull-ups, some examinees will not be able to execute even one. Thus it is not a
discriminating measure for some groups.

Modified push-ups may be used as an alternative test for female examinees.
These push-ups are performed with the knees touching the floor instead of the
feet, as seen in the full-length push-up. This test is depicted in Figures 19-25
and 19-26.

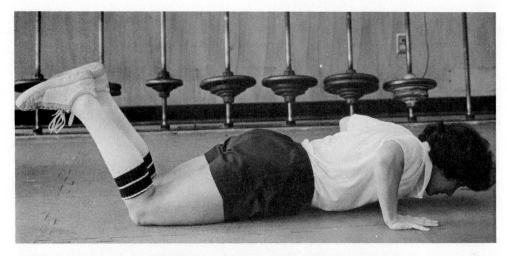

FIGURE 19-25 *Modified push-up with arms flexed.*

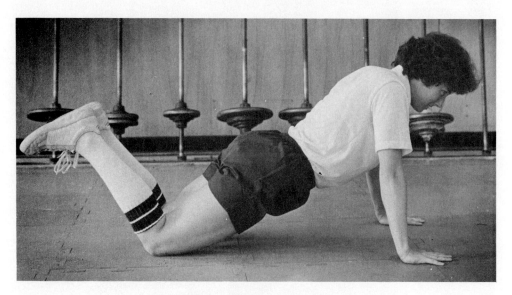

FIGURE 19-26 *Modified push-up with arms extended.*

If gymnastics equipment is available, the parallel bars can be used to test repeated executions of the dip. The parallel bars on a weight-training machine can
also be used for this purpose (see Figures 19-27 and 19-28). The dip is performed
by lowering the body until the elbow forms a 90-degree angle. A simpler version
of endurance testing using the dip is a modified test using a single bar. The
lower bar of the uneven bars can be used for this purpose. The body and arms

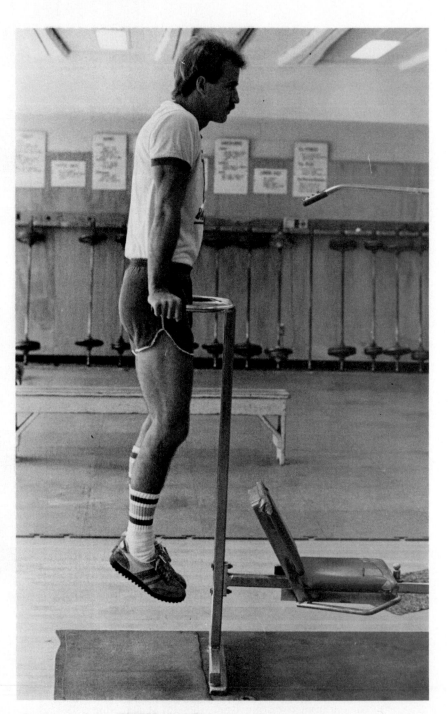

FIGURE 19-27 *Dip—arms fully extended.*

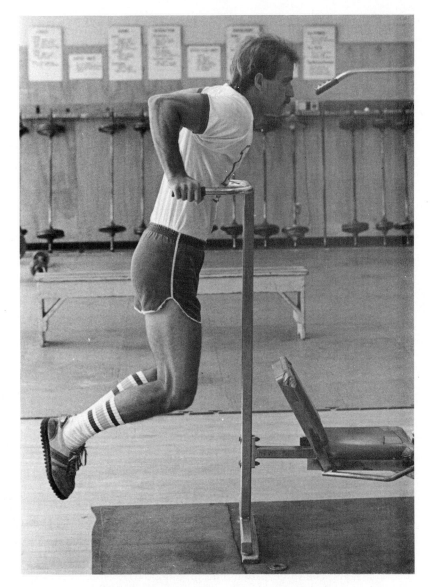

FIGURE 19-28 *Dip—elbow at 90-degree angle.*

are fully extended on the bar. The dip is performed by lowering the body on the bar until the elbows are at right angles. Then full extension takes place.

POWER TESTING

Power is the ability to generate maximum force in a minimum amount of time. Several practical tests of explosive power are quite popular in the physical edu-

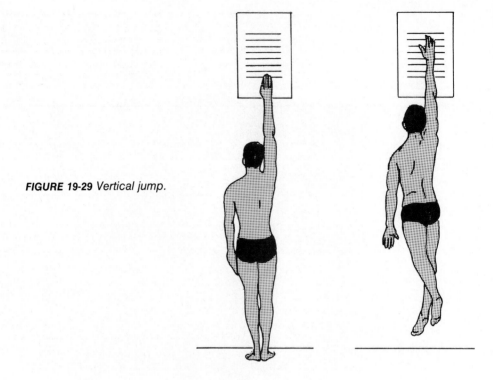

FIGURE 19-29 *Vertical jump.*

cation field. Two examples are the standing long jump, described in Chapter 17, and the Vertical Jump Test, described below.

Vertical Jump Test (Sargent, 1921)

Test Objective To measure the explosive power of the leg extensors.

Description For the **vertical jump,** the examinee stands with the dominant arm extended, as shown in Figure 19-29, holding a piece of chalk to mark the wall. The feet are flat on the floor. The examinee should reach as high as possible, making a mark on the measuring board. Then a preparatory position should be taken for the jump, which is a squat position with the feet still flat on the floor. The subject should jump as high as possible, touching the board again with the chalk at the height of the jump. Three trials are taken.

Test Area Measuring board (self-constructed or purchased commercially), marked in half inches, attached to the wall (if possible, the board should be attached 6 inches out from the wall so the examinee does not scrape the arm or side of the body while jumping), chalk and damp cloth (or eraser), yardstick, and scorecards.

Scoring For each trial, the score is the distance between the two chalk marks, measured to the nearest half inch. The test score is the best trial score.

TABLE 19-3 *Vertical Jump scoring table*

	100	90	80	70	60	50	40	30	20	10	0
Boys and girls 9-10-11	16	15	14	12	11	10	9	7	4	2	0
Boys 12-13-14	20	18	17	16	14	13	11	9	5	2	0
Girls 12-13-14	16	15	14	13	12	11	10	8	4	2	0
Boys 15-17	25	24	23	21	19	16	12	8	5	2	0
Girls 15-17	17	16	15	14	13	11	8	6	3	2	0
Men 18-34	26	25	24	23	19	16	13	9	8	2	0
Women 18-34	14	13	13	12	10	8	6	4	2	1	0

From Friermood, H.T.
Raw scores are located in the chart in accordance with age and sex, and percentile scores are located across the top.

Validity $r_{xy} = 0.78$, using a criterion test of four power events in track and field.

Reliability $r_{xx'} = 0.93$; objectivity coefficients > 0.90 have been reported.

Norms Norms for the vertical jump test are included in Table 19-3.

Comments The following are four of the many versions of the test:

1. Instead of using a piece of chalk, magnesium chalk can be placed on the fingertips of the hand on the wall side; or the fingertips can be dipped in water; or a stepladder can be placed adjacent to the measuring board, and an assistant can measure the height from this position. If chalk is used, the chalk marks must be removed, preferably with a damp cloth, after each trial.
2. Instead of facing the wall to take the initial measurement, the subject can stand with one side to the wall, with toes touching the wall.
3. Instead of standing flat footed to take the initial measurement, the subject stands on tip-toes.
4. The measurement is taken to the nearest quarter of an inch instead of the nearest half inch.

This test can be administered to 30 students in 45 minutes. If desired, the score can be adjusted so that body weight is taken into account.

SUMMARY

The measurement of muscular strength and endurance requires careful attention to the position of the examinee and the execution of the movement. Serious injuries can occur if proper protocol is not followed. The spotters must be thoroughly trained and remain attentive throughout the testing. The safety of the examinee must receive top priority. Test selection depends on the type of equipment available. Several strength and endurance tests require little or no equipment. Although tests using sophisticated and expensive equipment may be more valid, the practical versions are satisfactory for field testing.

LEARNING EXPERIENCES

1. To understand strength and endurance testing more fully, enroll in a weight-training class. This will familiarize you with the proper positions, the safety considerations, and the use of appropriate equipment. If it is not possible to enroll in such a course, observe a class two or three times at your campus or a private fitness club.
2. Ask a qualified classmate to administer an arm press and a leg press test to you. Be sure this person is thoroughly familiar with the protocol. Compare your scores to the norms in this chapter.
3. Administer the Vertical Jump Test to everyone in your class. Obtain the weight of each classmate as well. Correlate vertical jump scores with weight. Is there a substantial enough relationship to warrant using body weight to adjust vertical jump scores? How might this sort of adjustment be made?

REFERENCES

Baumgartner, T.A., and Jackson, A.S. 1982, 1987. Measurement for evaluation in physical education. Dubuque IA: Wm C Brown Group.

Clarke, H.H. 1966. Muscular strength and endurance in man. Englewood Cliffs, NJ: Prentice Hall, Inc.

Clarke, H.H. 1966. Application of measurement to health and physical education. Englewood Cliffs, NJ: Prentice Hall, Inc.

Heyward, V.H. 1984. Designs for fitness. Minneapolis: Burgess Publishing Co.

Jackson, A. 1986. Strength measurement: controlling for individual differences. Journal of Physical Education, Recreation and Dance, 57(6):82-84.

Jackson, A., Watkins, M., and Patton, R. 1980. A factor analysis of twelve selected maximal isotonic strength performances on the universal gym. Medicine and Science in Sports and Exercise, 12:274-277.

Jackson, A.S., and Smith, L. 1974. The validation of an evaluation system for weight-training. Unpublished study presented at the AAHPER Convention, March 1977, Anaheim, CA.

Johnson, B.L. 1966. Isometric strength tests. Northeast Louisiana University, Monroe.

Johnson, B.L., and Nelson, J.K. 1974. Practical measurements for evaluation in physical education. Minneapolis: Burgess Publishing Co.

Pollock, M.L., Wilmore, J.H., and Fox, S.M. 1978. Health and fitness through physical activity. New York: John Wiley & Sons.

Sargent, D.A. 1921. Physical test of a man. American Physical Education Review, 26(4):188-194.

ANNOTATED READINGS

Heyward, V.H. 1984. Assessment of muscular strength and endurance. In Designs for fitness. Minneapolis: Burgess Publishing Co.

Describes devices for measuring strength and muscular endurance; discusses problems associated with the assessment of static and dynamic muscle strength and endurance; analyzes calisthenic-type strength and endurance tests.

Katch, F.I., and McArdle, W.D. 1983. Conditioning for muscular strength. In Nutrition, weight control and exercise, ed. 2, Philadelphia: Lea & Febiger.

Describes three exercise systems for developing muscular strength—weight training, isometric training, and isokinetic training; includes sections on muscular adaptations with strength training, strength training for women, and circuit weight training; presents step-by-step procedure for planning a workout; provides instruction on selecting proper weights.

Leighton, J.R. 1983. Fitness, body development, and sports conditioning through weight training. Springfield, IL: Charles C Thomas, Publisher.

Provides beginning and advanced exercise programs for both men and women using free weights, multistation exercise machines, and variable resistence equipment; discusses conditioning for a variety of activities, such as golf, racquet sports, and soccer.

Sharkey, B.J. 1984. Physiology of fitness, ed. 2, Champaign, IL: Human Kinetics Publishers, Inc.

Includes section on muscular fitness training; presents test for fitness, training programs, in the appendix; covers the latest information on fitness.

20

Tests of Balance and Flexibility

KEY WORDS *Watch for these words as you read the following chapter:*

balance	flexibility	posture
dynamic balance	flexometer	static balance
elgon	goniometer	task specificity

Performance of any motor skill is dependent, to some extent, on one's balance and flexibility. Years ago, physical educators thought that people possessed a general ability to balance and another general ability reflecting overall flexibility. In other words, if a person could balance well on one body part, it was assumed that he or she could balance well on any body part. Based on this rationale, the development of practical tests of balance was quite straightforward. Only one balance test, for example, was needed to measure overall balance ability. Over the last two decades, however, research on both balance and flexibility has not substantiated the concept of general abilities. Rather, each of these abilities tends to be specific to a body part. This means that a person who is flexible at a hip joint is not necessarily flexible in the shoulder joint. Yet we have all seen gymnasts who are flexible in all joints. Does this not point to a general ability? Probably not. More likely, it reflects **task specificity,** a high level of flexibility in many specific abilities. Task specificity suggests that not only is the ability specific to a particular body part but also to a particular task.

These research results complicate the measurement of balance and flexibility considerably, unless one's interest lies only with measurement at a specific site. Yet many tests of these two attributes have been developed in the physical education field. While none is valid as a test of general balance or flexibility, some are useful in more specific settings. Although precise measures of both attributes are available, these are not emphasized in this textbook, since they are impractical for the typical school and private club setting. Several that might be useful in a nonschool setting are briefly described.

MEASURING BALANCE

Balance is the ability to maintain equilibrium. Even before a great deal of research was conducted on the nature of balance, it was deduced that two types of balance exist—**static balance,** the ability to maintain equilibrium in a stationary position, and **dynamic balance,** the ability to maintain equilibrium while in motion.

A physical educator or exercise scientist might be interested in measuring balance for a variety of reasons. Achievement of minimal balance standards might be a goal in a physical education instructional unit, such as posture/body mechanics or gymnastics. Balance tests might be used in assessing the movement patterns of young children and in evaluating the status of special education children. The measurement of balance is useful in assessing potential in gymnastics, diving, and other forms of physical activity that require balance skills. This topic is of great interest in the elderly population, where maintaining equilibrium is essential in the prevention of injury occurring as a result of falls. Several tests are described for each type of balance.

Examples of Tests of Static Balance

Bass Stick Test (lengthwise) (Bass, 1939)

Test Objective To measure the ability to balance in a stationary, upright position using a small base of support.

Description The examinee places the dominant foot lengthwise on a special stick, as shown in Figure 20-1. Both the ball of the foot and the heel should rest on the stick. The opposite foot is lifted from the floor and held in this position as long as possible. The stopwatch is started when the opposite foot leaves the floor and stopped when it touches the floor again, or when any part of the supporting foot touches the floor. Three trials are taken on each foot.

Test Area Smooth, flat floor.

Equipment Stick 1 inch wide, 1 inch high, and 12 inches long; stopwatch; and tape (to hold the stick to the floor).

Scoring The test score is the time for the best of three trials.

Validity Face validity.

Reliability $r_{xx'} = 0.90$

Norms Not reported for this test.

Comments If an examinee loses balance during the first 3 seconds of the trial, the trial may be restarted. This is a popular test in the field and is usually very motivating to the examinee, although it measures only a specific type of balance.

Bass Stick Test (crosswise) (Bass, 1939) Same as the Bass Stick Test (lengthwise) except that the foot is placed crosswise on the stick and the examinee balances on the ball of the foot (see Figure 20-2).

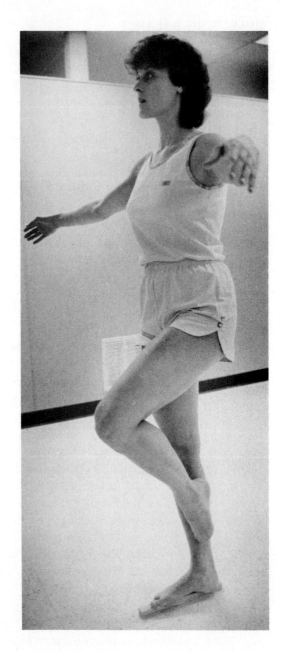

FIGURE 20-1 Bass Stick Test (lengthwise).

Stork Stand

Test Objective To measure the ability to balance in a stationary, upright position using a small base of support.

Description The examinee stands on the dominant foot, flat on the floor. The other foot is held so that it touches the inside of the supporting knee, as shown in Figure 20-3. The hands are placed on the hips. As soon as the proper position

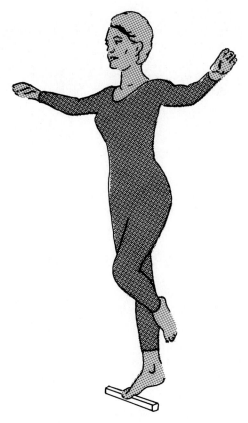

FIGURE 20-2 *Bass Stick Test (crosswise).*

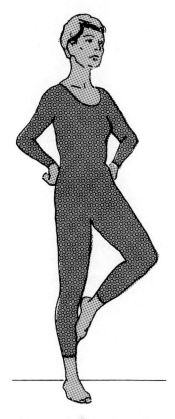

FIGURE 20-3 *Stork Stand Test.*

has been established, the stopwatch is started. The examinee holds the position as long as possible. When the nondominant foot is moved away from the knee, stop the watch. This constitutes one trial; three trials are taken.

Test Area Smooth, flat floor.

Equipment Stopwatch.

Scoring The best of three trials is the test score.

Validity Face validity.

Reliability $r_{xx'} = 0.85$, test-retest (as reported by Jensen and Hirst, 1980); $r_{xx'} = 0.85$, test-retest (as reported by Johnson and Nelson, 1979).

Norms Available for college men and women in Johnson and Nelson (1979) for a slightly different version of the test in which the examinee balances on the ball of the foot.

Comments The lack of a time limit is a drawback in administering the test. An examinee who can balance well in this position can hold this position for a lengthy period. If a group of students is being tested, this could be too time-consuming.

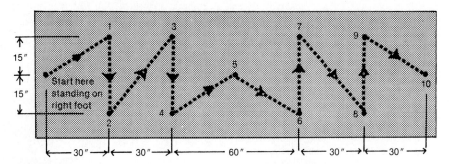

FIGURE 20-4 *Floor markings for the Johnson Modification of the Bass Test of Dynamic Balance.*

Examples of Tests of Dynamic Balance

Johnson Modification of the Bass Test of Dynamic Balance (Johnson and Leach, 1968)

Test Objective To measure dynamic balance.

Description Using the floor plan shown in Figure 20-4, the examinee begins with the right foot on the starting mark and leaps to the first tape mark, landing on the left foot and balancing on the ball of the foot as long as possible, up to 5 seconds. The examinee leaps to the next square, lands on the right foot, and tries to maintain balance for 5 seconds. This procedure is continued until the end of the floor pattern.

Test Area Smooth floor surface, 50 inches by 180 inches.

Equipment Stopwatch, tape measure, and floor tape.

Scoring For each successful landing on the tape mark, 5 points are scored; 1 point is scored for each second the examinee remains balanced on the mark, up to 5 seconds. It is possible to score 10 points at each tape mark and 100 points on the total test. The examinee is penalized 5 points for any of the following landing errors: not stopping after landing on the tape mark, touching the floor with any body part other than the supporting foot, and not covering the tape mark with the ball of the foot. If the examinee makes a landing error, the correct position can be resumed for the 5-second balance.

An additional 1-point penalty is given for the following errors during the 5-second balance: touching the floor with the heel of the hand or any body part other than the supporting foot and not holding the foot steady in the balance position. If the balance is lost, the examinee should return to the proper mark before leaping to the next mark.

Validity Face validity; $r_{xy} = 0.46$ using criterion of the original Bass Test of Dynamic Balance (as reported by Kirkendall, Gruber, and Johnson, 1980).

Reliability $r_{xx'} = 0.75$, test-retest.

Norms Norms are available for college women in Johnson and Nelson (1979).

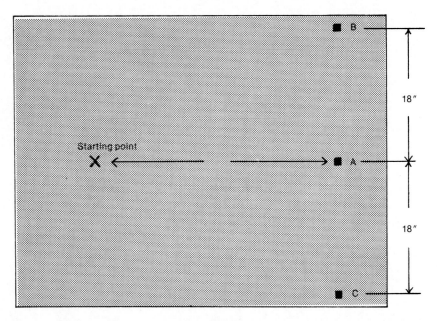

FIGURE 20-5 *Floor markings for the Modified Sideward Leap Test. Spot A is the landing point; spots B and C mark the placement of a small object.*

Comments While this is an interesting test, it is not a direct measure of dynamic balance. Usually, dynamic balance refers to balancing while the body (or body part) is moving. In this test, as in other tests of dynamic balance, the examinee moves but then stops and maintains a static balance.

Modified Sideward Leap (Scott and French, 1959)

Test Objective To measure dynamic balance.

Description The examinee begins on spot X, as shown in Figure 20-5, and places a small object on spots B and C. The starting position is assumed by standing on the left foot, with the right side toward spot A. The examinee takes a sideward leap to spot A, landing on the ball of the right foot, leans to spot B, and brushes the object off, using one hand. Balance on the ball of the foot should then be maintained for 5 seconds. Four trials are taken, two to each side.

Test Area Smooth floor surface, 50 inches by 50 inches.

Equipment Stopwatch; tape measure; floor tape; and a small, light object, such as a badminton shuttlecock.

Scoring The maximum number of points for each trial is 20:

1. 5 points for landing correctly on spot A.
2. 1 point for each second balance is held on spot A, up to 5 seconds.
3. 5 points for leaning and pushing object off spot B or C.
4. 1 point for each second balance is held on spot B or C, up to 5 seconds.

Validity Face validity.

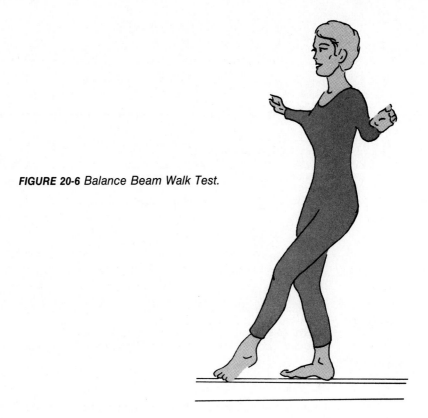

FIGURE 20-6 *Balance Beam Walk Test.*

Reliability $r_{xx'}$ = 0.66 to 0.88.

Norms Not reported for this specific test.

Comments Like the original version, this modification measures the ability to balance while performing other movements.

Balance Beam Walk (Jensen and Hirst, 1980*)

Test Objective To measure dynamic balance.

Description The examinee should stand on one end of the balance beam, slowly walk the full length of the beam (see Figure 20-6), pause for 5 seconds, turn around, and return to the starting position. Three trials are taken.

Test Area Smooth floor surface, 5 feet by 15 feet.

Equipment Balance beam and stopwatch.

Scoring Pass-fail.

Validity Face validity.

Reliability Not reported for this test.

---

*Although this test is described in Jensen and Hirst (1980), various versions of it have been in use for many years.

Norms Not reported for this test.

Comments There should be a time limit for this test; otherwise, the examinee could move at an excessively slow pace, consuming an unreasonable amount of time. Also, penalties should be identified for errors that occur throughout the test.

MEASURING FLEXIBILITY

Flexibility is the range of motion in a joint, specifically from a position of extension to flexion or the opposite movement. As noted previously, there is ample evidence that flexibility is specific to a given joint.

A flexibility test is included in all the recently revised national physical fitness tests. Low back flexibility is identified in these tests as an important factor in preventing low back pain. Many activities have a significant flexibility element, and flexibility is maintained and improved on a regular basis by individuals engaged in these activities. Flexibility tests are useful in monitoring the level of flexibility on a regular basis. Sufficient flexibility for the prevention of injury is essential, especially in the elderly population. Flexibility tests are widely used in today's society. In this chapter, both precise and practical measures of flexibility are discussed.

Precise Measures of Flexibility

Three devices are often mentioned when a precise measure of flexibility is desired. The **goniometer,** a 180-degree protractor with extended arms, provides the least precision of the three but is inexpensive and easy to use. The **flexometer** is an instrument with a weighted 360-degree dial and a weighted pointer (Leighton, 1942). Both the dial and pointer move independently and are affected by gravity. The flexometer is not affected by the length of the segments, and can be used to measure all body segments. Standard directions for measuring 30 segments are provided by Leighton (1955). The reliability of the flexometer has ranged from 0.901 to 0.983. The most sophisticated of the three, the **elgon,** is a goniometer with a potentiometer substituted for the protractor. Also known as an electrogoniometer, it records changes in degrees continuously throughout the movement. All three devices measure the movement of bodily segments in degrees. For more details, refer to Sigerseth's chapter in Montoye (1978).

Practical Tests of Flexibility

Because of the specific nature of flexibility tests, not many of the practical tests have a high degree of validity as measures of general flexibility, but some have a certain usefulness as measures of the flexibility of specific segments. However, caution must be used in the selection of flexibility tests, since certain measures require positioning the body in ways that might cause physical injury to some examinees.

Sit and Reach Test The Sit and Reach Test, described in detail in Chapter 16, is designed to measure flexibility of the low back and posterior thigh muscles. Although this is a reasonably practical test, it is not without problems. Flexibility is measured in centimeters (or, more recently, inches) rather than degrees. Performance on the test is somewhat dependent on the ratio of trunk length to lower body length. However, the test does provide comparative measurement. Furthermore, it requires little equipment, is inexpensive and easy to administer, and requires little time to administer. Students can learn to administer the test to each other. (See Chapter 16 for more information on this test, including abbreviated tables of norms.)

Kraus-Weber Floor Touch Test (Kraus and Hirschland, 1954*)

Test Objective To measure trunk flexibility or length of the back and hamstring muscles.

Description The examinee should assume an erect standing position in bare or stocking feet, with feet together. The arms should hang by the sides. With no prior warm-up bounces, the examinee should slowly lean downward, attempting to touch the floor with the fingertips (see Figure 20-7), and hold the floor-touch position for 3 seconds. The knees must be straightened throughout the test.

Test Area A small room.

Equipment Stopwatch.

Scoring As the test battery was originally devised, all test items were scored on a pass-fail basis. Using this procedure, if the floor touch is held for 3 seconds, the examinee passes the test. Otherwise, the examinee receives a fail. This system of scoring appears to be the most frequently used. Another scoring option uses numerical scores ranging from 0 to 10. If the floor touch position is held for 3 seconds, the examinee receives a score of 10. If the floor is not touched, 1 point is subtracted for every inch between the floor and the fingertips. If this distance is 10 inches or more, the score is 0.

Validity The validity of the Kraus-Weber Tests of Minimum Muscular Fitness is based on clinical evidence that patients with low back pain were unable to pass one or more of the Kraus-Weber test items. As their back conditions improved, their test results also improved.

Reliability Not reported for this specific test.

Norms Since the scoring is usually pass-fail, the use of norms is irrelevant.

Comments The test administrator might wish to hold the knees of the examinee being tested to insure that they remain straight throughout the test.

---

*This test is a part of the Kraus-Weber Tests of Minimum Muscular Fitness described in Chapter 16. The test battery includes six items.

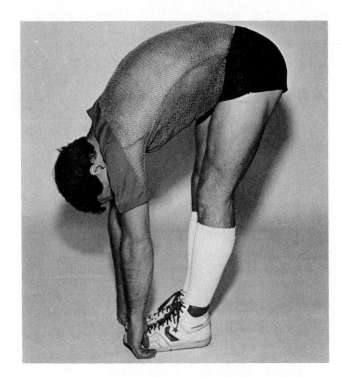

FIGURE 20-7 *Kraus-Weber Floor-Touch Test.*

Trunk Extension (Cureton, 1941)

Test Objective To measure the ability to hyperextend the trunk.

Description To assume the starting position of this test, the examinee should lie in a prone position on the mat. Both hands are placed on the lower back. A partner should hold the hips against the mat (see Figure 20-8). Using a tape measure, determine the distance from the mat to the suprasternal notch, the pronounced depression at the upper end of the sternum, at the base of the neck. Measure to the nearest quarter inch.

Test Area A small room.

Equipment Mat and tape measure.

Scoring To determine the test score, a standard measure of trunk length must first be taken. The examinee should sit with his or her back against the wall. Using a tape measure, determine the distance between the suprasternal notch and the floor or bench where the examinee is seated. Measure to the nearest quarter inch. Then, multiply the test measurement by 100 and divide by the standard measurement of trunk length to determine the test score (Jensen and Hirst, 1980).

Norms No national norms have been reported. In a local setting, the 50th

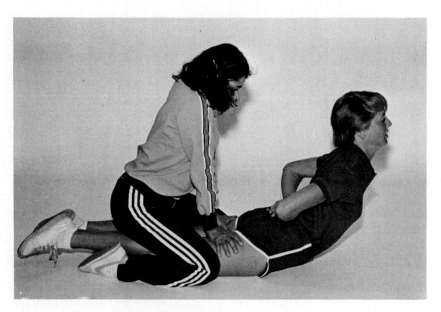

FIGURE 20-8 *Trunk Extension Test.*

percentile for college men was a score of 40; the 50th percentile for college women, a score of 38 (Johnson and Nelson, 1979).

Comments This test can be administered to an entire class of students in one class period.

Forward Bend of Trunk (Jensen and Hirst, 1980)

Test Objective To measure the flexion of the trunk and hips.

Description This test can be administered either on the floor or on a table. The examinee assumes a sitting position with feet against the wall, hip width apart. The knees must remain straight throughout the test. The hands are placed palms down on the mat, next to the upper thighs. The examinee should lean forward and downward as far as possible, reaching toward the heels of the feet (see Figure 20-9). Measure the vertical distance from the suprasternal notch to the floor and record the distance to the nearest quarter inch.

Test Area A small room with a smooth wall surface.

Equipment Mat (preferred) and tape measure.

Scoring The test score is the distance measured to the nearest quarter inch.

Validity Not reported for this specific test.

Reliability Not reported for this specific test.

Norms None available. Setting up a table of norms for one's own students is advisable.

Comments Keep in mind that lower scores (shorter distances) represent greater flexibility.

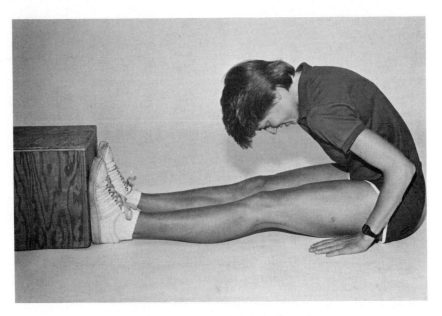

FIGURE 20-9 *Forward Bend of Trunk Test.*

MEASURING POSTURE

Although the measurement of posture is not a measure of balance or flexibility, these aspects certainly affect one's posture. **Posture** is defined as the alignment of the body and its segments.

New York State Posture Rating Test (New York State Education Department, 1966)

Test Objective To evaluate the posture of public school students grades 4 through 12.

Description The posture rating chart in Figure 20-10 is used to assess 13 areas of the body. Three profiles are shown for each area: the correct position, a slight deviation, and a pronounced deviation from the correct position. The examinee stands on a line in front of a screen. A plumb line is suspended just in front of the line. Another line is placed at right angles to the first line, extending 10 feet in front of the screen and perpendicular to it. The total distance from the screen to the line is 13 feet. The 13-foot point marks the location of the examiner.

The first six areas of the body are rated while the examinee stands facing the screen, with the plumb line bisecting the back of the head, the spine, and the legs and feet. The remaining seven areas are rated with the examinee's left side to the screen. The plumb line should fall along the ear, shoulder, hip, knee, and ankle.

Test Area Area 15 feet by 10 feet.

Equipment Screen, rating chart, and plumb line.

FIGURE 20-10 *Posture chart.*
By permission of the State Education Department, State University of New York, Albany.

GRADE	4	5	6	7	8	9	10	11	12
RATER'S INITIALS									
DATE OF TEST									

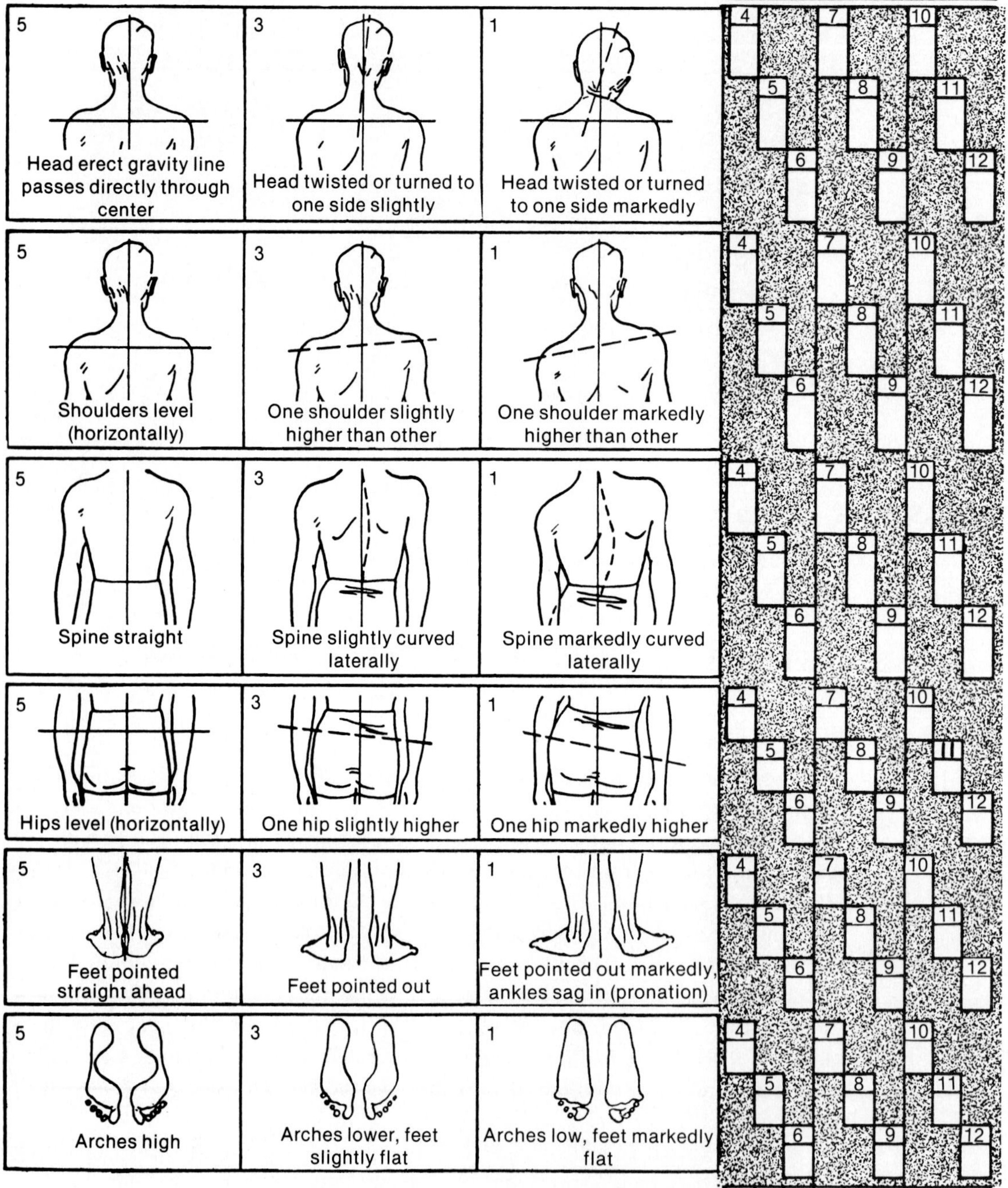

TOTAL PAGE ONE

FIGURE 20-10, cont'd

GRADE 4 | 5 | 6 | 7 | 8 | 9 | 10 | 11 | 12

TOTAL PAGE ONE

5 — Neck erect, chin in, head in balance directly above shoulders	3 — Neck slightly forward, chin slightly out	1 — Neck markedly forward, chin markedly out
5 — Chest elevated, breastbone furthest forward part of body	3 — Chest slightly depressed	1 — Chest markedly depressed (flat)
5 — Shoulders centered	3 — Shoulders slightly forward	1 — Shoulders markedly forward (shoulder blades protruding in rear)
5 — Upper back normally rounded	3 — Upper back slightly more rounded	1 — Upper back markedly rounded
5 — Trunk erect	3 — Trunk inclined to rear slightly	1 — Trunk inclined to rear markedly
5 — Abdomen flat	3 — Abdomen protruding	1 — Abdomen protruding and sagging
5 — Lower back normally curved	3 — Lower back slightly hollow	1 — Lower back markedly hollow

Scoring column grades: 4, 5, 6, 7, 8, 9, 10, 11, 12 (repeated for each item)

TOTAL RAW SCORE

To obtain total raw score:

1. Determine the score for each of the above 13 items as follows:
   5 points if description in left-hand column applies
   3 points if description in middle column applies
   1 point if description in right-hand column applies
2. Enter score for each item under proper grade in the scoring column
3. Add all 13 scores and place total in appropriate space

Scoring For the correct position, 5 points are scored; for a slight deviation, 3 points are scored; and for a pronounced deviation, 1 point is scored. The total point value is the student's score. Space to record the student's posture ratings in grades 4 through 12 is provided on the chart.

Validity Logical validity.

Reliability 0.93 to 0.98, for boys and girls at various grade levels.

Norms Norms are reported by sex and grade in the original source.

Comments This test has been in use in the physical education field for many years. It is fairly easy to administer, although prior training in using the chart is necessary. If a teacher administers the test, it can be quite time-consuming, since individual testing is necessary. For a rough screening of the students' posture, older students can be trained to use the chart. Having students test each other is an effective way of making them aware of good posture.

SUMMARY

Although it is evident that balance and flexibility are important attributes in the performance of a motor skill, the task-specific nature of each prohibits the use of one measure for each attribute. Because an individual may be flexible in one joint and not another, each joint must be measured separately to determine flexibility. The most valid measures are those requiring expensive equipment, trained personnel, and individual testing that is usually time-consuming. Practical tests of balance and flexibility have several drawbacks, but some of them can be useful to measure a specific segment of the body if carefully selected.

LEARNING EXPERIENCES

1. Administer the Stork Stand Test to at least 10 people. This can be done outside class, as long as you have a stopwatch or a watch with a second hand. Plot the trials for each person. Does each person improve as the number of trials increases? Analyze this test in terms of logical validity.
2. Take the Sit and Reach Test in your class or laboratory session. Summarize the data for males and females separately, including the means and standard deviations or medians and interpercentile ranges. Plot a frequency distribution for each gender.
3. Select a partner and review the posture chart in Figure 20-10. Use the chart to evaluate the posture of at least two other people. Ask each one to assume his or her normal posture at first, then his or her best posture. Rate both postures independently. Discuss the ratings with your partner after the assessment has been completed. Where discrepancies exist between ratings, discuss the differences. If there are major differences between ratings, rate the same examinees again.

REFERENCES

Bass, R.I. 1939. An analysis of the components of semi-circular canal function and of static and dynamic balance. Research Quarterly, **10**:33-42.

Cureton, T.K. 1941. Flexibility as an aspect of physical fitness. Research Quarterly Supplement, **12**:388-389.

Jensen, C.R., and Hirst, C.C. 1980. Measurement in physical education and athletics. New York: Macmillan Publishing Co., Inc.

Johnson, B.L., and Leach, J. 1968. A modification of the Bass Test of Dynamic Balance, unpublished study, Commerce: East Texas State University.

Johnson, B.L., and Nelson, J.K. 1979. Practical measurements for evaluation in physical education. Minneapolis: Burgess Publishing Co.

Kirkendall, D.R., Gruber, J.J., and Johnson, R.E. 1986. Measurement of evaluation for physical educators. Champaign, IL: Human Kinetics Publishers, Inc.

Kraus, H., and Hirschland, R.P. 1954. Minimum muscular fitness tests in school children. Research Quarterly, **25**:177-188.

Leighton, J.R. 1942. A simple objective and reliable measure of flexibility. Research Quarterly, **13**:205-216.

Leighton, J.R. 1955. An instrument and technique for the measurement of range and joint motion. Archives of Physical Medicine and Rehabilitation, **36**:571-578.

New York State Education Department. 1966. New York State Physical Fitness Test for Boys and Girls Grades 4-12. New York: New York State Education Department.

Scott, M.G., and French, E. 1959. Measurement and evaluation in physical education. Dubuque, IA: Wm C Brown Group.

Sigerseth, P.O. 1978. Flexibility. In Montoye, H.J., editor. An introduction to measurement in physical education and exercise science. Boston: Allyn & Bacon, Inc.

ANNOTATED READINGS

American Alliance for Health, Physical Education, Recreation and Dance. 1980. Health-Related Physical Fitness Test manual. Reston, VA:AAHPERD.

Reviews exercises for improving the flexibility of the low back region; presents exercises in terms of progressive difficulty; can be used as an aid to diagnose, as well as the basis for development of flexibility; provides excellent photographs of starting and exercise positions.

Corbin, C.B., and Noble, L. 1985. Flexibility—a major component of physical fitness. In Cundiff, D.E., editor. Implementation of health fitness exercise programs. Reston, VA: American Alliance for Health, Physical Education, Recreation and Dance.

Defines static and dynamic flexibility; discusses the joint specificity of flexibility; reviews measurement techniques; analyzes the relationship between flexibility and good health and flexibility and performance in sport; recommends techniques for improving flexibility.

Sigerseth, P.O. 1978. Flexibility. In Montoye, H.J., editor. An introduction to measurement in physical education. Boston: Allyn & Bacon, Inc.

Required reading for physical educators interested in precise measures of flexibility at each joint; describes the use of the Leighton flexometer to measure 30 joint movements at the neck, trunk, shoulder joint, elbow joint, radial-ulnar, wrist joint, hip joint, knee, and ankle joint; recommends exercises for improving flexibility.

Simri, U. 1974. Assessment procedures for human performance. In Larson, L.A., editor. Fitness, health, and work capacity; international standards for assessment. New York: Macmillan Publishing Co., Inc.

Presents international standards for measuring flexibility; recommends a test of forward flexion of the trunk (for a practical setting), as this movement is one of greatest importance in human movement; in a clinical setting, Simri recommends that the flexibility of each joint should be treated separately.

21 Tests of Motor Ability

KEY WORDS *Watch for these words as you read the following chapter:*

motor ability	motor educability	trait
motor capacity	task specificity	

During the early part of the twentieth century, a number of educators and psychologists explored the measurement of intelligence. Intelligence was viewed as an innate ability that could be measured by using intelligence tests and deriving an intelligence quotient (IQ). At the same time physical educators drew a parallel to motor behavior and surmised that there must be an innate ability to perform motor tasks. This was commonly referred to as motor ability. A few of the more prominent motor ability tests in the physical education field are described here. This chapter is an expanded version of a paper by M.J. Safrit and T.M. Wood entitled "The Use of Motor Ability Tests to Achieve Sex Fair Ability Groupings" (1982).

To understand motor ability tests better, the concepts on which they were based are reviewed first. Motor ability, motor educability, and motor capacity, while somewhat related in meaning, are distinct terms, which, to the confusion of the practitioner, have often been used interchangeably in motor ability literature. **Motor ability** is defined as "a present aptitude for physical skills" (Alden, Horton, and Caldwell, 1932), which includes strength and coordination as they appear in everyday motor habits (Howe, 1930). Similarly, McCloy (1934) distinguishes between general motor ability—motor capability at a given time—and general **motor capacity**—one's potential motor capability. Humiston (1937), taking a different approach, describes motor ability as the "ability to get around in situations demanding the use of big muscles—the ability to shift the body from one place to another" (p. 182). Scott and French (1959) link motor ability and motor educability in describing motor ability as "achievement in basic motor skills, or it may be interpreted as a more general term combining the concepts of motor educability and achievement" (p. 343). **Motor educability** is defined as the ease with which one learns motor skills (Singer, 1975).

When this information is synthesized, it appears that motor capacity refers to an individual's potential ability to perform motor skills, motor ability reflects an individual's present ability to perform motor skills, and motor educability deals with an individual's ability to learn new motor skills. Singer (1975) and Kirkendall, Gruber, and Johnson (1980) present other descriptions of motor ability. Singer (1975) describes motor ability as indicating present athletic ability and as denoting "the immediate state of the individual to perform in a wide range of motor skills" (p. 107). Kirkendall and associates suggest that motor ability is "a general quality that can facilitate more specific performances" (p. 213).

The extent to which motor ability is innate is unknown. Certainly a person is born with certain genetic features that affect the ability to perform motor skills. However, environment also plays an important role in the ability to execute motor tasks. Ability can be improved through learning. These issues continue to intrigue and baffle scientists. If the true nature—and indeed the existence—of something called motor ability is not clearly understood, how can it be measured? This confusion about the concept of motor ability did not exist to the same extent when the classic tests of motor ability were developed. Lacking scientific evidence to the contrary, the developers of these tests used a logical analysis as the basis for test construction.

Perhaps the most difficult challenge in constructing a test of motor ability was the determination of motor ability elements. Clarke (1976) lists nine elements frequently considered in constructing tests of motor ability: arm-eye coordination, muscular power, agility, muscular strength, muscular endurance, circulorespiratory endurance, flexibility, speed, and foot-eye coordination. Other lists have been generated over the years, but the benefits of examining lists of this type are limited, since each test developer identifies a different set of elements representing motor ability. This paradox has never been resolved, although it is obviously contradictory to discuss "general" motor ability and then to describe the components of motor ability in a magnitude of different ways. Generally, however, several common elements were found in the various sets of components.

The development of motor ability tests has come to a complete halt in the last two decades for several reasons. First, many exercise scientists and physical educators have questioned the existence of a general motor ability. This is a result of the research evidence indicating that ability may be task specific. Second, the construct validity of these tests has never been established. Third, legitimate questions can be raised about the extent to which this ability, if it exists, is affected by genetics in contrast to the environment.

Although there are many questions concerning the use of motor ability tests, they are discussed in this text because they have played an important historic role in the exercise science profession. Students should be familiar with one or two of the most widely used motor ability tests. Although no final answer on the value of motor ability tests has been attained and their use is now questionable, the elimination of the concept entirely is not a foregone conclusion. Examples of several motor ability tests are included at the end of the chapter. Because of their careful development and widespread use, these tests are often viewed as classics in the field. (See Chapter 10 for information on motor ability tests for children.)

CRITIQUE OF MOTOR ABILITY TESTS

The underlying assumption of the existence of a trait called motor ability has never been substantiated through a rigorously developed network of scientific evidence. Moreover, the use of the label **trait** in describing motor ability suggests that this ability is an enduring and unchanging dimension of motor behavior. Yet it is evident that the items included in the motor ability tests can be improved with practice; thus these items cannot measure innate motor ability. Of course, the same problems face researchers in the areas of intelligence testing and affective measurement. Barrow and McGee (1980) observed that, even though motor ability improves with training, experience, and maturity, individual differences in students tend to remain the same throughout the school years. However, no documentation was provided in support of this observation.

At the height of popularity of motor test usage, the procedure used to validate motor ability tests was fairly standard. Basically, it involved administering a large number of tests thought to represent various components of motor ability. A much smaller group of test items was extracted from this larger set, usually on the basis of two factors: it could be administered to a large group of people in a reasonable amount of time; and it correlated highly with the large test set, suggesting that it measured the same thing. Although this approach to validation was considered sound at the time, it was not without problems. There was no evidence that the large test set actually measured motor ability and simply no way of knowing whether it did.

Thus, although some motor ability tests were carefully developed, legitimate questions can be raised about the validity of these batteries. Unless new evidence is uncovered regarding a general motor ability component, motor ability tests will continue to be neglected in the future.

SHOULD MOTOR ABILITY TESTS BE USED FOR ABILITY GROUPING?

Unfortunately, the validity of motor ability batteries is questionable, even though many physical educators intuitively feel these types of tests would be useful to group individuals for participation in a physical activity program. Clarke (1976) is a strong proponent of ability grouping by general abilities in a physical education program "where activities may vary either within a single class period from day to day, or where the same activity does not continue on consecutive days for more than a week or two at most" (p. 229). Methodological problems aside, what is the practical usefulness of motor ability tests for classifying students?

If people are to be grouped on the basis of performance, what type of test should be used? Regrettably, several factors work against the use of motor ability tests for classification purposes. As early as 1934, researchers began questioning the concept of general motor ability tests in favor of **task specificity,** a concept of ability being specific to a given task rather than general across tasks. Ragsdale and Breckenfield (1934) in an investigation of junior high school boys concluded that "it is probably incorrect to speak of general motor ability in the same sense that we speak of general intelligence. In this study we [Ragsdale and Breckenfield] have distinguished two general factors which we have called strength and speed in running" (p. 54). In a study of motor ability of college men, Hoskins (1934) reported low correlations between motor ability as measured by the Mc-Cloy Test and subjective ratings of athletic skill in several activities. In direct contrast, McCloy (1934) reported correlations of 0.92 between his track and field items and subjective ratings of basketball skill and 0.84 between these items and subjective ratings of soccer skill. A year later Jones (1935) obtained low correlations between several motor ability tests, while Seashore (1942) distinguished between fine and gross motor abilities. In the late 1950s the task-specificity concept gained impetus with the work of Franklin Henry. Henry (1958) argued:

> The theory of specific motor abilities implies that some individuals are gifted with many specific abilities and others with only a few; it follows that there will inevitably be significant correlations between total test battery scores when tests involving many abilities are lumped together. The general motor factor which thus makes its appearance is a sample, fundamentally, of how many specifics the individual has, and the general motor ability does not exist in this sense. (p. 127)

Support for Henry's argument came swiftly. Lotter (1961) found that neuromotor specificity of speed-of-movement ability of arms and legs was extremely high. Lotter stated that "task specificity . . . implies that it is largely a matter of chance whether an individual who has a relatively high (or low) ability in one motor task will have a high or low ability in another motor task unless the two tasks are so similar as to be practically identical" (p. 57).

Further evidence for task specificity can be found in studies that reveal that general motor ability test scores do not correlate highly with various sports skills. Singer (1975) prepared an excellent review of this literature. One example of such research is a study by Burdeshaw, Spagens, and Weis (1970), who used the Scott Motor Ability Test to classify 106 women as a low-motor-ability group. This group was subdivided into three groups: Group 1 received a basic skills course; Group 2, a sport course other than badminton; and Group 3, no special treatment. All groups were subsequently enrolled in a badminton course. Testing at the midpoint and end of the badminton course revealed no difference among groups. The authors concluded that the "results supported the theory of specificity in motor skills and did not support the worth of basic skills courses in facilitating subsequent performance in the specific skills of badminton" (p. 472). Current motor learning textbooks summarize the same literature and draw similar conclusions about motor ability. (See the references at the end of this chapter.)

Not only do motor ability tests appear to be inappropriate for ability grouping in general but they also do not resolve the problem of determining sex-fair ability groups. For many years the separation of males and females in physical education classes in the United States was a common practice, especially in junior and senior high schools and colleges. During the early part of the twentieth century, several affluent communities even provided separate gymnasiums and swimming pools for males and females. When Title IX legislation was adopted, many schools complied with this law by offering a substantial number of coeducational classes. This is a desirable practice, of course, for appropriate activities. However, Title IX does not specify that all physical education classes must be coeducational. In fact the law allows "separation by sex within physical education during competition in wrestling, boxing, ice hockey, football, basketball and other sports, the purpose or major activity of which involves bodily contact" (Federal Register, 1977, p. 24132). On the other hand, the more general and pervasive policy dictates the use of ability grouping in physical education with the understanding that group membership is determined on the basis of individual performance rather than sex. The important point is that a male or a female should not be assigned to a group in physical education merely on the basis of his or her sex, but rather on the basis of ability to perform the activity being taught.

Safrit and others (1980) presented an overview of the research on three gender differences in motor performance—physical performance differences, body structure and composition differences, and differences in cardiorespiratory function. Thus true gender differences exist for many forms of motor behavior. How are these considered when dealing with motor ability tests as a means of grouping?

Even if the use of motor ability tests for sex-fair ability grouping could be justified, physical educators would face the practical problem of developing valid motor ability tests for both sexes. When separate programs existed for males and females in the past, apparently developing separate motor ability instruments, one for each sex, seemed reasonable. Thus although a number of motor ability tests have been developed, none of these was designed to be administered to both sexes. Certainly ability grouping will not be sex-fair unless the same test is used to classify all students. The Illinois State Board of Education (1982) published a booklet containing practical tips on ability grouping and performance evaluation in physical education. The board recommends that motor ability tests not be used to group students by ability.

EXAMPLES OF MOTOR ABILITY TESTS

The concept of motor ability implies an enduring trait that indicates one's present ability for most athletic activities. Therefore, researchers in the first half of this century attempted to develop tests that measure this trait for the purposes of classifying individuals for instruction and of predicting future athletic success. The development of separate motor ability tests for male and female students beyond elementary school age has been a generally consistent trend. Only the Scott Motor Ability Test and the Barrow Motor Ability Test are described in detail here. A third test, developed by McCloy, is mentioned briefly because of its historic value.

McCloy's General Motor Ability Test *(McCloy, 1934)*

In recognition of Charles H. McCloy's contributions as a pioneer in measurement in the exercise science field, it is appropriate to place McCloy's General Motor Ability Test first. During his lifetime, McCloy exerted a major influence on test development by using scientific measurement in his own work. He constructed tests of motor capacity, motor educability, and motor ability, along with a variety of measures in other areas. The significant influence of this distinguished physical educator is now legendary. McCloy developed two motor ability test batteries, one for boys and one for girls.

Boys' Battery (Events vary according to age and experience of group)
1. Pull-ups or chinning
2. Sprint (50 to 100 yards)
3. Long jump (running or standing)
4. Running high jump
5. Weight throwing (shot put, basketball throw, or baseball throw)

$$\text{General Motor Ability Score} = 0.122 \text{ (track and field score)} - 0.3928 \text{ (chinning strength)}$$

To determine the track and field score, test items 2 through 5 are scored using McCloy's scoring tables and then summed. Chinning strength is calculated using the following formula:

$$\text{Chinning Strength} = \text{(No. of pullups)} (W/10 + H - 60)$$
$$\text{where } W = \text{weight in pounds}$$
$$H = \text{height in inches}$$

Girls' Battery
1. Modified pull-ups
2. Sprint

3. Long jump
4. Throw

General Motor Ability Score = 0.42 (track and field score) + 9.6 (number of pull-ups)

To determine the track and field score, test items 2 through 4 are scored using McCloy's tables and then summed.

Scott Motor Ability Test *(Scott, 1943)*

The Scott Motor Ability Test was developed to measure the motor ability of college women and high school girls. Two test batteries were formed, one containing four items and a shorter version with three items. The shorter battery is presented in this chapter, since it is almost as valid as the longer battery and is easier to administer. Both batteries can be administered indoors.

Test 1—Basketball Throw

Test Objective To measure arm and shoulder girdle strength and coordination.

Description The examinee stands behind the restraining line and throws the basketball as far as possible. Any type of throw may be used. Three trials are taken. If an examinee steps on or over the restraining line during or after the throw, the trial is not scored. The trial score is the distance recorded to the nearest foot. The test score is the best of the three trials.

Test Area Floor area 80 feet by 20 feet.

Equipment Several regulation basketballs, tape measure, floor tape, and scorecards.

Validity Test validity is 0.79, with the McCloy General Motor Ability Test used as the criterion; 0.78 when correlated with a composite criterion and subjective ratings.

Reliability The within-day reliability estimate is 0.89.

Comments No demonstration of the basketball throw is permitted. Examinees should be permitted to warm up, although the number of practice trials is not specified in the test directions. This test should be standardized, if practice trials are to be taken.

Test 2—Long Jump

The Long Jump Test is the same as the standing long jump test described in Chapter 17. By using the criteria specified in the previous section, validity coefficients of 0.79 and 0.78 were calculated. Reliability coefficients of 0.79 for college women and 0.91 for high school girls were reported.

Test 3—Obstacle Race

Test Objective To measure speed, agility, and general body coordination. The course used for this test is shown in Figure 21-1.

Description The examinee assumes a back-lying position with heels just behind the starting line. On the signal *Ready, Go!* she gets up quickly and begins

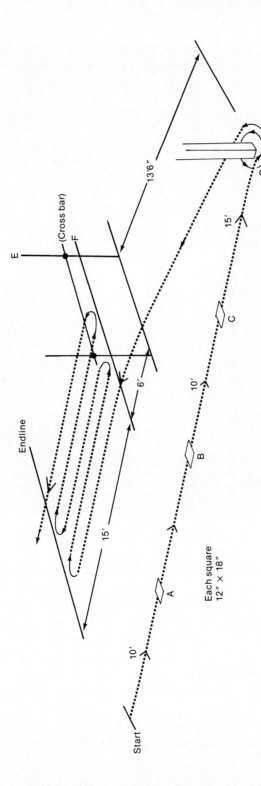

FIGURE 21-1 *Floor markings for the Scott Obstacle Race.*

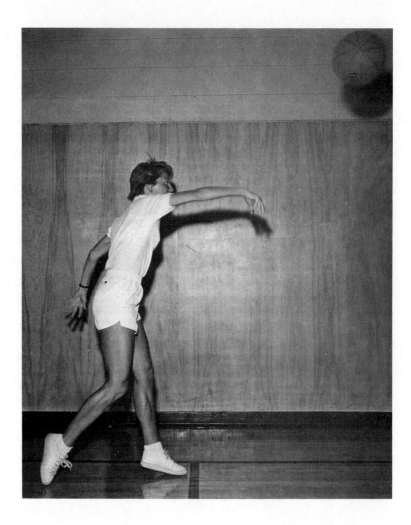

moving through the obstacle course. She runs to the first square (see Figure 21-1) and steps on the square with both feet. The same protocol is followed with the next two squares. She then runs to the jump standard, circles it twice, and races to the crossbar. She passes under the crossbar, attempting not to touch it, gets up, and runs to the end line as quickly as possible, touching this line with her hand. She runs back to line F, to the end line again, and to line F again, each time touching the line with her hand. Then she races across the endline to complete the test. One trial is administered. The score is the time required to complete the course.

Test Area Floor area 60 feet by 30 feet.

Equipment Stopwatch, jump standard, 6-foot crossbar and support poles, floor tape, and scorecards.

Validity By using the criteria described under the Basketball Throw for Distance, validity coefficients of 0.65 and 0.58 were calculated for a longer version of the test.

Reliability Test-retest reliability of 0.91 was reported.

Comments Although examinees should be instructed not to touch the crossbar, a foul is not constituted even if the bar is dislodged. It is assumed that the time will be lower as a result. The jump standard, however, cannot be touched. If it is, a foul is declared and the trial must be retaken. The test should be demonstrated, and examinees should be allowed to walk through the course before being tested. An assistant should be stationed between line F and the end line. When the examinee reaches line F, she should be reminded of each reverse turn and encouraged to run with maximum effort across the endline after the last turn. Otherwise, far too many examinees will not remember the correct sequence, thus invalidating the test. Also, examinees have a tendency to slow down as they approach the end line for the last time. The examinee should be reminded to run as fast as possible across the end line. Be sure individuals being tested are wearing proper shoes.

Test norms for college women and high school girls are shown in Tables 21-1 and 21-2. These norms have not been updated in recent years but can be used as rough guidelines of performance expectations.

Barrow Motor Ability Test *(Barrow, 1954)*

The Barrow Motor Ability Test is designed to measure the motor ability of college men and junior and senior high school boys. Two test batteries, one consisting of six items and a shorter version with three items, were developed. Only the shorter battery is included in this chapter, since it has high validity (r_{xy} = 0.92 when correlated with a composite of 29 test items measuring eight different components of motor ability). The shorter version can easily be administered indoors.

Test 1—Standing Long Jump The Standing Long Jump (SLJ) Test, used as a measure of explosive leg power, is described in Chapter 17. (See Standing Long Jump.) The test-retest reliability is 0.895, and the objectivity (comparing the two scorers) is 0.996. The validity, based on a comparison with the composite of 29 tests, is 0.759.

Test 2—Zigzag Run

Test Objective To measure agility. The course for the Zigzag Run (ZR) is shown in Figure 21-2.

Description The examinee assumes a ready position (standing) at the starting point. On the signal *Ready, Go!*, he runs the course in the designated manner as fast as possible. The cones should not be touched throughout the run. The examinee continues to run the course for a total of three times. As the finish line is crossed at the end of the first circuit, the timer stops the stopwatch. The score is

TABLE 21-1 *T-Scores for college women on Scott Motor Ability Test*

T-score	Basketball throw (feet)	Broad jump (inches)	Obstacle race (seconds)	T-score	Basketball throw (feet)	Broad jump (inches)	Obstacle race (seconds)
85	75	86	17.5-17.9	48		60	
84				47	34	59	25.0-25.4
83	71		18.0-18.4	46	33	58	
82				45	32	57	25.5-25.9
81		85		44	31		
80	70			43		56	26.0-26.4
79	69		18.5-18.9	42	30	55	
78	68	84		41		54	26.5-26.9
77	67	83		40	29	53	27.0-27.4
76	66			39	28	52	
75	65	82	19.0-19.4	38			27.5-27.9
74	64	81		37	27	51	28.0-28.4
73	62	80		36	26	50	
72	61	79	19.5-19.9	35		49	28.5-28.9
71	59			34	25	48	29.0-29.4
70	58	78	20.0-20.4	33		47	29.5-29.9
69	57	77		32		46	30.0-30.4
68	56	76		31		45	30.5-30.9
67	55	75	20.5-20.9	30	24	44	31.0-31.4
66	54	74		29		43	31.5-31.9
65	52			28	23	42	32.0-32.4
64	51	73	21.0-21.4	27	21	41	32.5-32.9
63	50	72		26		40	33.0-33.4
62	48	71	21.5-21.9	25	20	39	33.5-33.9
61	47			24		38	34.0-34.4
60	46	70		23		37	34.5-34.9
59	45	69	22.0-22.4	22		36	
58	44	68		21	19		35.0-35.4
57	43	67	22.5-22.9	20			
56	42			19		35	35.5-35.9
55	41	66	23.0-23.4	18			
54	40	65		17	18		
53	39	64	23.5-23.9	16			
52	38	63		15			
51	37		24.0-24.4	14			43.5-43.9
50	36	62		13		30	45.5-45.9
49	35	61	24.5-24.9				

Reprinted by permission of Dr. M. Gladys Scott.

TABLE 21-2 *T-Scores for high school girls on Scott Motor Ability Test*

T-score	Basketball throw (feet) (310)*	Broad jump (inches) (287)*	Obstacle race (seconds) (374)*	T-score	Basketball throw (feet) (310)*	Broad jump (inches) (387)*	Obstacle race (seconds) (374)*
80	71			49	35	70	
79		96		48		68	23.0-23.4
78				47	34	66	
77	68	94		46	33		23.5-23.9
76	66		18.5-18.9	45	32	64	
75	65			44	31		24.0-24.4
74	64	92		43		62	
73	63			43	30		24.5-24.9
72	61			41	29	60	
71	59	90		40	28		
70	55	88	19.0-19.4	39		58	25.0-25.4
69	54			38	27	56	
68	52	86		37		54	25.5-25.9
67	51		19.5-19.9	36	26		26.0-26.4
66	50			35		52	26.5-26.9
65	49			34	25	50	27.0-27.4
64	48	84	20.0-20.4	33			
63	47			32	24	47	27.5-27.9
62	46	82	20.5-20.9	31	23		
61		80		30		44	28.0-28.4
60	45			29	22		28.5-28.9
59	44	78	21.0-21.4	28			29.0-29.4
58	43			27	21		29.5-29.9
57	42	76	21.5-21.9	26		40	30.0-30.4
56	41			25	20		
55	40	74		24			30.5-31.4
54			22.0-22.4	23	19	36	31.5-32.4
53	39			22			32.5-34.9
52		72		21	16		
51	37		22.5-22.9	20			35.0-36.0
50	36						

Reprinted by permission of Dr. M. Gladys Scott.
*Size of normative group.

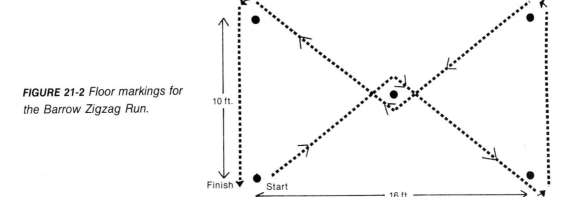

FIGURE 21-2 *Floor markings for the Barrow Zigzag Run.*

the time recorded to the nearest tenth of a second. If the cones are moved during the run, the trial is retaken.

Test Area Floor area 30 feet by 50 feet.

Equipment Stopwatch, five traffic cones, floor tape, and scorecards.

Validity Test validity is 0.736 based on a comparison of the test with a composite of 29 tests measuring eight different components of motor ability.

Reliability Test-retest reliability is 0.795. Test objectivity, comparing two timers, is 0.996.

Comments Before test day the run should be demonstrated, and the examinees should be allowed to walk or jog through the course. An assistant should be stationed near the finish line to remind the test taker to run the course three times and not to slow down until he has crossed the finish line. Proper shoes should be required.

Test 3—Medicine Ball Put

Test Objective To measure arm and shoulder girdle strength. The examinee is required to put a 6-pound medicine ball as far as possible.

Description For the Medicine Ball Put (MBP), the examinee stands between two restraining lines 15 feet apart. The medicine ball is held in one hand, close to the point where the shoulder joins the neck. The ball is thrust outward as far as possible. If a boy steps on or over the restraining line during or after the put, the trial is not scored. Three trials are taken. The score is the best of three throws, recorded to the nearest foot.

Test Area Floor area 90 feet by 25 feet.

Equipment Two or three 6-pound medicine balls, tape measure, floor tape, and scorecards.

Validity The validity of the test is 0.736, based on a comparison of the test with a composite of 29 tests measuring eight different components of motor ability.

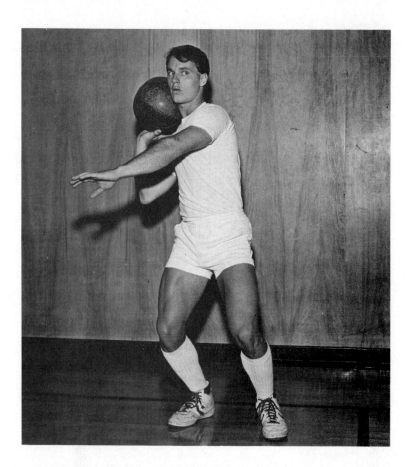

TABLE 21-3 *GMAS categories for college men (three-item test)*

Category	P.E. majors	Nonmajors
Excellent	197-higher	185-higher
Good	180-196	163-184
Average	161-179	138-162
Poor	143-160	116-137
Inferior	142-lower	115-lower

Reprinted by permission of Dr. H.M. Barrow.

Reliability The test-retest reliability is 0.893, and the objectivity for two scorers is 0.997.

Comments The regression equation for the General Motor Ability Score (GMAS) is 2.2(SBJ) + 1.6(ZR) + 1.2(MBP). Use Table 21-3 to interpret the GMAS.

TABLE 21-4 *T-scores for college men*

T-score	Standing broad jump (inches)	Zigzag run (seconds)	Medicine ball put (feet)	T-score
80	113 Up	20.8 Down	58 Up	80
75	109-112	21.6-20.9	55-57	75
70	105-108	22.4-21.7	52-54	70
65	101-104	23.1-22.5	48-51	65
60	97-100	23.9-23.2	45-47	60
55	93-96	24.7-24.0	42-44	55
50	89-92	25.5-24.8	39-41	50
45	85-88	26.3-25.6	35-38	45
40	81-84	27.1-26.4	32-34	40
35	77-80	27.8-27.2	29-31	35
30	73-76	28.6-27.9	26-28	30
25	69-72	29.4-28.7	23-25	25
20	68 Down	29.5 Up	22 Down	20

Reprinted by permission of Dr. H.M. Barrow.

TABLE 21-5 *Standing Broad Jump T-scores for high school and junior high school boys*

T-score	Grade 7	Grade 8	Grade 9	Grade 10	Grade 11
80	90 Up	97 Up	103 Up	105 Up	112 Up
75	86-89	92-96	98-102	101-104	107-111
70	82-85	88-91	93-97	97-100	103-106
65	77-81	83-87	88-92	92-96	97-102
60	73-76	78-82	83-87	88-91	93-96
55	69-72	73-77	79-82	83-87	88-92
50	65-68	69-72	74-78	79-82	83-87
45	61-64	64-68	69-73	75-78	78-82
40	56-60	59-63	64-68	71-74	74-77
35	52-55	54-58	59-63	66-70	69-73
30	48-51	50-53	54-58	62-65	64-68
25	44-47	45-49	49-53	58-61	59-63
20	43 Down	44 Down	48 Down	57 Down	58 Down

Reprinted by permission of Dr. H.M. Barrow.

TABLE 21-6 *Zigzag Run T-scores for high school and junior high school boys*

	Grade				
T-score	7	8	9	10	11
80	20.1 Down	17.8 Down	20.2 Down	21.6 Down	21.5 Down
75	21.4-20.2	19.5-17.9	21.3-20.3	22.7-21.7	22.6-21.6
70	22.7-21.5	21.2-19.6	22.4-21.4	23.8-22.8	23.7-22.7
65	24.0-22.8	22.8-21.3	23.5-22.5	24.8-23.9	24.7-23.8
60	25.2-24.1	24.5-22.9	24.6-23.6	25.8-24.9	25.8-24.8
55	26.5-25.3	26.2-24.6	25.7-24.7	26.9-25.9	26.8-25.9
50	27.8-26.6	27.8-26.3	26.8-25.8	27.9-27.0	27.8-26.9
45	29.0-27.9	29.5-27.9	27.9-26.9	28.9-28.0	28.9-27.9
40	30.3-29.1	31.2-29.6	29.0-28.0	29.9-29.0	29.9-29.0
35	31.6-30.4	32.8-31.3	30.1-29.1	31.0-30.0	31.0-30.0
30	32.8-31.7	34.5-32.9	31.2-30.2	32.1-31.1	32.0-31.1
25	34.1-32.9	36.2-34.6	32.3-31.3	33.1-32.2	33.0-32.1
20	34.2 Up	36.3 Up	32.4 Up	33.2 Up	33.1 Up

Reprinted by permission of Dr. H.M. Barrow.

TABLE 21-7 *Medicine Ball Put T-scores for high school and junior high school boys*

	Grade				
T-score	7	8	9	10	11
80	43 Up	45 Up	49 Up	50 Up	54 Up
75	38-42	43-44	46-48	47-49	51-53
70	35-37	40-42	44-45	44-46	48-50
65	33-34	37-39	41-43	42-43	46-47
60	30-32	34-36	38-40	39-41	43-45
55	27-29	31-33	35-37	37-38	40-42
50	25-26	28-30	32-34	34-36	37-39
45	22-24	25-27	29-31	32-33	34-36
40	19-21	23-24	27-28	29-31	31-33
35	17-18	20-22	24-26	27-28	28-30
30	14-16	17-19	21-23	24-26	25-27
25	12-13	14-16	18-20	22-23	22-24
20	11 Down	13 Down	17 Down	21 Down	21 Down

Reprinted by permission of Dr. H.M. Barrow.

Each throw must be measured directly from the landing point to the middle of the closest restraining line. Scoring may be facilitated by the stretching out of a tape measure and leaving it there to measure each throw. The tape must be moved for each put, however. It is possible to use floor tapes, but they must be laid out in arcs so that the proper distance will be measured no matter where the ball lands. Norms for all three tests are included in Tables 21-4 (college men) and 21-5 through 21-7 (junior and senior high school boys).

SUMMARY

The issues associated with the concept of motor ability and its measurement were once a major focus in the physical education field. This emphasis has been diminished by the experimental findings that ability seemed to be specific to a given motor task rather than across tasks. Nonetheless, at the time motor ability tests were being constructed, the measurement techniques were quite sophisticated and served as models for subsequent test development in other aspects of physical education and exercise science. Currently, the tests have limited usefulness, either as measures of general motor ability or as a means of ability grouping.

LEARNING EXPERIENCES

1. From the library, select one of the older textbooks in measurement and evaluation in physical education (published before 1950). Review the sections on the measurement of motor ability, motor capacity, and motor educability. Examine the test items in each type of test. In what ways are the three types of tests different? Write a report on your analysis.
2. Set up a Scott Obstacle Race and the Barrow Zigzag Run Test in a laboratory or gymnasium setting. The women in your class should take the Scott test; the men should take the Barrow test. Calculate the mean, standard deviation, and T-scores for each gender, and compare these values with the norms in Table 21-1 (Scott Test) and Table 21-4 (Barrow Test).

REFERENCES

Alden, F.D., Horton, M.O., and Caldwell, G.M. 1932. A motor ability test for university women in the classification of entering students into homogenous groups. Research Quarterly, 3(1):85-120.

Barrow, H.M. 1954. Test of motor ability for college men. Research Quarterly, 25(3):253-260.

Barrow, H.M., and McGee, R. 1980. A practical approach to measurement in physical education. Philadelphia: Lea & Febiger.

Burdeshaw, D., Spagens, J.E., and Weis, P.A. 1970. Evaluation of general versus specific instruction of badminton skills to women of low motor ability. Research Quarterly, 41(4):472-477.

Clarke, H.H. 1976. Application of measurement to health and physical education. Englewood Cliffs, NJ: Prentice-Hall Inc.

Henry, F.M. 1958. Specificity versus generality in learning motor skills. Proceedings of the College Physical Education Association, 61:127.

Hoskins, R.N. 1934. The relationship of measurements of general motor capacity to the learning of specific psychomotor skills. Research Quarterly, 5(1):63-72.

Howe, E.C. 1930. The precision and validation of physical fitness. Research Quarterly, 1(2):90-96.

Humiston, D. 1937. A measurement of motor ability in college women. Research Quarterly, 8(2):181-185.

Illinois State Board of Education. 1982. Tips and techniques: ability grouping and performance evaluation in physical education. Springfield, IL: Illinois State Board of Education.

Jones, L.M. 1935. A factorial analysis of ability in fundamental motor skills. In Contributions to Education. New York: Teachers College, Columbia University.

Kirkendall, D.R., Gruber, J.J., and Johnson, R.E. 1987. Measurement and evaluation for physical educators. Champaign, IL: Human Kinetics Publishers.

Lotter, W.S. 1961. Specificity or generality of speed of systematically related movements. Research Quarterly, 32(1):55-62.

McCloy, C.H. 1934. The measurement of general motor capacity and general motor ability. Research Quarterly, March Suppl.:46-61.

Ragsdale, C.E., and Breckenfield, I.J. 1934. The organization of physical and motor traits in junior high school boys. Research Quarterly, 5(3):47-55.

Safrit, M.J., and Wood, T.M. 1982. The use of motor ability tests to achieve sex fair ability groups. In Tips and techniques: ability grouping and performance evaluation in physical education. Springfield, IL: Illinois State Board of Education.

Safrit, M.J., and others, 1980. Issues in setting motor performance standards. Quest, 32(2):152-162.

Scott, M.G. 1939. The assessment of motor abilities of college women through objective tests. Research Quarterly, 10(3):63-83.

Scott, M.G., and French, E. 1959. Measurement and evaluation in physical education. Dubuque, IA: Wm C Brown Group.

Seashore, H.G. 1942. Some relationships of fine and gross motor abilities. Research Quarterly, 13(3):259-274.

Singer, R.N. 1975. Motor learning and performance: an application to physical education skills. London: Collier Macmillan Ltd.

United States Department of Health, Education, and Welfare, 1977. Federal Register, 40(108), June 4.

ANNOTATED READINGS

Keogh, J., and Sugden, D. 1985. Movement skill development. New York: Macmillan Publishing Co., pp. 182-194.

Includes a chapter on movement abilities; attempts to identify children's movement abilities; views ability not as a general trait but rather represented as components of ability, including factors such as balance, general flexibility, speed, and strength.

Magill, R.A. 1985. Motor learning: concepts and applications, ed. 2, Dubuque, IA: Wm C Brown Group, pp. 252-281.

Includes a chapter on individual differences; notes that individual differences research does not support the notion of a "general motor ability"; points out that this research has identified various motor abilities that characterize individuals; describes a task analysis process to identify abilities underlying a motor skill; uses the tennis serve as an example.

Oxendine, J.B. 1984. Psychology of motor learning, ed. 2, Engelwood Cliffs, NJ: Prentice-Hall, Inc. pp. 315-332.

Includes a chapter on the dimensions of human differences; discusses the lack of support for the view of motor ability as a general trait; notes that general motor ability tests have proved to have little validity in determining one's overall capacity or potential in motor skills.

Sage, G.E. 1984. Motor learning and control. Dubuque, IA: Wm C Brown Group, pp. 273-283.

Includes a chapter on motor abilities and motor behavior; discusses the notion of a general motor ability as one of the most persistent bits of folklore in physical education and coaching; reviews the development of motor ability tests and the reasons they are not valid indicators of an underlying trait thought to be general motor ability; recommends a classification system of motor abilities.

Schmidt, R.A. 1982. Motor control and learning. Champaign, IL: Human Kinetics Publishers, Inc., pp. 379-433.

Includes a chapter on individual differences and capabilities; discusses the concept of general motor ability and notes that considerable doubt can be cast on the general motor ability hypothesis; demonstrates that research has not supported this hypothesis; reinforces the view that motor abilities are specific to a particular task.

Singer, R.N. 1975. Motor learning and human performance, ed. 2, New York: Macmillan Publishing Co., pp. 213-306.

Refers to tests of motor capacity, motor fitness, and motor ability; notes that a strong relationship between motor ability and athletic performance has not been demonstrated; suggests that if a general motor ability really exists, it must be verified in future research.

Part Ten

Measures of Related Abilities

22

Tests of Affective Behavior

KEY WORDS *Watch for these words as you read the following chapter:*

affect	Likert scale	semantic differential scale
attitude	perceived exertion scale	social behavior
forced-choice item	reactive effect	sportsmanship
interests	response distortion	weak measure

Exercise scientists and physical educators are not only interested in performance in physical activity and sport but also the way participants feel about their performance. As William P. Morgan, a noted sports psychologist, has put it—the body also has a head. It is well known that many factors impact on motor behavior. Only some of these factors are physical. Other factors, such as self-esteem, attitude, and psychological traits, also have a bearing on performance. These latter factors represent examples of affective behavior.

An **affect** is a sociological or psychological characteristic manifested in a feeling or behavior. Affective behaviors of interest to the physical educators include attitudes, interests, values, psychological traits, and emotional states of the individual. Physical educators have tended to be most interested in the development of inventories to measure the attitudes of individuals toward physical education or physical activity. Other inventories have been constructed to assess the psychological characteristics of an individual in a sport or physical activity; however, the majority of these instruments have been employed by researchers rather than by physical education teachers and exercise specialists.

An **attitude** is a feeling one has about a specific attitude object, such as a situation, a person, an activity, and so forth. The interest in the measurement of attitudes toward physical education or physical activity is not surprising, since it is often assumed that an individual with a positive attitude toward physical education will be more inclined to participate in physical activity. Although this line of reasoning is intuitively appealing, it has been shown repeatedly that attitudes do not reflect behavior. When people are asked about their attitude toward physical activity in general, most will express a positive view, yet many of these individuals have sedentary lifestyles.

In private fitness clubs as well as physical education classes, the belief that unfavorable attitudes toward physical activity can be altered with a good instructional program has provided a rationale for the measurement of attitudes. In view of the favorable attitudes generally expressed toward physical activity, this rationale loses much of its impact, and the practical significance of changing an individual's attitude from favorable to more favorable is minimal.

Another affective behavior frequently measured in the physical education field is **interests,** which reflect one's likes and dislikes about various forms of physical activity, programming, scheduling, and so forth. In a school setting, **sportsmanship** is often stressed. In fact, some teachers grade each student on sportsmanship, although they may not measure this characteristic in a systematic, objective manner. (This is discussed in more detail later in the chapter.) Several instruments have been developed to measure **social behavior,** which encompasses the relationships among peers in a physical education setting. Of longstanding interest in the field are the measures of psychological characteristics, such as stress, anxiety, and a variety of elements of personality, which should be tested by a person trained in psychology.

Several shortcomings are associated with the use of affective inventories. Investigators may attempt to change affective behavior by imposing an intervention on the examinees during a designated period. A pretest of the affective behavior is administered before the intervention and a posttest afterward. However, the second administration of the inventory might be affected by a **reactive effect** from the first testing session. For instance, examinees may remember how they responded to the items during the first administration, or their affective behavior might change because of the first test session. For example, some may have given very little thought to their feelings about physical activity, especially in a broad context. Once they are exposed to new ideas, they may begin to examine their feelings carefully, leading to a solidification of attitudes. The next time the inventory is administered, they may change their response to certain items. In these cases, the score would reflect a change in affect, but it is not due to the planned intervention, as an investigator might conclude.

A second deficiency of many instruments measuring affective behavior is the possibility of **response distortion.** For example, examinees may not always respond with total honesty to these measures, faking good or bad responses, answering in a socially desirable way, or distorting responses in other ways. The more sophisticated inventories measuring affective behavior frequently include items designed to detect the tendency of examinees to distort items.

TYPES OF MEASURES

To construct a measure of affective behavior, the type of affect must be carefully defined so that a table of specifications can be developed, as described in Chapter 15. The number of items for each category is decided on the basis of the importance of each. (Remember that the number of items represents the weighting of each category.) At this stage a decision must be made on the type of item to use—generally, rating scales, forced-choice inventories, and questionnaires.

Likert Scale

The **Likert Scale** requires an expression of the individual's degree of agreement or disagreement with a series of affective statements. Kenyon's Attitude Toward Physical Activity Inventory uses a Likert scale. One of the items on this inventory is the statement, "I would gladly put in the necessary years of daily hard training for the chance to try out for the U.S. Olympic team." Response choices are the following: very strongly agree, strongly agree, agree, undecided, disagree, strongly disagree, and very strongly disagree. The examinee responds by circling the desired response on the answer sheet. A five-step version of a Likert scale is shown below:

1	2	3	4	5
Strongly disagree	Disagree	Undecided	Agree	Strongly agree

If the statement is positively worded (as in the Kenyon statement in the above paragraph), the number circled by the examinee is the score for that item. If the statement is negatively worded, the scoring procedure must be reversed. The circled number must be subtracted from the highest possible number plus 1. For example, assume an examinee circles 4 in response to a negatively worded statement (e.g., "Only highly skilled athletes should participate in vigorous physical activity"). If an examinee circles 4, this indicates agreement with the statement but negative view of vigorous physical activity. Thus, 4 is subtracted from 5 (the highest possible number) and added to 1. This calculation $(5-4+1)$ equals 2, accurately reflecting the examinee's negative perception.

Likert scales typically include five or seven steps. However, a two-step format (agree - disagree) may also be encountered, as well as scales including 10 or more steps. Increasing the number of scale steps increases the reliability of the item, up to a point. Most raters are not capable of using a large number of steps; therefore, it is probably best not to exceed seven categories.

Semantic Differential Scale

The **semantic differential scale** involves the rating of concepts using bipolar adjectives with scales anchored at the extremes. Bipolar adjectives represent opposite meanings, such as good-bad, strong-weak, and active-passive. An example of the semantic differential scale used to assess one's attitude toward physical activity is shown in the boxed material opposite. (Later in the chapter, the Children's

---

Semantic differential scale used to measure attitudes toward physical activity

Physical activity

Left								Right	Dimension
Pleasant								Unpleasant	(E)
Relaxed								Tense	(A)
Passive								Active	(A)
Unsuccessful								Successful	(E)
Delicate								Rugged	(P)
Fast								Slow	(A)
Good								Bad	(E)
Weak								Strong	(P)
Heavy								Light	(P)

Attitude Toward Physical Activity Scale, which uses the semantic differential scale, is described.)

The bipolar adjectives can readily be adapted to evaluate numerous concepts, and individuals can easily evaluate several different concepts using the same rating form. The examinee is asked to mark one of seven points best reflecting his or her feelings about the concept. The score for each item ranges from 1 to 7 if the positive adjective in the pair is listed to the right, and from 7 to 1 if the positive adjective is placed to the right.

Note that a letter—E, A, or P—appears to the right of each item, representing the three dimensions of a concept that can be measured with a semantic differential. Evaluation represents the "goodness" of the concept. This dimension is often viewed as a reflection of attitude. Activity reflects the action associated with the concept, while Potency involves the strength of the concept. The Evaluation (E) dimension is best described by the good-bad adjective pair; the Activity (A) dimension, by the fast-slow pair; and the Potency (P) dimension by the strong-weak pair. At least three items should be included under each dimension. Both positive and negative items should be placed in each column. When more than one dimension is being measured, the adjective pairs should be randomly ordered so that pairs representing each dimension are dispersed throughout the instrument. When using the semantic differential with young children, adjectives should be selected that match their reading comprehension level. This can be determined by a reading specialist.

The letters representing dimensions are displayed in the boxed material for illustrative purposes only. Although the test user should know the correct dimension for each item, this information should not be included on the test form.

Other Types of Scales

When the Likert scale or the semantic differential scale is used, the respondent indicates agreement or disagreement with a statement or preference for specific meanings of a particular concept. Statements that must be answered true or false provide another example of agree-disagree scales. The Physical Estimation and Attraction Scale, described later in this chapter, uses true-false responses. This scale is similar in style to the **forced-choice item.** With scales of forced-choice items, the examinee is required to choose among two or more alternatives that appear equally favorable or unfavorable. Discrimination and preference values of the items are determined, and the alternatives are combined in such a manner as to equalize these values.

Rating scales such as the type described in Chapter 14 are also used to measure affective behavior. For example, a five-point scale could be used to measure sportsmanship, with a descriptor specifically dealing with sportsmanship listed under each point. The desired elements of sportsmanship would be included under point 5, and the undesirable elements, under point 1. The points in between would reflect various stages of sportsmanship.

Another method for measuring affective behavior is a questionnaire. Typically, the examinee responds to questions by selecting a response from a set of options. An example of this type of instrument is the Health-Related Physical Fitness Opinionnaire (Safrit and Wood, 1983). Users and nonusers of the AAH-PERD Health-Related Physical Fitness Test are asked about their opinions of the test and how it compares with the Youth Fitness Test.

Another type of scale used in exercise science is the **perceived exertion scale** (Borg, 1973), which assesses the examinee's perception of his or her physical exertion during exercise. It is described later in this chapter.

Weak Measures

Sometimes a well-developed standardized test is not available to measure an affect of interest. On the other hand, a suitable test may have been published, but it may be too technical or excessively time-consuming to administer in a practical setting. Sometimes it is desirable to develop a short test that can be administered quickly and easily. The test user may be interested in making a decision that will not have a long-term impact on the examinees. Thus, estimating the reliability and validity of the test may not be possible, although it would be desirable. This type of measure would be viewed as weak. **A weak measure** is a measure with inadequate evidence of validity and reliability. When a measure is used to make a short-term decision about an examinee that could be readily modified, weak measures can be quite useful in the absence of a valid indicator. For example, a physical education teacher may include a goal of developing physical fitness. Time may be allotted for daily participation in jogging to meet an objective for cardiorespiratory function. Formative evaluation procedures may

---

Weak measure of student attitude toward jogging

How did you feel about jogging today?

Awful   1   2   3   4   5   6   7   Great

---

be used to monitor progress toward the predetermined standard. Since many teachers identify concomitant concerns associated with each major objective, testing attitudes toward this form of physical activity on a regular basis may be desirable. Although positive attitudes do not ensure participation in vigorous physical activity, a negative attitude would cause some concern, since it might reflect an unwillingness to engage in aerobic activities in the future.

A simple rating scale could be devised to obtain feedback on the students' attitudinal dispositions, as shown in the boxed material above. Although this is a weak measure, it can be justified if used on a continuing basis to provide a rough estimate of attitude. Students could be forced to run for 12 minutes during every class period; if they dislike this activity, however, they might develop negative attitudes toward physical fitness—even toward physical education—which may be retained.

Students would be asked to circle the number that best represents their feelings. Little time is required to obtain this information, since students can record a response as they leave class. They are asked not to mark the form in any other way, thus assuring anonymity. One word of caution: One should avoid collecting this type of data on only one day of the week. If the data were always collected on Fridays, the students' perceptions might be affected by the forthcoming weekend or by fatigue from the previous school week. A random selection of days is preferable. The averages of the responses for all students can be calculated every week and plotted, as in Figure 22-1.

Since a rating of 4 represents the neutral point on the scale, it is desirable if the average falls above that point. If more students felt awful about jogging than great, some type of intervention is necessary. Initially, the physical education staff might talk to them to find out why they have negative feelings.

USES OF AFFECTIVE MEASURES

Measures of affective behavior within the realm of sport and physical activity have been used in at least three ways: to assess the affective behavior of individual students in physical education classes, to assess the level of affective behavior for a class, and to control or manipulate some aspect of affective behavior in conducting a research study.

Considering the affective behavior of an individual student first, educators

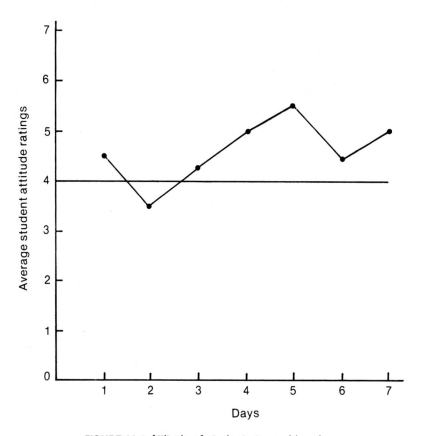

FIGURE 22-1 *Attitude of students toward jogging.*

most frequently express concerns about attitudes toward physical education, sportsmanship and self-concept. Many physical education teachers feel a student's attitude should be an important component of his or her grade. Usually the teacher is most interested in the student's attitude toward participation in physical education classes, that is, the behavior of the student in class. Sometimes attitude is judged on the basis of the answers to these questions: Is appropriate uniform worn? Does the student try in class? Does the student shower at the end of class? (See Chapter 9 for a discussion of whether factors such as these should be considered in determining a student's grade.)

Very few well-developed instruments are available to assess the affective behavior of an individual student in a physical education setting. Although a number of tests have been developed in the field, they were constructed years ago when the standards for test development were not as rigorous as today's. Several affective measures used in the exercise science field are included at the end of this chapter to provide examples of this test market.

Most of the affective inventories in the field should be used only to examine group behavior. It would be appropriate to administer an attitude inventory to a physical education class, calculate the mean (or median) and standard deviation (or interpercentile range) of the class data, and use this information as part of the evaluation of the physical education program in the school. If on the average the class attitude is negative, the physical education teacher could attempt to create a more positive environment. On the other hand, it would be inappropriate to use an individual's score on the inventory to determine his or her grade on attitude toward physical education.

EXAMPLES OF AFFECTIVE MEASURES

While many instruments have been developed to measure the affective behavior of interest to the exercise scientist, few have been developed according to the rigorous standards set for the construction of educational and psychological tests (American Psychological Association, 1985). In most cases, while reliabilities have been acceptable, content validity and construct validity have been inadequate and frequently overlooked. Examples of four types of instruments are included in this section: stress and anxiety, social behavior, attitudes, and sportsmanship and leadership.

Stress and Anxiety

Stress Inventory (Miller and Allen, 1982)

Test Objective To measure an individual's level of stress.

Test Description The inventory is presented in the boxed material on p. 542.

Comments The inventory provides information on a variety of stress indicators and, in this respect, would have logical validity. Obviously the examinee who marks "YES" by many items would be viewed as having a high level of stress. A low-stress individual would respond "NO" to most of the items. It would be unusual for an individual to mark "NO" by all items, since everyone functions with a certain level of stress. For information on other aspects of this inventory, including reliability, validity and scoring, refer to the original source.

Sport Competition Anxiety Test (Martens, 1977)

Test Objective To measure individual differences in the construct of competitive sport anxiety; to measure competitive A (anxiety) trait, which is defined as "a construct that describes individual differences in the tendency to perceive competitive situations as threatening and to respond to these situations with A (anxiety) state reactions of varying intensity" (Martens, 1977, p. 36).

Description The Sport Competition Anxiety Test for Children (SCAT-C) is presented in Table 22-1.

Materials Test forms and pencils.

Scoring Items 2, 3, 5, 8, 9, 12, 14, and 15 are scored using the following key:

1 = Hardly ever   2 = Sometimes   3 = Often

Stress inventory

Answer yes or no to each of the following questions:

Yes   No

___ ___ 1. Do you often experience headaches or backaches?

___ ___ 2. When sitting in a chair and talking to someone, do you continually move in the chair to seek a comfortable position?

___ ___ 3. When retiring for the night, are you unable to fall asleep immediately?

___ ___ 4. Do you often grind your teeth when you are confronted with an unpleasant experience?

___ ___ 5. Do you easily become angry or frustrated when you are faced with a problem for which there is no immediate solution?

___ ___ 6. Do you often complain of being tired?

___ ___ 7. Does your face often hold expressions of intense concentration?

___ ___ 8. Do you often drum your fingers aimlessly or forcibly to express irritation?

___ ___ 9. Does your posture appear stiff when you sit or walk?

___ ___ 10. Are you unable to concentrate on one problem at a time?

___ ___ 11. Are you unable to relax voluntarily?

___ ___ 12. Do you often experience nervousness and uneasy feelings?

___ ___ 13. Do you become upset when your plans are interrupted or must be changed?

___ ___ 14. Are you highly competitive in sports, in your test grades, in your daily responsibilities?

___ ___ 15. Are you time-conscious?

___ ___ 16. Do you experience extreme dissatisfaction and anxiety when you fail to achieve success in your endeavors?

___ ___ 17. Are you an aggressive person?

___ ___ 18. Are you often too busy to allow time for physical activity?

___ ___ 19. Do you plan your day's activities and often budget your time?

___ ___ 20. Are you critical of yourself when you make a mistake?

___ ___ 21. Do you feel "uptight" at the end of the day?

___ ___ 22. Are you impatient when others are late for an appointment with you?

___ ___ 23. Do you often set high goals or levels of achievement for yourself?

___ ___ 24. Do you experience bad moods often?

___ ___ 25. Are you unyielding when others disagree with your beliefs or convictions?

From Miller, D.K., and Allen, T.E.

TABLE 22-1 *Sport competition anxiety test for children*

Illinois competition questionnaire
Form C

Directions: We want to know how you feel about *competition*. You know what competition is. We all compete. We try to do better than our brother or sister or friend at something. We try to score more points in a game. We try to get the best grade in class or win a prize that we want. We all compete in sports and games. Below are some sentences about how boys and girls feel when they compete in sports and games. Read each statement below and decide if *you* HARDLY EVER, or SOMETIMES, or OFTEN feel this way when you compete in sports and games. Mark A if your choice is HARDLY EVER, mark B if you choose SOMETIMES, and mark C if you choose OFTEN. There are no right or wrong answers. Do not spend too much time on any one statement. *Remember:* choose the word that describes how you *usually* feel when competing in *sports and games.*

	Hardly ever	Some-times	Often
1. Competing against others is fun.	A ☐	B ☐	C ☐
2. Before I compete I feel uneasy.	A ☐	B ☐	C ☐
3. Before I compete I worry about not performing well.	A ☐	B ☐	C ☐
4. I am a good sportsman when I compete.	A ☐	B ☐	C ☐
5. When I compete I worry about making mistakes.	A ☐	B ☐	C ☐
6. Before I compete I am calm.	A ☐	B ☐	C ☐
7. Setting a goal is important when competing.	A ☐	B ☐	C ☐
8. Before I compete I get a funny feeling in my stomach.	A ☐	B ☐	C ☐
9. Just before competing I notice my heart beats faster than usual.	A ☐	B ☐	C ☐
10. I like rough games.	A ☐	B ☐	C ☐
11. Before I compete I feel relaxed.	A ☐	B ☐	C ☐
12. Before I compete I am nervous.	A ☐	B ☐	C ☐
13. Team sports are more exciting than individual sports.	A ☐	B ☐	C ☐
14. I get nervous wanting to start the game.	A ☐	B ☐	C ☐
15. Before I compete I usually get uptight.	A ☐	B ☐	C ☐

From Martens, R.

Items 6 and 11 are scored using the following key:

1 = Often   2 = Sometimes   3 = Hardly ever

Items 1, 4, 7, 10, and 13, the remaining items, are not scored; they are included in the inventory as spurious items, to direct attention to elements of competition other than anxiety.

Validity Content validity was claimed on the basis of the assessment by six judges of the content validity and grammatical clarity of the items. Extensive evidence of construct validity is presented in Martens monograph. The details of these studies are beyond the scope of this book; however, the general ap-

TABLE 22-2 *Normative data for sport competition anxiety test*

	SCAT-C Norms for normal children, grades 4-6				
	Male			Female	
Raw score	Standard score	Percentile		Standard score	Percentile
30	744	99		734	99
29	722	99		711	99
28	700	99		688	98
27	678	97		666	97
26	656	95		643	92
25	634	90		620	88
24	612	87		597	85
23	590	84		575	80
22	568	77		552	74
21	546	71		529	67
20	524	63		507	56
19	502	56		484	48
18	480	46		461	39
17	458	41		438	31
16	436	33		416	24
15	415	28		393	16
14	393	21		370	14
13	371	13		347	10
12	349	9		325	6
11	327	2		302	2
10	305	1		279	1

From Martens, R.

proaches to construct validity included studies of group differences. High scorers on the SCAT-C were expected to manifest higher A states in stressful competetive situations than low scorers on the SCAT-C.

Reliability Test-retest reliability was determined for both sexes of grades 5 and 6 and 8 and 9. Within-day reliability coefficients ranged from 0.85 to 0.93. Test-retest reliabilities ranged from 0.61 to 0.87. When $R_{xx'}$ was calculated to estimate reliability, the range of coefficients was 0.68 to 0.89.

Norms Both standard scores and percentile norms for normal children, grades 4 to 6 and grades 7 to 9, are presented in Table 22-2.

TABLE 22-2 *Normative data for sport competition anxiety test—cont'd*

SCAT-C Norms for normal children, grades 7-9

Raw score	Male		Female	
	Standard score	Percentile	Standard score	Percentile
30	730	99	688	99
29	709	99	669	97
28	687	99	649	96
27	665	97	630	91
26	644	93	610	88
25	622	90	591	84
24	601	85	571	76
23	579	79	552	70
22	558	73	532	63
21	536	66	513	53
20	515	59	493	49
19	493	51	473	42
18	472	43	454	35
17	450	37	434	30
16	429	30	415	26
15	407	24	395	19
14	386	18	376	17
13	364	12	356	12
12	342	8	337	9
11	321	4	317	5
10	299	2	298	2

Comments This test is easy to administer in a group setting. However, the Martens monograph should be reviewed before using SCAT so that the theoretical framework generating this instrument is understood.

Social Behavior

Cowell Social Adjustment Index (Cowell, 1958)

Test Objective To measure the extent of students' social adjustment, both positive and negative, within their social group.

Description Forms A and B of the scale are shown in Table 22-3. Each student is rated by the teacher. A mark is placed in the cell that best reflects the degree to which the behavior is judged to be displayed.

Materials Test forms and pencils.

TABLE 22-3 *Cowell social adjustment index*

Form A

Instructions: Think carefully of the student's behavior in group situations; check each behavior trend according to its degree of descriptiveness.

Behavior trends	Descriptive of student			
	Markedly (+3)	Somewhat (+2)	Only slightly (+1)	Not at all (0)
1. Enters heartily and with enjoyment into the spirit of social intercourse.				
2. Frank, talkative and sociable, does not stand on ceremony.				
3. Self-confident and self-reliant, tends to take success for granted, strong initiative, prefers to lead.				
4. Quick and decisive in movement, pronounced or excessive energy output.				
5. Prefers group activities, work or play, not easily satisfied with individual projects.				
6. Adaptable to new situations, makes adjustments readily, welcomes change.				
7. Is self-composed, seldom shows signs of embarrassment.				
8. Tends to elation of spirits, seldom gloomy or moody.				
9. Seeks a broad range of friendships, not selective or exclusive in games and the like.				
10. Hearty and cordial, even to strangers, forms acquaintanceships very easily.				

From Cowell, C.C.

Scoring The total index score is the sum of the points for the 10 items in Form A minus the sum of the points for the 10 items in Form B.

Validity $r_{xy} = 0.63$, using the Pupil Who's Who Ratings as a criterion measure; $r_{xy} = 0.50$, using the Pupil Personal Distance Ballot.

Reliability $r_{xx'} = 0.82$.

Norms Norms are available for junior high school boys in the original source.

Comments This index was developed by Charles Cowell, a well-known physical educator and long-time faculty member at Purdue University. It can be used with boys and girls, ages 12 to 17.

Blanchard Behavior Rating Scale (Blanchard, 1936)

Test Objective To measure the character and personality of the students.

TABLE 22-3 *Cowell social adjustment index—cont'd*

Form B

Instructions: Think carefully of the student's behavior in group situations; check each behavior trend according to its degree of descriptiveness.

Behavior trends	Descriptive of student			
	Markedly (−3)	Somewhat (−2)	Only slightly (−1)	Not at all (0)
1. Somewhat prudish, awkward, easily embarrassed in his social contacts.				
2. Secretive, seclusive, not inclined to talk unless spoken to.				
3. Lacking in self-confidence and initiative, a follower.				
4. Slow in movement, deliberative, or perhaps indecisive. Energy output moderate or deficient.				
5. Prefers to work and play alone, tends to avoid group activities.				
6. Shrinks from making new adjustments, prefers the habitual to the stress of reorganization required by the new.				
7. Is self-conscious, easily embarrassed, timid, or "bashful."				
8. Tends to depression, frequently gloomy or moody.				
9. Shows preference for a narrow range of intimate friends and tends to exclude others from his association.				
10. Reserved and distant except to intimate friends, does not form acquaintanceships readily.				

TABLE 22-4 *Blanchard behavior frequency rating scale*

Personal information	Frequency of observation					
	No opportunity to observe	Never	Seldom	Fairly often	Frequently	Extremely often / Score
Leadership						
1. He is popular with classmates		1	2	3	4	5
2. He seeks responsibility in the classroom		1	2	3	4	5
3. He shows intellectual leadership in the classroom....		1	2	3	4	5
Positive active qualities						
4. He quits on tasks requiring perseverance		5	4	3	2	1
5. He exhibits aggressiveness in his relationship with others		1	2	3	4	5
6. He shows initiative in assuming responsibility in unfamiliar situations		1	2	3	4	5
7. He is alert to new opportunities		1	2	3	4	5
Positive mental qualities						
8. He shows keenness of mind		1	2	3	4	5
9. He volunteers ideas		1	2	3	4	5
Self-control						
10. He grumbles over decisions of classmates		5	4	3	2	1
11. He takes a justified criticism by teacher or classmate without showing anger or pouting		1	2	3	4	5

From Blanchard, B.E.

Description The scale shown in Table 22-4 is used by the teacher to evaluate students in classes. For each item the teacher circles the item that best reflects his or her judgment of the student's behavior. A form is used for each student.

Materials Test forms and pencils.

Scoring The total score is the sum of the numbers that have been circled for all 24 items. The maximum number of points attainable is 120.

Validity $r_{xy} = 0.93$, using the criterion of the average of the correlations of each item with the remainder of the items measuring the same trait.

Reliability $r_{xx'} = 0.71$; this coefficient actually represents the correlation between the scores of teacher and student raters (interrater agreement).

TABLE 22-4 *Blanchard behavior frequency rating scale—cont'd*

Personal information	No opportunity to observe	Never	Seldom	Fairly often	Frequently	Extremely often	Score
Cooperation							
12. He is loyal to his group		1	2	3	4	5	
13. He discharges his group responsibilities well		1	2	3	4	5	
14. He is cooperative in his attitude toward the teacher.		1	2	3	4	5	
Social action standards							
15. He makes loud-mouthed criticisms and comments ..		5	4	3	2	1	
16. He respects the rights of others		1	2	3	4	5	
Ethical social qualities							
17. He cheats		5	4	3	2	1	
18. He is truthful		1	2	3	4	5	
Qualities of efficiency							
19. He seems satisfied to "get by" with tasks assigned .		5	4	3	2	1	
20. He is dependable and trustworthy.............................		1	2	3	4	5	
21. He has good study habits...		1	2	3	4	5	
Sociability							
22. He is liked by others		1	2	3	4	5	
23. He makes a friendly approach to others in the group		1	2	3	4	5	
24. He is friendly..		1	2	3	4	5	

Norms No norms were reported. Local norms can easily be calculated for several classes, a school, or a school district. Norms developed at the local level are often the most useful, since the tests are more likely to measure the curricular goals of the school system.

Comments This scale can be used with boys and girls, ages 12 to 17. The form in Table 22-4 can be adapted by changing the "he" to "she." The general nature of some of the test items may lead to considerable bias in the ratings. For example, note item 24: "He is friendly." What behaviors would a teacher expect to observe for a rating of 5? A rating of 2? Would another teacher make identical judgments of the same student?

Attitudes

Attitude Toward Physical Activity Inventory (Kenyon, 1968 a,b)

Test Objective To measure six dimensions of the attitude construct of active and passive involvement in physical activity.

Description The test items in the Health and Fitness Scale, one of the six dimensions of involvement in physical activity, are shown in Table 22-5. Both the men's and women's versions of the Attitude Toward Physical Activity (ATPA) Inventory can be obtained by writing Dr. Kenyon at the address on p. 553.

The six dimensions and a brief description of each are presented below:

Social Experience Physical activity is valued as medium for social relationships.

Health and Fitness Physical activity is valued because it contributes to the improvement of physical fitness and health.

Pursuit of Vertigo Physical activity is valued as a means of providing an element of risk to the participant.

Aesthetic Experience Physical activity is valued as a means of providing an artistic element to the participant, to experience the beauty of the movement.

Catharsis Physical activity is valued for its cleansing nature, as a release of tension.

Ascetic Experience Physical activity is valued as means of self-sacrifice requiring dedication to strenuous training.

Materials Test forms, scoring key, and pencils.

Scoring Each scale of the ATPA inventory is scored separately. Thus each examinee will receive six scores, one for each scale. The six scores should not be summed in an attempt to obtain a single indicator of attitude toward physical activity. Since the profile of six scores most accurately describes the examinee's attitude, a total of the scores is difficult to interpret.

A response to an item can range from Very Strongly Disagree to Very Strongly Agree, using a 7-point scale. The maximum number of points that can be scored for each dimension is presented in Table 22-6.

Keep in mind that the scoring must be reversed on several items before summing the dimension score. Note, for example, one of the Health and Fitness Scale items: "Being strong and highly fit is not the most important thing in my life." An examinee who strongly agrees with this statement would record a score of 7 on the item. However, since the statement is worded negatively, his or her score should be converted to a score of 1 to convey the expression of a negative attitude toward physical fitness. Adhere closely to the scoring key when scoring the instrument.

TABLE 22-5 *Health and fitness scale items*

VSA	SA	A	U	D	SD	VSD	Of all physical activities, those whose purpose is primarily to develop physical fitness would *not* be my first choice.
VSA	SA	A	U	D	SD	VSD	I would usually choose strenuous physical activity over light physical activity, if given the choice.
VSA	SA	A	U	D	SD	VSD	A large part of our daily lives must be committed to vigorous exercise.
VSA	SA	A	U	D	SD	VSD	Being strong and highly fit is *not* the most important thing in my life.
VSA	SA	A	U	D	SD	VSD	The time spent doing daily calisthenics could probably be used more profitably in other ways.
VSA	SA	A	U	D	SD	VSD	Strength and physical stamina are the most important prerequisites to a full life.
VSA	SA	A	U	D	SD	VSD	I believe calisthenics are among the less desirable forms of physical activity.
VSA	SA	A	U	D	SD	VSD	People should spend 20 to 30 minutes a day doing vigorous calisthenics.
VSA	SA	A	U	D	SD	VSD	Of all physical activities, my first choice would be those whose purpose is primarily to develop and maintain physical fitness.
VSA	SA	A	U	D	SD	VSD	Vigorous daily exercises are absolutely necessary to maintain one's general health.

Reprinted by permission of Kenyon, G.S., University of Lethbridge, Lethbridge, Alberta, Canada.

TABLE 22-6 *Maximum scores for ATPA dimensions*

	Men	Women
Social	70 (10 items)	56 (8 items)
Health and fitness	70 (10 items)	77 (11 items)
Vertigo	70 (10 items)	63 (9 items)
Aesthetic	70 (10 items)	63 (9 items)
Catharsis	63 (9 items)	63 (9 items)
Ascetic	70 (10 items)	56 (8 items)

TABLE 22-7 *Within-day reliability coefficients for ATPA*

	Male	Female	N
Social			
United States	0.782	0.794	120
England	0.783	0.790	120
Health and fitness			
United States	0.866	0.883	120
England	0.782	0.840	120
Pursuit of vertigo			
United States	0.910	0.883	120
England	0.867	0.806	120
Aesthetic			
United States	0.865	0.915	120
England	0.851	0.839	120
Catharsis			
United States	0.859	0.873	120
England	0.884	0.868	120
Ascetic			
United States	0.874	0.892	120
England	0.780	0.789	120

From Pooley, J.C.

Validity The six dimensions of attitude toward physical activity as hypothe-sized by Kenyon were verified using factor analytic procedures. Expert opinion also confirmed that the six dimensions adequately represented attitude toward active and passive involvement in physical activity. Several studies of construct validity have been conducted, using the group differences approach. Generally, athletes and nonathletes differed on the scales, as did males and females.

Reliability The within-day reliability coefficients for males and females on all six dimensions are given in Table 22-7.

Norms Although means and standard deviations have been reported in studies too numerous to report in this textbook, no norms have been developed. However, an annotated bibliography by Kenyon and Andrews includes most of these studies up to 1981. References that became available after 1981 are included in the System of Information Retrieval for Leisure and Sport (SIRLS),* a retrieval system at the University of Waterloo.

Comments This is an excellent inventory, developed by an outstanding sport sociologist in the field. It can be used in a practical as well as a research setting and is appropriate for males and females of high school through college age.

Children's Attitude Toward Physical Activity Inventory (Simon and Smoll, 1974)

Test Objective To measure children's attitude toward vigorous physical activity.

Description The Children's Attitude Toward Physical Activity (CATPA) was modeled after the ATPA, described in the previous section. A semantic differential scale was used, with each dimension calculated on the basis of eight pairs of bipolar adjectives, which are used to assess the value of each domain. The items for the social dimension of CATPA are shown on p. 554.

Materials Test forms and pencils.

Scoring Each of the six CATPA scales is scored separately. The bipolar adjectives of each pair are separated by a 7-point continuum, and the numerical values assigned to each of the eight adjective pairs are summed for the score on a single dimension. The maximum score for each domain is 56.

Validity It was assumed that the six ATPA dimensions were equally representative for young children. Except for the ascetic dimension, dimension names on the CATPA are the same as those used for the ATPA. The wording of the dimension descriptions was changed to be more appropriate for young children. In a study of construct validity, children's scores on the CATPA were significantly related to active involvement in physical activity but had no relationship to motor skill proficiency.

Reliability $R_{xx'} = 0.80 - 0.89$, within-day estimates; $R_{xx'} = 0.44 - 0.62$, test-retest estimates.

Norms Not reported for this specific test.

Comments This inventory is useful for program evaluation in the elementary and junior high schools.

Physical Estimation and Attraction Scale (Sonstroem, 1974)

Test Objective To measure the motivational properties of physical self-esteem (Estimation) and interest in vigorous physical activity.

---

*The bibliography and more information on references available after 1981 can be obtained by writing to G.S. Kenyon, University of Lethbridge, Lethbridge, Alberta, Canada T1K 3M4.

Items for social dimension of CATPA

What does the idea in the box mean to you?

PHYSICAL ACTIVITY AS A SOCIAL EXPERIENCE Physical activities that give you a chance to meet new people and be with your friends.

Always Think About the Idea in the Box.

1. Good ____ : ____ : ____ : ____ : ____ : ____ : ____ Bad
      1   2   3   4   5   6   7

2. Of no use ____ : ____ : ____ : ____ : ____ : ____ : ____ Useful
      1   2   3   4   5   6   7

3. Not pleasant ____ : ____ : ____ : ____ : ____ : ____ : ____ Pleasant
      1   2   3   4   5   6   7

4. Bitter ____ : ____ : ____ : ____ : ____ : ____ : ____ Sweet
      1   2   3   4   5   6   7

5. Nice ____ : ____ : ____ : ____ : ____ : ____ : ____ Awful
      1   2   3   4   5   6   7

6. Happy ____ : ____ : ____ : ____ : ____ : ____ : ____ Sad
      1   2   3   4   5   6   7

7. Dirty ____ : ____ : ____ : ____ : ____ : ____ : ____ Clean
      1   2   3   4   5   6   7

8. Steady ____ : ____ : ____ : ____ : ____ : ____ : ____ Nervous
      1   2   3   4   5   6   7

From Simon, J.A., and Smoll, F.L.

Description The Physical Estimation and Attraction Scale (PEAS) consists of a random ordering of 11 neutral items, 50 Attraction items, and 33 Estimation items. Sample items are presented on p. 555, and the full-length test along with the scoring key can be obtained from Dr. Sonstroem at the University of Rhode Island. There are two response choices: true, if the examinee agrees with the statement, and false, if not. Many of the items are of the forced-choice type, requiring the examinee to choose one activity over another.

Materials Test forms, pencils, and scoring key.

Scoring For each correct response 1 point is scored.

Validity A number of studies of construct validity have been conducted (Sonstroem, 1978). High and low fit boys differed significantly in their scores on both the Estimation and Attraction dimensions of the PEAS. Moderate relationships were reported between Estimation scores and a fitness index and between Esti-

---

Sample items from PEAS

Estimation items

Item 6.   My body is strong and muscular compared to other boys my age.
Item 26.   I am better coordinated than most people I know.
Item 33.   I am a good deal stronger than most of my friends.

Attraction items

Item 4.   I would much rather play softball than go for a ride in a car.
Item 17.   I like to be in sports that don't require a great amount of running.
Item 34.   I would rather play poker than softball.

From Sonstroem, R.J. Reprinted by permission of the author, University of Rhode Island, Kingston.

TABLE 22-8 *Summary statistics for PEAS*

Group	Scale	N	Mean	Standard deviation
Boys, grades 9-12	Estimation	187	20.40	6.60
	Attraction	187	35.52	8.99
Boys, high school	Estimation	106	22.2	5.75
Boys, junior high school	Estimation	112	21.96	6.29

mation scores and self-esteem. (Remember that the Estimation dimension taps one's physical self-esteem.)

Reliability $r_{xx'} = 0.87$, Attraction scale, within-day estimate; $r_{xx'} = 0.87$, Estimation scale, within-day estimate; and $r_{xx'} = 0.90$, total scale, test-retest estimate.

Norms No norms were reported. Summary data from Sonstroem's studies are given in Table 22-8.

Comments Although the scale has been used with male and female adults and adolescent boys, validity has been determined primarily for the latter sample. Since responses to PEAS items can be distorted and the scores influenced by response sets, the use of a distortion scale is advisable. A scale for this purpose should be provided by the test developer. Response distortion, one of the key words in this chapter, was described in the introductory section. If a distortion scale is available, an examinee scoring below a predetermined score on the scale is perceived as distorting his or her responses to the test of affect. Because of the low score on the distortion scale, the score on the affective test is viewed as invalid.

Wear Attitude Scale (Wear, 1955)

Test Objective To measure attitudes toward physical education.

Description Two forms of the scale, A and B, were developed. Form A is shown in the boxed material below and on p. 557. The students are instructed to respond to the scale according to their perceptions of physical education as an activity course taught during a regular class period. The five possible responses are strongly agree, agree, undecided, disagree, and strongly disagree. Students

---

Form A of the Wear Attitude Scale

1. If for any reason a few subjects have to be dropped from the school program, physical education should be one of the subjects dropped.
2. Physical education activities provide no opportunities for learning to control the emotions.
3. Physical education is one of the more important subjects in helping to establish and maintain desirable social standards.
4. Vigorous physical activity works off harmful emotional tensions.
5. I would take physical education only if it were required.
6. Participation in physical education makes no contribution to the development of poise.
7. Because physical skills loom large in importance in youth, it is essential that a person be helped to acquire and improve such skills.
8. Calisthenics taken regularly are good for one's general health.
9. Skill in active games or sports is not necessary for leading the fullest kind of life.
10. Physical education does more harm physically than it does good.
11. Associating with others in some physical education activity is fun.
12. Physical education classes provide situations for the formulation of attitudes, which make one a better citizen.
13. Physical education situations are among the poorest for making friends.
14. There is not enough value coming from physical education to justify the time consumed.
15. Physical education skills make worthwhile contributions to the enrichment of living.

From Wear, C.L.

should answer anonymously, or they should be informed that their responses will not affect their physical education grades.

Materials Test forms and pencils.

Scoring The total score is the sum of the scores of the 30 items. Positively worded items are scored 5-4-3-2-1, and negatively worded items are scored 1-2-3-4-5. High scores reflect positive attitudes toward physical education.

Validity Face validity.

Reliability $r_{xx'} = 0.94$, Form A; and $r_{xx'} = 0.96$, Form B.

Comments The Wear Attitude Scale, one of the classic scales of attitudes toward physical education, has been widely used and cited. Although the psychometric properties could be strengthened by today's standards, the scale stood for many years as one of the best affective measures in physical education.

Form A of the Wear Attitude Scale—cont'd

16. People get all the physical exercise they need in just taking care of their daily work.
17. All who are physically able will profit from an hour of physical education each day.
18. Physical education makes a valuable contribution toward building up an adequate reserve of strength and endurance for everyday living.
19. Physical education tears down sociability by encouraging people to attempt to surpass each other in many of the activities.
20. Participation in physical education activities makes for a more wholesome outlook on life.
21. Physical education adds nothing to the improvement of social behavior.
22. Physical education class activities will help to relieve and relax physical tensions.
23. Participation in physical education activities helps a person to maintain a healthful emotional life.
24. Physical education is one of the more important subjects in the school program.
25. There is little value in physical education as far as physical well-being is concerned.
26. Physical education should be included in the program of every school.
27. Skills learned in physical education class do not benefit a person.
28. Physical education provides situations for developing character qualities.
29. Physical education makes for more enjoyable living.
30. Physical education has no place in modern education.

Sportsmanship and Leadership

Lakie Attitude Toward Athletic Competition Scale (Lakie, 1964)

Test Objective To measure player's attitudes toward competition.

Description Lakie's scale is shown in the boxed material below and on p. 559. Examinees are instructed to read each item carefully and circle the number of the response best reflecting their judgment of the action described.

Lakie Attitude Toward Athletic Competition Scale

The following situations describe behavior demonstrated in sports. Circle the category that indicates your feeling toward the behavior described in each of the situations.

1. Strongly approve 2. Approve 3. Undecided 4. Disapprove 5. Strongly disapprove

1 2 3 4 5   1. During a football game team A has the ball on its own 45-yard line, fourth down and 1 yard to go for a first down. The coach of team A signals to the quarterback the play that he wants the team to run.

1 2 3 4 5   2. Team A is the visiting basketball team; and each time a member of the team is given a free shot, the home crowd sets up a continual din of noise until the shot has been taken.

1 2 3 4 5   3. Tennis player A frequently calls out, throws up his arms, or otherwise tries to indicate that his opponent's serve is out of bounds when it is questionable.

1 2 3 4 5   4. In a track meet, team A enters a man in the mile run who is to set a fast pace for the first half of the race and then drop out.

1 2 3 4 5   5. In a football game, team B's quarterback was tackled repeatedly after handing off and after he was out of the play.

1 2 3 4 5   6. Sam, playing golf with his friends, hit a drive into the rough. He accidentally moved the ball with his foot; although not improving his position, he added a penalty stroke to his score.

1 2 3 4 5   7. A basketball player was caught out of position on defense; and rather than allow his opponent to attempt a field goal, he fouled him.

1 2 3 4 5   8. Player A during a golf match made quick noises and movements when player B was getting ready to make a shot.

From Lakie, W.L.

1 2 3 4 5   9. School A has a powerful but quite slow football team. The night before playing a smaller but faster team, they allowed the field sprinkling system to remain on, causing the field to be heavy and slow.

1 2 3 4 5   10. A basketball team used player A to draw the opponent's high scorer into fouling situations.

1 2 3 4 5   11. The alumni of College A pressured the Board of Trustees to lower the admission and eligibility requirements for athletes.

1 2 3 4 5   12. Team A, by use of fake injuries, was able to stop the clock long enough to get off the play that resulted in the winning touchdown.

1 2 3 4 5   13. A tennis player was given the advantage of a bad call in a close match. He then "evened up" the call by intentionally hitting the ball out of bounds.

1 2 3 4 5   14. The coach of basketball team A removed his team from the floor in protest of an official's decision.

1 2 3 4 5   15. Between seasons a coach moved from College A to College B, and he then persuaded three of College A's athletes to transfer to College B.

1 2 3 4 5   16. After losing a close football game, the coach of the losing team publicly accused the game officials of favoritism when the game movies showed the winning touchdown had been scored by using an illegal maneuver.

1 2 3 4 5   17. College C lowered the admission requirements for boys awarded athletic scholarships.

1 2 3 4 5   18. Team A's safety man returned a punt for a touchdown. Unseen by the officials, he had stepped out of bounds in front of his team's bench. His coach notified the officials of this fact.

1 2 3 4 5   19. A college with very few athletic scholarships to offer gives athletes preference on all types of campus jobs.

1 2 3 4 5   20. Several wealthy alumni of College C make a monthly gift to several athletes who are in need of financial assistance.

1 2 3 4 5   21. College K has a policy of not allowing any member of a varsity squad to associate with the visiting team until the contest or meet is completed.

1 2 3 4 5   22. The Board of Trustees of College C fired the football coach and gave as the reason for his dismissal his failure to win a conference championship during the past five years.

Materials Test forms and pencils.

Scoring Total the scores for each item. Use the reverse order (5-4-3-2-1) to score negative items. The higher the score, the more competitive the player. A high score reflects a desire to win at any cost. The scale includes 22 items; thus, the highest possible score is 110 points.

Validity Face validity.

Reliability $r_{xx'} = 0.81$.

Norms Not reported for this specific test.

Comments The Lakie Attitude Scale is similar in type to a number of other measures, mostly unpublished, that have been developed in the field. Attitudes about competition have changed over the years, and some actions that are acceptable today were viewed as poor sportsmanship many years ago. It is difficult to develop this type of instrument without including items that seem to have quite obvious answers.

Nelson Sports Leadership Questionnaire (Nelson, 1966)

Test Objective To measure leadership in athletic settings.

Description Two questionnaires were designed, one for coaches and one for members of athletic teams. (See both sections of the boxed material on pp. 561-563.) The coach's questionnaire has 14 items; the player's, 20 items. On the team members' forms the examinee must list a first choice (under No. 1) and a second choice (under No. 2) of team members, excluding his or her own name. A team member's name can be used any number of times. Examinees are asked not to sign the questionnaire.

Materials Test forms and pencils.

Scoring List the names of team members appearing on a questionnaire. Allocate 5 points to a name appearing under No. 1 and 3 points to a name appearing under No. 2. Add the number of points for each player. These points can be summed by players, across all questionnaires. Players can then be ranked according to total points or average number of points.

Validity Face validity; construct validity, by comparing leaders and nonleaders.

Reliability $r_{xx'} = 0.96$, ninth-grade football players; $r_{xx'} = 0.78$, varsity college basketball players. Both of these estimates were reported in Johnson and Nelson (1974).

Norms Not reported for this specific test.

Comments Test directions should be typed onto the questionnaire. It can be used for males and females, junior high school through college level. A modified version of the player's questionnaire is presented in Johnson and Nelson (1974, p. 396). In this version the terms are not restricted to a specific sport; thus it has more widespread applicability.

Nelson Sports Leadership Questionnaire (coaches)

The same names can be used any number of times, and in all cases give your first and second choice for each question.

1. Who are the most popular men on your squad?
   1. _____ 2. _____
2. Which players on the team know the most basketball, in terms of strategy, team play, etc.?
   1. _____ 2. _____
3. Of all the players on your team, who exhibits the most poise on the floor during the crucial parts of the game?
   1. _____ 2. _____
4. Who are the "take charge" men on your squad?
   1. _____ 2. _____
5. Who are the most consistent ball handlers on your squad?
   1. _____ 2. _____
6. Who are the most consistent shooters on your squad?
   1. _____ 2. _____
7. Who are the most valuable players on your squad?
   1. _____ 2. _____
8. Who are the two players who play "most for the team"?
   1. _____ 2. _____
9. Which players have the most overall ability on the squad?
   1. _____ 2. _____
10. Who are the most likable players on the squad?
    1. _____ 2. _____
11. Which players do you think would make the best coaches?
    1. _____ 2. _____
12. If you were not present for practice, which players would you place in charge of the practice?
    1. _____ 2. _____
13. Who are the players endowed with leadership qualities?
    1. _____ 2. _____
14. Who are the players least endowed with leadership ability?
    1. _____ 2. _____

From Nelson, D.O.

Nelson Sports Leadership Questionnaire (players)

Do not sign your name to the questionnaire. Fill in the name or names of the squad member that, in your opinion, best fits the question. Give your first and second choice in all cases. *Do not use your own name* on any of the answers. The names of the same players can be used any number of times, and your answers will be kept confidential.

1. If you were on a trip and had a choice of the players you would share the hotel room with, who would they be?
   1. _____   2. _____
2. Who are the most popular men on the squad?
   1. _____   2. _____
3. Who are the best scholars on the squad?
   1. _____   2. _____
4. Which players on the team know the most basketball, in terms of strategy, team play, etc.?
   1. _____   2. _____
5. If the coach were not present for a workout, which players would be the most likely to take charge of the practice?
   1. _____   2. _____
6. Which players would you listen to first if the team appeared to be disorganized during a crucial game?
   1. _____   2. _____
7. Your team is behind 1 point with 10 seconds remaining in the game and you could pass to anyone on the squad. Who would it be?
   1. _____   2. _____
8. Of all the players on your team, who exhibits the most poise on the floor during the crucial parts of the game?
   1. _____   2. _____

From Nelson, D.O.

Other Measures

Perceived Exertion (Borg, 1973)

Test Objective To assess one's perception of his or her physical exertion during exercise.

Description The scale is shown in the boxed material on p. 563. At regular intervals during exercise the examinee is asked to select a rating that reflects his or her perception of physical exertion. At some point the activity may be terminated when a certain rating is reached; this is dependent on the protocol being used. Typically, other data are also considered before terminating exercise. The

---

Nelson Sports Leadership Questionnaire (players)—cont'd

9. Who are the "take charge" men on your team?
   1. _____   2. _____

10. Who are the most consistent ball handlers on your squad?
    1. _____   2. _____

11. Who are the most consistent shooters on your squad?
    1. _____   2. _____

12. Who are the most valuable players on your squad?
    1. _____   2. _____

13. Who are the most unselfish players who are interested most in the team as a whole and who play most "for the team"?
    1. _____   2. _____

14. Which players have the most overall ability of the squad?
    1. _____   2. _____

15. Who are the most likable players on the squad?
    1. _____   2. _____

16. Which players on your team have influenced you the most?
    1. _____   2. _____

17. Which players have actually helped you the most?
    1. _____   2. _____

18. Which players do you think would make the best coaches?
    1. _____   2. _____

19. Which players do you most often look to for leadership?
    1. _____   2. _____

20. Who are the hardest workers on the squad?
    1. _____   2. _____

Perceived exertion scale

6	14
7 Very, very light	15 Hard
8	16
9 Very light	17 Very hard
10	18
11 Fairly light	19 Very, very hard
12	20
13 Somewhat hard	

From Borg, G.A.V.

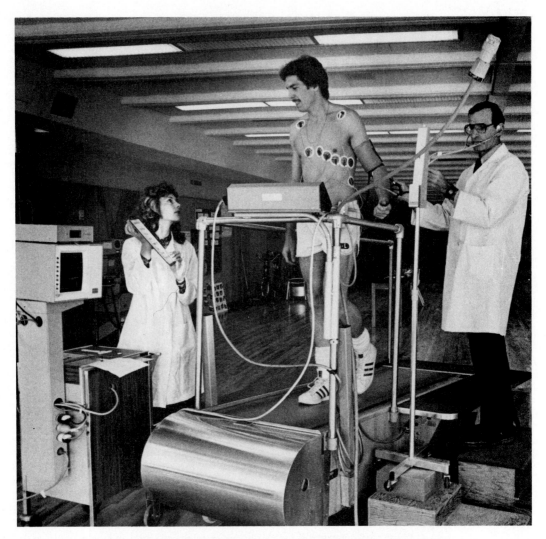

Use of Perceived Exertion Scale during stress test on treadmill.

photograph preceding the test description shows the perceived exertion scale being used in conjunction with a stress test on a treadmill.

Comments Borg has developed a new version of the perceived exertion scale that has ratio properties (Borg, 1982). In a review of the study and application of perceived exertion, Pandolf (1983) discusses the new scale and recommends that its use be limited to research. "Although this new scale may be more advantageous for studies requiring ratio scaling methods, Borg concluded that his old 15 point scale is still the best for applied studies" (Pandolf, 1983, p. 129).

SUMMARY

Measures of affective behavior are designed to measure attitudes, interests, values, psychological traits, social behavior, and emotional states of the individual. Many types of affective behavior are of interest to the physical educator, coach, and exercise specialist. Although a number of instruments have been developed to measure affective behavior in the field, many of these measures do not have strong psychometric underpinnings. However, they may have some usefulness if used as an indicator of a characteristic of a group of examinees rather than of an individual person. They might also be useful in a formative evaluation context. Few instruments are available that would be suitable in a research setting.

LEARNING EXPERIENCES

1. Analyze the Lakie Attitude Toward Athletic Competition Scale. First, take the test and determine your score. Identify the aspects of competition that are measured by this scale by naming each aspect of competition and listing the items falling under each. Are some aspects of competition overemphasized in this scale? If so, which ones? Are some aspects underemphasized? If so, which ones? Do you think this scale is useful in today's competitive settings? Give a thorough rationale for your answer.

2. Develop a rating scale to measure attitudes toward an official in a game. Use a 5-4-3-2-1 rating scale and write a descriptor for each point value. Each descriptor should reflect behaviors rather than a general phrase, such as 5 = excellent attitude, 4 = good attitude, and so forth. What behaviors would you expect to see in a person who is given a rating of 5? A rating of 1? This means that you must write several short phrases for each descriptor.

REFERENCES

American Psychological Association. 1985. Standards for educational and psychological tests. Washington, DC.

Blanchard, B.E. 1936. A behavior frequency rating scale for the measurement of character and personality traits in a physical education classroom situation. Research Quarterly, **7:**56-66.

Borg, G.A.V. 1973. Perceived exertion: a note on "history" and methods. Medicine and Science in Sports, **5:**90-93.

Borg, G.A.V. 1982. Psychophysical bases of perceived exertion. Medicine and Science in Sports and Exercise, **14:**377-381.

Cowell, C.C. 1958. Validating an index of social adjustment for high school use. Research Quarterly, **29:**7-18.

Johnson, B.L. and Nelson, J.K. 1974. Practical measurements for evaluation in physical education. Minneapolis: Burgess Publishing Co.

Kenyon, G.S. 1968a. A conceptual model for characterizing physical activity. Research Quarterly, **39:**96-105.

Kenyon, G.S. 1968b. Six scales for assessing attitudes toward physical activity. Research Quarterly, **39:**566-574.

Lakie, W.L. 1964. Expressed attitudes of various groups of athletes toward athletic competition. Research Quarterly, **35:**497-503.

Martens, R. 1977. Sport Competition Anxiety Test. Champaign, IL: Human Kinetics Publishers.

Miller, D.K., and Allen, T.E. 1982. Fitness: a lifetime commitment, ed 2. Minneapolis: Burgess Publishing Co.

Nelson, D.O. 1966. Nelson Sports Leadership Questionnaire. Research Quarterly, 37:268-275.

Pandolf, K.B. 1983. Advances in the study and application of perceived exertion. In Terjung, R.L., editor: Exercise and sport science reviews. Philadelphia: The Franklin Institute Press.

Pooley, J.C. 1971. The professionalism of physical education in the United States and England, Unpublished doctoral dissertation, University of Wisconsin, Madison.

Safrit, M.J., and Wood, T.M. 1983. The Health-Related Fitness Opinionnaire: a pilot survey. Research Quarterly for Exercise and Sport, 54:204-207.

Simon, J.A., and Smoll, F.L. 1974. An instrument for assessing children's attitude toward physical activity. Research Quarterly, 45:21-27.

Sonstroem, R.J. 1974. Attitude testing: examining certain physiological correlates of physical activity. Research Quarterly, 45:93-103.

Sonstroem, R.J. 1978. Physical estimation and attraction scales: rationale and research. Medicine and Science in Sports, 10:97-102.

Wear, C.L. 1955. Construction of equivalent forms of an attitude scale. Research Quarterly, 26:113-119.

ANNOTATED READINGS

Jones, J.G. 1975. An effective evaluation of an outdoor education experience. Journal of Physical Education and Recreation, 46:54-55.

Describes the construction of two test forms to evaluate ten outdoor activities in terms of student enjoyment, desire to continue the activity, and perceived learning; presents descriptive statistics for both forms of the test; concludes that the outdoor experience primarily emphasizes skill development and improved attitudes toward outdoor living.

Frye, P.A. 1983. Measurement of psychosocial aspects of physical education. Journal of Physical Education, Recreation and Dance, 54(8):26-27.

Discusses the principles and practices of measurement and evaluation as applied to psychosocial characteristics; suggests using available tests to draw inferences about group rather than individual behavior.

McGee, R. 1977. Measuring affective behavior in physical education. Journal of Physical Education and Recreation, 48:29-30.

Notes that affective domain deserves special attention by physical educators; recommends that affective measures such as self-concept, attitude, and social adjustment not be used for grading; should provide student with opportunity to know self better; discusses four instruments and their current usage in the field.

Weise, C.E., and Schick, J. 1982. Affective measurement in physical education: doing well and feeling good. Journal of Physical Education, Recreation and Dance, 53(2):15-25, 86.

Offers a series of articles on measuring affective behavior in physical education; presents discussion of the pros and cons of evaluation in the affective domain; includes uses and abuses of affective measurement.

Glossary

AAHPER Youth Fitness Test: Battery of six test items measuring primarily performance-related physical fitness, although two of the items are measures of health-related fitness

AAHPERD Physical Best Test: Five-item test battery designed to measure physical performance, particularly health-related physical fitness

accountability: Provision of evidence that predetermined goals and objectives have been met

achievement: Ability level of an examinee at a designated point

affect: Sociological or psychological characteristic manifested in a feeling or behavior, such as attitude, interest, and sportsmanship

affective domain: Levels of emotional behavior, including attitudes, interests, and various personality characteristics

alternatives: Set of responses in a multiple choice item; correct alternative is the *answer;* incorrect alternatives are *distractors*

anomaly: Unusual; irregular; contrary to general rule

athletic performance–related physical fitness: Type of physical fitness that enhances performance in sports and other forms of physical activity; different from health-related physical fitness, although health-related fitness may also benefit performance

attitude: Feeling one has about a specific attitude object, such as a situation, a person, or an activity

balance: Ability to maintain equilibrium

BASIC language: Beginners All-Purpose Symbolic Instruction Code; a computer language

basic movement patterns: Types of movement that emerge developmentally, usually at a young age, such as running, jumping, and throwing

behavioral objective: Objective stated in terms of the behavior the student will exhibit when the objective is successfully attained

bicycle ergometer: Stationary bicycle that can be operated at a variety of workloads; used to measure physical work capacity

bit: Smallest amount of information that can be identified by a computer; can specify either of two alternatives, one or zero

body composition: Combination of bone, muscle mass, and fatty tissue

booting: Loading a program into the computer's memory

byte: Equals one character, which is a letter, number, or punctuation mark; made up of eight bits or two nibbles

cable tensiometer: Device used to measure static strength; cable tension is determined

---

*The definitions of words marked with an asterisk (*) are taken from the Rules and Regulations for PL 94-192 published in the Federal Register.

†The definitions of words marked with a dagger are taken from the American Alliance for Health, Physical Education, Recreation and Dance, 1980.

"from the force needed to create offset on a riser in a cable stretched between two points" (Clarke, 1976:124)

carotid artery: Artery in the neck, along the side of the "Adam's apple"; often used to measure pulse rate

CATALOG: BASIC command to list the files on a disk

central processing unit: A microchip or portion of a microchip that controls peripherals and memory

central tendency: Center of distribution of test scores

cerebral palsy: Neuromuscular disability resulting from brain damage

checklist of objectives: Set of symbols to rate major objectives; often used in elementary schools

circumference measure: Measure of the outer surface of a body part, such as the upper arm; sometimes used to estimate body fatness

cognitive domain: Intellectual behavior ranging from a low level (memorization of facts) to a higher level (application of these facts) in some way

compatibles: Computer hardware that uses software written for another, often more expensive, computer

competency-based evaluation: Approach to evaluation in which a desired level of competency is identified, and examinees designated as competent must be able to meet or exceed this level

component model of intratask development: Identification of developmental characteristics of body parts in performing a task

components of skill: Elements of the skill that are essential to its correct execution

computer literacy: Possession of sufficient knowledge about computers to deal adequately with the computer age

concurrent validity: Degree to which a predictor test correlates with a criterion test

condition (in an objective): Situation in which behavior is expected to occur

congenital: Condition present at birth

construct validity: Degree to which a test measures an attribute or a trait that cannot be directly measured

content (in an objective): Material or skill the student is expected to learn

content validity: Degree to which the sample of test items, tasks, or questions on a test are representative of some defined universe or "domain" of content (American Psychological Association, 1985)

contingency coefficient: Method of determining the validity of a mastery test

contingency table: Table with numbers in each cell determined by jointly considering the two joint categories

contrasting groups method: Determination of valid cutoff point by comparing students expected to master an objective with those not expected to master it

correction for guessing: Alteration of test score based on number of items answered incorrectly

correlation: Relationship between two variables

correlation coefficient: Statistical procedure for estimating the relationship between two variables, X and Y *criterion:* Standard of behavior

criterion-referenced test: Test with a predetermined standard of performance that is tied to a specified domain of behavior

criterion-related validity: Extent to which a test measures the true or criterion behavior of examinees, usually determined by correlational procedures

criterion test: Highly valid test of the attribute to be measured; cannot be used in a practical setting because of its complexity, expense, and need for specially trained testers; standard against which a practical test is compared

cumulative frequency (cf): Column in frequency distribution table obtained by summing the frequencies from the bottom to the top of the column; the number at the top of the column equals *N*, the number of scores; represents the number of examinees scoring at or below a given interval

cumulative percent (c%): Column in frequency distribution table obtained by dividing the cumulative frequency by *N* and multiplying by 100; represents the percentage of examinees scoring at or below a given interval

curriculum objective: Translation of long-term objective into specific behavior expected after exposure to a curriculum

deaf: Severe hearing loss

decision validity: Accuracy of classification of masters and nonmasters

DELETE (program): BASIC command to erase a file from a disk

descriptive statistics: Statistics used to describe a set of data

disabled: Because of an impairment, the individual is limited or restricted in executing some skills, performing specific jobs or tasks, or participating in certain activities (American Alliance for Health, Physical Education, Recreation and Dance)

disk (floppy): Round sheet of plastic coated with iron oxide and inserted in a protective, black jacket; a means of storing data

disk drive: Device for storing data; means of communication between disk and central processor

disk operating system (DOS): Means of communicating between the disk in disk drive and the central processor

display: Information appearing on screen of monitor

domain: Range of all possible criterion behaviors

domain-referenced validity: Extent to which the tasks sampled by the test adequately represent the total domain of tasks

dynamic balance: Ability to maintain equilibrium while in motion

dynamic strength: Force exerted by a muscle group as a body part moves through space

dynamometer: Device used to measure static strength and endurance

educable: Capable of learning or being educated, as in educable mentally retarded

electromechanical instrument: Device (such as Cybex II) used to measure static and dynamic strength, endurance, and power

elgon: Goniometer with a potentiometer substituted for the protractor; also known as electrogoniometer; used to measure flexibility

enter key: Key on the keyboard used to enter commands into the computer

essay item: Item requiring examinee to construct a response at least several sentences long *evaluation:* Interpretation of a test score

evaluation objective: Short-term objective reflecting a change in behavior that has occured over a short period

face validity: Having the appearance of validity, but not formally validated

field test: Practical but valid substitute for a more complex laboratory test

Flexed-Arm Hang Test: Measures arm and shoulder girdle strength; usually designated for girls

flexibility: Range of movement about a joint, from a position of extension to flexion or the opposite movement

flexometer: Instrument with a weighted 360-degree dial and a weighted pointer, used to measure flexibility; both the dial and the pointer move indpendently as affected by gravity

forced-choice item: Item requiring examinee to choose among two or more alternatives that appear equally favorable or unfavorable

formative evaluation: Evaluation that occurs throughout a training period or instructional unit

formatting a disk: Preparing a disk for use; must be applied to new disks before using

frequency (f): Number of scores in an interval; sum of tallies in an interval

frequency distribution: Method of organizing test scores into mutually exclusive intervals

frequency polygon: Line graph of the frequency distribution, with score limits on the horizontal axis and frequency of cases on the vertical axis

game statistics: Record of events occurring during a game, such as number of shots attempted, percentage of successful shots, and so forth

gates: Pictorial representation of bits; open gate represents a "yes" choice; closed gate represents a "no" choice

goniometer: Protractor of 180 degrees with extended arms; used to measure flexibility

grade: Mark assigned to a student based on his or her performance on one or more tests

halo effect: Rater bias that may can occur when the rater is unduly influenced by previous performances of the examinee

handicapped†: Because of an impairment or disability, the individual is adversely affected psychologically, emotionally, or socially

hardware: Physical components of the computer, such as keyboard and monitor

health-related physical fitness: See Physical fitness (health-related)

histogram: Bar graph of the frequency distribution, with score limits on the horizontal axis and frequency of cases on the vertical axis

HOME: BASIC command to clear the screen

hydrostatic weighing: Assessment of body composition by weighing a person underwater

impaired†: Individual who has an identifiable organic or functional condition; some part of the body or a portion of an anatomical structure is actually missing; one or more parts of the body do not function properly; may be temporary or permanent

improvement: Change in behavior occurring between an initial and a final testing period

index of discrimination: Ratio of high to low scorers on the total test who answer a given item correctly

Individualized Education Program (IEP): Written plan of instruction, including evaluation procedures, developed for each student receiving special education

individually based norms: Norms based on the distribution of scores of individual examinees; type of norms used in the AAHPER Youth Fitness Test

initializing a disk: Preparing a disk for use, specifically on an Apple computer

instructed/uninstructed approach: Determination of valid cutoff point by comparing an instructed group with an uninstructed group

interclass reliability coefficient: Method of estimating reliability ($r_{xx'}$) using correlation procedures

interests: Affect reflecting one's likes and dislikes about various matters, such as physical activity, programming, and scheduling

interjudge objectivity: Consistency in scoring between two or more independent judgments of the same performance

interpercentile range: Measure of variability used in conjunction with the median; can be represented by a variety of ranges as long as equal portions of each end of the distribution are eliminated

interval (i): Range of scores identified to form categories of a frequency distribution

intraclass reliability coefficient: Method of estimating reliability ($R_{xx'}$) using analysis of variance

intrajudge objectivity: Consistency in scoring when one person scores the same test two or more times

intratask analysis: Identification of stages of development of a task from the time the task is first attempted to the time it is performed at a mature or an adult level

item analysis: Method for determining the usefulness of each individual item as a part of the total test

item difficulty: Proportion of examinees answering the item correctly

item function: Percentage of examinees selecting an alternative as the correct response, whether it is correct or not

kappa coefficient (k): Method of determining the reliability of a mastery test where change is taken into account

keyboard: Used to transmit information to computer; similar to keyboard of typewriter

kilobyte (k): 1024 bytes

Kraus-Weber Test: Test of minimal functioning of the low back area

level of behavior: Level of the process (cognitive, affective, or psychomotor) the learner uses in attaining an objective

Likert scale: Scale measuring degree of agreement or disagreement with a series of affective statements

LIST: BASIC command to list each line of the program in RAM

LOAD (program): A BASIC command to take a specified program from the disk and put it into RAM

logical validity: Extent to which a test measures the most important components of skill required to perform the motor task adequately

long-range goals: Long-term global goals that describe the end product of a complete education

mastery learning: Model of instruction whereby frequent feedback is given to the learner and a large percentage of learners can attain at least minimal success in a unit of instruction

mastery test: Type of criterion-referenced test in which examinees are classified as masters or nonmasters

matching item: Item containing two columns of words or phrases, with the right-hand column used as alternatives to match with the material in the left-hand column

maximal oxygen uptake: Maximal amount of oxygen an individual can transport and use during exercise. Max $\dot{V}o_2$: Symbol for maximal oxygen uptake; often expressed as ml/kg/min, or milliliters per kilogram of body weight per minute

mean: Arithmetic average of a set of scores; a measure of central tendency

measure: When used as a noun, refers to an instrument or technique used to obtain information (usually a score) about an attribute of a person or an object; when used as a verb, refers to the process of obtaining the score

measurement: Process of assigning a number to an attribute of a person or an object; the process of obtaining test scores

median: Score dividing the distribution such that 50% of the scores fall above that point and 50% fall below; the 50th percentile

mentally retarded*: Significantly subaverage, general intellectual functioning existing concurrently with deficits in adaptive behavior and manifested in the developmental period, which adversely affects a child's education performance

MET: Energy value; a multiple of the resting metabolism; one MET equals average energy expenditure at rest

microchip: Tiny silicon chip containing many microscopic switches or gates; an electrical charge opens some switches and closes others, creating a pattern simulating human logic

mode: Most frequently occurring score in the distribution; a measure of central tendency

modem: Device allowing a computer to communicate over telephone lines and other communication media

monitor: Television set, often specially manufactured to be connected to a computer

motor ability: Originally, the innate ability to perform motor skills; more commonly, the ability to perform motor skills

motor capacity: Individual's capacity to perform motor skills

motor educability: Individual's ability to learn new motor skills

multiple choice item: Test item that is answered using one of three or more alternatives

muscular endurance: "The ability of the muscle to maintain submaximum force levels for extended periods" (Heyward, 1984:5)

muscular strength: "The maximum force or tension that can be produced by the muscle group" (Heyward, 1984:4)

needs assessment: Comparison of actual status of target group with desired status on some attribute to determine program needs

NEW: BASIC command to erase everything stored in RAM

normal curve: Bell-shaped curve with known properties

norm-referenced test: Test used to compare an examinee's score with the scores of other similar examinees

objective test: Test with highly precise scoring system, yielding little error

objectivity: Precision with which test is scored

orthopedically impaired*: Severe orthopedic impairment that adversely affects a child's educational performance; includes impairments caused by a congenital anomaly (e.g., clubfoot, absence of some member), impairments caused by disease (e.g., poliomyelitis), and impairments from other causes (e.g., cerebral palsy, leukemia)

paraplegia: Paralysis of the legs and lower part of the body

pass-fail method: Method of grading using two grade categories

Pearson product-moment correlation coefficient: Statistical technique used to determine the relationship between two sets of measures of the same individuals

perceived exertion scale: Scale used to assess the examinee's perception of his or her physical exertion during exercise

percentage method: Method of grading based on the assignment of a percentage to each grade category; a norm-referenced approach to grading

percentage-correct method: Method of grading based on the percentage of test items or trials successfully completed; a criterion-referenced approach to grading

percentile: Score value for a specified percentage of cases in a distribution of scores

percentile norms: Norms calculated by converting raw scores to percentiles

percentile rank: Percentage of cases falling at or below a specified score in a distribution

peripheral: Device that can send information to the computer as well as receive information from it

physical fitness (health-related)†: Multifaceted continuum extending from birth to death; affected by physical activity; ranges from optimal abilities in all aspects of life to severely limiting disease and dysfunction

posture: Alignment of the body and its segments

power: Ability to generate maximum force in a minimum amount of time

predictive validity: Appropriateness of a test as a predictor of behavior

predictor: Test or variable that predicts a criterion behavior

program evaluation: Assessment of the extent to which a program has met predetermined objectives

proportion of agreement (P): Method of determining the reliability of a criterion-referenced test

psychomotor domain: Motor behavior ranging from a low level, reproducing a skill, to higher levels in which the skill is used creatively in a game setting

Pull-Ups Test: Measures arm and shoulder girdle strength; usually designated for boys

pulse rate: Estimation of heart rate; often made by placing the tips of two or three fingers on the skin above an artery and counting the beats

qualitative measurement: Predominantly judgmental approach to measurement

quantitative measurement: Objective approach to measurement in which a number is assigned to the attribute of interest

range: Spread of scores; in a distribution, the bottom score subtracted from the top score plus 1

random access memory (RAM): Primary memory of a computer; information can be stored in RAM as well as retrieved and modified

rank difference correlation coefficient: Statistical technique used to calculate the correlation coefficient when the scores are ranked

rating scale: Scale used to subjectively assess performance

raw score: Score obtained by an examinee on a test

reactive effect: Change in affect resulting from heightened awareness because of the experience of taking an inventory measuring the affective behavior

read only memory (ROM): Computer memory in which information is stored once, usually by the manufacturer; cannot be changed

real limits: Upper and lower limits of intervals in a frequency distribution representing the entire area between intervals; do not represent score units actually obtained on the test

reflexes: Inborn, genetically endowed, involuntary behaviors

reliability: Dependability of scores, their relative freedom from error; the consistency of an individual's performance on a test

reliability (criterion-referenced): Consistency of classification of masters and nonmasters

response distortion: Invalid response because of failure to respond to an item, usually an affective measure, with total honesty

RUN *(program):* BASIC command to execute a specified program

SAVE *(program):* BASIC command to take a specified program out of RAM and put it onto the disk for storage

score limits: Upper and lower limits of intervals in a frequency distribution represented in raw score units, that is, the actual scores obtained on the test

semantic differential scale: Rating of concepts with scales anchored at the extremes with bipolar adjectives

short-answer item: Test item including a statement with one or more blank spaces to be filled in by the examinee

Shuttle Run Test: Measures speed and change of direction

Sit-Ups Test: Measures abdominal strength

skewness: Shape of the curve when the majority of the scores falls at one end of the distribution, with the remainder of the scores tapering off as reflected in the long tail of the distribution

skinfold caliper: Device for measuring skinfold thickness

skinfold thickness: Thickness of a fold of skin when lifted away from the muscle; used to estimate body fatness

social behavior: Behavior displayed in dealing with others, such as relationships among peers

software: Set of instructions that makes the computer function in some desired way

speech impairment*: Communication disorder, such as stuttering, impaired articulation, language impairment, or voice impairment, which adversely affects a child's educational performance

split-half reliability estimate: Reliability estimate determined by dividing the test into halves and correlating scores on the two half-tests

sportsmanship: Behaviors considered appropriate for sports participants and spectators; for example, fair play, following rules, and showing respect for officials

standard deviation: Square root of the average of the squared deviations of scores from the mean; a measure of variability

standard deviation method: Method of grading based on the standard deviation of the distribution of scores; a norm-referenced approach to grading

standard error of measurement: Estimate of the absolute error of an individual's score

standard of performance: Degree to which the student is expected to meet the objective

standard score: Score standardized by taking the deviation of the score from the mean and dividing it by the standard deviation

standard score method: Same as the standard deviation method of grading; use of z-scores

Standing Long Jump Test: Measures explosive leg power

static balance: Ability to maintain equilibrium in a stationary position

static strength: Force exerted against an immovable resistance

statistics: Methodology for analyzing a set of test scores

stem: Introductory question or statement in a multiple choice item

step test: Field test of cardiorespiratory function in which the examinee steps up and down on a bench until a predetermined heart rate is reached

subjective test: Test with imprecise scoring system, usually because of differences in the judgment of scorers

subjectivity: Use of individual judgment in evaluating motor performance

summative evaluation: Evaluation that takes place at the end of a training period or instructional unit

systematic decrease in scores: Gradual decrease in test scores from trial to trial, often because of fatigue or loss of motivation

systematic increase in scores: Gradual increase in test scores from trial to trial, often because of practice or learning

table of specifications: Table of the categories of cognitive behavior (knowledge) to be tested; categories are weighed according to their importance

tally: Mark placed adjacent to an interval in a frequency distribution representing a score in the interval

task specificity: Concept that ability to perform a task is specific to the task

taxonomy: Classification scheme

terminal behavior: Behavior a student is expected to display upon successful attainment of the objective

test: Instrument or technique used to obtain information (usually a score) about an attribute of a person or object

test battery: Group of tests designed to measure complex abilities in sport and physical activity

test user: Individual who selects and/or administers the test

Title IX: Legislation providing for equality by gender in many areas, including physical education programs

trait: Enduring and unchanging characteristic

true-false item: Test item that is answered using one of two alternatives

T-scores: Distribution of standard scores with a mean of 50 and a standard deviation of 10; a conversion of the z-score distribution

validity: Soundness of the interpretations of a test; the extent to which a test measures what it is supposed to measure

validity coefficient: Correlation coefficient representing the relationship between a test and a criterion measure

variability: Spread of scores in a distribution

variance: Squared deviations of scores from the mean; indicator of the variability or spread of a set of scores

vertical jump: Jump executed as high as possible in a vertical direction; reflects explosive power of leg extensor muscles

visually handicapped*: Visual impairment which, even with correction, adversely affects a child's educational performance; includes both partially seeing and blind children

weak measure: Measure lacking adequate evidence of validity and reliability

weight (of grade): Number designating the importance of a grade; higher number reflects greater importance

weight-training machine: Device used to measure muscular strength and endurance

50-Yard Dash Test: Measures speed

600-Yard Run: Measures cardiorespiratory function

z-scores: Most basic of standard score distributions, with a mean of 0 and a standard deviation of 1; used as the basis for many other standard score transformations

Appendixes

A   Critical Values of the Correlation Coefficient

B   Units of Measure

C   The F and t Distributions

D   Sources for Selected Sports Skills Tests

E   Programs for Apple IIe Computer

    1 SFCALC program
    2 GRADES program
    3 DIRECTIONS program
    4 PERCENTILE program
    5 CHANGE program

F   NCYFS Norms

G   Sources of Tests and Skinfold Calipers

Appendix A

Critical Values of the Correlation Coefficient

df = n-2	α = .10	.05	.02	.01
1	.988	.997	.9995	.9999
2	.900	.950	.980	.990
3	.805	.878	.934	.959
4	.729	.811	.882	.917
5	.669	.754	.833	.874
6	.622	.707	.789	.834
7	.582	.666	.750	.798
8	.549	.632	.716	.765
9	.521	.602	.685	.735
10	.497	.576	.658	.708
11	.476	.553	.634	.684
12	.458	.532	.612	.661
13	.441	.514	.592	.641
14	.426	.497	.574	.623
15	.412	.482	.558	.606
16	.400	.468	.542	.590
17	.389	.456	.528	.575
18	.378	.444	.516	.561
19	.369	.433	.503	.549
20	.360	.423	.492	.537
21	.352	.413	.482	.526
22	.344	.404	.472	.515
23	.337	.396	.462	.505
24	.330	.388	.453	.496
25	.323	.381	.445	.487
26	.317	.374	.437	.479
27	.311	.367	.430	.471
28	.306	.361	.423	.463
29	.301	.355	.416	.456
30	.296	.349	.409	.449
35	.275	.325	.381	.418
40	.257	.304	.358	.393
45	.243	.288	.338	.372
50	.231	.273	.322	.354
60	.211	.250	.295	.325
70	.195	.232	.274	.302
80	.183	.217	.256	.283
90	.173	.205	.242	.267
100	.164	.195	.230	.254

Appendix A is taken from Table V.A. of Fisher and Yates, Statistical methods for research workers, published by Oliver & Boyd, Edinburgh. By permission of the authors and publishers.

Appendix B

Units of Measure

Distance	
1 inch	= 2.54 centimeters (cm) = 25.4 millimeters (mm) = 0.0254 meters (m)
1 foot	= 30.48 cm = 304.8 mm = 0.304 m
1 yard	= 91.44 cm = 914.4 mm = 0.914 m
1 mile	= 5280 ft = 1760 yd = 1609.35 m = 1.61 kilometers (km)
1 cm	= 0.3937 in
1 m	= 39.37 in = 3.28 ft = 1.09 yd = 100 cm = 1000 mm
1 km	= 0.62 mi = 1000 m

Weights	
1 ounce (oz)	= 0.0625 lb = 28.35 grams (g) = 0.028 kg
1 pound (lb)	= 16 oz = 454 g = 0.454 kg
1 g	= 0.035 oz = 0.0022 lb = 0.001 kg
1 kg	= 35.27 oz = 2.2 lb = 1000 g

Appendix C

The F Distribution

alpha = .05

V_1 = d.f. of numerator V_2 = d.f. of denominator

V_2 \ V_1	1	2	3	4	5	6	7	8	9	10
1	161.4	199.5	215.7	224.6	230.2	234.0	236.8	238.9	240.5	241.9
2	18.51	19.00	19.16	19.25	19.30	19.33	19.35	19.37	19.38	19.40
3	10.13	9.55	9.28	9.12	9.01	8.94	8.89	8.85	8.81	8.79
4	7.71	6.94	6.59	6.39	6.26	6.16	6.09	6.04	6.00	5.96
5	6.61	5.79	5.41	5.19	5.05	4.95	4.88	4.82	4.77	4.74
6	5.99	5.14	4.76	4.53	4.39	4.28	4.21	4.15	4.10	4.06
7	5.59	4.74	4.35	4.12	3.97	3.87	3.79	3.73	3.68	3.64
8	5.32	4.46	4.07	3.84	3.69	3.58	3.50	3.44	3.39	3.35
9	5.12	4.26	3.86	3.63	3.48	3.37	3.29	3.23	3.18	3.14
10	4.96	4.10	3.71	3.48	3.33	3.22	3.14	3.07	3.20	2.98
11	4.84	3.98	3.59	3.36	3.20	3.09	3.01	2.95	2.90	2.85
12	4.75	3.89	3.49	3.26	3.11	3.00	2.91	2.85	2.80	2.75
13	4.67	3.81	3.41	3.18	3.03	2.92	2.83	2.77	2.71	2.67
14	4.60	3.74	3.34	3.11	2.96	2.85	2.76	2.70	2.65	2.60
15	4.54	3.68	3.29	3.06	2.90	2.79	2.71	2.64	2.59	2.54
16	4.49	3.63	3.24	3.01	2.85	2.74	2.66	2.59	2.54	2.49
17	4.45	3.59	3.20	2.96	2.81	2.70	2.61	2.55	2.49	2.45
18	4.41	3.55	3.16	2.93	2.77	2.66	2.58	2.51	2.46	2.41
19	4.38	3.52	3.13	2.90	2.74	2.63	2.54	2.48	2.42	2.38
20	4.35	3.49	3.10	2.87	2.71	2.60	2.51	2.45	2.39	2.35
21	4.32	3.47	3.07	2.84	2.68	2.57	2.49	2.42	2.37	2.32
22	4.30	3.44	3.05	2.82	2.66	2.55	2.46	2.40	2.34	2.30
23	4.28	3.42	3.03	2.80	2.64	2.53	2.44	2.37	2.32	2.27
24	4.26	3.40	3.01	2.78	2.62	2.51	2.42	2.36	2.30	2.25
25	4.24	3.39	2.99	2.76	2.60	2.49	2.40	2.34	2.28	2.24
26	4.23	3.37	2.98	2.74	2.59	2.47	2.39	2.32	2.27	2.22
27	4.21	3.35	2.96	2.73	2.57	2.46	2.37	2.31	2.25	2.20
28	4.20	3.34	2.95	2.71	2.56	2.45	2.36	2.29	2.24	2.19
29	4.18	3.33	2.93	2.70	2.55	2.43	2.35	2.28	2.22	2.18
30	4.17	3.32	2.92	2.69	2.53	2.42	2.33	2.27	2.21	2.16
40	4.08	3.23	2.84	2.61	2.45	2.34	2.25	2.18	2.12	2.08
60	4.00	3.15	2.76	2.53	2.37	2.25	2.17	2.10	2.04	1.99
120	3.92	3.07	2.68	2.45	2.29	2.17	2.09	2.02	1.96	1.91
∞	3.84	3.00	2.60	2.37	2.21	2.10	2.01	1.94	1.88	1.83

E.S. Pearson and H.O. Hartley. Biometrika tables for statisticians. New York: Cambridge University Press, 1966. Vol. 1. By permission of the authors and publisher.

alpha = .05

V_1 / V_2	12	15	20	24	30	40	60	120	∞
1	243.9	245.9	248.0	249.1	250.1	251.1	252.2	253.3	254.3
2	19.41	19.43	19.45	19.45	19.46	19.47	19.48	19.49	19.50
3	8.74	8.70	8.66	8.64	8.62	8.59	8.57	8.55	8.53
4	5.91	5.86	5.80	5.77	5.75	5.72	5.69	5.66	5.63
5	4.68	4.62	4.56	4.53	4.50	4.46	4.43	4.40	4.36
6	4.00	3.94	3.87	3.84	3.81	3.77	3.74	3.70	3.67
7	3.57	3.51	3.44	3.41	3.38	3.34	3.30	3.27	3.23
8	3.28	3.22	3.15	3.12	3.08	3.04	3.01	2.97	2.93
9	3.07	3.01	2.94	2.90	2.86	2.83	2.79	2.75	2.71
10	2.91	2.85	2.77	2.74	2.70	2.66	2.62	2.58	2.54
11	2.79	2.72	2.65	2.61	2.57	2.53	2.49	2.45	2.40
12	2.69	2.62	2.54	2.51	2.47	2.43	2.38	2.34	2.30
13	2.60	2.53	2.46	2.42	2.38	2.34	2.30	2.25	2.21
14	2.53	2.46	2.39	2.35	2.31	2.27	2.22	2.18	2.13
15	2.48	2.40	2.33	2.29	2.25	2.20	2.16	2.11	2.07
16	2.42	2.35	2.28	2.24	2.19	2.15	2.11	2.06	2.01
17	2.38	2.31	2.23	2.19	2.15	2.10	2.06	2.01	1.96
18	2.34	2.27	2.19	2.15	2.11	2.06	2.02	1.97	1.92
19	2.31	2.23	2.16	2.11	2.07	2.03	1.98	1.93	1.88
20	2.28	2.20	2.12	2.08	2.04	1.99	1.95	1.90	1.84
21	2.25	2.18	2.10	2.05	2.01	1.96	1.92	1.87	1.81
22	2.23	2.15	2.07	2.03	1.98	1.94	1.89	1.84	1.78
23	2.20	2.13	2.05	2.01	1.96	1.91	1.86	1.81	1.76
24	2.18	2.11	2.03	1.98	1.94	1.89	1.84	1.79	1.73
25	2.16	2.09	2.01	1.96	1.92	1.87	1.82	1.77	1.71
26	2.15	2.07	1.99	1.95	1.90	1.85	1.80	1.75	1.69
27	2.13	2.06	1.97	1.93	1.88	1.84	1.79	1.73	1.67
28	2.12	2.04	1.96	1.91	1.87	1.82	1.77	1.71	1.65
29	2.10	2.03	1.94	1.90	1.85	1.81	1.75	1.70	1.64
30	2.09	2.01	1.93	1.89	1.84	1.79	1.74	1.68	1.62
40	2.00	1.92	1.84	1.79	1.74	1.69	1.64	1.58	1.51
60	1.92	1.84	1.75	1.70	1.65	1.59	1.53	1.47	1.39
120	1.83	1.75	1.66	1.61	1.55	1.50	1.43	1.35	1.25
∞	1.75	1.67	1.57	1.52	1.46	1.39	1.32	1.22	1.00

alpha = .01

V_1 / V_2	1	2	3	4	5	6	7	8	9	10
1	4052	4999.5	5403	5652	5764	5859	5928	5981	6022	6056
2	98.50	99.00	99.17	99.25	99.30	99.33	99.36	99.37	99.39	99.40
3	34.12	30.82	29.46	28.71	28.24	27.91	27.67	27.49	27.35	27.23
4	21.20	18.00	16.69	15.98	15.52	15.21	14.98	14.80	14.66	14.55
5	16.26	13.27	12.06	11.39	10.97	10.67	10.46	10.29	10.16	10.05
6	13.75	10.92	9.78	9.15	8.75	8.47	8.26	8.10	7.98	7.87
7	12.25	9.55	8.45	7.85	7.46	7.19	6.99	6.84	6.72	6.62
8	11.26	8.65	7.59	7.01	6.63	6.37	6.18	6.03	5.91	5.81
9	10.56	8.02	6.99	6.42	6.06	5.80	5.61	5.47	5.35	5.26
10	10.04	7.56	6.55	5.99	5.64	5.39	5.20	5.06	4.94	4.85
11	9.65	7.21	6.22	5.67	5.32	5.07	4.89	4.74	4.63	4.54
12	9.33	6.93	5.95	5.41	5.06	4.82	4.64	4.50	4.39	4.30
13	9.07	6.70	5.74	5.21	4.86	4.62	4.44	4.30	4.19	4.10
14	8.86	6.51	5.56	5.04	4.69	4.46	4.28	4.14	4.03	3.94
15	8.68	6.36	5.42	4.89	4.56	4.32	4.14	4.00	3.89	3.80
16	8.53	6.23	5.29	4.77	4.44	4.20	4.03	3.89	3.78	3.69
17	8.40	6.11	5.18	4.67	4.34	4.10	3.93	3.79	3.68	3.59
18	8.29	6.01	5.09	4.58	4.25	4.01	3.84	3.71	3.60	3.51
19	8.18	5.93	5.01	4.50	4.17	3.94	3.77	3.63	3.52	3.43
20	8.10	5.85	4.94	4.43	4.10	3.87	3.70	3.56	3.46	3.37
21	8.02	5.78	4.87	4.37	4.04	3.81	3.64	3.51	3.40	3.31
22	7.95	5.72	4.82	4.31	3.99	3.76	3.59	3.45	3.35	3.26
23	7.88	5.66	4.76	4.26	3.94	3.71	3.54	3.41	3.30	3.21
24	7.82	5.61	4.72	4.22	3.90	3.67	3.50	3.36	3.26	3.17
25	7.77	5.57	4.68	4.18	3.85	3.63	3.46	3.32	3.22	3.13
26	7.72	5.53	4.64	4.14	3.82	3.59	3.42	3.29	3.18	3.09
27	7.68	5.49	4.60	4.11	3.78	3.56	3.39	3.26	3.15	3.06
28	7.64	5.45	4.57	4.07	3.75	3.53	3.36	3.23	3.12	3.03
29	7.60	5.42	4.54	4.04	3.73	3.50	3.33	3.20	3.09	3.00
30	7.56	5.39	4.51	4.02	3.70	3.47	3.30	3.17	3.07	2.98
40	7.31	5.18	4.31	3.83	3.51	3.29	3.12	2.99	2.89	2.80
60	7.08	4.98	4.13	3.65	3.34	3.12	2.95	2.82	2.72	2.63
120	6.85	4.79	3.95	3.48	3.17	2.96	2.79	2.66	2.56	2.47
∞	6.63	4.61	3.78	3.32	3.02	2.80	2.64	2.51	2.41	2.32

alpha = .01

V_1 / V_2	12	15	20	24	30	40	60	120	∞
1	6106	6157	6209	6235	6261	6287	6313	6339	6366
2	99.42	99.43	99.45	99.46	99.47	99.47	99.48	99.49	99.50
3	27.05	26.87	26.69	26.60	26.50	26.41	26.32	26.22	26.13
4	14.37	14.20	14.02	13.93	13.84	13.75	13.65	13.56	13.46
5	9.89	9.72	9.55	9.47	9.38	9.29	9.20	9.11	9.02
6	7.72	7.56	7.40	7.31	7.23	7.14	7.06	6.97	6.88
7	6.47	6.31	6.16	6.07	5.99	5.91	5.82	5.74	5.65
8	5.67	5.52	5.36	5.28	5.20	5.12	5.03	4.95	4.86
9	5.11	4.96	4.81	4.73	4.65	4.57	4.48	4.40	4.31
10	4.71	4.56	4.41	4.33	4.25	4.17	4.08	4.00	3.91
11	4.40	4.25	4.10	4.02	3.94	3.86	3.78	3.69	3.60
12	4.16	4.01	3.86	3.78	3.70	3.62	3.54	3.45	3.36
13	3.96	3.82	3.66	3.59	3.51	3.43	3.34	3.25	3.17
14	3.80	3.66	3.51	3.43	3.35	3.27	3.18	3.09	3.00
15	3.67	3.52	3.37	3.29	3.21	3.13	3.05	2.96	2.87
16	3.55	3.41	3.26	3.18	3.10	3.02	2.93	2.84	2.75
17	3.46	3.31	3.16	3.08	3.00	2.92	2.83	2.75	2.65
18	3.37	3.23	3.08	3.00	2.92	2.84	2.75	2.66	2.57
19	3.30	3.15	3.00	2.92	2.84	2.76	2.67	2.58	2.49
20	3.23	3.09	2.94	2.86	2.78	2.69	2.61	2.52	2.42
21	3.17	3.03	2.88	2.80	2.72	2.64	2.55	2.46	2.36
22	3.12	2.98	2.83	2.75	2.67	2.58	2.50	2.40	2.31
23	3.07	2.93	2.78	2.70	2.62	2.54	2.45	2.35	2.26
24	3.03	2.89	2.74	2.66	2.58	2.49	2.40	2.31	2.21
25	2.99	2.85	2.70	2.62	2.54	2.45	2.36	2.27	2.17
26	2.96	2.81	2.66	2.58	2.50	2.42	2.33	2.23	2.13
27	2.93	2.78	2.63	2.55	2.47	2.38	2.29	2.20	2.10
28	2.90	2.75	2.60	2.52	2.44	2.35	2.26	2.17	2.06
29	2.87	2.73	2.57	2.49	2.41	2.33	2.23	2.14	2.03
30	2.84	2.70	2.55	2.47	2.39	2.30	2.21	2.11	2.01
40	2.66	2.52	2.37	2.29	2.20	2.11	2.02	1.92	1.80
60	2.50	2.35	2.20	2.12	2.03	1.94	1.84	1.73	1.60
120	2.34	2.19	2.03	1.95	1.86	1.76	1.66	1.53	1.38
∞	2.18	2.04	1.88	1.79	1.70	1.59	1.47	1.32	1.00

Critical Values of t

greater than T → more significance
to be significant

df	Level of significance for one-tailed test					
	.10	.05	.025	.01	.005	.0005
	Level of significance for two-tailed test					
	.20	.10	.05	.02	.01	.001
1	3.078	6.314	12.706	31.821	63.657	636.619
2	1.886	2.920	4.303	6.965	9.925	31.598
3	1.638	2.353	3.182	4.541	5.841	12.941
4	1.533	2.132	2.776	3.747	4.604	8.610
5	1.476	2.015	2.571	3.365	4.032	6.859
6	1.440	1.943	2.447	3.143	3.707	5.959
7	1.415	1.895	2.365	2.998	3.499	5.405
8	1.397	1.860	2.306	2.896	3.355	5.041
9	1.383	1.833	2.262	2.821	3.250	4.781
10	1.372	1.812	2.228	2.764	3.169	4.587
11	1.363	1.796	2.201	2.718	3.106	4.437
12	1.356	1.782	2.179	2.681	3.055	4.318
13	1.350	1.771	2.160	2.650	3.012	4.221
14	1.345	1.761	2.145	2.624	2.977	4.140
15	1.341	1.753	2.131	2.602	2.947	4.073
16	1.337	1.746	2.120	2.583	2.921	4.015
17	1.333	1.740	2.110	2.567	2.898	3.965
18	1.330	1.734	2.101	2.552	2.878	3.922
19	1.328	1.729	2.093	2.539	2.861	3.883
20	1.325	1.725	2.086	2.528	2.845	3.850
21	1.323	1.721	2.080	2.518	2.831	3.819
22	1.321	1.717	2.074	2.508	2.819	3.792
23	1.319	1.714	2.069	2.500	2.807	3.767
24	1.318	1.711	2.064	2.492	2.797	3.745
25	1.316	1.708	2.060	2.485	2.787	3.725
26	1.315	1.706	2.056	2.479	2.779	3.707
27	1.314	1.703	2.052	2.473	2.771	3.690
28	1.313	1.701	2.048	2.467	2.763	3.674
29	1.311	1.699	2.045	2.462	2.756	3.659
30	1.310	1.697	2.042	2.457	2.750	3.646
40	1.303	1.684	2.021	2.423	2.704	3.551
60	1.296	1.671	2.000	2.390	2.660	3.460
120	1.289	1.658	1.980	2.358	2.617	3.373
	1.282	1.645	1.960	2.326	2.576	3.291

Abridged from Table III of Fisher, *Statistical methods for research workers*, published by Oliver and Boyd, Ltd., Edinburgh. By permission of the author and the publisher.

Appendix D

Sources for Selected Sports Skills Tests

ARCHERY

American Association for Health, Physical Education and Recreation. 1967. Archery skills test manual. Washington, D.C.: AAHPER.

Bohn, R.W. 1962. An achievement test in archery, Unpublished master's thesis, The University of Wisconsin, Madison.

Hyde, E.I. 1937. An achievement scale in archery. Research Quarterly, 8:109-116.

Shifflett, B., and Schuman, B. 1982. A criterion-referenced test for archery. Research Quarterly for Exercise and Sport, 53:330-335.

Zabick, R.M., and Jackson, A.S. 1969. Reliability of archery achievement. Research Quarterly, 40:254-255.

BADMINTON

French, E., and Stalter, E. 1949. Study of skill tests in badminton for college women. Research Quarterly, 20:257-272.

Greiner, M.R. 1964. Construction of a short serve test for beginning badminton players. Master's thesis, The University of Wisconsin, Madision. (Microcard PE 670, University of Oregon, Eugene.)

Hale, P.A. 1970. Construction of a long serve test for beginning badminton players (singles). Master's thesis, The University of Wisconsin, Madison. (Microcard PE 1133, University of Oregon, Eugene.)

Hicks, J.V. 1967. The construction and evaluation of a battery of five badminton skill tests, Unpublished doctoral dissertion, Texas Women's University, Denton, Tex.

Johnson, B.L., and Nelson, J.K. 1979. Badminton smash test. In Practical measurements for evaluation in physical education. Minneapolis: Burgess Publishing Co.

Lockhart, A., and McPherson, F.A. 1949. The development of a test of badminton playing ability. Research Quarterly, 20:402-405.

McDonald, E.D. 1968. The development of a skill test for the badminton high clear. Master's thesis, Southern Illinois University, Carbondale, Ill. (Microcard PE 1083, University of Oregon, Eugene.)

Miller, F.A. 1951. A badminton wall volley test. Research Quarterly, 22:208-213.

Poole, J., and Nelson, J. 1970. Construction of a badminton skills test battery, Unpublished manuscript, Louisiana State University, Baton Rouge.

Scott, M.G. 1941. Achievement examinations in badminton. Research Quarterly, 12:242-253.

Scott, M.G., and Fox, M. 1959. Long serve test. In Measurement and evaluation in physical education. Dubuque, Iowa: Wm C Brown Group.

Thorpe, J., and West, C. 1969. A test game sense in badminton. Perceptual and Motor Skills, 28:159-169.

BASEBALL

Kelson, R.E. 1953. Baseball classification plan for boys. Research Quarterly, 24:304-309.

Rodgers, E.G., and Heath, M.L. 1931. An experiment in the use of knowledge and skill tests in playground baseball. Research Quarterly, 2:113-131.

BASKETBALL

American Association for Health, Physical Education and Recreation. 1966. Basketball skills tests manual for boys. Washington, D.C.: AAHPER.

American Association for Health, Physical Education and Recreation. 1966. Basketball skills test manual for girls. Washington, D.C.: AAHPER.

Barrow, H.M. 1959. Basketball skill test. The Physical Educator, **16**:26.

Dyer, J.T., Schurig, J.C., and Apgar, S.L. 1939. A basketball motor ability test for college women and secondary school girls. Research Quarterly, **10**:128-147.

Edgren, H.D. 1932. An experiment in the testing of ability and progress in basketball. Research Quarterly, **3**:159-171.

Glassow, R.B., Colvin, V., and Schwartz, M.M. 1938. Studies measuring basketball playing ability of college women. Research Quarterly, **9**:60-68.

Hopkins, D.R. 1977. Factor analysis of selected basketball skill test. Research Quarterly, **48**:535-540.

Hopkins, D.R., Shick, J. and Plack, J.J. 1984. Basketball for boys and girls: skills test manual. Reston, Va.: American Alliance for Health, Physical Education, Recreation and Dance.

Johnson, L.W. 1976. Objective tests in basketball for high school boys. In Clarke, H.H. Application of measurement to health and physical education. Englewood Cliffs, N.J.: Prentice-Hall, Inc.

Kay, H.K. 1966. A statistical analysis of the profile technique for the evaluation of competetive basketball performance, Unpublished master's thesis, University of Alberta, Edmonton, Canada.

Knox, R.K. 1947. Basketball ability tests. Scholastic Coach, **17**:45.

Lambert, A.T. 1969. A basketball skill test for college women, Unpublished master's thesis, University of North Carolina, Greensboro.

Latchaw, M. 1954. Measuring selected motor skills in fourth, fifth, and sixth grades. Research Quarterly, **25**:439-499.

Lehsten, N. 1948. A measure of basketball skills in high school boys. The Physical Educator, **4**:103-106.

Leilich, A. 1980. Leilich basketball test. In Barrow, H.M., and R., McGee. A practical approach to measurement in physical education, ed. 3, Philadelphia: Lea & Febiger.

Miller, W.K. 1954. Achievement levels in basketball skills for women physical education majors. Research Quarterly, **25**:450-455.

Schwartz, H. 1937. Knowledge and achievement tests in girls' basketball on the senior high school level. Research Quarterly, **8**:152-156.

Stroup, F. 1955. Game results as a criterion for validating basketball skill tests. Research Quarterly, **26**:353-357.

Thornes, M.B. 1963. An analysis of a basketball shooting test and its relation to other basketball skill tests. Master's thesis, The Univeristy of Wisconsin, Madison. (Microcard PE 694, University of Oregon, Eugene.)

Young, G., and Moser, H. 1934. A short battery of tests to measure playing ability in women's basketball. Research Quarterly, **5**:3-23.

BOWLING

Martin, J.L. 1960. Bowling norms for college men and women. Research Quarterly, **31**:113-116.

Martin, J., and Keogh, J. 1964. Bowling norms for college students in elective physical education classes. Research Quarterly, **35**:325-327.

Olson, J.K., and Liba, M.R. 1967. A device for evaluating spot bowling ability. Research Quarterly, **38**:193-210.

Phillips, M., and Summers, D. 1950. Bowling norms and learning curves for college women. Research Quarterly, **21**:377-385.

Schunk, C. 1969. Test questions for bowling. Philadelphia: W.B. Saunders Co.

FENCING

Bowar, M.G. 1961. A test of general fencing ability, Unpublished master's thesis, University of Southern California, Los Angeles.

Cooper, C.K. 1968. The development of a fencing skill test for measuring achievement of beginning collegiate women fencers in using the advance, beat, and lunge. Unpublished master's thesis, Western Illinois University, Macomb.

Fein, J.T. 1964. Construction of skill tests for beginning collegiate women fencers, Unpublished master's thesis, University of Iowa, Iowa City.

Safrit, M.J. 1962. Construction of a skill test for beginning fencers, Unpublished master's thesis, The University of Wisconsin, Madison.

Schultz, J.K. 1940. Construction of an achievement scale in fencing for women, Unpublished master's thesis, University of Washington, Seattle.

Wyrick, W. 1958. A comparison of the effectiveness of two methods of teaching beginning fencing to college women, Unpublished master's thesis, The Woman's College of the University of North Carolina, Greensboro.

FIELD HOCKEY

Chapman, N.L. 1982. Chapman ball control test-field hockey. Research Quarterly for Exercise and Sport, **53**:239-242.

Friedel, J.W. 1956. The development of a field hockey skill test for high school girls. Master's thesis, Illinois State University, Normal. (Microcard PE 289, University of Oregon, Eugene.)

Illner, J.A. 1968. The construction and validation of a skill test for the drive in field hockey. Master's thesis, Southern Illinois University, Carbondale. (Microcard PE 1075, University of Oregon, Eugene.)

Perry, E.L. 1969. An investigation of field hockey skill tests for college women, Unpublished master's thesis, Pennsylvania State University, University Park.

Schmithals, M., and French, E. 1940. Achievement tests in field hockey for college women. Research Quarterly, **11**:84-92.

Strait, C.J. 1960. The construction and evaluation of a field hockey skills test, Unpublished master's thesis, Smith College, Northampton, Mass.

FOOTBALL

American Association for Health, Physical Education and Recreation. 1960. Football skills test manual. Washington, D.C.: AAHPER.

Borleske, S.E. 1937. Achievement of college men in touch football. In F.W. Cozens, editor. Ninth annual report of the committee on curriculum research of the college physical education association. Research Quarterly, **8**:73-78.

McElroy, H.N. 1938. A report on some experimentation with a skill test. Research Quarterly, **9**:83-88.

GOLF

Brown, H.S. 1969. A test battery for evaluating golf skills. Texas Association for Health, Physical Education and Recreation Journal, pp. 4-5, 28-29.

Clevett, M.A. 1931. An experiment in teaching methods of golf. Research Quarterly, **2**:104-112.

Cochrane, J.F. 1960. The construction of indoor golf skills test as a measure of golfing ability, Unpublished master's thesis, University of Minnesota, Minneapolis.

Cotten, D., Thomas, J.R., and Plaster, T. 1972. A plastic ball test for golf iron skill, Unpublished study presented at the American Association for Health, Physical Education and Recreation Convention Houston, March 1972.

McKee, M.E. 1950. A test for the full swinging shot in golf. Research Quarterly, **21**:40-46.

Nelson, J.K. 1979. An achievement test in golf. In Johnson, B.L., and Nelson, J.K. Practical measurements for evaluation in physical education. Minneapolis: Burgess Publishing Co.

Shick, J., and Berg, N. 1983. Indoor golf skill test for junior high boys. Research Quarterly for Exercise and Sport, **54**:75-78.

Vanderhoof, E.R. 1956. Beginning golf achievement tests. Master's thesis, State University of Iowa, Iowa City. (Microcard PE 306, University of Oregon, Eugene.)

Watts, H. 1942. Construction and evaluation of a target on testing the approach shot in golf. Unpublished master's thesis, The University of Wisconsin, Madison.

West, C., and Thorpe, J. 1968. Construction and validation of an eight-iron approach test. Research Quarterly, **39**:1115-1120.

GYMNASTICS

Bowers, C.O. 1965. Gymnastics skill test for beginning to low intermediate girls and women. Master's thesis, The Ohio State University, Columbus. (Microcard PE 734, University of Oregon, Eugene.)

Faulkner, J., and Loken, N. 1962. Objectivity of judging at the national collegiate athletic association gymnastic meet: a ten-year follow-up study. Research Quarterly, **33**:485-486.

HANDBALL

Cornish, C. 1949. A study of measurement of ability in handball. Research Quarterly, **20**:215-222.

Griffith, M.A. 1960. An objective method of evaluating ability in handball singles, Unpublished master's thesis, The Ohio State University, Columbus.

Montoye, H.J., and Brotzmann, J. 1951. An investigation of the validity of using the results of a doubles tournament as a measure of handball ability. Research Quarterly, **22**:214-218.

Pennington, G.G., and others. (1967). A measure of handball ability. Research Quarterly, **38**:247-253.

ICE HOCKEY

Merrifield, H.H., and Walford, G.A. 1969. Battery of ice hockey skill tests. Research Quarterly, **40**:146-152.

ICE SKATING

Carriere, D.L. 1969. An objective figure skating test for use in beginning classes, Unpublished master's thesis, University of Illinois, Urbana.

Leaming, T.W. 1959. A measure of endurance of young speed skaters, Unpublished master's thesis, University of Illinois, Urbana.

Recknagel, D. 1945. A test for beginners in skating. Journal of Health and Physical Education, **26**:91-92.

LACROSSE

Hodges, C.V. 1967. Construction of an objective knowledge test and skill tests in lacrosse for college women. Master's thesis, University of North Carolina, Greensboro. (Microcard PE 1974, University of Oregon, Eugene.)

Lutze, M.C. 1963. Achievement tests in beginning lacrosse for women, Unpublished master's thesis, State University of Iowa, Iowa City.

Wilke, B.J. 1967. Achievement tests for selected lacrosse skills of college women, Unpublished master's thesis, University of North Carolina, Greensboro.

RACQUETBALL

Hensley, L.D., East, W.B. and Stillwell, J.L. 1979. A racquetball skills test. Research Quarterly, **50**:114-118.

Karpman, M., and Isaacs, L.D. 1979. An improved racquetball skills test. Research Quarterly, **50**:526-527.

SKIING

Rogers, H.M. 1960. Construction of objectively scored skill tests for beginning skiers, Unpublished master's thesis, University of Colorado, Boulder.

Wolfe, J.E., and Merrifield, H.H. Predictability of beginning skiing success from basic skill tests in college age females, Paper presented at the National American Association for Health, Physical Education and Recreation Convention in Detroit, April, 1971.

SOCCER

Bailey, C.I., and Teller, F.L. 1969. Test questions for soccer. Philadelphia: W.B. Saunders Co.

Bontz, J. 1942. An experiment in the construction of a test for measuring ability in some of the fundamental skills used by fifth and sixth grade children in soccer, Unpublished master's thesis, State University of Iowa, Iowa City.

Heath, M.L., and Rodgers, E.G. 1932. A study in the use of knowledge and skill tests in soccer. Research Quarterly, **3**:33-43.

Johnson, J.R. 1963. The development of a single-item test as a measure of soccer skill. Microcarded master's thesis, University of British Columbia, Vancouver.

McDonald, L.G. 1951. The construction of a kicking skill test as an index of general soccer ability, Unpublished master's thesis, Springfield College, Springfield, Mass.

McElroy, H.N. 1938. A report on some experimentation with a skill test. Research Quarterly, **9**:82-88.

Mitchell, J.R. 1980. Mitchell modification of the McDonald soccer skill test. In Barrow, H.M., and McGee, R. A practical approach to measurement in physical education, ed. 3, Philadelphia: Lea & Febiger.

Schaufele, E.F. 1980. Schaufele soccer volleying test. In Barrow, H.M., and McGee, R. A practical approach to measurement in physical education, ed. 3, Philadelphia: Lea & Febiger.

Tomlinson, R. 1964. Soccer skill test. Soccer-speedball guide—July 1964-July 1966.

Washington, D.C.: Division of Girls and Women's Sports, American Association for Health, Physical Education and Recreation.

Warner, G.F.H. 1950. Warner soccer test. Newsletter of the National Soccer Coaches Association of America, **6**:13-22.

Whitney, A.H., and Chapin, H. 1946. Soccer skill testing for girls. Soccer-speedball guide—July 1946-July 1948. Washington, D.C.: National Section on Women's Athletics, American Association for Health, Physical Education and Recreation.

SOFTBALL

American Association for Health, Physical Education and Recreation. 1967. Softball skills test manual for boys. Washington, D.C.: AAHPER.

American Association for Health, Physical Education and Recreation. 1967. Softball skills test manual for girls. Washington, D.C.: AAPHER.

Broer, M.R. 1958. Reliability of certain skill tests for junior high school girls. Research Quarterly, **29**:139-143.

Davis, R. 1959. The development of an objective softball batting test for college women. In Scott, M.G., and French, E. Measurement and evaluation in physical education. Dubuque, Iowa: Wm C Brown Group.

Dexter, G. 1957. Checklist for rating softball batting skills. Teachers guide to physical education for girls in high school. Sacramento, Calif.: California State Department of Education.

Elrod, J.M. 1969. Construction of a softball skill test battery for high school boys, Unpublished master's thesis, Louisiana State University, Baton Rouge.

Fox, M.G., and Young, O.G. 1954. A test of softball batting ability. Research Quarterly, **25**:26-27.

Fringer, M.N. 1980. Fringer softball battery. In Barrow, H.M., and McGee, R. A practical approach to measurement in physical education, ed. 2, Philadelphia, Lea & Febiger.

Kehtel, C.H. 1958. The development of a test to measure the ability of a softball player to field a ground ball and successfully throw it at a target, Unpublished master's thesis, University of Colorado, Boulder.

O'Donnell, D.J. 1960. Validation of softball skill tests for high school girls, Unpublished master's thesis, Indiana University, Bloomington.

Research Committee, Central Association for Physical Education of College Women. 1959. Fielding test. In Scott, M.G., and French, E. Measurement and evaluation in physical education. Dubuque, Iowa: Wm C Brown Group.

Safrit, M.J. 1974. Wisconsin softball pitching test: summative evaluation. Softball guide: January, 1974-January, 1976. Washington, D.C.: Division of Girls' and Women's Sports, American Association for Health, Physical Education and Recreation.

Safrit, M.J., and Pavis, A. 1969. Overarm throw skill testing. In Felshin, J., and O'Brien, C., editors. Selected softball articles. Washington, D.C.: Division of Girls' and Women's Sports, American Association for Health, Physical Education and Recreation.

Scott, M.G., and French, E. 1959. Softball repeated throws test. In Scott, M.G., and French, E. Measurement and evaluation in physical education. Dubuque, Iowa: Wm C Brown Group.

Shick, J. 1970. Battery of defensive softball skills tests for college women. Research Quarterly, **41**:82-87.

Sopa, A. 1967. Construction of an indoor batting skills test for junior high school girls, Unpublished master's thesis, The University of Wisconsin, Madison.

Thomas, J. 1947. Skill tests. In Softball-volleyball guide—July 1947-July 1949. Washington, D.C.: National Section on Women's Athletics, American Association for Health, Physical Education and Recreation.

SPEEDBALL

Buchanan, R.E. 1942. A study of achievement tests in speedball for high school girls, Unpublished master's thesis, State University of Iowa, Iowa City.

Smith, G. 1980. Speedball skills tests for college women. In Barrow, H.M., and McGee, R. A practical approach to measurement in physical education, ed. 3, Philadelphia: Lea & Febiger.

STUNTS AND TUMBLING

Cotteral, B., and Cotteral D. 1936. Scale for judging quality of performance in stunts and tumbling. The teaching of stunts and tumbling. New York: The Ronald Press Co.

Edwards, V.M. 1969. Test questions for tumbling. Philadelphia: W.B. Saunders Co.

SWIMMING AND DIVING

Bennett, L.M. 1942. A test of diving for use in beginning classes. Research Quarterly, **13**:109-115.

Chapman, P.A. 1965. A comparison of three methods of measuring swimming stroke proficiency. Master's thesis, The University of Wisconsin, Madison. (Microcard PE 738, University of Oregon, Eugene.)

Fox, M.G. 1957. Swimming power test. Research Quarterly, **28**:233-237.

Fried, C.R. 1983. An examination of the test characteristics of the 12-minute aerobic swim test, Unpublished master's thesis, University of Wisconsin, Madison.

Hewitt, J.E. 1948. Swimming achievement scales for college men. Research Quarterly, **19**:282-289.

Hewitt, J.E. 1949. Swimming achievement scale scores for high school swimming. Research Quarterly, **20**:170-179.

Jackson, A., Jackson, A.S., and Frankiewiez, R.G. 1979. The construct and concurrent validity of a 12-minute crawl stroke swim as a field test of swimming endurance. Research Quarterly for Exercise and Sport, **50**:641-648.

Jackson, A.S., and Pettinger, J. 1969. The development and discriminant analysis of swimming profiles of college men. Proceedings of the 72nd annual meeting, National College Physical Education Association for Men.

Munt, M.R. 1964. Development of an objective test to measure the efficiency of the front crawl for college women, Unpublished master's thesis, The University of Michigan, Ann Arbor.

Rosentswieg, J.A. 1968. A revision of the power swimming test. Research Quarterly **39**:818-819.

Wilson, C.T. 1934. Coordination tests in swimming. Research Quarterly, **5**:81-88.

Wilson, M.R. 1971. Wilson achievement test for intermediate swimming. In Barrow, H.M., and McGee, R., editors. A practical approach to measurement in physical education, ed. 2, Philadelphia: Lea & Febiger.

TABLE TENNIS

Mott, J.A., and Lockhart, A. 1946. Table tennis backboard test. Journal of Health and Physical Education, **17**:550-552.

TENNIS

Avery, C.A., Richardson, P.A., and Jackson, A.W. 1979. A practical tennis serve test: measurement of skill under simulated game conditions. Research Quarterly for Exercise and Sport, **50**:554-564.

Avery, C., Richardson, P., and Jackson, A. 1981. Response to McGhee's discussion. Research Quarterly for Exercise and Sport, **52**:296-297.

Benton, R. 1963. Teaching tennis by testing. In Davis, D., editor. Selected tennis and badminton articles. Washington, D.C.: Division of Girls' and Women's Sports, American Association for Health, Physical Education and Recreation.

Broer, M.R., and Miller, D.M. 1950. Achievement tests for beginning and intermediate tennis. Research Quarterly, **21**:301-313.

Cobane, E. 1962. Test for the service. In Tennis and badminton guide—June 1962-June 1964. Washington, D.C.: Division of Girls' and Women's Sports, American Association for Health, Physical Education and Recreation.

DiGennaro, J. 1969. Construction of forehand drive, backhand drive, and service tennis tests. Research Quarterly, **40**:496-501.

Dyer, J.T. 1938. Revision of the backboard test of tennis ability. Research Quarterly, **9**:25-31.

Edwards, J. 1965. A study of three measures of the tennis serve. Master's thesis. The University of Wisconsin, Madison. (Microcard PE 746, University of Oregon, Eugene.)

Felshin, J., and Spencer, E. 1963. Evaluation procedures for tennis. In Davis, D., editor. Selected tennis and badminton articles. Washington, D.C.: Division of Girls' and Women's Sports, American Association for Health, Physical Education and Recreation.

Fox, K. 1953. A study of the validity of the Dyer backboard test and the Miller forehand-backhand test for beginning tennis players. Research Quarterly, **24**:1-8.

Hewitt, J.E. 1965. Revision of the Dyer backboard tennis test. Research Quarterly, **36**:153-157.

Hewitt, J.E. 1966. Hewitt's tennis achievement test. Research Quarterly, **37**:231-236.

Hewitt, J.E. 1968. Classification tests in tennis. Research Quarterly, **39**:552-555.

Hubbell, N.C. 1960. A battery of tennis skill tests for college women, Unpublished master's thesis, Texas Women's University, Denton.

Hulac, G.M. 1971. Hulac rating scale for the tennis serve. In Barrow, H.M., and McGee, R., editors. A practical approach to measurement in physical education, ed. 2, Philadelphia: Lea & Febiger.

Hulbert, B.A. 1966. A study of tests for the forehand drive in tennis. Master's thesis, The University of Wisconsin, Madison. (Microcard PE 818, University of Oregon, Eugene.)

Johnson, J. 1957. Tennis serve of advanced women players. Research Quarterly, **28**:123-131.

Johnson, J. 1963. Tennis knowledge test. In Davis, D., editor. Selected tennis and badminton articles. Washington, D.C.: Division of Girls' and Women's Sports, American Association for Health, Physical Education and Recreation.

Kemp, J., and Vincent, M.F. 1968. Kemp-Vincent rally test of tennis skill. Research Quarterly, **39**:1000-1004.

Malinak, N.R. 1961. The construction of an objective measure of accuracy in the performance of the tennis serve, Unpublished master's thesis, University of Illinois, Urbana.

McGhee, R. 1981. Discussion of "A practical tennis serve test: measurement of skill under simulated game conditions." Research Quarterly for Exercise and Sport, **52**:294-295.

Purcell, K. 1981. A tennis forehand-backhand drive skill test which measures ball control and stroke firmness. Research Quarterly for Exercise and Sport, **52**:238-245.

Ronning, H.E. 1959. Wall tests for evaluating tennis ability. Master's thesis, Washington State University, Pullman. (Microcard PE 441, University of Oregon, Eugene.)

Scott, M.G. 1941. Achievement examinations for elementary and intermediate tennis classes. Research Quarterly, **7**:40-49.

Scott, M.G. and French, E. 1959. Scott-French revision of the Dyer wallboard test. In Scott, M.G., and French, E. Measurement and evaluation in physical education. Dubuque, Iowa: Wm C Brown Group.

Shepard, G.J. 1972. The tennis drive skills test. Tennis-badminton-squash guide. Washington, D.C.: Division of Girls' and Women's Sports, American Association for Health, Physical Education and Recreation.

VOLLEYBALL

American Association for Health, Physical Education and Recreation. 1967. Volleyball skills test manual. Washington, D.C.: American Association for Health, Physical Education and Recreation.

Bassett, G., Glassow, R.B., and Locke, M. 1937. Studies in testing volleyball skills. Research Quarterly, **8**:60-72.

Blackman, C.J. 1968. The development of a volleyball test for the spike, Unpublished master's thesis, Southern Illinois University, Carbondale.

Brady, C.F. 1945. Preliminary investigation of volleyball playing ability. Research Quarterly, **16**:14-17.

Broer, M.A. 1958. Reliability of certain skill tests for junior high school girls. Research Quarterly, **29**:139-145.

Brumbach, W.B. 1979. Brumbach service test. In Johnson, B.L. and Nelson, J.K. Practical measurements for evaluation in physical education. Minneapolis: Burgess Publishing Co.

Clifton, M. 1962. Single hit volley test for women's volleyball. Research Quarterly, **33**:208-211.

Crogan, C. 1943. A simple volleyball classification test for high school girls. The Physical Educator, **4**:34-37.

Cunningham, P., and Garrison, J. 1968. High wall volley test for women. Research Quarterly, **39**:486-490.

French, E.L., and Cooper, B.I. 1937. Achievement tests in volleyball for high school girls. Research Quarterly, **8**:150-157.

Helman, R.M. 1971. Development of power volleyball skill tests for college women. Paper presented at the Research Section of the 1971 American Association for Health, Physical Education and Recreation National Convention, Detroit.

Jackson, P.L. 1966. A rating scale for discriminating relative playing performance of skilled female volleyball players. Master's thesis, University of Alberta, Edmonton, Canada. (Microcard PE 931. University of Oregon, Eugene.)

Kessler A. 1968. The validity and reliability of the Sandefur volleyball spiking test, Unpublished master's thesis, California State College, Long Beach.

Kronqvist, R.A., and Brumbach, W.B. 1968. A modification of the Brady volleyball skill test for high school boys. Research Quarterly, **39**:116-120.

Latchaw, M. 1954. Measuring selected motor skills in fourth, fifth, and sixth grades. Research Quarterly, **25**:439-449.

Liba, M.R., and Stauff, M.R. 1963. A test for the voleyball pass. Research Quarterly, **34**:56-63.

Londeree, B.R., and Eicholtz, E.C. 1970. Reliabilities of selected volleyball skill tests. Paper presented at the Research Section of the 1970 American Association for Health, Physical Education Recreation National Convention, Seattle.

Lopez, D. 1957. Serve test. In Volleyball guide—July 1957-July 1959. Washington, D.C.: Division of Girls' and Women's Sport, American Association for Health, Physical Education and Recreation.

Mohr, D.R., and Haverstick, M.J. 1955. Repeated volleys tests for women's volleyball. Research Quarterly, **26**:179-184.

Russell, N., and Lange, E. 1940. Achievement tests in volleyball for junior high school girls. Research Quarterly, **11**:33-41.

Ryan, M.F. 1969. A study of tests for the volleyball serve. Master's thesis, The University of Wisconsin, Madison. (Microcard PE 1040, University of Oregon, Eugene.)

Slaymaker, T., and Brown, V.H. 1969. Test questions for power volleyball. Philadelphia: W.B. Saunders Co.

Snavely, M. 1960. Volleyball skill tests for girls. In Lockhart, A. editor. Selected volleyball articles. Washington, D.C.: Division of Girls' and Women's Sports, American Association for Health, Physical Education and Recreation.

Thorpe, J., and West, C. 1967. A volleyball skills chart with attainment levels for selected skills. Volleyball guide—July 1967-July 1969. Washington, D.C.: Division of Girls' and Women's Sports, American Association for Health, Physical Education and Recreation.

Watkins, A. 1960. Skill testing for large groups. In Lockhart, A. editor. Selected volleyball articles. Washington, D.C.: Division of Girls' and Women's Sports, American Association for Health, Physical Education and Recreation.

West, C. 1957. A comparative study between height and wall volley test scores as related to volleyball playing ability of girls and women, Unpublished master's thesis, The Women's College of the University of North Carolina, Greensboro.

WRESTLING

Sickels, W.L. 1980. Sickels amateur wrestling ability rating form. In Barrow, H.M., and McGee, R. A practical approach to measurement in physical education, ed. 3, Philadelphia: Lea & Febiger.

Yetter, H. 1963. A test of wrestling aptitude: a preliminary explanation, Unpublished master's thesis, University of Wisconsin, Madison.

Appendix E—Programs for Apple IIe Computer

(1) SFCALC PROGRAM*

Input data: Name, age, weight, and three skinfold measures
Males: chest, abdomen, and thigh
Females: triceps, thigh, and suprailium
Output data: Percent body fat and ideal weight
LIST

```
10   REM PROGRAM "SFCALC"
20   REM
30   REM PROGRAMMED BY TERRY M. WOOD
40   REM
50   REM DEPARTMENT OF PHYSICAL EDUCATION
60   REM UNIVERSITY OF WISCONSIN, MADISON
70   REM
80   REM COPYRIGHT 1982
85   REM
86   REM THIS PROGRAM ASSUMES A PRINTER IN SLOT #1
87   REM
90   HOME
100  VTAB (6)
110  PRINT TAB(8)"SKINFOLD-CALC: A PROGRAM"
120  VTAB (8)
130  PRINT TAB(5)"TO CALCULATE PERCENT BODY FAT"
140  VTAB (10)
150  PRINT TAB(10)"AND IDEAL BODY WEIGHT"
160  VTAB (13)
170  PRINT TAB(13)"COPYRIGHT, 1982"
180  VTAB (15)
190  PRINT TAB(4)"TERRY WOOD, DEPT. OF P.E. AND DANCE"
200  VTAB (17)
210  PRINT TAB(5)"UNIVERSITY OF WISCONSIN-MADISON"
220  VTAB (20)
230  INPUT "DO YOU WISH TO CONTINUE? 1=YES 2=NO";CTN
240  IF CTN = 1 THEN GOTO 290
250  IF CTN = 2 THEN GOTO 1740
260  PRINT
270  PRINT "THAT WAS NOT A 1 OR A 2!"
280  GOTO 230
290  HOME
```

---

*The SFCALC program is reproduced by permission of Terry M. Wood, Ph.D., Department of Physical Education, Oregon State University, Corvallis.

```
300   VTAB (4)
310   PRINT "SKINFOLD-CALC IS AN INTERACTIVE PROGRAM."
320   PRINT "WHEN THE PROGRAM ASKS YOU TO SUPPLY"
330   PRINT "INFORMATION, TYPE IN THE APPROPRIATE"
340   PRINT "RESPONSE AND THEN PRESS 'RETURN'."
350   VTAB (11)
360   INPUT "DO YOU WISH TO CONTINUE? 1=YES 2=NO";CTN
370   IF CTN = 1 THEN GOTO 420
380   IF CTN = 2 THEN GOTO 1740
390   PRINT
400   PRINT "THAT WAS NOT A 1 OR A 2!"
410   GOTO 360
420   HOME
430   VTAB (4)
440   INPUT "HOW MANY SUBJECTS ARE IN YOUR SAMPLE? ";N
450   IF N > = 1 THEN GOTO 500
460   PRINT
470   PRINT "SINCE THERE ARE NO SUBJECTS, THIS RUN"
480   PRINT "IS TERMINATED!"
490   GOTO 1730
500   HOME
510   VTAB (4)
520   PRINT "DATA MUST BE FROM MALES OR FROM FEMALES,"
530   PRINT "BUT NOT FROM BOTH."
540   PRINT "ARE YOUR SUBJECTS MALES OR FEMALES?"
550   INPUT "1=MALES 2=FEMALES";SEX
560   IF (SEX = 1) OR (SEX = 2) THEN GOTO 600
570   PRINT
580   PRINT "THAT WAS NOT A 1 OR A 2!"
590   GOTO 540
600   HOME
610   VTAB (4)
620   PRINT "WHEN CALCULATING IDEAL BODY WEIGHT WHAT"
630   PRINT "PERCENT BODY FAT WILL YOU CONSIDER"
640   PRINT "NORMAL FOR YOUR POPULATION? YOU MUST"
650   PRINT "TYPE A NUMBER GREATER THAN ZERO."
660   PRINT "FOR EXAMPLE, TYPE A 23 IF YOU WANT 23"
670   PRINT "PERCENT."
680   PRINT
690   INPUT "WHAT PERCENT DO YOU WANT? ";PCF
700   IF PCF > 0 THEN GOTO 740
710   PRINT
720   PRINT "THE NUMBER MUST BE GREATER THAN ZERO!"
730   GOTO 690
```

```
740   HOME
750   VTAB (4)
760   PRINT "NEXT YOU MUST INPUT THE DATA FOR EACH"
770   PRINT "SUBJECT SEPARATELY. TO DO THIS TYPE IN"
780   PRINT "THE SUBJECT'S FULL NAME, AGE (YEARS),"
790   PRINT "WEIGHT (LBS.), AND THREE SKINFOLD"
800   PRINT "MEASURES ON SEPARATE LINES."
810   PRINT "PRESS 'RETURN' AFTER EACH LINE."
820   PRINT "SKINFOLD MEASURES MUST BE CHEST, ABDOMEN,"
830   PRINT "AND THIGH FOR MALES AND TRICEPS,"
840   PRINT "THIGH, AND SUPRAILIUM FOR FEMALES."
850   PRINT "THE COMPUTER WILL 'BEEP' TO LET YOU"
860   PRINT "KNOW WHEN TO START TYPING THE NEXT": PRINT "LINE OF
      DATA."
870   PRINT "PLEASE LIMIT THE NAME FOR EACH SUBJECT": PRINT "TO 18
      CHARACTERS INCLUDING SPACES."
880   PRINT
890   INPUT "TO START DATA INPUT TYPE A 1 AND PRESS 'RETURN' ";CTN
900   IF CTN = 1 GOTO 940
910   PRINT
920   PRINT "THAT WAS NOT A 1!"
930   GOTO 890
940   S = − 16336
950   PRINT
960   DIM NAME$(N) ,AGE(N) ,WT(N) ,ASF(N) ,BSF(N) ,CSF(N)
970   IF SEX = 2 GOTO 1190
980   FOR I = 1 TO N
990   GOSUB 1690
1000  PRINT "NAME FOR SUBJECT #";I
1010  INPUT NAME$(I): PRINT
1020  GOSUB 1690
1030  PRINT "AGE (YEARS) FOR SUBJECT #";I
1040  INPUT AGE(I): PRINT
1050  GOSUB 1690
1060  PRINT "WEIGHT (LBS.) FOR SUBJECT #";I
1070  INPUT WT(I): PRINT
1080  GOSUB 1690
1090  PRINT "CHEST SKINFOLD FOR SUBJECT #";I
1100  INPUT ASF(I): PRINT
1110  GOSUB 1690
1120  PRINT "ABDOMEN SKINFOLD FOR SUBJECT #";I
1130  INPUT BSF(I): PRINT
1140  GOSUB 1690
1150  PRINT "THIGH SKINFOLD FOR SUBJECT #";I
```

```
1160   INPUT CSF(I): PRINT
1170   NEXT I
1180   GOTO 1390
1190   FOR I = 1 TO N
1200   GOSUB 1690
1210   PRINT "NAME FOR SUBJECT #";I
1220   INPUT NAME$(I): PRINT
1230   GOSUB 1690
1240   PRINT "AGE (YEARS) FOR SUBJECT #";I
1250   INPUT AGE(I): PRINT
1260   GOSUB 1690
1270   PRINT "WEIGHT (LBS.) FOR SUBJECT #";I
1280   INPUT WT(I): PRINT
1290   GOSUB 1690
1300   PRINT "TRICEPS SKINFOLD FOR SUBJECT #";I
1310   INPUT ASF(I): PRINT
1320   GOSUB 1690
1330   PRINT "THIGH SKINFOLD FOR SUBJECT #";I
1340   INPUT BSF(I): PRINT
1350   GOSUB 1690
1360   PRINT "SUPRAILIUM SKINFOLD FOR SUBJECT #";I
1370   INPUT CSF(I): PRINT
1380   NEXT I
1390   HOME
1395   VTAB (4): PRINT "DON'T FORGET TO TURN YOUR PRINTER ON!":
       PRINT: PRINT "PRESS ANY KEY TO START PRINTING"
1396   GET CC$
1400   PR# 1
1405   PRINT CHR$ (9);"8ON"
1410   VTAB (4)
1415   PRINT: PRINT
1420   PRINT "HERE ARE THE RESULTS FOR YOUR SUBJECTS:"
1430   PRINT: PRINT "THE DATA INPUT FOR EACH SUBJECT WERE: ":
       PRINT
1440   PRINT "NAME";: HTAB 30: PRINT "AGE";: POKE 36,40: PRINT
       "WEIGHT";: POKE 36,50: PRINT "SF1";: POKE 36,57: PRINT "SF2";:
       POKE 36,64: PRINT "SF3"
1450   PRINT
1460   FOR I = 1 TO N: PRINT NAME$(I);: HTAB 31: PRINT AGE(I);: POKE 36,41:
       PRINT WT(I);: POKE 36,50: PRINT ASF (I);: POKE 36,57: PRINT BSF(I);:
       POKE 36,64: PRINT CSF(I)
1470   NEXT I
1480   PRINT : PRINT : PRINT "THE % BODY FAT AND IDEAL WEIGHT FOR
       EACH SUBJECT ARE:": PRINT
```

```
1490   PRINT "NAME";: HTAB 30: PRINT "% BODY FAT";: POKE 36,50: PRINT
       "IDEAL WT.": PRINT
1500   IF SEX = 2 GOTO 1600
1510   FOR J = 1 TO N
1520   SUM = 0
1530   SUM = ASF(J) + BSF(J) + CSF(J)
1540   BD = 1.10938 − 0.0008267 * SUM + 0.0000016 * SUM ^ 2 − 0.0002574 *
       AGE(J)
1550   FT = (4.95 / BD − 4.5) * 100
1560   WEIGHT = (WT(J) − (WT(J) * FT) / 100) / (1 − PCF / 100)
1570   PRINT NAME$(J);: HTAB 30: PRINT FT;: POKE 36,50: PRINT WEIGHT
1580   NEXT J
1590   GOTO 1730
1600   FOR K = 1 TO N
1610   SUM = 0
1620   SUM = ASF(K) + BSF(K) + CSF(K)
1630   BD = 1.0994921 − 0.0009929 * SUM + 0.0000023 * SUM ^ 2 − 0.0001392
       * AGE(K)
1640   FT = (4.95 / BD − 4.5) * 100
1650   WEIGHT = (WT(K) − (WT(K) * FT) / 100) / (1 − PCF / 100)
1660   PRINT NAME$(K);: HTAB 30: PRINT FT;: POKE 36,50: PRINT WEIGHT
1670   NEXT K
1680   GOTO 1730
1690   FOR SND = 1 TO 20
1700   SOUND = PEEK (S) − PEEK (S) + PEEK (S) − PEEK (S)
1710   NEXT SND
1720   RETURN
1730   CLEAR : PR# 0: HOME
1732   PRINT: PRINT "DO YOU WISH TO RESTART THE PROGRAM?": INPUT
       "1=YES 2=NO ";CTN
1733   IF CTN = 1 THEN GOTO 420
1734   IF CTN = 2 THEN GOTO 1740
1735   PRINT : PRINT "THAT WAS NOT A 1 OR A 2!": GOTO 1732
1740   PRINT : PRINT : PRINT "GOODBYE!"
1750   END
```

(2) GRADES PROGRAM

This is an expanded version of the GRADES Program in Chapter 5. This program allows
you to print the results for each student.

```
 1   HOME
 2   SPEED = 100
 9   HTAB 3: PRINT "THIS IS A PROGRAM TO CALCULATE FINAL"
10   HTAB 3: PRINT "GRADES FOR A UNIT OF INSTRUCTION."
11   HTAB 3: PRINT "YOU WILL BE ASKED TO PROVIDE THE"
```

```
12   HTAB 3: PRINT "FOLLOWING DATA FOR YOUR STUDENTS:"
13   HTAB 3: PRINT "NUMBER OF STUDENTS, NUMBER OF GRADES"
14   HTAB 3: PRINT "FOR EACH STUDENT, AND THE WEIGHTS FOR"
15   HTAB 3: PRINT "EACH GRADE.": PRINT : FOR N = 1 TO 5000: NEXT N
16   HTAB 3: PRINT "IF ALL OF THE GRADES ARE OF EQUAL"
17   HTAB 3: PRINT "WEIGHT, ASSIGN A WEIGHT OF 1 TO EACH"
18   HTAB 3: PRINT "ONE. THAT IS, IF EACH GRADE IS AS"
19   HTAB 3: PRINT "IMPORTANT AS ANY OTHER GRADE, THEY"
20   HTAB 3: PRINT "SHOULD BE WEIGHTED THE SAME.": PRINT : FOR N
     = 1 TO 5000: NEXT N
21   HTAB 3: PRINT "ONCE YOU HAVE ENTERED THE DATA"
22   HTAB 3: PRINT "APPLYING TO ALL STUDENTS (NUMBER OF"
23   HTAB 3: PRINT "STUDENTS, NUMBER OF GRADES, AND"
24   HTAB 3: PRINT "WEIGHTS), THE COMPUTER WILL ASK YOU"
25   HTAB 3: PRINT "FOR THE NAME AND LETTER GRADES"
26   HTAB 3: PRINT "FOR EACH STUDENT.": PRINT : FOR N = 1 TO 5000:
     NEXT N
27   HTAB 3: PRINT "YOU CAN USE PLUSSES AND MINUSES"
28   HTAB 3: PRINT "WITH ALL GRADES EXCEPT AN F.": PRINT : FOR N
     = 1 TO 5000: NEXT N
32   HTAB 3: PRINT "REMEMBER TO PRESS THE RETURN KEY"
33   HTAB 3: PRINT "EACH TIME YOU TYPE INFORMATION INTO"
34   HTAB 3: PRINT "THE COMPUTER.": PRINT
35   FOR N = 1 TO 5000: NEXT N
44   HOME
45   PRINT : PRINT : PRINT
46   SPEED = 225
47   INPUT "HOW MANY STUDENTS?  ";S
48   PRINT
50   INPUT "HOW MANY GRADES FOR EACH STUDENT?  ";N
60   PRINT
65   DIM N$(S),GD(N,3),LG$(S,N),AG$(S),AG(S),T(S),T$(S)
70   LET ADD = 0
120  FOR X = 1 TO N
130  PRINT "WEIGHT FOR TEST";X;: INPUT ":  ";GD(X,2)
134  PRINT
135  ADD = ADD + GD(X,2)
140  NEXT X
150  FOR Y = 1 TO S
155  PRINT
156  PRINT Y;"−STUDENT NAME:";
158  INPUT N$(Y)
160  PRINT
200  FOR X = 1 TO N
```

```
210    INPUT "GRADE?";GD$(X)
211    IF GD$(X) = "A+" THEN GD(X,1) = 12
212    IF GD$(X) = "A" THEN GD(X,1) = 11
213    IF GD$(X) = "A−" THEN GD(X,1) = 10
214    IF GD$(X) = "B+" THEN GD(X,1) = 9
215    IF GD$(X) = "B" THEN GD(X,1) = 8
216    IF GD$(X) = "B−" THEN GD(X,1) = 7
217    IF GD$(X) = "C+" THEN GD(X,1) = 6
218    IF GD$(X) = "C" THEN GD(X,1) = 5
219    IF GD$(X) = "C−" THEN GD(X,1) = 4
220    IF GD$(X) = "D+" THEN GD(X,1) = 3
221    IF GD$(X) = "D" THEN GD(X,1) = 2
222    IF GD$(X) = "D−" THEN GD(X,1) = 1
223    IF GD$(X) = "F" THEN GD(X,1) = 0
310    GD(X,3) = GD(X,1) * GD(X,2)
315    LG$(Y,X) = GD$(X)
319    NEXT X
320    PRINT
321    PRINT N$(Y);"'S GRADES ARE:";
322    FOR X = 1 TO N
323    PRINT " ";LG$(Y,X);
324    NEXT X
325    PRINT
326    PRINT
327    INPUT "DO YOU WANT TO CHANGE ANYTHING? YES/NO ";A$
328    IF A$ = "YES" THEN GOTO 155
329    PRINT
330    LET SUM = 0
340    FOR X = 1 TO N
350    SUM = SUM + GD(X,3)
360    NEXT X
370    PRINT
375    T = SUM / ADD
381    IF T < 12.1 THEN T$ = "A+"
382    IF T < 11.5 THEN T$ = "A"
383    IF T < 10.5 THEN T$ = "A−"
384    IF T < 9.5 THEN T$ = "B+"
385    IF T < 8.5 THEN T$ = "B"
386    IF T < 7.5 THEN T$ = "B−"
387    IF T < 6.5 THEN T$ = "C+"
388    IF T < 5.5 THEN T$ = "C"
389    IF T < 4.5 THEN T$ = "C−"
390    IF T < 3.5 THEN T$ = "D+"
391    IF T < 2.5 THEN T$ = "D"
```

```
392   IF T < 1.5 THEN T$ = "D−"
393   IF T < .5 THEN T$ = "F"
394   AG(Y) = T
395   AG$(Y) = T$
396   NEXT Y
397   INPUT "DO YOU WANT A COPY OF THE RESULTS? YES/NO";B$
398   IF B$ = "NO" THEN GOTO 403
399   PRINT
400   INPUT "PLEASE TURN ON THE PRINTER AND PRESS RETURN. ";C$
401   INPUT "TEST NAME OR NUMBER: ";Z$
402   PR# 1: HOME
403   PRINT Z$: PRINT
404   FOR Y = 1 TO S
405   PRINT Y;"−STUDENT NAME:";N$(Y)
407   PRINT TAB(4) "GRADES: ";
408   FOR X = 1 TO N
409   PRINT LG$(Y,X);
410   IF X < N THEN PRINT ",";
412   NEXT X
420   PRINT
430   PRINT TAB(4)"AVERAGE GRADE:"AG(Y)
450   PRINT TAB(4)"AVERAGE LETTER GRADE: ";AG$(Y)
480   PRINT
482   PR# 0
485   INPUT "PRESS RETURN TO CONTINUE ";R$: PRINT
486   IF B$ = "NO" OR B$ = "N" THEN GOTO 490
487   PR# 1
490   NEXT Y
495   PR# 0
496   PRINT "DO YOU WANT TO START THE"
497   PRINT
498   INPUT "PROGRAM AGAIN? YES/NO ";D$
500   IF D$ = "YES" OR D$ = "Y" THEN RUN 44
510   FLASH
515   PRINT : PRINT : PRINT : PRINT
520   PRINT "THE PROGRAM IS OVER."
530   NORMAL
540   END
550   RUN 44
```

(3) DIRECTIONS PROGRAM

(Directions to using TSCORES Program)

```
  5   PRINT: PRINT
 10   PRINT "DIRECTIONS FOR TSCORES";
```

```
 12   PRINT: PRINT
 15   PRINT "1. LIMITED TO 60 STUDENTS";
 20   PRINT: PRINT
 25   PRINT "2. AVERAGE UP TO 5 SCORES";
 30   PRINT: PRINT
 35   PRINT "3. LINES 1320 − 1360 ASSIGN LETTER GRADE TO TSCORES";
 40   PRINT: PRINT
 45   PRINT "4. YOU CAN CHANGE LETTER GRADES";
 50   PRINT: PRINT
 55   PRINT "5. AVERAGE TSCORES OPTION WILL CALCULATE MEAN
      AND STANDARD DEVIATION FOR ANY SET OF SCORES";
100   END
```

TSCORES PROGRAM*

```
 10   REM DESIGNED TO CALCULATE T-SCORES OR AVERAGE T-SCORES
 20   L = 1
 30   DIM S1(60,10),T(60),NM$(60),S9(60),M(60),T9(60),G$(60)
 40   REM PAINT SCREEN
 50   S9 = 0:M = 0:D = 0:T1 = 0:T2 = 0
 60   A = 0
 70   HOME: VTAB 4: PRINT "********** MAIN MENU **********"
 80   VTAB 8: PRINT TAB(5);"1⟩ AVERAGE A SET OF T-SCORES"
 90   VTAB 10: PRINT TAB(5); "2⟩ CALCULATE RAW DATA INTO T-SCORES"
100   VTAB 12: PRINT TAB(5); "3⟩ END PROGRAM"
110   VTAB 20: PRINT "ENTER SELECTION ⟨1,2,3⟩": GET S
120   IF S < 1 OR S > 3 THEN GOTO 110
130   IF S = 1 THEN GOTO 160
140   IF S = 2 THEN GOTO 770
150   IF S = 3 THEN GOTO 1640
160   REM AVG SET OF T-SCORES
170   HOME: INPUT "NUMBER OF STUDENTS: ";X1
180   VTAB 4: INPUT "NUMBER OF SCORES PER STUDENT: ";X2
190   HOME: PRINT "ENTER NAME AND SCORES"
200   PRINT: PRINT
210   FOR I = 1 TO X1
220   PRINT "NAME";I;" ";
230   INPUT NM$(I)
240   FOR J = 1 TO X2
250   PRINT TAB(3);"SCORE";J;" ";
260   INPUT S1(I,J)
270   NEXT J
280   X3 = 0
```

*The DIRECTIONS and TSCORES programs are reproduced by permission of Diane Ross, Ph.D., Department of Physical Education, California State University, Fullerton.

```
290   NEXT I
300   HOME: PRINT "WOULD YOU LIKE TO VIEW THESE SCORES"
310   INPUT "⟨Y/N⟩";Y$
320   IF Y$ = "N" THEN GOTO 420
330   FOR I = L TO X1
340   PRINT I;" ";NM$(I)
350   FOR J = 1 TO X2
360   PRINT TAB(3);S1(I,J)
370   NEXT J
380   L1 = I
390   X3 = X3 + (X2 + 1)
400   IF X3 = 18 OR X3 = 20 THEN GOTO 420
410   NEXT I
420   INPUT "ARE THESE SCORES CORRECT ⟨Y/N⟩";Y$
430   IF Y$ = "Y" AND X3 = 0 THEN GOTO 500
440   IF Y$ = "Y" AND X3 ⟨ ⟩ 0 THEN GOTO 1650
450   INPUT "STUDENT'S NO. TO BE CHANGED (0 TO END) ";Z
460   IF Z = 0 AND X3 = 0 THEN GOTO 500
470   IF Z = 0 AND X3 ⟨ ⟩ 0 THEN GOTO 1650
480   GOSUB 950
490   GOTO 420
500   FOR I = 1 TO X1
510   FOR J = 1 TO X2
520   LET T(I) = S1(I,J) + T(I)
530   NEXT J
540   NEXT I
550   FOR I = 1 TO X1
560   LET M(I) = T(I) / X2
570   LET M(I) = INT (M(I) * 10 + .5) / 10
580   T9(I) = M(I):A = 1
590   GOTO 1320
600   NEXT I
610   HOME: INPUT "WOULD YOU LIKE A HARD COPY ⟨Y/N⟩";Y$
620   IF Y$ = "Y" THEN Q = 1
630   IF Y$ = "N" THEN Q = 0
640   HOME: PRINT CHR$ (4);"PR#";Q
650   S = 0
660   PRINT TAB(5);"NAME"; TAB(28);"MEAN"; TAB(34);"GRADE"
670   PRINT TAB(5);"= = = ="; TAB(28);"= = = ="; TAB(34);"= = = ="
680   FOR I = 1 TO X1
690   IF I = 20 OR I = 40 AND Q = 0 THEN INPUT "PRESS RETURN";Y$
700   PRINT NM$(I); TAB(28);M(I); TAB(36);G$(I)
710   NEXT I
720   IF Q = 1 THEN PRINT CHR$(4);"PR#0"
```

```
730   PRINT: IF Q = 0 THEN INPUT "PRESS RETURN";Q$
740   FOR I = 1 TO X1:T(I) = M(I) = 0: NEXT I
750   X1 = X2 = 0
760   GOTO 50
770   REM CALCULATE T-SCORES
780   M = 0:D = 0:T1 = 0:T2 = 0
790   HOME
800   INPUT "NUMBER OF STUDENTS: ";N
801   FOR I = 1 TO N:T9(I) = S9(I) = 0: NEXT I
820   PRINT: PRINT
830   FOR I = 1 TO N
840   PRINT "NAME";I;" ";
850   INPUT NM$(I)
860   PRINT SPC(3);"SCORE:";
870   INPUT S9(I)
880   NEXT I
890   FOR I = 1 TO N
900   IF I = 20 OR I = 40 THEN GOSUB 1090
910   PRINT I;" ";NM$(I); TAB(30);S9(I)
920   NEXT I
930   IF I 〈 〉 20 AND I 〈 〉 40 THEN GOSUB 1090
940   GOTO 1180
950   REM SUBROUTINE TO CORRECT SCORES FOR AVG.
960   HOME: VTAB 6
970   PRINT NM$(Z)
980   FOR K = 1 TO X2
990   PRINT TAB(3);"SCORE";K;"=";S1(Z,K)
1000  NEXT K
1010  PRINT: PRINT
1020  INPUT "INPUT SCORE # TO BE CHANGED (0 TO END) ";N9
1030  IF N9 < 0 OR N9 > X2 THEN GOTO 1020
1040  IF N9 = 0 THEN GOTO 1080
1050  PRINT: PRINT "OLD SCORE= ";S1(Z,N9);" ";
1060  INPUT "NEW SCORE= ";S1(Z,N9)
1070  VTAB 20: PRINT "PRESS RETURN": GET Q$
1080  RETURN
1090  REM SUBROUTINE TO CORRECT SCORES FOR T-SCORES
1100  PRINT: PRINT "ARE THESE SCORES CORRECT <Y/N> ";
1110  INPUT Y$
1120  IF Y$ = "Y" THEN 1170
1130  INPUT "NO. TO CORRECT ";N1
1140  PRINT "OLD: ";S9(N1); TAB(15);
1150  INPUT "NEW: ";S9(N1)
1160  GOTO 1100
```

```
1170   RETURN
1180   FOR I = 1 TO N
1190   LET T1 = T1 + S9(I)
1200   LET T2 = T2 + S9(I) ^ 2
1210   NEXT I
1220   M = T1 / N
1230   D = SQR (((T2 − ((T1 ^ 2) / N)) / N))
1250   FOR I = 1 TO N
1260   T9(I) = 50 + (10 / D) * (S9(I) − M)
1270   LET T9(I) = INT (T9(I) * 10 + .5) / 10
1280   NEXT I
1300   REM PUT GRADE TO T-SCORE
1310   FOR I = 1 TO N
1320   IF T9(I) > = 60 THEN G$(I) = "A"
1330   IF T9(I) > = 50 AND T9(I) < = 59.9 THEN G$(I) = "B"
1340   IF T9(I) > = 40 AND T9(I) < = 49.9 THEN G$(I) = "C"
1350   IF T9(I) > = 30 AND T9(I) < = 39.9 THEN G$(I) = "D"
1360   IF T9(I) < = 29.9 THEN G$(I) = "F"
1370   IF A = 1 THEN GOTO 600
1380   NEXT I
1390   HOME: INPUT "WOULD YOU LIKE A HARDCOPY <Y/N> ";Y$
1400   IF Y$ = "Y" THEN Q = 1
1410   IF Y$ = "N" THEN Q = 0
1420   PRINT CHR$ (4);"PR#";Q
1430   PRINT TAB(3);"NAME"; TAB(20);"SCORE"; TAB(27);"T-SCORE";
       TAB(36);"GRADE"
1440   PRINT TAB(3);"= = = ="; TAB(20);"= = = = ="; TAB
       (27);"= = = = = = ="; TAB(36);"= = = = ="
1450   PRINT
1460   FOR I = 1 TO N
1470   PRINT NM$(I); TAB(22);S9(I); TAB(29);T9(I); TAB(38);G$(I)
1480   IF Q = 0 AND I = 20 OR I = 40 THEN INPUT "PRESS RETURN";Q$
1490   NEXT I
1495   PRINT
1496   FLASH
1500   INPUT "PRESS RETURN";Q$
1505   NORMAL
1510   PRINT: PRINT "CLASS MEAN = "; INT (M * 10 + .5) / 10
1520   PRINT "CLASS STAN. DEV. = "; INT (D * 10 + .5) / 10
1530   PRINT CHR$ (4);"PR#0"
1540   PRINT: INPUT "NEW RAW SCORES <Y/N> ";Y$
1550   IF Y$ = "N" THEN GOTO 50
1560   T1 = 0:T2 = 0:D = 0:M = 0
1570   FOR I = 1 TO N:T9(I) = S9(I) = 0: NEXT I
```

```
1580   FOR I = 1 TO N
1590   PRINT NM$(I)
1600   PRINT TAB(3);"SCORE";:INPUT S9(I)
1610   NEXT I
1620   GOSUB 1100
1630   GOTO 1180
1640   HOME : END
1650   X3 = 0
1660   L = L1 + 1
1670   IF L > X1 THEN 500
1680   GOTO 330
```

(4) PERCENTILE PROGRAM*

(to form table of percentiles)

```
       LIST
   5   HOME
  10   READ N
  20   FOR I = 1 TO N
  30   READ X
  40   X1 = X1 + X
  50   X2 = X2 + X ^ 2
  60   NEXT I
  70   M = X1 / N
  80   S = ((X2 − X1 ^ 2 / N) / (N − 1)) ^ .5
  81   D(1) = 3.00 * S:D(2) = 1.64 * S:D(3) = 1.38 * S:D(4) = 1.04 * S:D(5) = .84
       * S:D(6) = .67 * S:D(7) = .52 * S:D(8) = .39 * S:D(9) = .25 * S:D(10) = .13
       * S
  85   VTAB 4: PRINT "THE 99.9TH PERCENTILE IS";M + D(1)
  90   P = 95
 100   FOR I = 2 TO 10
 110   PRINT: PRINT "THE";P; "THE PERCENTILE IS";M + D(I)
 112   P = P − 5
 115   NEXT I
 120   PRINT: PRINT "THE 50TH PERCENTILE IS";M
 124   PRINT
 125   VTAB 24: INPUT "PRESS RETURN ";A$
 130   P = 45
 135   HOME
```

---

*To see how this program works, enter RUN PERCENTILES. To insert a new set of scores, enter:

```
       LIST
 200   DATA (number of scores)
 210   DATA (enter each score, followed by a comma)
       RUN
```

The results can be used to form a table of percentile ranks.

```
140  FOR I = 10 TO 2 STEP − 1
150  PRINT : PRINT "THE";P;"THE PERCENTILE IS ";M − D(I)
155  P = P − 5
160  NEXT I
170  PRINT : PRINT "THE 0.1TH PERCENTILE IS";M − D(I)
180  PRINT : PRINT "MEAN: ";M
190  PRINT "SD :";S;
200  DATA 10
210  DATA 20,30,35,32,31,25,26,28,19,24
```

(5) CHANGE PROGRAM*

(to calculate improvement scores)

```
 1   HOME
 3   PRINT
     "= = = = = = = = = = = = = = = = = = = = = = = = = = = = = = = = = = = = ="
 4   PRINT : PRINT : PRINT
 5   PRINT "THIS PROGRAM IS DESIGNED TO CALCULATE IMPROVE-
     MENT SCORES FOR PAIRS OF INITIAL (PREINSTRUCTIONAL) AND
     FINAL (POST-INSTRUCTIONAL SCORES)."
 6   PRINT : PRINT : PRINT : PRINT : PRINT "PRESS RETURN": GET A$
 8   HOME : VTAB 4: PRINT "HOW MANY STUDENTS ARE IN THE CLASS?"
 9   INPUT N
11   SUMX = 0:FLAG = 0
12   SUMY = 0
13   SX2 = 0
14   SY2 = 0
15   ADDXY = 0
16   SMAX = 30.
18   HOME : VTAB 8: PRINT "WHAT IS THE MAXIMUM PERFORMANCE
     SCORE----IF IT IS UNKNOWN ENTER A '0' "
19   INPUT RMAX
25   DIM X(100),Y(100)
30   HOME : VTAB 3
35   FOR I = 1 TO N
37   PRINT "SCORE 1 FOR SUBJECT"; I;" = ";
38   INPUT X(I)
39   PRINT "SCORE 2 FOR SUBJECT"; I;" = ";
40   INPUT Y(I)
70   XX = XX + X(I)
80   YY = YY + Y(I)
90   XSQ = X(I) ^ 2
```

---

*Reproduced by permission of Whitfield B. East, Ph.D., Department of Physical Education, East Tennessee State University.

```
100   YSQ = Y(I) ^ 2
110   SX2 = SX2 + XSQ
120   SY2 = SY2 + YSQ
130   CROSSXY = X(I) * Y(I)
140   ADDXY = ADDXY + CROSSXY
145   PRINT : PRINT
150   NEXT I
154   REM
155   REM COMPUTE THE PEARSON CORRELATION COEFFICIENT
156   REM
160   NUM = (N * ADDXY) − (XX * YY)
170   DEM = SQR (((N * SX2) − (XX ^ 2)) * ((N * SY2) − (YY ^ 2)))
180   R = NUM/DEM
184   Z = 0
185   HOME : VTAB 8: PRINT "DO YOU WANT A PRINTED COPY OF YOUR
      RESULTS − Y/N"
188   GET A$: IF A$ = "Y" THEN Z = 1
190   IF A$ = "N" THEN Z = 0
199   REM
200   REM COMPUTE THE MEANS AND STANDARD DEVIATIONS FOR THE
      INITIAL AND FINAL SCORES
201   REM
205   MEANX = XX/N
210   MNY = YY/N
215   SDX = SQR (((N * SX2) − XX ^ 2) / (N * (N − 1)))
220   STDY = SQR (((N * SY2) − YY ^ 2) / (N * (N − 1)))
222   HOME : PR# Z
223   VTAB 4: PRINT " MEANS AND STANDARD DEVIATIONS":
      PRINT "_____"
224   PRINT : PRINT
225   PRINT "MEAN FOR INITIAL SCORES = ";MEANX
230   PRINT "MEAN FOR FINAL SCORES = ";MNY
232   PRINT : PRINT : PRINT
235   PRINT "STANDARD DEV FOR INITIAL = ";SDX
240   PRINT "STANDARD DEV FOR FINAL = ";STDY
243   GOSUB 700
245   BETA = (R * (STDY / SDX))
250   IF RMAX > 0 GOTO 260
255   RMAX = (MNY + (3 * STDY))
260   ALPH = ((LOG (SMAX + 1)) / RMAX)
298   REM
299   REM
300   REM COMPUTE EXPONENTIAL IMPROVEMENT SCORES
301   REM
```

```
302   REM
305   DIM IMPROV(100),YRES(100)
310   FOR I = 1 TO N
315   IMPROV(I) = ((LOG (( EXP (ALPH * BETA) * ( EXP (ALPH * X(I)) − EXP
      (ALPH * MEANX))) + EXP (ALPH * MNY))) / ALPH)
320   YRES (I) = ((Y(I) − X(I)) / (IMPROV(I) − X(I))) * 100.
325   NEXT I
350   HOME : PR#Z: PRINT : PRINT : PRINT : PRINT
355   PRINT "RAW SCORES PREDICTED PERCENT"
360   PRINT
365   PRINT "SUB INITIAL FINAL FINAL IMPROVEMENT"
370   PRINT
371   M = 0:FLAG = 1
375   Q = N / 10.:TTL = 10:Q% = N / 10.:LFT = N − (10 * Q%)
377   IF Q% <> Q THEN Q% = Q% + 1
378   FOR I = 1 TO Q%: IF I = Q% THEN TTL = LFT
379   FOR J = 1 TO TTL:M = M + 1: PR# Z
380   W = LEN ( STR$ (M)): HTAB 1: PRINT SPC ( 3 − W);M;
381   W = LEN ( STR$ (X(M))): HTAB 4: PRINT SPC ( 6 − W + 1);X(M):
382   W = LEN ( STR$ (Y(M))): HTAB 11: PRINT SPC ( 6 − W + 1);Y(M):
383   IMPROV(M) = INT (IMPROV(M) * 100 + .5) / 100.
384   W = LEN (STR$ (INT (IMPROV(M)))) + 3
385   HTAB 19: PRINT SPC (8 − W + 1); IMPROV(M);
386   YRES(M) = INT (YRES(M) * 100 + .5) / 100.
387   W = LEN ( STR$ (INT (YRES(M)))) + 3
388   HTAB 28: PRINT SPC ( 9 − W + 1);YRES (M)
389   NEXT J
390   GOSUB 700: VTAB 8: CALL − 958: PRINT : PRINT : PR# Z: NEXT I
398   PR# Z
399   HOME : PRINT : PRINT : PRINT : PRINT : HOME : PR# Z
400   HOME : HTAB 10: PRINT "IMPROVEMENT SCORES": HTAB 8:
      PRINT"_____"
410   FLAG = 3:CT = 0
415   FOR I = 1 TO N
417   PRINT : PRINT
418   CT = CT + 1
420   PRINT I;"INITIAL SCORE";: HTAB 27: PRINT X(I)
425   PRINT "FINAL SCORE";: HTAB 27: PRINT Y(I)
430   PRINT "PREDICTED FINAL SCORE";: HTAB 27: PRINT IMPROV(I)
435   PRINT "PERCENT IMPROVEMENT";: HTAB 27: PRINT YRES(I)
440   ON CT = FLAG GOSUB 750: PR# Z: NEXT I
600   GOTO 800
700   PR# 0: VTAB 23: PRINT "PRESS 'RETURN' TO CONTINUE"
710   GET A$: IF FLAG = 0 THEN GOTO 725
```

```
715   RETURN
725   HOME : PRINT: PRINT : PRINT : PRINT : HOME : RETURN
750   PR# 0: VTAB 23: PRINT "PRESS 'RETURN' TO CONTINUE"
755   GET Z$:CT = 0: HOME : RETURN
800   END
```

Appendix F

NCYFS Norms

TABLE A-1 NCYFS norms by age for the one-mile walk/run—boys (in minutes and seconds)

Percentile	10	11	12	13	14	15	16	17	18
99	6:55	6:21	6:21	5:59	5:43	5:40	5:31	5:14	5:33
90	8:13	7:25	7:13	6:48	6:27	6:23	6:13	6:08	6:10
80	8:35	7:52	7:41	7:07	6:58	6:43	6:31	6:31	6:33
75	8:48	8:02	7:53	7:14	7:08	6:52	6:39	6:40	6:42
70	9:02	8:12	8:03	7:24	7:18	7:00	6:50	6:46	6:57
60	9:26	8:38	8:23	7:46	7:34	7:13	7:07	7:10	7:15
50	9:52	9:03	8:48	8:04	7:51	7:30	7:27	7:31	7:35
40	10:15	9:25	9:17	8:26	8:14	7:50	7:48	7:59	7:53
30	10:44	10:17	9:57	8:54	8:46	8:18	8:04	8:24	8:12
25	11:00	10:32	10:13	9:06	9:10	8:30	8:18	8:37	8:34
20	11:25	10:55	10:38	9:20	9:28	8:50	8:34	8:55	9:10
10	12:27	12:07	11:48	10:38	10:34	10:13	9:36	10:43	10:50

From the National Children and Youth Fitness Study.

TABLE A-2 NCYFS norms by age for the one-mile walk/run—girls (in minutes and seconds)

Percentile	10	11	12	13	14	15	16	17	18
99	7:55	7:14	7:20	7:08	7:01	6:59	7:03	6:52	6:58
90	9:09	8:45	8:34	8:27	8:11	8:23	8:28	8:20	8:22
80	9:56	9:35	9:30	9:13	8:49	9:04	9:06	9:10	9:27
75	10:09	9:56	9:52	9:30	9:16	9:28	9:25	9:26	9:31
70	10:27	10:10	10:05	9:48	9:31	9:49	9:41	9:41	9:36
60	10:51	10:35	10:32	10:22	10:04	10:20	10:15	10:16	10:08
50	11:14	11:15	10:58	10:52	10:32	10:46	10:34	10:34	10:51
40	11:54	11:46	11:26	11:22	10:58	11:20	11:08	10:59	11:27
30	12:27	12:33	12:03	11:55	11:35	11:53	11:49	11:43	11:58
25	12:52	12:54	12:33	12:17	11:49	12:18	12:10	12:03	12:14
20	13:12	13:17	12:53	12:43	12:10	12:48	12:32	12:30	12:37
10	14:20	14:35	14:07	13:45	13:13	14:07	13:42	13:46	15:18

From the National Children and Youth Fitness Study.

TABLE A-3 *NCYFS norms by age for the timed bent-knee sit-ups—boys (number in 60 seconds)*

Percentile	10	11	12	13	14	15	16	17	18
99	60	60	61	62	64	65	65	68	67
90	47	48	50	52	52	53	55	56	54
80	43	43	46	48	49	50	51	51	50
75	40	41	44	46	47	48	49	50	50
70	38	40	43	45	45	46	48	49	48
60	36	38	40	41	43	44	45	46	44
50	34	36	38	40	41	42	43	43	43
40	32	34	35	37	39	40	41	41	40
30	30	31	33	34	37	37	39	39	38
25	28	30	32	32	35	36	38	37	36
20	26	28	30	31	34	35	36	35	35
10	22	22	25	28	30	31	32	31	31

From the National Children and Youth Fitness Study.

TABLE A-4 *NCYFS norms by age for the timed bent-knee sit-ups—girls (number in 60 seconds)*

Percentile	10	11	12	13	14	15	16	17	18
99	50	53	66	58	57	56	59	60	65
90	43	42	46	46	47	45	49	47	47
80	39	39	41	41	42	42	42	41	42
75	37	37	40	40	41	40	40	40	40
70	36	36	39	39	40	39	39	39	40
60	33	34	36	35	37	36	37	37	38
50	31	32	33	33	35	35	35	36	35
40	30	30	31	31	32	32	33	33	33
30	27	28	30	28	30	30	30	31	30
25	25	26	28	27	29	30	30	30	30
20	24	24	27	25	27	28	28	29	28
10	20	20	21	21	23	24	23	24	24

From the National Children and Youth Fitness Study.

TABLE A-5 *NCYFS norms by age for the sit-and-reach—boys (in inches)*

Percentile	10	11	12	13	14	15	16	17	18
99	18.0	18.5	18.5	19.5	20.0	21.5	22.0	21.5	22.0
90	16.0	16.5	16.0	16.5	17.5	18.0	19.0	19.5	19.5
80	15.0	15.5	15.0	15.0	16.0	17.0	18.0	18.0	18.0
75	14.5	15.0	15.0	15.0	15.5	16.5	17.0	17.5	17.5
70	14.5	14.5	14.5	14.5	15.0	16.0	17.0	17.0	17.0
60	14.0	14.0	13.5	13.5	14.0	15.0	16.0	16.0	16.0
50	13.5	13.0	13.0	13.0	13.5	14.0	15.0	15.5	15.0
40	12.5	12.5	12.0	12.5	13.0	13.5	14.0	14.5	14.5
30	12.0	12.0	11.5	12.0	12.0	12.5	13.5	13.5	13.5
25	11.5	11.5	11.0	11.0	11.0	12.0	13.0	13.0	13.0
20	11.0	11.0	10.5	10.5	11.0	11.5	12.0	12.5	12.5
10	10.0	9.5	8.5	9.0	9.0	9.5	10.0	10.5	10.0

The 1980 AAHPERD norms used a 0 point of 23 cm, but NCYFS used 12 inches. To adjust the 0 point and to change inches to centimeters, use the following formula: Score in centimeters = (Score in inches × 2.54) − 7.48. From the National Children and Youth Fitness Study.

TABLE A-6 *NCYFS norms by age for the sit-and-reach—girls (in inches)*

Percentile	10	11	12	13	14	15	16	17	18
99	20.5	20.5	21.0	22.0	22.0	23.0	23.0	23.0	22.5
90	17.5	18.0	19.0	20.0	19.5	20.0	20.5	20.5	20.5
80	16.5	17.0	18.0	19.0	19.0	19.0	19.5	19.5	19.5
75	16.5	16.5	17.0	18.0	18.5	19.0	19.0	19.0	19.0
70	16.0	16.5	17.0	17.5	18.0	18.5	19.0	19.0	18.5
60	15.0	15.5	16.0	17.0	17.5	18.0	18.0	18.0	18.0
50	14.5	15.0	15.5	16.0	17.0	17.0	17.5	18.0	17.5
40	14.0	14.0	15.0	15.5	16.0	17.0	17.0	17.0	17.0
30	13.0	13.5	14.5	14.5	15.0	16.0	16.5	16.0	16.0
25	13.0	13.0	14.0	14.0	15.0	15.5	16.0	15.5	15.5
20	12.0	13.0	13.5	13.5	14.0	15.0	15.5	15.0	15.0
10	10.5	11.5	12.0	12.0	12.5	13.5	14.0	13.5	13.0

The 1980 AAHPERD norms used a 0 point of 23 cm, but NCYFS used 12 inches. To adjust the 0 point and to change inches to centimeters, use the following formula: Score in centimeters = (Score in inches × 2.54) − 7.48 From the National Children and Youth Fitness Study.

TABLE A-7 NCYFS norms by age for the triceps skinfold—boys (in millimeters)

Percentile	10	11	12	13	14	15	16	17	18
99	5	4	4	4	4	4	4	4	4
90	7	7	6	6	5	5	5	5	5
80	8	7	8	7	6	6	6	6	6
75	8	8	8	7	7	7	6	6	6
70	9	9	9	8	7	7	7	7	7
60	10	10	10	9	8	8	7	7	8
50	11	11	11	10	9	9	8	8	8
40	13	12	12	11	10	10	9	9	10
30	14	14	14	13	11	11	11	11	11
25	15	15	15	14	12	12	11	12	12
20	16	16	17	15	13	13	12	13	13
10	20	20	21	20	18	18	16	15	16

From the National Children and Youth Fitness Study.

TABLE A-8 NCYFS norms by age for the triceps skinfold—girls (in millimeters)

Percentile	10	11	21	13	14	15	16	17	18
99	5	6	6	6	6	7	7	8	7
90	7	8	9	9	9	10	10	11	10
80	9	9	10	10	11	12	12	12	12
75	10	10	10	11	12	13	12	13	13
70	10	10	11	11	12	13	13	14	13
60	11	12	12	13	14	15	14	15	14
50	12	13	13	14	15	16	15	17	15
40	14	15	14	15	16	17	17	18	17
30	15	16	16	17	18	19	18	20	19
25	16	17	17	18	19	20	19	21	20
20	17	19	18	20	20	21	20	21	21
10	21	23	22	24	23	25	24	24	23

From the National Children and Youth Fitness Study.

TABLE A-9 *NCYFS norms by age for the sum of triceps and subscapular skinfolds—boys (in millimeters)*

Percentile	10	11	12	13	14	15	16	17	18
99	9	9	9	9	9	10	10	10	11
90	12	12	12	11	12	12	12	13	13
80	13	13	13	13	13	13	13	14	14
75	14	14	14	13	13	14	14	14	15
70	15	15	15	14	14	14	14	15	15
60	16	16	16	15	15	15	15	16	17
50	17	18	17	17	17	17	17	17	18
40	20	20	20	19	18	18	18	19	19
30	22	23	22	21	21	20	20	21	22
25	24	25	24	23	22	22	22	22	24
20	25	26	28	25	25	24	23	24	25
10	35	36	38	34	33	32	30	30	30

From the National Children and Youth Fitness Study.

TABLE A-10 *NCYFS norms by age for the sum of triceps and subscapular skinfolds—girls (in millimeters)*

Percentile	10	11	12	13	14	15	16	17	18
99	10	11	11	12	12	13	13	16	14
90	13	14	15	15	17	19	19	20	19
80	15	16	17	18	19	21	21	22	21
75	16	17	18	19	20	23	22	23	22
70	17	18	18	20	21	24	23	24	23
60	18	19	21	22	24	26	24	26	25
50	20	21	22	24	26	28	26	28	27
40	22	24	24	26	28	30	28	31	28
30	25	28	27	29	31	33	32	34	32
25	27	30	29	31	33	34	33	36	34
20	29	33	31	34	35	37	35	37	36
10	36	40	40	43	40	43	42	42	42

From the National Children and Youth Fitness Study.

TABLE A-11 *NCYFS norms by age for the chin-up—boys (number completed)*

Percentile	10	11	12	13	14	15	16	17	18
99	13	12	13	17	18	18	20	20	21
90	8	8	8	10	12	14	14	15	16
80	5	5	6	8	9	11	12	13	14
75	4	5	5	7	8	10	12	12	13
70	4	4	5	7	8	10	11	12	12
60	2	3	4	5	6	8	10	10	11
50	1	2	3	4	5	7	9	9	10
40	1	1	2	3	4	6	8	8	9
30	0	0	1	1	3	5	6	6	7
25	0	0	0	1	2	4	6	5	6
20	0	0	0	0	1	3	5	4	5
10	0	0	0	0	0	1	2	2	3

From the National Children and Youth Fitness Study.

TABLE A-12 *NCYFS norms by age for the chin-up—girls (number completed)*

Percentile	10	11	12	13	14	15	16	17	18
99	8	8	8	5	8	6	8	7	6
90	3	3	2	2	2	2	2	2	2
80	2	1	1	1	1	1	1	1	1
75	1	1	1	1	1	1	1	1	1
70	1	1	1	0	1	1	1	1	1
60	0	0	0	0	0	0	0	0	0
50	0	0	0	0	0	0	0	0	0
40	0	0	0	0	0	0	0	0	0
30	0	0	0	0	0	0	0	0	0
25	0	0	0	0	0	0	0	0	0
20	0	0	0	0	0	0	0	0	0
10	0	0	0	0	0	0	0	0	0

From the National Children and Youth Fitness Study.

Appendix G

Sources of Tests and Skinfold Calipers

CHAPTER 10

The following references are excellent sources of additional tests of motor behavior for children. Each reference includes an analytical critique of selected tests to assist the teacher in identifying appropriate tests.

Haubenstricker, J.L. 1977. A critical review of selected perceptual-motor tests and scales currently used in the assessment of motor behavior. In Landers, D., and Christina, R., editors. Psychology of motor behavior and sport—1977. Champaign, Ill.: Human Kinetics Publishers, Inc.

Herkowitz, J. 1977. Instruments which assess the efficiency/maturity of children's fundamental motor pattern performance. In Landers, D., and Christina, R., editors. Psychology of motor behavior and sport—1977. Champaign, Ill.: Human Kinetics Publishers, Inc.

Herkowitz, J. 1978. Assessing the motor development of children: presentation and critique of tests. In Ridenour, M., editor. Motor development: issues and applications. Princeton, N.J.: Princeton Book Co., Publishers.

McGee, R. 1984. Evaluation of processes and products. In Logsden, B., editor. Physical education for children: a focus on the teaching process. Philadelphia: Lea & Febiger.

CHAPTER 11

Sensorimotor tests
Quick Neurological Screening Test
Academic Therapy Publications
20 Commercial Boulevard
Novato, CA 94949

Frostig Developmental Test of Visual
    Perception
Consulting Psychologist Press, Inc.
577 College Avenue
Palo Alto, CA 94360

Motor development tests
California State University Motor
Development Checklist
Janet A. Seaman
California State University
5151 State University Drive
Los Angeles, CA 90032

Bayley Scales of Motor Development
Psychological Corporation
757 Third Avenue
New York, NY 10017

Motor ability tests
Six Category Gross Motor Test
B.J. Cratty
*Perceptual Motor Behavior and
    Educational Processes*
Springfield, Ill.:
Charles C Thomas, Publisher, 1969

Basic Motor Ability Test—Revised
D. Arnheim and A. Sinclair
The Clumsy Child
St. Louis: The C.V. Mosby Co., 1979

CHAPTER 16

FAT-O-METER: Health Education Services Corp., 7N015 York Road, Bensenville, IL 60106

SLIM GUIDE: Creative Health Products, 9135 General Ct., Plymouth, MI 48170

PHYSIQUE METER: Dr. H. Co., P.O. Box 266, Chesterfield, MO 63017

HARPENDEN: Quinton Instrument Co., 2121 Terry Avenue, Seattle, WA 98121

LANGE: J.A. Preston Corp., 71 Fifth Ave., New York, NY 10013

Credits and Acknowledgments

Chapter 2 Summarizing a Set of Test Scores

P. 23—Courtesy Midvale Elementary School, Madison, Wis.; 33—Courtesy Measurement Laboratory, Department of Physical Education and Dance, University of Wisconsin, Madison.

Chapter 3 Describing a Distribution of Test Scores

P. 55—From Text Service Notebook 148, 1980. p. 1: The Psychological Corporation; 68—Courtesy Midvale Elementary School, Madison, Wis.

Chapter 5 Microcomputer Applications

P. 99—By permission of Johnny Hart and Field Enterprises, Inc.

Chapter 6 Validity and Reliability of Norm-Referenced Tests

P. 114—Courtesy Measurement Laboratory, Department of Physical Education and Dance, University of Wisconsin, Madison; 117—From Handbook for AAHPER Cooperative Physical Education Tests. Copyright © 1971 by Educational Testing Service. All rights reserved. Reproduced by permission; 126—From Morgan, W.P., and Johnson, R.W. 1978. Personality characteristics of successful and unsuccessful oarsmen, International Journal of Sports Psychology 9:119-133. By permission of the publisher; 127—From Morgan, W.P., and Raven, P.B. 1985. Prediction of distress for individuals wearing industrial respirators. Am. Ind. Hyg. Assoc. J. 46(7):363-368.

Chapter 7 Validity and Reliability of Criterion-Referenced Tests

P. 143, 152–Courtesy Midvale Elementary School, Madison, Wis.

Chapter 8 Tests and Testing

P. 157—Courtesy Measurement Laboratory, Department of Physical Education and Dance, University of Wisconsin, Madison; 159—Modified from Imwold, C.H., Rider, R.A., and Johnson, D.J. 1982. Journal of Teaching in Physical Education, 2:13-18; 167—Courtesy Biodynamics Laboratory, Department of Physical Education and Dance, University of Wisconsin, Madison.

Chapter 9 Grading in Physical Education

P. 170—Reprinted by permission of United Feature Syndicate, Inc. 192—Reprinted by permission of Hafeman, D.A., Ph.D., Superintendent, Madison Metropolitan School District, Madison, Wis.

Chapter 10 Measuring Motor Performance in Children

P. 200—From Seefeldt, V., and Haubenstricker, J. 1982. Patterns, phases, or stages: an analytical model for the study of developmental movement. In Kelso, J.A.S., and Clark, J.E., editors. The development of movement control and coordination. London: John Wiley & Sons, Ltd. By permission of the publisher; 201, 223—Redrawn from Robertson, M.A., and Halverson, L.E. 1984. Courtesy Motor Development and Child Study Laboratory, University of Wisconsin, Madison: 202, 203, 205, 206-210, 212, 214—Reprinted by permission of the American Alliance for Health, Physical Education, Recreation and Dance, 1900 Association Drive, Reston, VA 22091: 204-205, 206-207, 209, 211—From Scott, M.G., and French, E. 1959. Measurement and evaluation in physical education. Dubuque, Iowa: Wm C Brown Group. By permission of Scott, M.G., Ph.D.; 210-215—From Johnson, R.D. 1962. Measurements of achievement in fundamental skills of elementary school children. Research Quarterly 33:94-103. Reprinted by permission of the American Alliance for Health, Physical Education, Recreation and Dance, 1900 Association Drive, Reston, VA 22091; 217—Courtesy American Medical Association. Copyright © 1978; 218—Courtesy of Dale A. Ulrich, 1989; 220-221—Reprinted by permission of Ross Laboratories. Adapted from Hamill, P.V.V., Drižd, T.A., Johnson, C.L., et al.: Physical growth: National Center for Health Statistics percentiles. Am. J. Clin. Nurtr. 32:607-629, 1979. Data from the National Center for Health Statistics (NCHS), Hyattsville, Md.

Chapter 11 Adapting Tests and Measurements for Special Populations

P. 229, 239, 249—Courtesy Measurement and Biodynamics Laboratories. Department of Physical Education and Dance, University of Wisconsin, Madison; 232, 234, 235, 252—Courtesy Janet A. Seaman, Professor, California State University, Los Angeles; 246, 247, 248—From Winnick, J.P., and Short, F.X. 1982. The Physical Fitness of Sensory and Orthopedically Impaired Youth. By permission of Joseph P. Winnick, 246, 250, 251—Courtesy Dale A. Ulrich, 1989.

Chapter 12 A Review of Testing Procedures
P. 262, 266, 275—Courtesy Biodynamics Laboratory, Department of Physical Education and Dance, University of Wisconsin, Madison; 263-264—From Vic Tanny International of Wisconsin. By permission of Dr. Paul Ward, Dr. Frank I. Katch, and Mr. Bernard F. Palluck, Vice President and Area Director; procedures were formulated by Dr. Ward; percent fat regression equation was developed by Drs. Katch and McArdle; 265—From the Olympic Health and Racquet Club. By permission of Ray Fraley; 267—From the Exercise Resource Facility, CUNA Mutual Insurance Group, Madison, Wis. By permission of Katie Munns; 268, 269, 270-274—Courtesy Sentry World Headquarters, Stevens Point, Wis.; 276-277—Golding, L.A., Myers, C.R., and Sinning, W.E. editors. 1982. National Board of YMCA of the USA. Chicago. Copies available YMCA of the USA, Program Resources, 6400 Shafer Court, Rosemont, IL 60018. By permission of the YMCA.

Chapter 14 Constructing Sports Skills Tests
P. 304, 310—Courtesy Measurement Laboratory, Department of Physical Education and Dance, University of Wisconsin, Madison.

Chapter 15 Constructing Knowledge Tests
P. 323, 324—From Haskins, M.J. 1971. Evaluation in physical education. Dubuque, Iowa. Wm C Brown Group. By permission of the author; 331—From Ebel, R.L. 1965. Measuring educational achievement. Englewood Cliffs, N.J.: Prentice-Hall, Inc. By permission of the publisher.

Chapter 16 Tests of Health-Related Physical Fitness
P. 337—Courtesy Biodynamics Laboratory, University of Wisconsin, Madison; 342—Reproduced from Physical Best. Reston, VA: AAHPERD, 1988. Reprinted by permission of the American Alliance of Health, Physical Education, Recreation, and Dance, 1900 Association Drive, Reston, VA 22091; 343—From The Chrysler Fund-AAU Physical Fitness Program. 1987. The Chrysler Fund-Amateur Athletic Union: Bloomington, IN; 345—Reproduced from Fit Youth Today Program Manual. 1988. Austin, TX: American Health and Fitness Foundation. By permission of the publisher; 346, 347, 348-349—Reproduced from FITNESSGRAM User's Manual. 1987. Dallas: Institute for Aerobics Research. By permission of the publisher; 352—Reproduced from the Presidential Physical Fitness Award Program: Instructor's Guide. 1987. Washington, D.C. President's Council on Physical Fitness and Sports. By permission of the publisher; 365—Reprinted with permission from the Journal of Physical Education, Recreation and Dance, 58(9):100, 1987. The Journal is a publication of the American Alliance for Health, Physical Education, Recreation and Dance, 1900 Association Drive, Reston, VA 22091; 354, 373—From Health-Related Physical Fitness Test Manual. Reston, VA: AAHPERD, 1980. By permission of the AAHPERD; 351, 357, 368-369, 371, 372, 375, 376, 378—From the National Children and Youth Fitness Study I. 1985. Public Health Service, Office of Disease Prevention and Health Promotion, U.S. Department of Health and Human Services: Washington, D.C. 20201; 356, 362, 363, 364, 366, 370, 374, 375—From the National Children and Youth Fitness Study II, 1987. U.S. Department of Health and Human Services: Washington, D.C. 20201; 373—Courtesy Measurement Laboratory, Department of Physical Education and Dance, University of Wisconsin, Madison; 379, 381—Reprinted with permission from the Journal of Physical Education, Recreation and Dance, 59(4): 79, 1988. The Journal is a publication of the American Alliance for Health, Physical Education, Recreation and Dance, 1900 Association Drive, Reston, VA 22091; From Pate, R., and Corbin, C. 1981. A taxonomy of physical fitness objectives. Implications for curriculum, Journal of Physical Education and Recreation 52(1):36. Reprinted by permission of the American Alliance for Health, Physical Education, Recreation and Dance, 1900 Association Drive, Reston, VA 22091; 386—From Nutrition Weight Control and Exercise, by Katch, F.I., and McArdle, W.D. 1983. ed. 2. By permission of Lea & Febiger; 390—Courtesy Pollock, M.L. and the W.B. Saunders Co. From Pollock, M.L., Wilmore, J.M., and Fox, S.M. 1984. Exercise in health and disease: evaluation and prescription for prevention and rehabilitation. Philadelphia: W.B. Saunders Co.; 391—From Pollack, M.L., Schmidt, D.H., and Jackson, A.S. 1980. Measurement of cardiorespiratory fitness and body composition in the clinical setting. Comprehensive Therapy 6(9):12-27. By permission of the Laux Co., Inc., Harvard, Massachusetts.

Chapter 17 Tests of Performance-Related Physical Fitness
P. 398, 402-405, 419—Courtesy Measurement Laboratory, Department of Physical Education and Dance, University of Wisconsin, Madison; 400-401, 410, 411, 412, 413, 414, 415, 416, 417—From Youth Fitness Test Manual. Washington, D.C.: AAHPER, 1976. Used by permission; 408-409—Reprinted by permission of the American Alliance for Health Physical Education, Recreation and Dance, 1900 Association Drive, Reston, VA

22091; 400-418—Modified from Youth Fitness Test Manual. Washington, D.C.: AAHPERD, 1976. Reprinted by permission of the American Alliance for Health, Physical Education, Recreation and Dance, 1900 Association Drive, Reston, VA 22091; 425, 427—From Spray, J.A. 1977. Interpreting group or class performances using AAHPER Youth Fitness Test Norms. Journal of Physical Education and Recreation 48:56-57. By permission of the publisher; 426—From Table 1 in Spray, J.A. 1977. Interpreting group or class performances using AAHPER Youth Fitness Test Norms. Journal of Physical Education and Recreation. 48:56-57. Reprinted by permission of the American Alliance for Health, Physical Education, Recreation and Dance, 1900 Association Drive, Reston, VA 22091.

Chapter 18 Tests of Sports Skills
P. 437—From Archery for boys and girls: Skills test manual. 1967. Washington, D.C.: AAHPER. Reprinted by permission of the American Alliance for Health, Physical Education, Recreation and Dance, 1900 Association Drive, Reston, VA 22091; 438, 440—Redrawn from Johnson, B.L., and Nelson, J.K. 1979. Practical measurements for evaluation in physical education. Minneapolis: Burgess Publishing Co. By permission of Nelson, J.K., Ph.D.; 439—In Scott, M.G., and French, E. 1959. Measurement and evaluation in physical education. Dubuque, Iowa: Wm C Brown Group. By permission of Scott, M.G., Ph.D.; 443, 444, 445, 446, 447-450—From Hopkins, D.R., Shick, J., and Plack, J.J. 1984. Basketball for boys and girls: skills test manual. Reston, VA.: AAHPERD. Reprinted by permission of the American Alliance for Health, Physical Education, Recreation and Dance, 1900 Association Drive, Reston, VA 22091; 451—From Chapman, N.L. 1982. Chapman ball control

test-field hockey. Research Quarterly for Exercise and Sport 53(3):239-242. Reprinted by permission of the American Alliance for Health, Physical Education, Recreation and Dance, 1900 Association Drive, Reston VA 22091; 453—From AAHPER. 1966. Football: skills test manual. Washington, D.C.: AAHPER. Reprinted by permission of the American Alliance for Health, Physical Education, Recreation and Dance, 1900 Association Drive, Reston, VA 22091; 454—From Shick, J., and Berg, N.G. 1983. Indoor golf skill test for junior high school boys. Research Quarterly for Exercise and Sport 54(1):75-78. Reprinted by permission of the American Alliance for Health, Physical Education, Recreation and Dance, 1900 Association Drive, Reston, VA 22091; 457—From Shick, J. 1970. Battery of softball skills tests for college women. Research Quarterly 42:82-87. Reprinted by permission of the American Alliance for Health, Physical Education, Recreation and Dance, 1900 Association Drive, Reston, VA 22091; 459-460—From Hewitt, J.E. 1966. Hewitt's tennis achievement test. Research Quarterly 31:231-237. Reprinted by permission of the American Alliance for Health, Physical Education, Recreation and Dance, 1900 Association Drive, Reston, VA 22091; 462, 463—From Purcell, K. 1981. A tennis forehand-backhand drive skill test which measures ball control and stroke firmness. Research Quarterly for Exercise and Sport 52(2):238-245. Reprinted by permission of the American Alliance for Health, Physical Education, Recreation and Dance, 1900 Association Drive, Reston, VA 22091; 464—From Brady, G.F. 1945. Preliminary investigation of volleyball playing ability. Research Quarterly 16:14-17. Reprinted by permission of the American Alliance for Health, Physical Education, Recreation and Dance, 1900 Association Drive, Reston, VA 22091; 465—From Brumbach, W.B. 1967. Beginning volleyball, a

syllabus for teachers, revised edition. Eugene, Ore.: Wayne Baker Brumbach. By permission of the author.

Chapter 19 Tests of Muscular Strength and Endurance
P. 475—Pollock, M.L., and others. 1978. Health and fitness through physical activity. New York: John Wiley & Sons. By permission of the publisher; 477—Heyward, V.H. 1984. Designs for Fitness. Minneapolis: Burgess Publishing Co. By permission of the publisher; 495—Friermood, H.T. 1967. "Volleyball Skills Contest for Olympic Development," in United States Volleyball Association, Annual Official Volleyball Rules and Reference Guide of the U.S. Volleyball Association, Berne, Ind.: USVBA Printer, pp. 134-135. By permission of H.T. Friermood and the U.S. Volleyball Association. †Raw scores are located in the chart in accordance with age and sex, and percentile scores are located across the top.

Chapter 20 Tests of Balance and Flexibility
P. 510-511—By permission of the State Education Department, State University of New York, Albany.

Chapter 21 Tests of Motor Ability
P. 524-525—Reprinted by permission of Dr. M. Gladys Scott, Emerita Professor, University of Iowa, Iowa City; 522, 526—Courtesy Measurement Laboratory, Department of Physical Education and Dance, University of Wisconsin, Madison; 527-529—Reprinted by permission of Dr. Harold M. Barrow, Emeritus Professor, Wake Forest University, North Carolina.

Chapter 22 Tests of Affective Behavior
P. 542—From Miller, D.K., and Allen, T.E. 1982. Fitness: a lifetime commitment, ed. 2. Minneapolis: Burgess Publishing Co. Reprinted by permission of the publisher; 543, 544-545—From Martens, R. 1977.

Sport Competition Anxiety Test. Champaign, Ill.: Human Kinetics Publishers. By permission of the publisher; 546-547—From Cowell, C.C. 1958. Validity: an index of social adjustment for high school use. Research Quarterly 29:7-18. Reprinted by permission of the American Alliance for Health, Physical Education, Recreation and Dance, 1900 Association Drive, Reston, VA 22091; 548-549—From Blanchard, B.E. 1936. A behavior frequency rating scale for the measurement of character and personality traits in physical education classroom situations. Research Quarterly 7:56-66. Reprinted by permission of the American Alliance for Health, Physical Education, Recreation and Dance, 1900 Association Drive, Reston, VA 22091; 551—Reprinted by permission of Kenyon, G.S., University of Lethbridge, Lethbridge, Alberta, Canada; 552—From Pooley, J.C. 1971. The professional socialization of physical education students in the United States and England. Unpublished doctoral dissertation, The University of Wisconsin, Madison. By permission of the author; 554—From Simon, J.A., and Smoll, F.L. 1974. An instrument for assessing children's attitudes toward physical activity. Research Quarterly 45:21-27. By permission of the authors; 555—From Sonstroem, R.J. 1974. Attitude testing: examining certain psychological correlates of physical activity. Research Quarterly 39:566-574. Reprinted by permission of the author, University of Rhode Island, Kingston; 556-557—From Wear, C.L. 1955. Construction of equivalent forms of an attitude scale. Research Quarterly 26:113-119. Reprinted by permission of the American Alliance for Health, Physical Education, Recreation and Dance, 1900 Association Drive, Reston, VA 22091; 558-559—From Lakie, W.L. 1964. Expressed attitudes of various groups of athletes toward athletic competition. Research Quarterly 35:497-503. Reprinted by permission of the American Alliance for Health, Physical Education, Recreation and Dance, 1900 Association Drive, Reston, VA 22091; 561-563—From Nelson, D.O. 1966. Nelson Sports Leadership Questionnaire. Research Quarterly 37:268-275. Reprinted by permission of the author; 563—From Borg, G.A.V. 1973. Perceived exertion: a note on "history" and methods. Medicine and Science in Sports 5:90-93. Reproduced by permission of the publisher; 564—Courtesy Biodynamics Laboratory, Department of Physical Education and Dance, University of Wisconsin, Madison.

Index